Handbook of Clinical Psychiatry

Handbook of Clinical Psychiatry

Editor: Angela Giles

AMERICAN
MEDICAL PUBLISHERS
www.americanmedicalpublishers.com

AMERICAN
MEDICAL PUBLISHERS
www.americanmedicalpublishers.com

Cataloging-in-Publication Data

Handbook of clinical psychiatry / edited by Angela Giles.
p. cm.
Includes bibliographical references and index.
ISBN 979-8-88740-143-0
1. Clinical psychology. 2. Psychiatry. 3. Psychology, Applied. I. Giles, Angela.
RC467 .H36 2023
616.89--dc23

American Medical Publishers,
41 Flatbush Avenue,
1st Floor, New York,
NY 11217, USA

ISBN 979-8-88740-143-0 (Hardback)

Contents

Preface

The world is advancing at a fast pace like never before. Therefore, the need is to keep up with the latest developments. This book was an idea that came to fruition when the specialists in the area realized the need to coordinate together and document essential themes in the subject. That's when I was requested to be the editor. Editing this book has been an honour as it brings together diverse authors researching on different streams of the field. The book collates essential materials contributed by veterans in the area which can be utilized by students and researchers alike.

Psychiatry is a field of medicine that aims to study, prevent and treat mental illness in human beings. It includes various maladaptations associated with cognition, behavior, perceptions and mood. It helps in treating and managing mental illnesses that are traditionally classified into three types, namely, personality disorders, mental illnesses and severe learning disabilities. The main pillars of psychotherapy used in the treatment of psychological disorders are psychoanalysis, humanistic psychology and behaviorism. A psychiatric assessment can be conducted to determine the mental and physical health of a person. This typically involves questioning the individual and gathering information from a variety of sources including associates, emergency medical personnel, relatives, psychiatric rating scales, health and social care professionals and law enforcement personnel. The mental and physical examination is useful in determining or ruling out other disorders that could be contributing to the psychiatric problems. This book explores all the important aspects of psychiatry in the present day scenario. It aims to understand the clinical perspectives of psychiatry. This book will prove to be immensely beneficial to students and researchers in this field.

Each chapter is a sole-standing publication that reflects each author´s interpretation. Thus, the book displays a multi-facetted picture of our current understanding of application, resources and aspects of the field. I would like to thank the contributors of this book and my family for their endless support.

Editor

1

Is it Possible to Predict the Future in First-Episode Psychosis?

Jaana Suvisaari[1], Outi Mantere[1,2,3,4], Jaakko Keinänen[1,4], Teemu Mäntylä[1,5,6], Eva Rikandi[1,5,6], Maija Lindgren[1], Tuula Kieseppä[1,4] and Tuukka T. Raij[1,5]*

[1] Mental Health Unit, National Institute for Health and Welfare, Helsinki, Finland, [2] Department of Psychiatry, McGill University, Montreal, QC, Canada, [3] Bipolar Disorders Clinic, Douglas Mental Health University Institute, Montreal, QC, Canada, [4] Department of Psychiatry, Faculty of Medicine, University of Helsinki, Helsinki, Finland, [5] Department of Neuroscience and Biomedical Engineering, and Advanced Magnetic Imaging Center, Aalto NeuroImaging, Aalto University School of Science, Espoo, Finland, [6] Department of Psychology and Logopedics, University of Helsinki, Helsinki, Finland

***Correspondence:**
Jaana Suvisaari
jaana.suvisaari@thl.fi

The outcome of first-episode psychosis (FEP) is highly variable, ranging from early sustained recovery to antipsychotic treatment resistance from the onset of illness. For clinicians, a possibility to predict patient outcomes would be highly valuable for the selection of antipsychotic treatment and in tailoring psychosocial treatments and psychoeducation. This selective review summarizes current knowledge of prognostic markers in FEP. We sought potential outcome predictors from clinical and sociodemographic factors, cognition, brain imaging, genetics, and blood-based biomarkers, and we considered different outcomes, like remission, recovery, physical comorbidities, and suicide risk. Based on the review, it is currently possible to predict the future for FEP patients to some extent. Some clinical features—like the longer duration of untreated psychosis (DUP), poor premorbid adjustment, the insidious mode of onset, the greater severity of negative symptoms, comorbid substance use disorders (SUDs), a history of suicide attempts and suicidal ideation and having non-affective psychosis—are associated with a worse outcome. Of the social and demographic factors, male gender, social disadvantage, neighborhood deprivation, dysfunctional family environment, and ethnicity may be relevant. Treatment non-adherence is a substantial risk factor for relapse, but a small minority of patients with acute onset of FEP and early remission may benefit from antipsychotic discontinuation. Cognitive functioning is associated with functional outcomes. Brain imaging currently has limited utility as an outcome predictor, but this may change with methodological advancements. Polygenic risk scores (PRSs) might be useful as one component of a predictive tool, and pharmacogenetic testing is already available and valuable for patients who have problems in treatment response or with side effects. Most blood-based biomarkers need further validation. None of the currently available predictive markers has adequate sensitivity or specificity used alone. However, personalized treatment of FEP will need predictive tools. We discuss some methodologies, such as machine learning (ML), and tools that could lead to the improved prediction and clinical utility of different prognostic markers in FEP. Combination of different markers in ML models with a user friendly interface, or novel findings from e.g., molecular genetics or neuroimaging, may result in computer-assisted clinical applications in the near future.

Keywords: first-episode psychosis, remission, recovery, comorbidities, mortality, prediction

INTRODUCTION

Naturalistic follow-up studies have found highly divergent outcomes in first-episode psychosis (FEP) (1, 2). While an episodic course is the most common (1) and the majority of patients with FEP initially achieve remission (2), a minority experience early sustained recovery (3), or have an antipsychotic treatment-resistant illness from the onset of the illness (4). The challenge for the clinician treating patients with FEP is how to predict these different disease trajectories and make the best treatment choices for individual patients.

A growing concern in recent years has been the multiple physical comorbidities in people with schizophrenia and other psychotic disorders (5) and the premature mortality caused by these comorbidities (6, 7). Antipsychotic medication contributes to these problems by causing weight gain, impaired glucose tolerance and dyslipidemias. However, antipsychotics differ in their propensity to cause these side effects (8), and there is also considerable individual variation in the sensitivity to these side-effects. Moreover, other factors, possibly even shared etiological mechanisms, contribute to the development of comorbidities like diabetes (9). The personalized treatment of FEP would benefit from biomarkers identifying the patients at greatest risk for medication side effects and comorbidities.

While cardiovascular and pulmonary diseases are overall the most important causes of premature mortality (6), in the first years of illness increased mortality is mainly caused by suicide (10). Suicide prevention is one of the key goals in the treatment of FEP (11), and yet another important outcome for which the clinician needs to identify relevant risk factors.

In addition to these main areas where outcome prediction is needed—remission, recovery, physical comorbidities, and suicide risk—some domains in the psychosis phenotype, for example cognitive functioning, can be considered both as predictors of the long-term course and as relevant long-term outcomes.

This selective review aims to provide a synthesis of the current literature on outcome prediction for FEP. We also discuss some methodologies and tools that could enhance possibilities to predict the future in FEP.

OUTCOME PREDICTION: CURRENT EVIDENCE

Clinical and Sociodemographic Factors

Remission in FEP refers to symptomatic remission; the Remission in Schizophrenia Working Group defined it as maintaining a symptom level of mild or less regarding positive, negative, and disorganized symptoms over a 6-month period (12). Recovery is a broad concept that should take both clinical symptoms and psychosocial functioning into account, with subjective recovery being an important component (13). While the Remission in Schizophrenia Working Group criteria for remission have achieved gold standard status in research, no uniform criteria exist for recovery. In a recent meta-analysis of longitudinal FEP studies, the pooled proportion of patients achieving remission after an average of 5.5 years follow-up was 58%, and studies conducted in more recent years found higher remission rates (2). However, the proportion achieving recovery after an average of 7.2 years follow-up was only 38%, and this was lower in both more recent studies and in studies with longer follow-up times (2). After 2 years of follow-up, the proportion achieving recovery was stable, suggesting that the poor outcome trajectory is already apparent during the early stages of illness (2). Recovery rates were also lower in studies requiring a longer duration of good functioning and the absence of symptoms (2). Schizophrenia was associated with lower remission and recovery rates than other psychotic disorders (2).

Clinical features related to the first psychotic episode were surprisingly poor predictors of remission and recovery in the meta-analysis by Lally et al. (2). Remission status was not predicted by the severity of psychotic symptoms at baseline, the duration of untreated psychosis (DUP), treatment adherence, employment status, or marital status (2). In another meta-analysis focusing on relapse risk following the first psychotic episode, significant risk factors were medication non-adherence, persistent substance use disorder (SUD), the carer's critical comments and poor premorbid adjustment (14). In the Etiology and Ethnicity in Schizophrenia and Other Psychoses (AESOP) study, patients with an initial diagnosis of non-affective psychosis, patients living in a deprived area, and male patients had a poorer 10-year outcome than other patients (1). Some ethnic minorities had a worse outcome, which was partly explained by social disadvantage (15). In another large longitudinal FEP study, deterioration in premorbid social functioning, DUP of ≥26 weeks, a core schizophrenia spectrum disorder and no remission within the first 3 months all predicted a longer time in psychosis during a 10-year follow-up (16). Regarding shorter-term outcomes, unemployment, poor education, functional deficits, unmet psychosocial needs, previous depressive episodes, male sex, and suicidality predicted poor 1-year outcomes in a machine learning (ML) study that utilized data from the European First Episode Schizophrenia Trial (17).

Recent studies have reported inconsistent findings regarding the effects of the discontinuation of antipsychotic treatment after achieving remission of FEP. A meta-analysis of treatment discontinuation vs. maintenance treatment strategies in FEP clearly showed that the relapse risk is higher in the discontinuation group (18). In a recent register-based follow-up study, the discontinuation of antipsychotic medication was a strong predictor of both rehospitalization and premature mortality even after several years of continuous outpatient antipsychotic treatment (19). While one study found that early dose reduction or the discontinuation of antipsychotic treatment following a 6-month remission were both associated with a better long-term outcome (20), another recent randomized clinical trial (RCT) found that discontinuation after 1 year of antipsychotic maintenance treatment was associated with a poorer 10-year clinical outcome (21). However, in the AESOP study, 12.5% of FEP patients had early sustained recovery with no relapses over a 10-year follow-up period, and their median duration of antipsychotic treatment was only 53 days (3). Predictors of early sustained remission were female gender, being employed, being in a relationship, having have a short DUP, and having mania or a brief psychotic disorder diagnosis (3). Unfortunately, all these predictors are relatively common and not specific enough to evaluate who would possibly benefit from antipsychotic discontinuation after FEP.

About a quarter of FEP patients are treatment-resistant, that is, they show little or no improvement in psychotic symptoms after two consecutive treatments with different antipsychotics of adequate dose and duration (4, 22). The majority of treatment-resistant patients are treatment resistant from the onset of illness (4, 22). In two large FEP studies, treatment resistance was predicted by a younger age at onset, a schizophrenia diagnosis, negative symptoms, and a longer DUP (4, 22).

Insight and Resilience

Insight has been of special interest as a predictor of the outcome of FEP, as defects in insight may possibly arise from the same functional and structural brain pathology as psychosis itself (23, 24). Cognitive insight at baseline, including measures of both self-reflectiveness and self-certainty, has been shown to predict overall psychopathology at 1-year follow-up (25). However, after a 4-year follow-up, only the self-reflectiveness subscale was associated with symptom remission (26). In FEP, cognitive insight has been associated with cortical thickness (27), and the self-certainty subscale has been associated with changes in a frontal network (28). However, greater insight has also predicted suicidality after FEP (29).

Impaired clinical insight, which is somewhat separable from cognitive insight, has been associated with poorer social functioning, more re-hospitalizations and treatment non-adherence (30). In one study, the best predictors of relapse within 2 years after FEP were cannabis use before relapse and poor insight (insight being measured at a 2-month follow-up) (31). Poor insight may prolong the DUP (32) and predict non-adherence to medication treatment in FEP patients (33), although the results in prospective studies with FEP samples are somewhat mixed with regards to treatment adherence (34). Interestingly, baseline self-rated insight and objective insight at 6 weeks predicted hospital readmission in a sample consisting mostly of first-episode non-affective psychosis patients, whereas baseline objective insight and self-rated insight at 6 weeks were not significant predictors (35). Clinical insight changes over time in FEP, and likewise its correlation with symptoms and psychosocial functioning is not consistent in the early course of illness and the later course of illness (36). In a 3-year follow-up of a large FEP cohort, improvement in insight in the early course of illness was associated with increasing depressive symptoms, but this association disappeared later (36). Improving insight was associated with improving psychosocial functioning in the early course of the illness, but later the relationship became more complex (36). This reflects a complex social identity process that occurs after a first psychotic episode, in which insight is more than just a simple trait or state feature (36).

Resilience, a personality trait manifesting in a response to adversity, also plays a role in recovery, as it implies successful adaptation despite difficult experiences. Resilience is linked to psychological well-being or positive mental health, which is increasingly seen as an important treatment target on its own and which tends to be at a low level, particularly for patients with active delusions (37). Fully recovered patients with first episode schizophrenia—defined as patients living independently, working or studying, having absent or stably mild symptoms for 2 years, and having social contacts and participation—showed a significant increase in resilience at 4-year follow-up (20, 38). These results indicate that individual differences in resilience will differently affect the recovery process (20), stressing the importance of taking resilience into account in outcome studies and using resilience-building strategies. Measures of resilience and psychological well-being might be important as outcome predictors, but currently they have rarely been studied in large FEP cohorts.

Cognition

Cognitive deficits are common in FEP throughout all phases of the illness, including impairment in working memory, processing speed, verbal and visual learning, reasoning, and social cognition. Cognitive deficits are already present during the prodromal phases of the illness (39) and are not correlated with the DUP (40). Although it is widely believed that symptom fluctuation usually does not affect cognitive performance (41), an association between the level of negative symptoms and cognitive deficits has been reported several times, with cognitive performance improving when negative symptoms ease off (42).

There does not seem to be a cognitive decline in the first years of illness (39), a possible exception being progressive verbal memory deterioration (42). However, with longer follow-up times, cognitive functioning may continue to decline following the first episode. Over a lifespan, periods of cognitive deterioration in schizophrenia appear to be a period before the first episode and another at approximately 65 years of age (43). In the long term, people with schizophrenia are also at increased risk of dementia (11). Dementia is a very long-term outcome and not very relevant for the treatment of FEP. Recent research suggests that the increased risk of dementia may be mediated through comorbidities like cardiovascular disease (CHD) (44), whereas there is no genetic correlation between schizophrenia and Alzheimer's disease (45).

Cognitive functioning at the beginning of the psychotic illness may predict the illness course and functional outcome such as self-care, work performance and social functioning (46). Remission and relapses of FEP within the first 2 years of illness may be predicted by verbal fluency, memory and social cognition, and persistent negative symptoms and functional outcomes may be predicted by verbal memory (47). Social cognition has been found to specifically predict everyday community functioning, such as independent living skills, and social and work functioning (48). Of the social cognitive domains, the theory of mind might be an especially important treatment target due to its associations with functional outcome (48). In one study, FEP patients with preserved intelligence quotient (IQ) at psychosis onset had better outcomes at 3 years than other patients in terms of disorganization and negative symptoms, index admissions, and occupational outcome (49). Severe cognitive impairment by the time of the first psychotic episode may thus predict a more severe illness. Deficits in cognitive functions may affect adherence, insight, social skills, and one's overall capacity to take care of oneself thus, leading to a worse symptomatic and functional outcome. On the other hand, premorbid adjustment, motivation, negative symptoms, and insight may moderate the impact of cognition on these functional outcomes (46).

The functional outcome of FEP has also been predicted with premorbid cognitive reserve (50, 51). Higher premorbid IQ and educational attainment may help a person to cope with the effects of the disease, thus affecting the neuropsychological, functional and clinical outcome of FEP. High cognitive reserve may help the individual use compensatory abilities and is associated with better insight (49).

Brain Imaging

Brain imaging methods have been used to differentiate patients from healthy controls and to predict the long-term outcome of FEP. In recent years, several studies have used either structural or functional brain imaging, sometimes together with clinical information and other biomarker information, to classify FEP patients or patients with clinical high-risk symptoms from healthy control subjects (52–58). Accuracies in these ML studies that use one imaging modality have ranged from 66% (52, 55) to 87% (53), and the combination of structural magnetic resonance imaging (MRI) and diffusion tensor imaging data has been reported to result in enhanced accuracy: 93% (54). These classification studies have built the grounds upon which to study whether FEP patients can be further classified into subgroups with different outcomes.

Early multivariate ML studies suggested that continuous and remitting courses of illness were predictable based on structural MRIs alone, with accuracies of 58% (59) and 70% (60). However, these findings were not replicated in other research centers nor in the data pooled across centers (60). In a follow-up study by Pina-Camacho and co-workers, brain volumetric measures did not enhance the classification accuracy of schizophrenia spectrum vs. other psychoses beyond the 81% classification accuracy achieved using clinical symptoms alone (61).

Most earlier brain imaging studies on outcome prediction have used univariate methods. Univariate findings which may predict outcomes include alterations in rhythmic activity in electroencephalogram (EEG) (62); a prefrontal MRI spectroscopic marker of neuronal integrity (63); striatal dopamine-2 receptor binding potential (64); the integrity of the frontotemporal white matter tracts (65); abnormal gyrification of the cerebral cortex (66, 67); white matter network organization (68); and the volumes of the ventricles (69) and the temporal lobe in general (70), and the volumes of the hippocampus (71, 72) and the superior temporal gyrus (73) in particular. For a review on structural MRI measures as predictors of outcome, see Dazzan et al. (74). Outcome prediction based on any of the univariate findings is too inaccurate to be clinically useful (75). An exception might turn out to be using a lack of elevated dopamine synthesis capacity, which has been associated with antipsychotic treatment resistance in two studies (76, 77). These findings, however, provide important information for more complex ML models with potential for clinically sufficient prediction accuracy.

Genetics

The etiological significance of genetic factors in psychotic disorders is substantial: the heritability of schizophrenia spectrum and bipolar disorders is around 65–85% (78–80). Numerous studies have correlated variants in schizophrenia candidate genes with phenotypic features, sometimes also with outcome measures. However, recent genetic studies have questioned the validity of previously suggested schizophrenia candidate genes (81, 82). Therefore, we focus here on the potential value of genome-wise significant findings from genome-wide association (GWA) studies and rare damaging variants identified from GWA or exome/whole genome sequencing studies in predicting the outcomes of psychosis.

The number of identified, genome-wide significant genetic loci associated with schizophrenia in GWA studies currently increases in proportion to sample size, being already over 100 in 2014 (83) and 145 in the most recently reported GWA study (84). Consequently, polygenic risk score (PRS) estimates derived from GWA studies have become increasingly accurate. They have been used to predict both treatment response and long-term outcome. A higher schizophrenia PRS has been associated with worse treatment response (85), a higher likelihood of being in clozapine treatment (86), more frequent hospital admissions (87), and more severe negative symptoms (88) in patients with schizophrenia. One fairly large study, however, failed to find an association between PRS and poor treatment response in schizophrenia (89). In patients with bipolar disorder, a high schizophrenia PRS is associated with an increased risk of having psychotic symptoms (88), particularly mood-incongruent psychotic symptoms (90). In a FEP study sample, the schizophrenia PRS was predictive of a future schizophrenia diagnosis (as opposed to the diagnosis of other psychotic disorders), although its discriminatory accuracy was relatively modest (91). The bipolar disorder PRS, in turn, is associated with having more severe manic symptoms in patients with schizophrenia, but also with psychotic symptoms in patients with bipolar disorder, and a PRS calculated from the variants shared between bipolar disorder and schizophrenia is associated with psychotic symptoms in bipolar disorder and more severe negative symptoms in schizophrenia (88). The schizophrenia PRS has been associated with lower hippocampal volume in FEP patients (92), but overall the associations between the schizophrenia PRS and psychosis endophenotypes are modest (93). The benefit of a PRS is that it is a stable trait feature. It could be a useful component of larger predictive algorithms in the future, but this still needs more research.

Besides the polygenic background of common variants which individually have a very small effect, rare variants have been identified which are present in a very small proportion of the population but have a substantially larger effect on schizophrenia/psychosis risk. The Psychiatric Genomics Consortium recently validated six deletions and two duplications of significant risk factors for schizophrenia, and identified several novel ones (94). However, while these copy number variants (CNVs) are associated with an up to 60-fold elevated risk of schizophrenia in case-control studies (94), general population-based studies have also identified people carrying the same CNVs who have normal functioning and only minimal problems in cognitive tests (95). In exome and whole-genome sequencing studies, the first rare mutations in single genes that are associated with a substantially increased schizophrenia risk have been identified (96, 97). In addition, it has been shown that there is a burden of rare variants in genes intolerant of loss-of-function variants in schizophrenia (98). It is likely that the number of identified rare mutations in single genes in schizophrenia will increase considerably in the near future, and more information will be available from the phenotypic spectrum associated with them.

A common feature in CNVs and rare mutations is an association with a variety of neurodevelopmental problems, including intellectual disability, and patients with schizophrenia who have these rare variants have worse cognitive functioning than other patients with schizophrenia (96–98). Therefore, genetic testing for these rare variants may be useful for FEP patients who have a history of neurodevelopmental problems, poor cognitive functioning, and neurological symptoms. In contrast, there is currently no evidence on whether these variants are also predictive of treatment response or the long-term outcome.

There is also evidence of specific genes that are associated with both antipsychotic treatment response and side-effect risk which differ from those associated with disease risk. Alleles in the dopamine D2 receptor and in the glutamate ionotropic receptor delta type subunit 2 (GRID2) are associated with antipsychotic treatment response (99), and several genetic variants that predispose to antipsychotic-induced weight gain have been identified (100). In addition, pharmacogenetic tests related to drug metabolism are already in clinical use (101).

Blood-Based Biomarkers

Besides genetics, other potential blood-based biomarkers for psychotic disorders have been studied extensively (102), and several reviews and meta-analyses have been published (102–106). Some of the main lines of research are presented below. In general, there is much more research on whether certain biomarkers cross-sectionally separate patients from healthy controls than there is research about the possible predictive value of the biomarkers in patient treatment.

The association of a dysregulated immune response and psychosis is well-established. Several pro-inflammatory cytokines are elevated in FEP patients (107–109), including drug-naïve patients (110). The changes are similar in the cerebrospinal fluid (CSF) and blood, and they occur across severe mental disorders (109). There are also changes in the levels of distinct lymphocyte subtypes (111). While meta-analyses initially suggested that antipsychotic medication might decrease pro-inflammatory activation (108), a later meta-analysis did not find a significant medication effect (110). Further signals of a change in immune response come from associations with markers of oxidative stress (112) and the activation of the complement system (113). While various markers of immune response have been found to correlate with clinical features, such as structural brain abnormalities, symptoms and cognitive deficits (114–116), less is known about their predictive value. These biomarkers are part of a dynamic signaling network, and we currently do not fully understand their temporal patterns and variation in early psychosis. For other medical conditions, concentrations of immunological molecules in different tissues have been shown to be quite rapidly changing (117), which is understandable given their role in the coordination of immune response. In early psychosis, there may also be other factors, like sleep deprivation (118), which may contribute to the pro-inflammatory activation. The question remains open regarding to what extent inflammation might be secondary to metabolic changes, or vice versa. More information is needed on such confounding factors before inflammatory markers can be introduced as diagnostic or prognostic biomarkers.

C-reactive protein (CRP) has been the most commonly used measure of inflammation. In the largest meta-analysis on CRP levels and psychotic disorders, CRP levels were increased in both drug-naïve and unmedicated patients, as well as after the onset of psychosis (119), although one study with only drug-naïve FEP patients did not detect any difference in CRP between cases and controls (120). In Mendelian randomization studies, genetic variants leading to increased CRP levels are not associated with an increased risk of schizophrenia (121, 122), suggesting that the association between elevated CRP and schizophrenia is not caused by a common genetic mechanism. CRP is associated with increased mortality risk but not with the risk of rehospitalization in patients with depression, bipolar disorder or schizophrenia (123). However, CRP has been studied and suggested as a biomarker for numerous acute and chronic diseases, and it remains to be studied whether its best value in treating patients with psychotic disorders would actually be found in assessing the risk of comorbidities (e.g., in cardiovascular risk assessment) (124).

The anti-N-methyl-D-aspartate-type glutamate receptor (anti-NMDAR) encephalitis can in some cases present with prominent psychotic symptoms (125, 126). The identification of encephalitis in patients with early psychosis is crucial, as over 75% of patients with classic anti-NMDAR encephalitis have substantial recovery with specific treatments, while antipsychotic treatment is not effective (125). Based on several reports, however, the diagnostic evaluation of autoimmune encephalitis in FEP can be focused on those presenting specific neurological symptoms (125). Other than anti-NMDAR antibodies, autoantibodies detected in autoimmune encephalitis seem to remain negative in patients with isolated early psychotic symptoms (127). However, a recent study found that patients with schizophrenia and NMDAR antibodies suffer from more severe symptoms than other patients with schizophrenia despite a negative test for encephalitis (128). Therefore, the role of autoantibodies as biomarkers of longer-term outcomes deserves attention in future studies.

Several endocrine markers have also been studied in FEP, but it is unclear whether they reflect primary changes or secondary effects. They correlate with inflammation and metabolic changes, and the link to early trauma and stress response is strong for all of them. For instance, Misiak et al. have reviewed evidence for increased levels of testosterone and dehydroepiandrosterone in FEP (129) and suggest that these alterations might be related to a stress response. In drug-naïve FEP patients, there is evidence for an increased level of morning cortisol, cortisol awakening response, and increased prolactin levels, all of which may refer to a dysregulated hypothalamic-pituitary-adrenal (HPA) axis (130). In clinical high-risk patients, elevated cortisol predicted transitioning to psychosis (131), and in FEP patients it is correlated with the severity of symptoms and aggression (102). Its predictive value is less clear (102). Increased leptin in psychosis is mostly explained by a medication effect on weight gain, and a meta-analysis did not find significant changes in drug-naïve patients (132).

Peripheral monoamines and their metabolites have been studied as candidate biomarkers for treatment response in FEP. Elevated levels of plasma homovanillic acid, the principal dopamine metabolite, and the norepinephrine metabolite 3-methoxy-4-hydroxyphenylglycol have been associated with a better treatment response in a few, relatively small, studies (102). Tryptophan metabolite kynurenine acid (KYNA) has been studied extensively in recent years. A meta-analysis found that KYNA levels are elevated in CSF, but not in plasma, in patients with schizophrenia (133), and KYNA elevation is linked to proinflammatory activation (134). In addition, ratios of different tryptophan metabolites have predicted treatment response in patients with schizophrenia (135).

In the search for biomarkers, "omics"-based methodologies are becoming widely used. Proteomic methods have been used to identify the biomarkers that differentiate FEP or first-episode schizophrenia patients from controls (104). There tends to be consistency between studies in the identified biological pathways, many of which have already been mentioned before; the most important were the acute-phase pathway, communication between innate and adaptive immune cells, lipid and glucose metabolism, blood formation and clotting, and the stress response (104). Studies using the metabolomics and lipidomics approaches in schizophrenia research were recently reviewed by Davison et al. (106). The most consistent findings across studies have been elevated 3-methoxy-4-hydroxyphenylglycol, glutamate, lipid peroxidation metabolites, and triglycerides (triacylglycerols), and decreased creatinine, vitamins (B6, D, E, and folate), phosphatidylcholines, phosphatidylethanolamines, and polyunsaturated fatty acids (106). Several groups have suggested biomarker panels that differentiate patients with schizophrenia from healthy controls, but there is little overlap in individual metabolites in these panels (106). Fewer studies have investigated whether these biomarkers have prognostic value. As examples of such studies, 3-hydroxykynurenine was predictive of symptom improvement in first-episode schizophrenia in one study (136), and the higher baseline levels of triacylglycerols with a low carbon number and double-bond count were predictive of weight gain in FEP in another study (137). Of note is that low levels in some biomarkers of nutrition, like vitamin D, require supplementation, and it may be relevant to monitor them as a part of the general health assessment of patients with FEP.

Increasingly, various biomarkers are combined into panels in order to have better predictive value, resembling the PRS of genetic studies. Typically, individual biomarkers and their analytical methods differ between research groups, and therefore this line of work is difficult to summarize. One example is given in the following. Sabine Bahn's group developed and validated a biomarker panel using five independent study samples (138). Their panel consisted of 26 analytes measuring lipid transport, inflammation, the immune system, hormonal signaling, growth factor signaling and the clotting cascade (138). The predictive power of the panel to identify patients who later developed psychosis from two independent at-risk cohorts was good (the area under the curve 0.82–0.90) (138). In the North American Prodrome Longitudinal Study, a classifier was built that was able to predict psychosis conversion with an accuracy of 0.90 using 15 analytes measuring lipid transport, immune system, hormonal signaling and the clotting cascade (139). Of note is that, while the profile of analytes were fairly similar in these two studies, only three individual analytes (interleukin 8, thyroid stimulating hormone, and factor VII) were the same in both panels (138, 139). While this example is not about prognostic biomarkers, it illustrates the challenges in replicating this type of biomarker panels.

Physical Comorbidities and Their Predictors

CVDs are a leading cause of excess mortality in schizophrenia (6, 7), and preventing CVD risk factors (such as impaired glucose tolerance and diabetes, obesity and dyslipidemia) in patients with FEP is an important target.

Weight gain affects a significant proportion of individuals using antipsychotic medication and is associated with almost all antipsychotics (8, 140). However, there is considerable individual variation in antipsychotic-induced weight gain. Various risk factors for antipsychotic-induced weight gain have been reported in the literature but only with limited consistency. Several studies have found that a young age and low BMI before antipsychotic treatment predict a larger increase in weight (141–144). Other reported risk factors for weight gain include female sex, a non-white ethnic background, negative symptoms, poor social functioning, and co-medications, while smoking and cannabis use have been associated with less weight gain (141–146). A dysregulated glucose metabolism may also mark an increased risk of weight gain (147, 148). Early weight gain predicted further weight increase in a longer follow-up (149). In a meta-analysis of the genetic factors affecting antipsychotic-induced weight gain, 13 single-nucleotide polymorphisms (SNPs) in nine genes were significant predictors, with the most significant effect sizes for SNPs in ADRA2A, DRD2, HTR2C, and MC4R (100). However, a PRS computed from the 6 SNPs with the largest effect on weight gain only explained 5.6% of the variance in weight gain in two cohorts of FEP patients, showing that the predictive value of genetic markers is modest (100). Combining the genetic findings with clinical risk factors for weight gain has resulted in modest improvements when compared to only using clinical factors. Whereas, in one study genetic data (SNPs from GWA studies of BMI and candidate gene studies) increased the prediction accuracy compared to using clinical data alone (150), in another study adding data from PRSs did not improve the prediction of weight gain compared to the clinical information (148).

Regarding impaired glucose tolerance and dyslipidemias, antipsychotic medication contributes to them, but many markers of prediabetes—including insulin resistance, impaired glucose tolerance, and elevated triglycerides—are more common in drug-naïve patients with FEP than in age- and gender-matched controls (130, 151, 152). Insulin resistance seems to precede obesity in FEP (153, 154), and antipsychotic-naïve FEP patients do not differ in BMI from controls (155). Antipsychotics have a more rapid effect on insulin sensitivity than on weight, which has also been shown in healthy volunteers exposed to antipsychotics (156). Furthermore, insulin resistance predicts more increase in weight in patients with FEP during the first year of antipsychotic treatment (147). A rare, unpredictable adverse effect of several second-generation antipsychotics is type 2 diabetes manifesting as diabetic ketoacidosis (9). Similarly, there are case reports of severe triglyceridemia and acute pancreatitis related to antipsychotics (157, 158). Predictors of progression to diabetes or the risk of severe dyslipidemias in FEP are currently lacking.

The overall risk of CVDs may not be elevated in drug-naïve patients with FEP but it already increases significantly during the first 6–12 months of antipsychotic treatment (159, 160). Besides the classical risk factors, also elevated total white blood cell count and CRP levels have been associated with increased CVD risk, and increased CRP levels have been associated with mortality in psychotic disorders (123, 161). Of the other predictors of mortality, smoking increases the mortality risk due to associated diseases and medical conditions (7, 162). Antipsychotic use is associated with a lower mortality risk in several studies (23, 163), but using doses of antipsychotics that exceed the recommended dose may increase CVD mortality (164). The prediction of CVD risk for people with severe mental illness is more accurate if the traditional risk factors—smoking, diabetes, hypertension, obesity, and dyslipidemia—are complemented with information on psychiatric diagnosis, the use of antipsychotics and antidepressants, and harmful alcohol use (165). Many studies have evaluated the CVD risk for patients with psychotic disorders compared to the risk for healthy controls using traditional algorithms like the Framingham risk score (166), but it has not been studied in large, prospective cohorts whether these risk algorithms should be tailored to patients with psychotic disorders.

Suicide Risk and its Predictors

Up to 90% of clinical high-risk patients report suicidal ideation, between 15 and 26% of FEP patients have made at least one suicide attempt by their first treatment contacts, and 2–11% attempt to end their lives over the first year after treatment onset (167). The risk for an attempt is highest during the month preceding treatment seeking and the first 2 months following that (10, 168). Suicide attempts in the early course of illness are characterized by methods of high lethality and include most of the suicide completions (168). Long-term follow-up studies and register studies also show that most suicides occur during the first 2 years after the onset of FEP (10, 169, 170).

The predictors of a higher suicide risk include the earlier age of onset; a history of previous suicide attempts; the severity of the symptoms of depression, anxiety, and psychosis; substance abuse; being male; a high IQ and better neurocognitive functioning; a high level of education; high socio-economic status; poor premorbid adjustment; living alone; a longer DUP; insight; and a family history of suicide (29, 167, 170, 171). Compliance with treatment has been demonstrated to reduce the suicide risk (171), whereas the highest OR for suicides has been found for patients with a previous history of suicide attempts and a history of alcohol abuse (172).

The neurobiology of suicidality was recently reviewed (173); the presented biological mechanisms have all also been of interest in the etiological research of early psychosis. Several investigators have also presented ML algorithms to identify suicidal patients in a retrospective setting. The prediction has been done based on the information from health records, either through an expert review (154) or using language analysis (155). Applications predicting the future in the predictive models could detect half of the suicide attempts and deaths during the next 60 days (156). These models were not developed specifically for FEP patients, however.

Substance Use

Continuing substance use is predictive of several adverse outcomes in FEP patients. It is associated with a higher risk of relapse and a poorer 10-year outcome, whereas patients who discontinued substance use within 2 years after the first psychotic episode had similar 10-year outcome as those who had no history of substance use (174). Sustained cannabis use in FEP patients is associated with higher relapse rates, longer hospital admissions, and more severe positive symptoms (175, 176). As reviewed above, substance abuse is a risk factor for suicidal behavior. In addition, smoking is a major risk factor for premature mortality in patients with psychosis, as it is in the general population (7, 162). To summarize, the outcome is worse across many domains in FEP patients with persistent SUD but not for those who discontinue substance use. Therefore, treating a comorbid SUD should be an integral part of treatment of FEP.

Limitations

In order to build reliable prediction tools, large and representative patient samples are needed. Clinical follow-up studies, which require good collaboration and interest from the participants, always have some attrition. In the Oslo Schizophrenia Recovery study, 10% of those fully recovered were no longer in any contact with mental health services (38). These individuals are easily lost in follow-up, which should be taken into account when estimating the recovery rates and predictors of remission and recovery (38). On the other hand, patients with prominent disorganized symptoms may be too ill to give an informed consent in the first place. In retrospective studies where complete information has been available (e.g., from a lifetime review of medical records), about 15–20% of patients with schizophrenia have had the disorganized subtype, which is characterized by poor functioning from the onset of illness and a considerably poorer long-term outcome compared to other schizophrenia subtypes (177, 178). If these patients are underrepresented in clinical studies which have intensive protocols and require the capacity to give informed consent, this could explain why disorganized symptoms have not emerged as notable outcome predictors in many studies. Register-based studies are able to overcome selective attrition, but clinical data available in health care registers is often superficial and the information available from those who have dropped out from treatment is limited, even in countries where different types of nationwide registers exist (e.g., registers on sociodemographic factors like work and income).

A problem related to blood-based biomarkers is that psychiatric research rarely fully considers what is already known about these biomarkers in other medical fields. Many suggested biomarkers have stronger research evidence from another medical field and are affected by various confounding factors, like stress, sleep, nutrition, smoking, exercise, and BMI. There may be substantial effects of antipsychotic and other psychotropic medication on various biomarkers, and these have not yet been fully characterized. On the other hand, some biomarkers may only be relevant for a specific subtype of FEP. These factors should be carefully examined before recommending any blood-based biomarker for clinical use.

FUTURE DIRECTIONS

Methodological advancements may lead to better biomarkers from one modality or to improved prediction by an optimal combination of various markers. Clinicians also need better tools for interpretation of predictive information.

Prediction Strategies and Tools

Disease risk calculators have been available in many medical fields for decades (179, 180) but are only now emerging in psychiatry. As an example, a risk calculator for predicting the psychosis conversion risk in patients with a clinical high-risk state was recently published (181). The calculator combined scores on prodromal symptom severity, decline in social functioning, and verbal learning and memory (181). However, with increasing predicted risk the sensitivity of the test became quite modest (181).

Outcome prediction tools for FEP do not currently exist. Two recent studies have used simulated data to illustrate an approach to developing such tools. Schubert et al. illustrated how multimodal sociodemographic, clinical, psychological, imaging, and other neurobiological information could be used to develop a prediction tool for the different disease trajectories of FEP (47). Schmidt et al. (105) suggested sequential testing as another method to improve outcome testing. They presented such a model in the context of clinical high-risk research, where it was shown that sequential testing, first with clinical markers and then with different biological markers—including MRI, EEG, and blood biomarkers—was able to markedly improve the accuracy of predicting future psychosis (105). Of the patients who showed increased risk in all three tests, only 2% did not convert to psychosis (105). The challenge of sequential testing is compromised sensitivity as each known test misses true converters. ML provides promising tools for increasing sensitivity.

Machine Learning

ML refers to various tools that learn to classify or score new data once given a training data set (182). Thus, it offers a technique with which to attain a computer-assisted clinical decision-making tool. In unsupervised ML, the algorithm differentiates naturally occurring classes in the data set. In supervised ML, the ML algorithm is given a known outcome, for example a diagnosis or a level of functioning. ML algorithms can handle enormous quantities of data and find, in addition to linear associations, non-linear associations, including those between an outcome and different combinations of data features (182). The resulting complexity of the model easily leads to overfitting, that is, high accuracy in the training set, but poor generalizability to independent data sets. The goal of ML analysis is to optimize the model so that the algorithm performs optimally, both in the training set and in an independent test set (182, 183).

There are multiple ML methods available, including neural networks and support vector machine. By some analogy to the brain's functioning, neural networks use a set of hierarchical layers that correspond to different levels of abstraction (182). A support vector machine finds the largest marginal between the data points that separates the defined outcomes (184). By using a matrix of similarities between data points (the kernel), high dimensional data sets, such as brain images, can be used efficiently even in small samples (184). ML tools are not restricted to a single modality, such as a clinical data set or a brain image, and different modalities can be combined. They may have complementary information, and emerging evidence suggests multimodal methods are likely to enhance accuracy (185). Results from ML analyses in a single modality can be used as either a concatenated or separate input to a new ML model, or they can be used in sequential testing.

Novel Imaging Methods

Non-invasive brain imaging methods are developing constantly. For example, an increase in MRI field strengths increases the signal-to-noise ratio and benefits translational research in FEP. New imaging methods can reveal new aspects of the brain (186). Such methods may provide complementary data that increase the accuracy of predictive models either alone or combined with other data.

In addition to the development of devices and radioligands, functional imaging may benefit from task development. Tasks are necessary in addition to resting-state imaging as they synchronize mental states and related brain functions, resulting in imaging signals that are comparable across subjects and time points. A limitation in common tasks—such as sensory, motor, or cognitive tasks—is that while they are well-controlled, they only activate a very limited set of brain circuitries. In contrast, psychotic disorders are related to multiple functional alterations across the brain (187). Therefore, predictive models would likely benefit from rich naturalistic stimuli—such as music, stories, or movies—that activate most of the brain across subjects in a synchronous manner (188, 189).

Biomarkers

Novel methodologies may lead to new biomarker discoveries. Methodologies are developing rapidly in genetics and various fields of "omics" research. An example of a novel strategy is untargeted screening for IgG reactivity to fragments of human proteins, which has identified potentially interesting novel autoantibodies in FEP (190). However, in order to have new biomarkers for clinical use, several steps are needed after initial discovery (191). As noted by Fond et al. (102), biomarkers need to be "accurate, reproducible, acceptable to the patient, easy to interpret, and have an adequate sensitivity and specificity." This means that the procedures for assays need to be optimized and their reproducibility within and between laboratories ensured (191). Possible important covariates affecting the biomarker level, like age or sex, need to be identified and taken into account (191). The frequency of true-positive and false-positive results must be determined in different clinical settings, after which the criteria for a positive screening test need to be defined (191). If biomarkers are combined as risk scores, this process is needed both for the individual components and the combined score (191). Finally, the cost-effectiveness of biomarkers needs to be demonstrated (191). For the great majority of biomarkers presented in this review, the critical steps regarding reproducibility and accuracy in clinical settings have not yet been accomplished.

The Validation of Multimodal Predictive Models

To be implemented clinically, multimodal predictive models need to be validated. Discovery studies tend to be small and need to be replicated in larger samples. Multicenter studies can provide the necessary evidence that a model functions independently of certain samples and investigators. It has been shown, however, that the high heterogeneity of a sample decreases the performance of the model in multicenter studies (192). Thus, the model may need to be finally optimized in the local population. Finally, it is not enough to predict the future for those with FEP, but the predictions need to serve the patients' needs. Thus, the ultimate goal is to show that validated predictive models help to enhance the outcomes of the patients in randomized controlled settings.

No predictive model can be deterministic as the future of many internal and environmental factors is impossible to predict. Thus, to optimize predictive models, they should be updated based on follow-up data. Such updates may not need costly examinations by the health care system. Knowledge about daily experiences can be collected by mobile applications (193) and information about changes in movements and communication can be collected from mobile phones without the need of a patient actively inputting the data. Such information may help to update the multimodal prediction models of the future.

User Interface

Multimodal prediction models need visualization tools in order to be clinically useful. Naturally, before such tools are incorporated into clinical practice, there has to be robust evidence that the prediction model itself is valid. An example of a computer-assisted clinical decision-making tool is the Disease State Index (DSI) and the Disease State Fingerprint tool, which were initially developed to predict Alzheimer's disease risk in elderly people with mild cognitive impairment and they have been expanded for use in differentiating the separate types of dementias (194–196). Two important features in the DSI are that full information from all potential predictors is not needed from an individual patient to use the prediction model and also that the visualization of different risk components is easy to interpret. Furthermore, the tool illustrates whether there are inconsistencies between different predictors, in other words if some outcome predictors point out to a poor, other predictors indicate a better outcome. Such tools would be very useful especially for enhancing the use of brain imaging and cognitive data in outcome prediction for FEP.

Conclusions

The personalized treatment of FEP will need predictive tools. At a group level, there are already many clinical parameters that predict different outcomes, but these should be transformed into an individual-level prediction, where patients typically have mixed features—some predicting a better outcome, others a worse outcome. Methodological advancements such as ML will help in developing multimodal prediction tools and in transforming the research findings into clinical practice. User-friendly interfaces are needed for such tools. The possibility to use such platforms with incomplete information is also important. At the same time, it has to be remembered that scientific breakthroughs are often unpredictable. The research field needs to ensure that novel findings, for example those emerging from genetic studies, are thoroughly investigated—it is possible that the biomarkers available within 10 years are completely outside the lists mentioned in this review.

AUTHOR CONTRIBUTIONS

All authors listed have made a substantial, direct and intellectual contribution to the work, and approved it for publication.

FUNDING

This work was supported by the Academy of Finland (grant #278171 to JS and #251155 to TR), the Sigrid Jusélius Foundation (JS, TR), the Finnish Cultural Foundation (TM, JS), the Jalmari and Rauha Ahokas Foundation (TM), the Doctoral Program Brain and Mind of the University of Helsinki (TM), the Finnish Medical Foundation (TR), the Yrjö Jahnsson Foundation (#6781 to ML), the Päivikki and Sakari Sohlberg Foundation (ML), the Juho Vainio Foundation (ML), State funding for university-level health research (Hospital District of Helsinki and Uusimaa #TYH2017128 to TK and #TYH2013332, #TYH2014228 to OM and TK) and the University of Helsinki (OM, TK, and JK).

REFERENCES

1. Morgan C, Lappin J, Heslin M, Donoghue K, Lomas B, Reininghaus U, et al. Reappraising the long-term course and outcome of psychotic disorders: the AESOP-10 study. *Psychol Med.* (2014) 44:2713–26. doi: 10.1017/S0033291714000282
2. Lally J, Ajnakina O, Stubbs B, Cullinane M, Murphy KC, Gaughran F, et al. Remission and recovery from first-episode psychosis in adults: systematic review and meta-analysis of long-term outcome studies. *Br J Psychiatry* (2017) 211:350–8. doi: 10.1192/bjp.bp.117.201475
3. Lappin JM, Heslin M, Lomas B, Jones PB, Doody GA, Reininghaus UA, et al. Early sustained recovery following first episode psychosis: evidence from the AESOP10 follow-up study. *Schizophr Res.* (2018) 199:341–45. doi: 10.1016/j.schres.2018.03.014
4. Demjaha A, Lappin JM, Stahl D, Patel MX, MacCabe JH, Howes OD, et al. Antipsychotic treatment resistance in first-episode psychosis: prevalence, subtypes and predictors. *Psychol Med.* (2017) 47:1981–9. doi: 10.1017/S0033291717000435
5. Eskelinen S, Sailas E, Joutsenniemi K, Holi M, Koskela TH, Suvisaari J. Multiple physical healthcare needs among outpatients with schizophrenia: findings from a health examination study. *Nord J Psychiatry* (2017) 71:448–54. doi: 10.1080/08039488.2017.1319497
6. Olfson M, Gerhard T, Huang C, Crystal S, Stroup TS. Premature mortality among adults with schizophrenia in the United States. *JAMA Psychiatry* (2015) 72:1172–81. doi: 10.1001/jamapsychiatry.2015.1737
7. Keinänen J, Mantere O, Markkula N, Partti K, Perälä J, Saarni SI, et al. Mortality in people with psychotic disorders in Finland: a population-based 13-year follow-up study. *Schizophr Res.* (2018) 192:113–8. doi: 10.1016/j.schres.2017.04.048
8. Leucht S, Cipriani A, Spineli L, Mavridis D, Orey D, Richter F, et al. Comparative efficacy and tolerability of 15 antipsychotic drugs in schizophrenia: a multiple-treatments meta-analysis. *Lancet* (2013) 382:951–62. doi: 10.1016/S0140-6736(13)60733-3
9. Suvisaari J, Keinänen J, Eskelinen S, Mantere O. Diabetes and schizophrenia. *Curr Diab Rep.* (2016) 16:16. doi: 10.1007/s11892-015-0704-4
10. Simon GE, Stewart C, Yarborough BJ, Lynch F, Coleman KJ, Beck A, et al. Mortality rates after the first diagnosis of psychotic disorder in adolescents and young adults. *JAMA Psychiatry* (2018) 75:254–60. doi: 10.1001/jamapsychiatry.2017.4437
11. Fedyszyn IE, Robinson J, Harris MG, Paxton SJ, Francey S, Edwards J. Suicidal behaviours during treatment for first-episode psychosis: towards a comprehensive approach to service-based prevention. *Early Interv Psychiatry* (2014) 8:387–95. doi: 10.1111/eip.12084
12. Andreasen NC, Carpenter WT Jr, Kane JM, Lasser RA, Marder SR, Weinberger DR. Remission in schizophrenia: proposed criteria and rationale for consensus. *Am J Psychiatry* (2005) 162:441–9. doi: 10.1176/appi.ajp.162.3.441
13. Temesgen WA, Chien WT, Bressington D. Conceptualizations of subjective recovery from recent onset psychosis and its associated factors: a systematic review. *Early Interv Psychiatry* (2018). doi: 10.1111/eip.12698. [Epub ahead of print].
14. Alvarez-Jimenez M, Priede A, Hetrick SE, Bendall S, Killackey E, Parker AG, et al. Risk factors for relapse following treatment for first episode psychosis: a systematic review and meta-analysis of longitudinal studies. *Schizophr Res.* (2012) 139:116–28. doi: 10.1016/j.schres.2012.05.00
15. Morgan C, Fearon P, Lappin J, Heslin M, Donoghue K, Lomas B, et al. Ethnicity and long-term course and outcome of psychotic disorders in a UK sample: the ÆSOP-10 study. *Br J Psychiatry* (2017) 211:88–94. doi: 10.1192/bjp.bp.116.193342
16. Friis S, Melle I, Johannessen JO, Røssberg JI, Barder HE, Evensen JH, et al. Early predictors of ten-year course in first-episode psychosis. *Psychiatr Serv.* (2016) 67:438–43. doi: 10.1176/appi.ps.201400558
17. Koutsouleris N, Kahn RS, Chekroud AM, Leucht S, Falkai P, Wobrock T, et al. Multisite prediction of 4-week and 52-week treatment outcomes in patients with first-episode psychosis: a machine learning approach. *Lancet Psychiatry* (2016) 3:935–46. doi: 10.1016/S2215-0366(16)30171-7
18. Thompson A, Winsper C, Marwaha S, Haynes J, Alvarez-Jimenez M, Hetrick S, et al. Maintenance antipsychotic treatment versus discontinuation strategies following remission from first episode psychosis: systematic review. *BJPsych Open* (2018) 4:215–25. doi: 10.1192/bjo.2018.17
19. Tiihonen J, Tanskanen A, Taipale H. 20-year nationwide follow-up study on discontinuation of antipsychotic treatment in first-episode schizophrenia. *Am J Psychiatry* (2018) 175:765–73. doi: 10.1176/appi.ajp.2018.17091001
20. Wunderink L, Nieboer RM, Wiersma D, Sytema S, Nienhuis FJ. Recovery in remitted first-episode psychosis at 7 years of follow-up of an early dose reduction/discontinuation or maintenance treatment strategy: long-term follow-up of a 2-year randomized clinical trial. *JAMA Psychiatry* (2013) 70:913–20. doi: 10.1001/jamapsychiatry.2013.19
21. Hui CLM, Honer WG, Lee EHM, Chang WC, Chan SKW, Chen ESM, et al. Long-term effects of discontinuation from antipsychotic maintenance following first-episode schizophrenia and related disorders: a 10 year follow-up of a randomised, double-blind trial. *Lancet Psychiatry* (2018) 5:432–42. doi: 10.1016/S2215-0366(18)30090-7
22. Lally J, Ajnakina O, Di Forti M, Trotta A, Demjaha A, Kolliakou A, et al. Two distinct patterns of treatment resistance: clinical predictors of treatment resistance in first-episode schizophrenia spectrum psychoses. *Psychol Med.* (2016) 46:3231–40. doi: 10.1017/S0033291716002014
23. Raij TT, Mäntylä T, Mantere O, Kieseppä T, Suvisaari J. Cortical salience network activation precedes the development of delusion severity. *Psychol Med.* (2016) 46:2741–8. doi: 10.1017/S0033291716001057
24. van der Meer L, Costafreda S, Aleman A, David AS. Self-reflection and the brain: a theoretical review and meta-analysis of neuroimaging studies with implications for schizophrenia. *Neurosci Biobehav Rev* (2010) 34:935–46. doi: 10.1016/j.neubiorev.2009.12.004
25. O'Connor JA, Wiffen BD, Di Forti M, Ferrato L, Joseph C, Kolliakou A, et al. Neuropsychological, clinical and cognitive insight predictors of outcome in a first episode psychosis study. *Schizophr Res.* (2013) 149:70–6. doi: 10.1016/j.schres.2013.06.005
26. O'Connor JA, Ellett L, Ajnakina O, Schoeler T, Kolliakou A, Trotta A, et al. Can cognitive insight predict symptom remission in a first episode psychosis cohort? *BMC Psychiatry* (2017) 17:54. doi: 10.1186/s12888-017-1210-9
27. Buchy L, Barbato M, MacMaster FP, Bray S, Clark D, Deighton S, et al. Cognitive insight is associated with cortical thickness in first-episode psychosis. *Schizophr Res.* (2016) 172:16–22. doi: 10.1016/j.schres.2016.02.026
28. Kuang C, Buchy L, Barbato M, Makowski C, MacMaster, FP, Bray S, et al. A pilot study of cognitive insight and structural covariance in first-episode psychosis. *Schizophr Res.* (2017) 179:91–6. doi: 10.1016/j.schres.2016.09.036
29. Coentre R, Talina MC, Góis C, Figueira ML. Depressive symptoms and suicidal behavior after first-episode psychosis: a comprehensive systematic review. *Psychiatry Res.* (2017) 253:240–8. doi: 10.1016/j.psychres.2017.04.010
30. Vohs JL, George S, Leonhardt BL, Lysaker PH. An integrative model of the impairments in insight in schizophrenia: emerging research on causal factors and treatments. *Expert Rev Neurother.* (2016) 16:1193–204. doi: 10.1080/14737175.2016.1199275
31. Bergé D, Mané A, Salgado P, Cortizo R, Garnier C, Gomez L, et al. Predictors of relapse and functioning in first-episode psychosis: a two-year follow-up study. *Psychiatr Serv.* (2016) 67:227–33. doi: 10.1176/appi.ps.201400316
32. Lysaker PH, Pattison ML, Leonhardt BL, Phelps S, Vohs JL. Insight in schizophrenia spectrum disorders: relationship with behavior, mood and perceived quality of life, underlying causes and emerging treatments. *World Psychiatry* (2018) 17:12–23. doi: 10.1002/wps.20508
33. Czobor P, Van Dorn RA, Citrome L, Kahn RS, Fleischhacker WW, Volavka J. Treatment adherence in schizophrenia: a patient-level meta-analysis of combined CATIE and EUFEST studies. *Eur Neuropsychopharmacol.* (2015) 25:1158–66. doi: 10.1016/j.euroneuro.2015.04.003
34. Velligan DI, Sajatovic M, Hatch A, Kramata P, Docherty JP. Why do psychiatric patients stop antipsychotic medication? A systematic review of reasons for nonadherence to medication in patients with serious mental illness. *Patient Prefer Adherence* (2017) 11:449–68. doi: 10.2147/PPA.S124658
35. Drake RJ, Nordentoft M, Haddock G, Arango C, Fleischhacker WW, Glenthøj B, et al. Modeling determinants of medication attitudes and poor adherence in early nonaffective psychosis: implications for intervention. *Schizophr Bull.* (2015) 41:584–96. doi: 10.1093/schbul/sbv015
36. Klaas HS, Clémence A, Marion-Veyron R, Antonietti JP, Alameda L, Golay P, et al. Insight as a social identity process in the evolution of psychosocial

functioning in the early phase of psychosis. *Psychol Med.* (2017) 47:718–29. doi: 10.1017/S0033291716002506

37. Freeman D, Startup H, Dunn G, Wingham G, Cernis E, Evans N, et al. Persecutory delusions and psychological well-being. *Soc Psychiatry Psychiatr Epidemiol.* (2014) 49:1045–50. doi: 10.1007/s00127-013-0803-y
38. Torgalsbøen AK, Fu S, Czajkowski N. Resilience trajectories to full recovery in first-episode schizophrenia. *Eur Psychiatry* (2018) 52:54–60. doi: 10.1016/j.eurpsy.2018.04.007
39. Bora E, Murray RM. Meta-analysis of cognitive deficits in ultra-high risk to psychosis and first-episode psychosis: do the cognitive deficits progress over, or after, the onset of psychosis? *Schizophr Bull.* (2014) 40:744–55. doi: 10.1093/schbul/sbt085
40. Bora E, Yalincetin B, Akdede BB, Alptekin K. Duration of untreated psychosis and neurocognition in first-episode psychosis: a meta-analysis. *Schizophr Res.* (2018) 193:3–10. doi: 10.1016/j.schres.2017.06.021
41. Rund BR, Barder HE, Evensen J, Haahr U, ten Velden Hegelstad W, Joa I, et al. Neurocognition and duration of psychosis: a 10-year follow-up of first-episode patients. *Schizophr Bull.* (2016) 42:87–95. doi: 10.1093/schbul/sbv083
42. Bozikas VP, Andreou C. Longitudinal studies of cognition in first episode psychosis: a systematic review of the literature. *Aust N Z J Psychiatry* (2011) 45:93–108. doi: 10.3109/00048674.2010.541418
43. Harvey PD. What is the evidence for changes in cognition and functioning over the lifespan in patients with schizophrenia? *J Clin Psychiatry* (2014) 75 (Suppl. 2):34–8. doi: 10.4088/JCP.13065su1.08
44. Lin CE, Chung CH, Chen LF, Chi MJ. Increased risk of dementia in patients with schizophrenia: a population-based cohort study in Taiwan. *Eur Psychiatry* (2018) 53:7–16. doi: 10.1016/j.eurpsy.2018.05.005
45. Brainstorm Consortium, Anttila V, Bulik-Sullivan B, Finucane HK, Walters RK, Bras J, et al. Analysis of shared heritability in common disorders of the brain. *Science* (2018) 360:eaap8757. doi: 10.1126/science.aap8757
46. Rajji TK, Miranda D, Mulsant BH. Cognition, function, and disability in patients with schizophrenia: a review of longitudinal studies. *Can J Psychiatry* (2014) 59:13–7. doi: 10.1177/070674371405900104
47. Schubert KO, Clark SR, Baune BT. The use of clinical and biological characteristics to predict outcome following First Episode Psychosis. *Aust N Z J Psychiatry* (2015) 49:24–35. doi: 10.1177/0004867414560650
48. Fett AK, Viechtbauer W, Dominguez MD, Penn DL, van Os J, Krabbendam L. The relationship between neurocognition and social cognition with functional outcomes in schizophrenia: a meta-analysis. *Neurosci Biobehav Rev.* (2011) 35:573–88. doi: 10.1016/j.neubiorev.2010.07.001
49. Leeson VC, Sharma P, Harrison M, Ron MA, Barnes TR, Joyce EM. IQ trajectory, cognitive reserve, and clinical outcome following a first episode of psychosis: a 3-year longitudinal study. *Schizophr Bull.* (2011) 37:768–77. doi: 10.1093/schbul/sbp143
50. Amoretti S, Bernardo M, Bonnin CM, Bioque M, Cabrera B, Mezquida G, et al. The impact of cognitive reserve in the outcome of first-episode psychoses: 2-year follow-up study. *Eur Neuropsychopharmacol.* (2016) 26:1638–48. doi: 10.1016/j.euroneuro.2016.07.003
51. van Winkel R, Myin-Germeys I, De Hert M, Delespaul P, Peuskens J, van Os J. The association between cognition and functional outcome in first-episode patients with schizophrenia: mystery resolved? *Acta Psychiatr Scand.* (2007) 116:119–24. doi: 10.1111/j.1600-0447.2007.01014.x
52. Bendfeldt K, Smieskova R, Koutsouleris N, Klöppel S, Schmidt A, Walter A, et al. Classifying individuals at high-risk for psychosis based on functional brain activity during working memory processing. *Neuroimage Clin.* (2015) 9:555–63. doi: 10.1016/j.nicl.2015.09.015
53. Borgwardt S, Koutsouleris N, Aston J, Studerus E, Smieskova R, Riecher-Rössler A, et al. Distinguishing prodromal from first-episode psychosis using neuroanatomical single-subject pattern recognition. *Schizophr Bull.* (2013) 39:1105–14. doi: 10.1093/schbul/sbs095
54. Peruzzo D, Castellani U, Perlini C, Bellani M, Marinelli V, Rambaldelli G, et al. Classification of first-episode psychosis: a multi-modal multi-feature approach integrating structural and diffusion imaging. *J Neural Transm (Vienna).* (2015) 122:897–905. doi: 10.1007/s00702-014-1324-x
55. Pettersson-Yeo W, Benetti S, Marquand AF, Dell'acqua F, Williams SC, Allen P, et al. Using genetic, cognitive and multi-modal neuroimaging data to identify ultra-high-risk and first-episode psychosis at the individual level. *Psychol Med.* (2013) 43:2547–62. doi: 10.1017/S003329171300024X
56. Rikandi E, Pamilo S, Mäntylä T, Suvisaari J, Kieseppä T, Hari R, et al. Precuneus functioning differentiates first-episode psychosis patients during the fantasy movie Alice in Wonderland. *Psychol Med.* (2017) 47:495–506. doi: 10.1017/S0033291716002609
57. Squarcina L, Perlini C, Peruzzo D, Castellani U, Marinelli V, Bellani M, et al. The use of dynamic susceptibility contrast (DSC) MRI to automatically classify patients with first episode psychosis. *Schizophr Res.* (2015) 165:38–44. doi: 10.1016/j.schres.2015.03.017
58. Squarcina L, Castellani U, Bellani M, Perlini C, Lasalvia A, Dusi N, et al. Classification of first-episode psychosis in a large cohort of patients using support vector machine and multiple kernel learning techniques. *Neuroimage* (2017) 145(Pt B):238–45. doi: 10.1016/j.neuroimage.2015.12.007
59. Zanetti MV, Schaufelberger MS, Doshi J, Ou Y, Ferreira LK, Menezes PR, et al. Neuroanatomical pattern classification in a population-based sample of first-episode schizophrenia. *Prog Neuropsychopharmacol Biol Psychiatry* (2013) 43:116–25. doi: 10.1016/j.pnpbp.2012.12.005
60. Nieuwenhuis M, Schnack HG, van Haren NE, Lappin J, Morgan C, Reinders AA, et al. Multi-center MRI prediction models: predicting sex and illness course in first episode psychosis patients. *Neuroimage* (2017) 145(Pt B):246–53. doi: 10.1016/j.neuroimage.2016.07.027
61. Pina-Camacho L, Garcia-Prieto J, Parellada M, Castro-Fornieles J, Gonzalez-Pinto AM, Bombin I, et al. Predictors of schizophrenia spectrum disorders in early-onset first episodes of psychosis: a support vector machine model. *Eur Child Adolesc Psychiatry* (2015) 24:427–40. doi: 10.1007/s00787-014-0593-0
62. Manchanda R, Norman R, Malla A, Harricharan R, Northcott S, Richard J. Electroencephalographic abnormalities and 5-year outcome in first-episode psychosis. *Can J Psychiatry* (2014) 59:285–8. doi: 10.1177/070674371405900508
63. Wood SJ, Berger GE, Lambert M, Conus P, Velakoulis D, Stuart GW, et al. Prediction of functional outcome 18 months after a first psychotic episode: a proton magnetic resonance spectroscopy study. *Arch Gen Psychiatry* (2006) 63:969–76. doi: 10.1001/archpsyc.63.9.969
64. Corripio I, Pérez V, Catafau AM, Mena E, Carrió I, Alvarez E. Striatal D2 receptor binding as a marker of prognosis and outcome in untreated first-episode psychosis. *Neuroimage* (2006) 29:662–6. doi: 10.1016/j.neuroimage.2005.07.038
65. Luck D, Buchy L, Czechowska Y, Bodnar M, Pike GB, Campbell JS, et al. Fronto-temporal disconnectivity and clinical short-term outcome in first episode psychosis: a DTI-tractography study. *J Psychiatr Res.* (2011) 45:369–77. doi: 10.1016/j.jpsychires.2010.07.007
66. Palaniyappan L, Marques TR, Taylor H, Handley R, Mondelli V, Bonaccorso S, et al. Cortical folding defects as markers of poor treatment response in first-episode psychosis. *JAMA Psychiatry* (2013) 70:1031–40. doi: 10.1001/jamapsychiatry.2013.203
67. Palaniyappan L, Marques TR, Taylor H, Mondelli V, Reinders AATS, Bonaccorso S, et al. Globally efficient brain organization and treatment response in psychosis: a connectomic study of gyrification. *Schizophr Bull.* (2016) 42:1446–56. doi: 10.1093/schbul/sbw069
68. Crossley NA, Marques TR, Taylor H, Chaddock C, Dell'Acqua F, Reinders AA, et al. Connectomic correlates of response to treatment in first-episode psychosis. *Brain* (2017) 140:487–96. doi: 10.1093/brain/aww297
69. Lieberman J, Chakos M, Wu H, Alvir J, Hoffman E, Robinson D, Bilder R. Longitudinal study of brain morphology in first episode schizophrenia. *Biol Psychiatry* (2001) 49:487–99. doi: 10.1016/S0006-3223(01)01067-8
70. Milev P, Ho BC, Arndt S, Nopoulos P, Andreasen NC. Initial magnetic resonance imaging volumetric brain measurements and outcome in schizophrenia: a prospective longitudinal study with 5-year follow-up. *Biol Psychiatry* (2003) 54:608–15. doi: 10.1016/S0006-3223(03)00293-2
71. de Castro-Manglano P, Mechelli A, Soutullo C, Landecho I, Gimenez-Amaya JM, Ortuño F, et al. Structural brain abnormalities in first-episode psychosis: differences between affective psychoses and schizophrenia and relationship to clinical outcome. *Bipolar Disord.* (2011) 13:545–55. doi: 10.1111/j.1399-5618.2011.00953.x

72. Sauras R, Keymer A, Alonso-Solis A, Díaz A, Molins C, Nuñez F, et al. Volumetric and morphological characteristics of the hippocampus are associated with progression to schizophrenia in patients with first-episode psychosis. *Eur Psychiatry* (2017) 45:1–5. doi: 10.1016/j.eurpsy.2017.06.006
73. Takahashi T, Wood SJ, Yung AR, Soulsby B, McGorry PD, Suzuki M, et al. Progressive gray matter reduction of the superior temporal gyrus during transition to psychosis. *Arch Gen Psychiatry* (2009) 66:366–76. doi: 10.1001/archgenpsychiatry.2009.12
74. Dazzan P, Arango C, Fleischacker W, Galderisi S, Glenthøj B, Leucht S, et al. Magnetic resonance imaging and the prediction of outcome in first-episode schizophrenia: a review of current evidence and directions for future research. *Schizophr Bull.* (2015) 41:574–83. doi: 10.1093/schbul/sbv024
75. Fusar-Poli P, Meyer-Lindenberg A. Forty years of structural imaging in psychosis: promises and truth. *Acta Psychiatr Scand.* (2016) 134:207–24. doi: 10.1111/acps.12619
76. Demjaha A, Murray RM, McGuire PK, Kapur S, Howes OD. Dopamine synthesis capacity in patients with treatment-resistant schizophrenia. *Am J Psychiatry* (2012) 169:1203–10. doi: 10.1176/appi.ajp.2012.12010144
77. Kim E, Howes OD, Veronese M, Beck K, Seo S, Park JW, et al. Presynaptic dopamine capacity in patients with treatment-resistant schizophrenia taking clozapine: an [(18)F]DOPA PET study. *Neuropsychopharmacology* (2017) 42:941–50. doi: 10.1038/npp.2016.258
78. Cannon TD, Kaprio J, Lönnqvist J, Huttunen M, Koskenvuo M. The genetic epidemiology of schizophrenia in a Finnish twin cohort. A population-based modeling study. *Arch Gen Psychiatry* (1998) 55:67–74.
79. Kieseppä T, Partonen T, Haukka J, Kaprio J, Lönnqvist J. High concordance of bipolar I disorder in a nationwide sample of twins. *Am J Psychiatry* (2004) 161:1814–21.
80. Lichtenstein P, Yip BH, Björk C, Pawitan Y, Cannon TD, Sullivan PF, et al. Common genetic determinants of schizophrenia and bipolar disorder in Swedish families: a population-based study. *Lancet* (2009) 373:234–9. doi: 10.1016/S0140-6736(09)60072-6
81. Farrell MS, Werge T, Sklar P, Owen MJ, Ophoff RA, O'Donovan MC, et al. Evaluating historical candidate genes for schizophrenia. *Mol Psychiatry* (2015) 20:555–62. doi: 10.1038/mp.2015.16
82. Johnson EC, Border R, Melroy-Greif WE, de Leeuw CA, Ehringer MA, Keller MC. No evidence that schizophrenia candidate genes are more associated with schizophrenia than noncandidate genes. *Biol Psychiatry* (2017) 82:702–8. doi: 10.1016/j.biopsych.2017.06.033
83. Schizophrenia Working Group of the Psychiatric Genomics Consortium. Biological insights from 108 schizophrenia-associated genetic loci. *Nature* (2014) 511:421–7. doi: 10.1038/nature13595
84. Pardiñas AF, Holmans P, Pocklington AJ, Escott-Price V, Ripke S, Carrera N, et al. Common schizophrenia alleles are enriched in mutation-intolerant genes and in regions under strong background selection. *Nat Genet.* (2018) 50:381–9. doi: 10.1038/s41588-018-0059-2
85. Li J, Yoshikawa A, Brennan MD, Ramsey TL, Meltzer HY. Genetic predictors of antipsychotic response to lurasidone identified in a genome wide association study and by schizophrenia risk genes. *Schizophr Res.* (2018) 192:194–204. doi: 10.1016/j.schres.2017.04.009
86. Frank J, Lang M, Witt SH, Strohmaier J, Rujescu D, Cichon S, et al. Identification of increased genetic risk scores for schizophrenia in treatment-resistant patients. *Mol Psychiatry* (2015) 20:150–1. doi: 10.1038/mp.2015.52
87. Meier SM, Agerbo E, Maier R, Pedersen CB, Lang M, Grove J, et al. High loading of polygenic risk in cases with chronic schizophrenia. *Mol Psychiatry* (2016) 21:969–74. doi: 10.1038/mp.2015.130
88. Bipolar Disorder and Schizophrenia Working Group of the Psychiatric Genomics Consortium. Genomic dissection of bipolar disorder and schizophrenia, including 28 subphenotypes. *Cell* (2018) 173:1705–15. doi: 10.1016/j.cell.2018.05.046
89. Wimberley T, Gasse C, Meier SM, Agerbo E, MacCabe JH, Horsdal HT. Polygenic risk score for schizophrenia and treatment-resistant schizophrenia. *Schizophr Bull.* (2017) 43:1064–9. doi: 10.1093/schbul/sbx007
90. Allardyce J, Leonenko G, Hamshere M, Pardiñas AF, Forty L, Knott S, et al. Association between schizophrenia-related polygenic liability and the occurrence and level of mood-incongruent psychotic symptoms in bipolar disorder. *JAMA Psychiatry* (2018) 75:28–35. doi: 10.1001/jamapsychiatry.2017.3485
91. Vassos E, Di Forti M, Coleman J, Iyegbe C, Prata D, Euesden J, et al. An examination of polygenic score risk prediction in individuals with first-episode psychosis. *Biol Psychiatry* (2017) 81:470–7. doi: 10.1016/j.biopsych.2016.06.028
92. Harrisberger F, Smieskova R, Vogler C, Egli T, Schmidt A, Lenz C, et al. Impact of polygenic schizophrenia-related risk and hippocampal volumes on the onset of psychosis. *Transl Psychiatry* (2016) 6:e868. doi: 10.1038/tp.2016.143
93. Ranlund S, Calafato S, Thygesen JH, Lin K, Cahn W, Crespo-Facorro B, et al. A polygenic risk score analysis of psychosis endophenotypes across brain functional, structural, and cognitive domains. *Am J Med Genet B Neuropsychiatr Genet.* (2018) 177:21–34. doi: 10.1002/ajmg.b.32581
94. Marshall CR, Howrigan DP, Merico D, Thiruvahindrapuram B, Wu W, Greer DS, et al. Contribution of copy number variants to schizophrenia from a genome-wide study of 41,321 subjects. *Nat Genet.* (2017) 49:27–35. doi: 10.1038/ng.3725
95. Kendall KM, Rees E, Escott-Price V, Einon M, Thomas R, Hewitt J, et al. Cognitive performance among carriers of pathogenic copy number variants: analysis of 152,000 UK Biobank subjects. *Biol Psychiatry* (2017) 82:103–10. doi: 10.1016/j.biopsych.2016.08.014
96. Singh T, Kurki MI, Curtis D, Purcell SM, Crooks L, McRae J, et al. Rare loss-of-function variants in SETD1A are associated with schizophrenia and developmental disorders. *Nat Neurosci.* (2016) 19:571–7. doi: 10.1038/nn.4267
97. Steinberg S, Gudmundsdottir S, Sveinbjornsson G, Suvisaari J, Paunio T, Torniainen-Holm M, et al. Truncating mutations in RBM12 are associated with psychosis. *Nat Genet.* (2017) 49:1251–4. doi: 10.1038/ng.3894
98. Singh T, Walters JTR, Johnstone M, Curtis D, Suvisaari J, Torniainen M, et al. The contribution of rare variants to risk of schizophrenia in individuals with and without intellectual disability. *Nat Genet.* (2017) 49:1167–73. doi: 10.1038/ng.3903
99. Zhang JP, Malhotra AK. Recent progress in pharmacogenomics of antipsychotic drug response. *Curr Psychiatry Rep.* (2018) 20:24. doi: 10.1007/s11920-018-0886-y
100. Zhang JP, Lencz T, Zhang RX, Nitta M, Maayan L, John M, et al. Pharmacogenetic associations of antipsychotic drug-related weight gain: a systematic review and meta-analysis. *Schizophr Bull.* (2016) 42:1418–37. doi: 10.1093/schbul/sbw058
101. Luzum JA, Pakyz RE, Elsey AR, Haidar CE, Peterson JF, Whirl-Carrillo M, et al. The Pharmacogenomics Research Network Translational Pharmacogenetics Program: outcomes and metrics of pharmacogenetic implementations across diverse healthcare systems. *Clin Pharmacol Ther.* (2017) 102:502–10. doi: 10.1002/cpt.630
102. Fond G, d'Albis MA, Jamain S, Tamouza R, Arango C, Fleischhacker WW, et al. The promise of biological markers for treatment response in first-episode psychosis: a systematic review. *Schizophr Bull.* (2015) 41:559–73. doi: 10.1093/schbul/sbv002
103. Goff DC, Romero K, Paul J, Mercedes Perez-Rodriguez M, Crandall D, Potkin SG. Biomarkers for drug development in early psychosis: current issues and promising directions. *Eur Neuropsychopharmacol.* (2016) 26:923–37. doi: 10.1016/j.euroneuro.2016.01.009
104. Sabherwal S, English JA, Föcking M, Cagney G, Cotter DR. Blood biomarker discovery in drug-free schizophrenia: the contribution of proteomics and multiplex immunoassays. *Expert Rev Proteomics* (2016) 13:1141–55. doi: 10.1080/14789450.2016.1252262
105. Schmidt A, Cappucciati M, Radua J, Rutigliano G, Rocchetti M, Dell'Osso L, et al. Improving prognostic accuracy in subjects at clinical high risk for psychosis: systematic review of predictive models and meta-analytical sequential testing simulation. *Schizophr Bull.* (2017) 43:375–88. doi: 10.1093/schbul/sbw098
106. Davison J, O'Gorman A, Brennan L, Cotter DR. A systematic review of metabolite biomarkers of schizophrenia. *Schizophr Res.* (2018) 195:32–50. doi: 10.1016/j.schres.2017.09.021
107. Goldsmith DR, Rapaport MH, Miller BJ. A meta-analysis of blood cytokine network alterations in psychiatric patients: comparisons between schizophrenia, bipolar disorder and depression. *Mol Psychiatry* (2016) 21:1696–709. doi: 10.1038/mp.2016.3

108. Miller BJ, Buckley P, Seabolt W, Mellor A, Kirkpatrick B. Meta-analysis of cytokine alterations in schizophrenia: clinical status and antipsychotic effects. *Biol Psychiatry* (2011) 70:663–71. doi: 10.1016/j.biopsych.2011.04.013
109. Wang AK, Miller BJ. Meta-analysis of cerebrospinal fluid cytokine and tryptophan catabolite alterations in psychiatric patients: comparisons between schizophrenia, bipolar disorder, and depression. *Schizophr Bull.* (2018) 44:75–83. doi: 10.1093/schbul/sbx035
110. Upthegrove R, Manzanares-Teson N, Barnes NM. Cytokine function in medication-naive first episode psychosis: a systematic review and meta-analysis. *Schizophr Res.* (2014) 155:101–8. doi: 10.1016/j.schres.2014.03.005
111. Miller BJ, Gassama B, Sebastian D, Buckley P, Mellor A. Meta-analysis of lymphocytes in schizophrenia: clinical status and antipsychotic effects. *Biol Psychiatry* (2013) 73:993–9. doi: 10.1016/j.biopsych.2012.09.007
112. Flatow J, Buckley P, Miller BJ. Meta-analysis of oxidative stress in schizophrenia. *Biol Psychiatry* (2013) 74:400–9. doi: 10.1016/j.biopsych.2013.03.018
113. Kopczynska M, Zelek W, Touchard S, Gaughran F, Di Forti M, Mondelli V, et al. Complement system biomarkers in first episode psychosis. *Schizophr Res.* (2017) 89:187. doi: 10.1016/j.schres.2017.12.012
114. Mäntylä T, Mantere O, Raij TT, Kieseppä T, Laitinen H, Leiviskä J, et al. Altered activation of innate immunity associates with white matter volume and diffusion in first-episode psychosis. *PLoS ONE* (2015) 10:e0125112. doi: 10.1371/journal.pone.0125112
115. Lesh TA, Careaga M, Rose DR, McAllister AK, Van de Water J, Carter CS, et al. Cytokine alterations in first-episode schizophrenia and bipolar disorder: relationships to brain structure and symptoms. *J Neuroinflamm.* (2018) 15:165. doi: 10.1186/s12974-018-1197-2
116. Fillman SG, Weickert TW, Lenroot RK, Catts SV, Bruggemann JM, Catts VS, et al. Elevated peripheral cytokines characterize a subgroup of people with schizophrenia displaying poor verbal fluency and reduced Broca's area volume. *Mol Psychiatry* (2016) 21:1090–8. doi: 10.1038/mp.2015.90
117. Helmy A, Carpenter KL, Menon DK, Pickard JD, Hutchinson PJ. The cytokine response to human traumatic brain injury: temporal profiles and evidence for cerebral parenchymal production. *J Cereb Blood Flow Metab.* (2011) 31:658–70. doi: 10.1038/jcbfm.2010.142
118. Chen WR, Liu HB, Sha Y, Shi Y, Wang H, Yin DW, Chen YD, Shi XM. Effects of statin on arrhythmia and heart rate variability in healthy persons with 48-hour sleep deprivation. *J Am Heart Assoc.* (2016) 5:e003833. doi: 10.1161/JAHA.116.003833
119. Fernandes BS, Steiner J, Bernstein HG, Dodd S, Pasco JA, Dean OM, et al. C-reactive protein is increased in schizophrenia but is not altered by antipsychotics: meta-analysis and implications. *Mol Psychiatry* (2016) 21:554–64. doi: 10.1038/mp.2015.87
120. Fernandez-Egea E, Bernardo M, Donner T, Conget I, Parellada E, Justicia A, et al. Metabolic profile of antipsychotic-naive individuals with non-affective psychosis. *Br J Psychiatry* (2009) 194:434–8. doi: 10.1192/bjp.bp.108.052605
121. Prins BP, Abbasi A, Wong A, Vaez A, Nolte I, Franceschini N, et al. Investigating the causal relationship of C-reactive protein with 32 complex somatic and psychiatric outcomes: a large-scale cross-consortium Mendelian randomization study. *PLoS Med.* (2016) 13:e1001976. doi: 10.1371/journal.pmed.1001976
122. Hartwig FP, Borges MC, Horta BL, Bowden J, Davey Smith G. Inflammatory biomarkers and risk of schizophrenia: a 2-sample Mendelian randomization study. *JAMA Psychiatry* (2017) 74:1226–33. doi: 10.1001/jamapsychiatry.2017.3191
123. Horsdal HT, Köhler-Forsberg O, Benros ME, Gasse C. C-reactive protein and white blood cell levels in schizophrenia, bipolar disorders and depression - associations with mortality and psychiatric outcomes: a population-based study. *Eur Psychiatry* (2017) 44:164–72. doi: 10.1016/j.eurpsy.2017.04.012
124. Ridker PM. A test in context: high-sensitivity C-reactive protein. *J Am Coll Cardiol.* (2016) 67:712–23. doi: 10.1016/j.jacc.2015.11.037
125. Kayser MS, Dalmau J. Anti-NMDA receptor encephalitis, autoimmunity, and psychosis. *Schizophr Res.* (2016) 176:36–40. doi: 10.1016/j.schres.2014.10.007
126. Pollak TA, Rogers JP, Nagele RG, Peakman M, Stone JM, David AS, et al. Antibodies in the diagnosis, prognosis, and prediction of psychotic disorders. *Schizophr Bull.* (2018). doi: 10.1093/schbul/sby021. [Epub ahead of print].
127. Mantere O, Saarela M, Kieseppä T, Raij T, Mäntylä T, Lindgren M, et al. Anti-neuronal anti-bodies in patients with early psychosis. *Schizophr Res.* (2018) 192:404–7. doi: 10.1016/j.schres.2017.04.027
128. Jézéquel J, Johansson EM, Dupuis JP, Rogemond V, Gréa H, Kellermayer B, et al. Dynamic disorganization of synaptic NMDA receptors triggered by autoantibodies from psychotic patients. *Nat Commun.* (2017) 8:1791. doi: 10.1038/s41467-017-01700-3
129. Misiak B, Frydecka D, Loska O, Moustafa AA, Samochowiec J, Kasznia J, et al. Testosterone, DHEA and DHEA-S in patients with schizophrenia: a systematic review and meta-analysis. *Psychoneuroendocrinology* (2018) 89:92–102. doi: 10.1016/j.psyneuen.2018.01.007
130. Pillinger T, D'Ambrosio E, McCutcheon R, D Howes O. Is psychosis a multisystem disorder? A meta-review of central nervous system, immune, cardiometabolic, and endocrine alterations in first-episode psychosis and perspective on potential models. *Mol Psychiatry* (2018). doi: 10.1038/s41380-018-0058-9. [Epub ahead of print].
131. Walker EF, Trotman HD, Pearce BD, Addington J, Cadenhead KS, Cornblatt BA, et al. Cortisol levels and risk for psychosis: initial findings from the North American prodrome longitudinal study. *Biol Psychiatry* (2013) 74:410–7. doi: 10.1016/j.biopsych.2013.02.016
132. Stubbs B, Wang AK, Vancampfort D, Miller BJ. Are leptin levels increased among people with schizophrenia versus controls? A systematic review and comparative meta-analysis. *Psychoneuroendocrinology* (2016) 63:144–54. doi: 10.1016/j.psyneuen.2015.09.026
133. Plitman E, Iwata Y, Caravaggio F, Nakajima S, Chung JK, Gerretsen P, et al. Kynurenic acid in schizophrenia: a systematic review and meta-analysis. *Schizophr Bull.* (2017) 43:764–77. doi: 10.1093/schbul/sbw221
134. Erhardt S, Schwieler L, Imbeault S, Engberg G. The kynurenine pathway in schizophrenia and bipolar disorder. *Neuropharmacology* (2017) 112(Pt B):297–306. doi: 10.1016/j.neuropharm.2016.05.020
135. Myint AM, Schwarz MJ, Verkerk R, Mueller HH, Zach J, Scharpé S, et al. Reversal of imbalance between kynurenic acid and 3-hydroxykynurenine by antipsychotics in medication-naïve and medication-free schizophrenic patients. *Brain Behav Immun.* (2011) 25:1576–81. doi: 10.1016/j.bbi.2011.05.005
136. Condray R, Dougherty GG Jr, Keshavan MS, Reddy RD, Haas GL, Montrose DM, et al. 3-Hydroxykynurenine and clinical symptoms in first-episode neuroleptic-naive patients with schizophrenia. *Int J Neuropsychopharmacol* (2011) 14:756–67. doi: 10.1017/S1461145710001689
137. Suvitaival T, Mantere O, Kieseppä T, Mattila I, Pöhö P, Hyötyläinen T, et al. Serum metabolite profile associates with the development of metabolic co-morbidities in first-episode psychosis. *Transl Psychiatry* (2016) 6:e951. doi: 10.1038/tp.2016.222
138. Chan MK, Krebs MO, Cox D, Guest PC, Yolken RH, Rahmoune H, et al. Development of a blood-based molecular biomarker test for identification of schizophrenia before disease onset. *Transl Psychiatry* (2015) 5:e601. doi: 10.1038/tp.2015.91
139. Perkins DO, Jeffries CD, Addington J, Bearden CE, Cadenhead KS, Cannon TD, et al. Towards a psychosis risk blood diagnostic for persons experiencing high-risk symptoms: preliminary results from the NAPLS project. *Schizophr Bull.* (2015) 41:419–28. doi: 10.1093/schbul/sbu099
140. Tek C, Kucukgoncu S, Guloksuz S, Woods SW, Srihari VH, Annamalai A. Antipsychotic-induced weight gain in first-episode psychosis patients: a meta-analysis of differential effects of antipsychotic medications. *Early Interv Psychiatry* (2016) 10:193–202. doi: 10.1111/eip.12251
141. Basson BR, Kinon BJ, Taylor CC, Szymanski KA, Gilmore JA, Tollefson GD. Factors influencing acute weight change in patients with schizophrenia treated with olanzapine, haloperidol, or risperidone. *J Clin Psychiatry* (2001) 62:231–8. doi: 10.4088/JCP.v62n0404
142. Strassnig M, Miewald J, Keshavan M, Ganguli R. Weight gain in newly diagnosed first-episode psychosis patients and healthy comparisons: one-year analysis. *Schizophr Res.* (2007) 93:90–8. doi: 10.1016/j.schres.2007.02.024
143. Saddichha S, Ameen S, Akhtar S. Predictors of antipsychotic-induced weight gain in first-episode psychosis: conclusions from a randomized, double-blind, controlled prospective study of olanzapine, risperidone, and haloperidol. *J Clin Psychopharmacol.* (2008) 28:27–31. doi: 10.1097/jcp.0b013e3181602fe6

144. Pérez-Iglesias R, Martínez-García O, Pardo-Garcia G, Amado JA, Garcia-Unzueta MT, Tabares-Seisdedos R, et al. Course of weight gain and metabolic abnormalities in first treated episode of psychosis: the first year is a critical period for development of cardiovascular risk factors. *Int J Neuropsychopharmacol.* (2014) 17:41–51. doi: 10.1017/S1461145713001053
145. Gebhardt S, Haberhausen M, Heinzel-Gutenbrunner M, Gebhardt N, Remschmidt H, Krieg JC, et al. Antipsychotic-induced body weight gain: predictors and a systematic categorization of the long-term weight course. *J Psychiatr Res.* (2009) 43:620–6. doi: 10.1016/j.jpsychires.2008.11.001
146. Scheffler F, Kilian S, Chiliza B, Asmal L, Phahladira L, du Plessis S, et al. Effects of cannabis use on body mass, fasting glucose and lipids during the first 12-months of treatment in schizophrenia spectrum disorders. *Schizophr Res.* (2018) 199:90–5. doi: 10.1016/j.schres.2018.02.050
147. Keinänen J, Mantere O, Kieseppä T, Mäntylä T, Torniainen M, Lindgren M, et al. Early insulin resistance predicts weight gain and waist circumference increase in first-episode psychosis – a one year follow-up study. *Schizophr Res.* (2015) 169:458–63. doi: 10.1016/j.schres.2015.11.002
148. Harrison RNS, Gaughran F, Murray RM, Lee SH, Cano JP, Dempster D, et al. Development of multivariable models to predict change in Body Mass Index within a clinical trial population of psychotic individuals. *Sci Rep.* (2017) 7:14738. doi: 10.1038/s41598-017-15137-7
149. Vandenberghe F, Gholam-Rezaee M, Saigí-Morgui N, Delacrétaz A, Choong E, Solida-Tozzi A, et al. Importance of early weight changes to predict long-term weight gain during psychotropic drug treatment. *J Clin Psychiatry* (2015) 76:e1417–23. doi: 10.4088/JCP.14m09358
150. Vandenberghe F, Saigí-Morgui N, Delacrétaz A, Quteineh L, Crettol S, Ansermot N, et al. Prediction of early weight gain during psychotropic treatment using a combinatorial model with clinical and genetic markers. *Pharmacogenet Genomics* (2016) 26:547–57. doi: 10.1097/FPC.0000000000000249
151. Greenhalgh AM, Gonzalez-Blanco L, Garcia-Rizo C, Fernandez-Egea E, Miller B, Arroyo MB, et al. Meta-analysis of glucose tolerance, insulin, and insulin resistance in antipsychotic-naïve patients with nonaffective psychosis. *Schizophr Res.* (2017) 179:57–63. doi: 10.1016/j.schres.2016.09.026
152. Pillinger T, Beck K, Stubbs B, Howes OD. Cholesterol and triglyceride levels in first-episode psychosis: systematic review and meta-analysis. *Br J Psychiatry* (2017) 211:339–49. doi: 10.1192/bjp.bp.117.200907
153. Liu ML, Zhang XT, Du XY, Fang Z, Liu Z, Xu Y, et al. Severe disturbance of glucose metabolism in peripheral blood mononuclear cells of schizophrenia patients: a targeted metabolomic study. *J Transl Med.* (2015) 13:226. doi: 10.1186/s12967-015-0540-y
154. Perry BI, McIntosh G, Weich S, Singh S, Rees K. The association between first-episode psychosis and abnormal glycaemic control: systematic review and meta-analysis. *Lancet Psychiatry* (2016) 3:1049–58. doi: 10.1016/S2215-0366(16)30262-0
155. Foley DL, Morley KI. Systematic review of early cardiometabolic outcomes of the first treated episode of psychosis. *Arch Gen Psychiatry* (2011) 68:609–16. doi: 10.1001/archgenpsychiatry.2011.2
156. Burghardt KJ, Seyoum B, Mallisho A, Burghardt PR, Kowluru RA, Yi Z. Atypical antipsychotics, insulin resistance and weight; a meta-analysis of healthy volunteer studies. *Prog Neuropsychopharmacol Biol Psychiatry* (2018) 83:55–63. doi: 10.1016/j.pnpbp.2018.01.004
157. Kimmel R, Levy MR. Profound hypertriglyceridemia and weight gain in the first week following initiation of olanzapine: a case report with implications for lipid monitoring guidelines. *Psychosomatics* (2013) 54:392–4. doi: 10.1016/j.psym.2012.10.005
158. Franco JM, Vallabhajosyula S, Griffin TJ. Quetiapine-induced hypertriglyceridaemia causing acute pancreatitis. *BMJ Case Rep.* (2015) 2015:bcr2015209571. doi: 10.1136/bcr-2015-209571
159. Srihari VH, Phutane VH, Ozkan B, Chwastiak L, Ratliff JC, Woods SW, et al. Cardiovascular mortality in schizophrenia: defining a critical period for prevention. *Schizophr Res.* (2013) 146:64–8. doi: 10.1016/j.schres.2013.01.014
160. Correll CU, Robinson DG, Schooler NR, Brunette MF, Mueser KT, Rosenheck RA, et al. Cardiometabolic risk in patients with first-episode schizophrenia spectrum disorders: baseline results from the RAISE-ETP study. *JAMA Psychiatry* (2014) 71:1350–63. doi: 10.1001/jamapsychiatry.2014.1314
161. Miller BJ, Kandhal P, Rapaport MH, Mellor A, Buckley P. Total and differential white blood cell counts, high-sensitivity C-reactive protein, and cardiovascular risk in non-affective psychoses. *Brain Behav Immun.* (2015) 45:28–35. doi: 10.1016/j.bbi.2014.12.005
162. Dickerson F, Origoni A, Schroeder J, Adamos M, Katsafanas E, Khushalani S, et al. Natural cause mortality in persons with serious mental illness. *Acta Psychiatr Scand.* (2018) 137:371–9. doi: 10.1111/acps.12880
163. Crump C, Winkleby MA, Sundquist K, Sundquist J. Comorbidities and mortality in persons with schizophrenia: a Swedish national cohort study. *Am J Psychiatry* (2013) 170:324–33. doi: 10.1176/appi.ajp.2012.12050599
164. Torniainen M, Mittendorfer-Rutz E, Tanskanen A, Björkenstam C, Suvisaari J, Alexanderson K, et al. Antipsychotic treatment and mortality in schizophrenia. *Schizophr Bull.* (2015) 41:656–63. doi: 10.1093/schbul/sbu164
165. Osborn DP, Hardoon S, Omar RZ, Holt RI, King M, Larsen J, et al. Cardiovascular risk prediction models for people with severe mental illness: results from the prediction and management of cardiovascular risk in people with severe mental illnesses (PRIMROSE) research program. *JAMA Psychiatry* (2015) 72:143–51. doi: 10.1001/jamapsychiatry.2014.2133
166. Foguet-Boreu Q, Fernandez San Martin MI, Flores Mateo G, Zabaleta Del Olmo E, Ayerbe García-Morzon L, Perez-Piñar López M, et al. Cardiovascular risk assessment in patients with a severe mental illness: a systematic review and meta-analysis. *BMC Psychiatry* (2016) 16:141. doi: 10.1186/s12888-016-0833-6
167. Ventriglio A, Gentile A, Bonfitto I, Stella E, Mari M, Steardo L, et al. Suicide in the early stage of schizophrenia. *Front Psychiatry* (2016) 7:116. doi: 10.3389/fpsyt.2016.00116
168. Ayesa-Arriola R, Alcaraz EG, Hernández BV, Pérez-Iglesias R, López Moríñigo JD, Duta R, et al. Suicidal behavior in first-episode non-affective psychosis: specific risk periods and stage-related factors. *Eur Neuropsychopharmacol.* (2015) 25:2278–88. doi: 10.1016/j.euroneuro.2015.09.008
169. Dutta R, Murray RM, Hotopf M, Allardyce J, Jones PB, Boydell J. Reassessing the long-term risk of suicide after a first episode of psychosis. *Arch Gen Psychiatry* (2010) 67:1230–7. doi: 10.1001/archgenpsychiatry.2010.157
170. Nordentoft M, Madsen T, Fedyszyn I. Suicidal behavior and mortality in first-episode psychosis. *J Nerv Ment Dis.* (2015) 203:387–92. doi: 10.1097/NMD.0000000000000296
171. Pompili M, Serafini G, Innamorati M, Lester D, Shrivastava A, Girardi P, Nordentoft M. Suicide risk in first episode psychosis: a selective review of the current literature. *Schizophr Res.* (2011) 129:1–11. doi: 10.1016/j.schres.2011.03.008
172. Robinson J, Harris MG, Harrigan SM, Henry LP, Farrelly S, Prosser A, et al. Suicide attempt in first-episode psychosis: a 7.4 year follow-up study. *Schizophr Res.* (2010) 116:1–8. doi: 10.1016/j.schres.2009.10.009
173. Lutz PE, Mechawar N, Turecki G. Neuropathology of suicide: recent findings and future directions. *Mol Psychiatry* (2017) 22:1395–412. doi: 10.1038/mp.2017.141
174. Weibell MA, Hegelstad WTV, Auestad B, Bramness J, Evensen J, Haahr U, et al. The effect of substance use on 10-year outcome in first-episode psychosis. *Schizophr Bull.* (2017) 43:843–51. doi: 10.1093/schbul/sbw179
175. Schoeler T, Monk A, Sami MB, Klamerus E, Foglia E, Brown R, et al. Continued versus discontinued cannabis use in patients with psychosis: a systematic review and meta-analysis. *Lancet Psychiatry* (2016) 3:215–25. doi: 10.1016/S2215-0366(15)00363-6
176. Bowtell M, Eaton S, Thien K, Bardell-Williams M, Downey L, Ratheesh A, et al. Rates and predictors of relapse following discontinuation of antipsychotic medication after a first episode of psychosis. *Schizophr Res.* (2018) 195:231–6. doi: 10.1016/j.schres.2017.10.030
177. Fenton WS, McGlashan TH. Natural history of schizophrenia subtypes. I. Longitudinal study of paranoid, hebephrenic, and undifferentiated schizophrenia. *Arch Gen Psychiatry* (1991) 48:969–77.
178. Suvisaari J, Perälä J, Saarni SI, Juvonen H, Tuulio-Henriksson A, Lönnqvist J. The epidemiology and descriptive and predictive validity of DSM-IV

delusional disorder and subtypes of schizophrenia. *Clin Schizophr Relat Psychoses* (2009) 2:289–97. doi.org/10.3371/CSRP.2.4.2
179. Allan GM, Garrison S, McCormack J. Comparison of cardiovascular disease risk calculators. *Curr Opin Lipidol.* (2014) 25:254–65. doi: 10.1097/MOL.0000000000000095
180. Sankar A, Beattie WS, Wijeysundera DN. How can we identify the high-risk patient? *Curr Opin Crit Care* (2015) 21:328–35. doi: 10.1097/MCC.0000000000000216
181. Cannon TD, Yu C, Addington J, Bearden CE, Cadenhead KS, Cornblatt BA, et al. An individualized risk calculator for research in prodromal psychosis. *Am J Psychiatry* (2016) 173:980–8. doi: 10.1176/appi.ajp.2016.15070890
182. Jordan MI, Mitchell TM. Machine learning: trends, perspectives, and prospects. *Science* (2015) 349:255–60. doi: 10.1126/science.aaa8415
183. Deo RC. Machine learning in medicine. *Circulation* (2015) 132:1920–30. doi: 10.1161/CIRCULATIONAHA.115.001593
184. Orrù G, Pettersson-Yeo W, Marquand AF, Sartori G, Mechelli A. Using Support Vector Machine to identify imaging biomarkers of neurological and psychiatric disease: a critical review. *Neurosci Biobehav Rev.* (2012) 36:1140–52. doi: 10.1016/j.neubiorev.2012.01.004
185. Kim J, Lee B. Identification of Alzheimer's disease and mild cognitive impairment using multimodal sparse hierarchical extreme learning machine. *Hum Brain Mapp.* (2018) 39:3728–41. doi: 10.1002/hbm.24207
186. Tago T, Toyohara J. Advances in the development of PET ligands targeting histone deacetylases for the assessment of neurodegenerative diseases. *Molecules* (2018) 23:E300. doi: 10.3390/molecules23020300
187. Crossley NA, Mechelli A, Ginestet C, Rubinov M, Bullmore ET, McGuire P. Altered hub functioning and compensatory activations in the connectome: a meta-analysis of functional neuroimaging studies in schizophrenia. *Schizophr Bull.* (2016) 42:434–42. doi: 10.1093/schbul/sbv146
188. Hasson U, Honey CJ. Future trends in Neuroimaging: neural processes as expressed within real-life contexts. *Neuroimage* (2012) 62:1272–8. doi: 10.1016/j.neuroimage.2012.02.004
189. Mäntylä T, Nummenmaa L, Rikandi E, Lindgren M, Kieseppä T, Hari R, et al. Aberrant cortical integration in first-episode psychosis during natural audiovisual processing. *Biol Psychiatry* (2018) 84:655–64. doi: 10.1016/j.biopsych.2018.04.014
190. Zandian A, Wingård L, Nilsson H, Sjöstedt E, Johansson DX, Just D, et al. Untargeted screening for novel autoantibodies with prognostic value in first-episode psychosis. *Transl Psychiatry* (2017) 7:e1177. doi: 10.1038/tp.2017.160
191. Frisoni GB, Boccardi M, Barkhof F, Blennow K, Cappa S, Chiotis K, et al. Strategic roadmap for an early diagnosis of Alzheimer's disease based on biomarkers. *Lancet Neurol.* (2017) 16:661–76. doi: 10.1016/S1474-4422(17)30159-X
192. Schnack HG, Kahn RS. Detecting neuroimaging biomarkers for psychiatric disorders: sample size matters. *Front Psychiatry.* (2016) 7:50. doi: 10.3389/fpsyt.2016.00050
193. Depp CA, Moore RC, Perivoliotis D, Holden JL, Swendsen J, Granholm EL. Social behavior, interaction appraisals, and suicidal ideation in schizophrenia: the dangers of being alone. *Schizophr Res.* (2016) 172:195–200. doi: 10.1016/j.schres.2016.02.028
194. Soininen H, Mattila J, Koikkalainen J, van Gils M, Hviid Simonsen A, Waldemar G, et al. Software tool for improved prediction of Alzheimer's disease. *Neurodegener Dis.* (2012) 10:149–52. doi: 10.1159/000332600
195. Hall A, Muñoz-Ruiz M, Mattila J, Koikkalainen J, Tsolaki M, Mecocci P, et al. Generalizability of the disease state index prediction model for identifying patients progressing from mild cognitive impairment to Alzheimer's disease. *J Alzheimers Dis.* (2015) 44:79–92. doi: 10.3233/JAD-140942
196. Muñoz-Ruiz MÁ, Hall A, Mattila J, Koikkalainen J, Herukka SK, Husso M, et al. Using the Disease State Fingerprint Tool for differential diagnosis of frontotemporal dementia and Alzheimer's Disease. *Dement Geriatr Cogn Dis Extra* (2016) 6:313–29. doi: 10.1159/000447122

2

Constructing the Immune Signature of Schizophrenia for Clinical Use and Research: An Integrative Review Translating Descriptives into Diagnostics

Rune A. Kroken [1,2,3], Iris E. Sommer [4,5], Vidar M. Steen [6,7], Ingrid Dieset [8,9,10] and Erik Johnsen [1,2,3]*

[1] Psychiatric Division, Haukeland University Hospital, Bergen, Norway, [2] Norwegian Centre for Mental Disorders Research, Haukeland University Hospital, Bergen, Norway, [3] Department of Clinical Medicine, University of Bergen, Bergen, Norway, [4] Department of Neuroscience and Department of Psychiatry, University Medical Center Groningen, University of Groningen, Groningen, Netherlands, [5] Department of Biological and Medical Psychology, University of Bergen, Bergen, Norway, [6] Department of Clinical Science, Norwegian Centre for Mental Disorders Research, KG Jebsen Centre for Psychosis Research, University of Bergen, Bergen, Norway, [7] Dr. E. Martens Research Group of Biological Psychiatry, Department of Medical Genetics, Haukeland University Hospital, Bergen, Norway, [8] Norwegian Centre for Mental Disorders Research, KG Jebsen Centre for Psychosis Research, Oslo University Hospital and University of Oslo, Oslo, Norway, [9] Division of Mental Health and Addiction, Acute Psychiatric Department, Oslo University Hospital, Oslo, Norway, [10] Faculty of Medicine, Institute of Clinical Medicine, University of Oslo, Oslo, Norway

Correspondence:
Rune A. Kroken
rune.kroken@helse-bergen.no

Schizophrenia is considered a syndrome comprised by several disease phenotypes, covering a range of underlying pathologies. One of these disease mechanisms seems to involve immune dysregulation and neuroinflammation. While the current dopamine receptor-blocking antipsychotic drugs decrease psychotic symptoms and prevent relapse in the majority of patients with schizophrenia, there is a huge need to explore new treatment options that target other pathophysiological pathways. Such studies should aim at identifying robust biomarkers in order to diagnose and monitor the immune biophenotype in schizophrenia and develop better selection procedures for clinical trials with anti-inflammatory and immune-modulating drugs. In this focused review, we describe available methods to assess inflammatory status and immune disturbances *in vivo*. We also outline findings of immune disturbances and signs of inflammation at cellular, protein, and brain imaging levels in patients with schizophrenia. Furthermore, we summarize the results from studies with anti-inflammatory or other immune-modulating drugs, highlighting how such studies have dealt with participant selection. Finally, we propose a strategy to construct an immune signature that may be helpful in selecting and monitoring participants in studies with immune modulating drugs and also applicable in regular clinical work.

Keywords: CRP-C-reactive protein, schizophrenia, inflammation, immunity, cytokine, anti-inflammatory drugs, monoclocal antibody, MRI

INTRODUCTION

Immune dysregulation in schizophrenia has been found in numerous studies comparing patients to healthy controls, and meta-analyses find that patients with schizophrenia, on a group level, show signs of a low-grade peripheral inflammation with upregulation of several proinflammatory cytokines (1–3) and C-reactive protein (CRP) (4). While the origin of these findings is not established, a major result from genome wide association studies (GWAS) has been a robust genetic association between schizophrenia and the major histocompatibility complex (MCH) locus on chromosome 6 (5). This genetic susceptibility can in part be explained by variants of complement factor 4 (C4), possibly linked to increased synaptic pruning during brain development (6). Furthermore, studies show increased risk of schizophrenia in individuals with prenatal exposure to influenza, although disputed (7), or with elevated titers of IgG antibodies to toxoplasma gondii (8), likely to work in concert with a genetic background (9). Interestingly, the pathological influence of prenatal infection may be an unspecific effect of having an inflammation response and increased cytokine levels more than a specific effect of a particular infectional agent (9). Moreover, studies of post-mortem brains of patients with schizophrenia suggest increased microglial activity (10). While these findings and others have broadened the knowledge of how immunity may influence ethio-pathological processes in schizophrenia, the advance of novel treatment algoritms for the individual patient would benefit from identification of robust immune-biomarkers for schizophrenia (11). In addition, theranostic biomarkers predicting effects of treatment with anti-inflammatory or immune-modulating drugs are needed (12) and descriptive group level findings must be translated into diagnostic assessment of the individual patient (11).

Although dopamine D2-receptor blocking antipsychotic drugs play a major role in the treatment of psychotic disorders (13), new treatment options are strongly needed, above all for the cognitive and negative symptoms of schizophrenia. D2-blockers offer symptomatic relief for delusions and hallucinations and efficient relapse prevention to a majority of users (14), but a disease-modifying effect in schizophrenia has not been found. Immune-modulating treatments might target pathological processes more proximal to the roots of the psychotic disorder than is the case for the current D2-receptor blocking drugs, and accordingly may be able to treat not only symptoms. Since 2002, there has been several pivotal studies exploring the potential effect of non-steroidal anti-inflammatory drugs (NSAIDS) (15), estrogens, statins, EPA/DHA fatty acids, davunetide, minocycline, and N-acetyl cysteine in schizophrenia (16). Furthermore, trials with monoclonal antibodies toward cytokines or cytokine receptors are emerging (17), which can specifically target one component of the immune system and may provide opportunities for precision medicine. This is a rapidly developing field (18), that now contains a range of well-established treatment options for various medical and neurological disorders, such as multiple sclerosis (MS). There is now a broad understanding that immune dysregulation may form an important part of the pathophysiology of schizophrenia and a whole range of drugs targeting specific parts of the immune system are already available. Following up on the studies with various anti-inflammatory acting drugs that have already been conducted, the stage is set for a new phase of drug studies in schizophrenia (19).

However, in order to maximize chances of showing effect in studies with immune-modulating drugs a schizophrenia inflammatory phenotype should be defined and delineated at the individual level both for research and clinical purposes. Several authors have highlighted that in most studies of inflammation in schizophrenia around 40% of the patients have some degree of inflammation (20–22). Assuming that immune dysregulation is involved in the pathoetiology of sub-groups with schizophrenia is in line with the notion that schizophrenia is a syndrome comprised by several disease phenotypes with a range of distinct underlying pathologies (23, 24). One of these disease mechanisms could be related to immunity, while others may be more influenced by compromised energy metabolism or synaptic dysfunctions (11). As several authors have noted already, we need robust biomarkers to diagnose immune dysregulation in schizophrenia and help selecting participants for trials with immune-modulating drugs. Further down the line, biomarkers are also needed in clinical settings in order to evaluate the individual patient for treatment. Promising indications of the possibilities that such a strategy represents derive from trials with immune-modulating drugs in depression. In two studies of infliximab which blocks tumor necrosis factor (TNF)-α in patients with major depression, treatment only benefited participants with CRP above a certain level (25, 26). Also, a schizophrenia trial stratifying results on degree of inflammation showed stronger treatment effects in the participants with increased inflammation (27).

Here we first review available methods to assess inflammatory status or immune disturbances. Findings of disturbances in immune cells, cytokines including mRNA, acute phase proteins, other molecular level methods and findings, and brain imaging methods will be outlined. Furthermore, we summarize the results from studies with anti-inflammatory or other immune-modulating drugs, highlighting how the studies have dealt with participant selection. Finally, we propose a strategy to construct an inflammatory signature that may be useful in selecting and monitoring participants in studies with immune modulating drugs and also applicable in the regular clinical work. We will start with a brief overview of the immune system.

IMMUNITY AND INFLAMMATION

The two categorically different parts of the immune systems are the innate system—that responds to pathogens in an unspecific way but does not produce lasting immunity—and the adaptive system which responds to specific antigens in a way that creates long-lasting recognition. The long-lasting recognition is produced through the creation of cell lines that give a specific antibody response. The cells of the innate system are the dendritic cells (DC), the macrophages, granulocytes, mast cells, and the natural killer (NK) cells, while the humoral responses of the

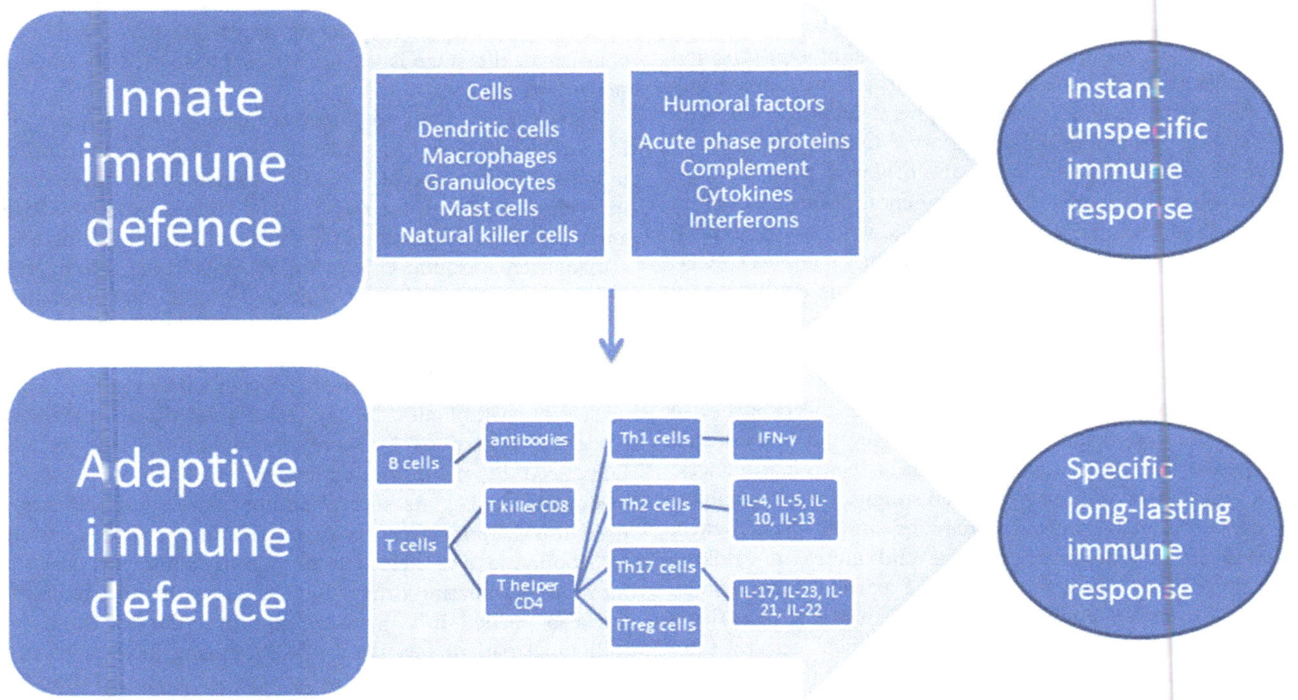

FIGURE 1 | The immune system—an overview.

innate system consist of the complement system, cytokines and interferons. The cells of the adaptive system are the B and T lymphocytes, while the antibodies are the humoral part of the adaptive system (28), see **Figure 1**. An important part of the innate response is the toll-like receptors (TLRs) located at the macrophages where they induce phagocytosis and production of albumin, fibrinogen, and serum amyloid A protein together with CRP—the acute phase proteins (29). A further acute response consists of the production of cytokines that stimulates T and B cells into producing responses specific to the given antigen. T cells are divided into subsets on the basis of their surface receptors, and the two main types are the cluster of differentiation (CD)4 T helper(h) cell, and the CD8—the T killer cells. The CD4 Th cells secrete a major portion of the cytokines of the body. Cytokines and chemokines are small molecules that act predominantly in the microenvironment of the cells that secrete them, while interleukin (IL)-1β, transforming growth factor (TGF) and TNF are exceptions to this and can also circulate through the body (28). Cytokines and chemokines have important roles in the communication between cells in the immune system, they can have stimulatory or inhibitory effects and their role may change depending on context. When the CD4 Th cell is activated, it can differentiate into Th1 and Th2 effector cells producing different types of cytokines. Th1 cells produce interferon (IFN)- γ which has strong pro-inflammatory properties, while the Th2 cells upon stimulation produces IL-4, IL-5, IL-10, IL-13 with mixed effects (30). CD4 Th cells can also differentiate into Th17 cells and induced regulatory T (iTreg) cells. Th17 produces several cytokines with a predominantly pro-inflammatory effect, IL-17, IL-23, IL-21, IL-22, and IL-17/IL-23 induce the IL-17/IL-23 immune axis (31).

Several specific cytokines need particular attention as they are consistently reported to be associated with schizophrenia. The **IL-1 family** consists of seven proteins displaying a predominantly pro-inflammmatory function: IL-1α, IL-1β, IL-18, IL-33, IL-36a, IL-36b, IL-36g, moreover three receptor antagonists IL-1Ra, IL-36Ra, IL-38, and one cytokine with anti-inflammatory actions; IL-37 (32). The IL-1 family are pleiotropic, and also have immunoregulatory and hematopoitic effects (28). IL-1 influences antigen presentation and non-specific lymphocyte function, and is closely linked to innate immunity (33). The IL-1 receptor type 1(RI) shows strong similarities to the TLR. Binding of IL-1 can initiate and strengthen the acute phase response by inducing fever that increases migration of leucocytes, by stimulating the acute phase proteins such as CRP, by activation of the hypothalamus-pituitary-adrenal (HPA) axis with cortisol regulating innate inflammation, and by inducing adhesion molecules that increase leucocyte recruitement (32). IL1 is mainly produced by activated macrophages, which is for instance activated by interferon (IFN)-γ and bacterial products (28, 32). **IL-6 is** produced by immune cells, adipocytes, skeletal muscle cells and vascular endothelial cells, and the IL-6 receptor is located on macrophages, lymphocytes, neutrophils and hepatocytes (34). IL-6 stimulates B cell differentation and activation of T cells in acute inflammation, and promotes the synthesis of CRP, fibrinogen and albumin in the acute response

(34). IL-6 influences the aforementioned differentiation of Th17 cells together with TGF-β, and constrains TGF-induced Treg cells differentiation (35). The fatigue, anorexia and fever associated with acute inflammations may be induced by IL-6 (36). However, IL6 also has a role in dampening the inflammatory response by reducing the production of IL-1β and TNF-α (37), and by inducing the production of IL-1 Ra (38) and the anti-inflammatory cytokine IL-10 (39). Recent results indicate that activation of IL-6 without a concomitant activation of IL-1β and TNF, for example during physical exercise, mostly induces anti-inflammatory actions (39). **TNF-α** is another pro-inflammatory cytokine with important functions in innate and adaptive immunity. It is produced in macrophages and monocytes, as well as in T-cells, adipocytes and smooth muscle cells and binds to tumor necrosis factor receptor type I (TNF-RI) and type II (TNF-RII). With the exception of erythrocytes, TNF-RI and TNF-RII are located on all cells of the body and are involved in pro-inflammatory pathways through the activation of nuclear factor-kB (40).

DYSREGULATED IMMUNE SYSTEM AND INFLAMMATION IN SCHIZOPHRENIA

There is a growing body of evidence implicating dysregulated immunity in schizophrenia from both *in-vitro* and *in-vivo* studies. In this overview we will limit the description to studies applying tissues and methods that can potentially become useful in the clinical assessments of patients. We will present relevant immune cells, cytokines and acute phase proteins, expression of cytokine genes, other proteins and metabolites, and finally brain imaging methods used to assess neuroinflammation, see **Figure 2**.

Assessments in Peripheral Tissues

Immune Cells

The immune cells are the cornerstones of the immune system, and it is rather unlikely that an immune disturbance of possible pathoetiological significance in schizophrenia would be present without a detectable immune cell signature. However, few studies have described immune cell disturbances so far. A meta-analysis of 16 studies of lymphocytes in schizophrenia vs. healthy controls (41) showed a significant increase in the percentage of CD4 and CD56 (natural killer cells) in acutely ill patients. Drug naïve first episode patients showed a significant increase in the levels of lymphocytes, CD3 (all T-cells) and CD4 levels, and the CD4/CD8 ratio. Absolute CD56 levels were suggested to be trait-dependent, while CD4/CD8 ratio could be state-dependent. A study of 18 patients with schizophrenia (17 treated with clozapine) vs. 18 healthy persons found elevated monocytes, NK cells, naïve B cells and CXCR5+ memory CD4 cells in the schizophrenia group, and decreased number of DC and several T cells populations. The authors find it plausible that clozapine treatment influenced the results (42). In a selective review by Bergink et al. (43) several studies report elevated monocyte counts in the periphery of patients with schizophrenia and higher gene expression for inflammatory cytokines in circulating monocytes. For circulating T cells three referred studies found reduced numbers of circulating lymphocytes, while one study found increased numbers of Th1, Th17, and suppressive natural T regulatory cells (44). In a study of 69 drug-naïve first episode patients with schizophrenia (FES) compared to 70 healthy controls, FES had significantly higher proportion of Th17 cells (45), and the proportion of Th17 cells correlated positively with PANSS total. Interestingly, after 4 weeks of treatment with risperidone, the proportion of Th17 cells decreased significantly. However, conflicting results regarding the Th17 axis have been published (30). It is clearly an advantage from a clinical point of view that immune cells can be assessed with well-established and readily available methods, for example flow-cytometry (46), and are routinely surveyed in the clinical treatment of various conditions, see for example the website of the Karolinska hospital where a full menu of lymphocyte immunphenotyping is offered (www.karolinska.se). Taken together, studies of lymphocytes as well as monocytes in patients with schizophrenia show very interesting differences compared to healthy controls, but more research is needed to evaluate immune cell counts such as lymphocyte immunophenotyping as theranostic biomarkers for immune dysregulation/inflammation in schizophrenia.

Cytokine Protein Levels in Serum

A major body of knowledge regarding immune dysfunction in schizophrenia derives from studies on cytokines in peripheral blood. During the last two decades, many studies have been performed and new ones are arriving (47). Others have summarized these results in systematic reviews and meta-analyses (1–3). The recent study by Rodrigues-Amorim et al. (3) also contains a very helpful summary of the function and clinical impact of the different cytokines. They included 99 studies with 8,234 participants and found that peripheral levels of the following cytokines differed between patients with schizophrenia and healthy controls in more than 50% of the included studies, listed according to falling prevalence among the studies: IL-6, TNF-α, IL-10, IFN-γ, IL-1β, IL-8, IL-2, IL-1RA, furthermore the gene polymorphisms for TNF-α 1800629, IL-6 rs1800795, and IL-1β rs16944, and elevated expression levels of IL-6, TNFR1, TNFR2, and IL-1β mRNAs (3). It is important to emphasize that the identified changes are smaller in magnitude compared to findings from for example inflammation in rheumatoid artritis and other auto-immune disorders, and collectively it is referred to as a low-grade inflammation (48).

Drug-naïve FES

IL-1β, soluble (s)IL-2receptor(R), IL-6, and TNF-α were significantly elevated in a meta-analysis of 23 studies with 570 subjects with drug-naïve FES vs. 683 controls (1). Also non-significant changes of IL-2, IL-4, and IFN-γ were identified. An earlier meta-analysis with 14 studies in FES (2) found IL-1β, sIL-2R, IL-6, IL-12, TNF-α, IFN-γ, TGF-β to be increased in FES vs. controls. Furthermore, in a study of 12 ultra-high risk (UHR) individuals compared to 16 healthy controls IL-17 was significantly decreased and IL-6 increased in the UHR group (49). The finding of low-grade peripheral inflammation in a

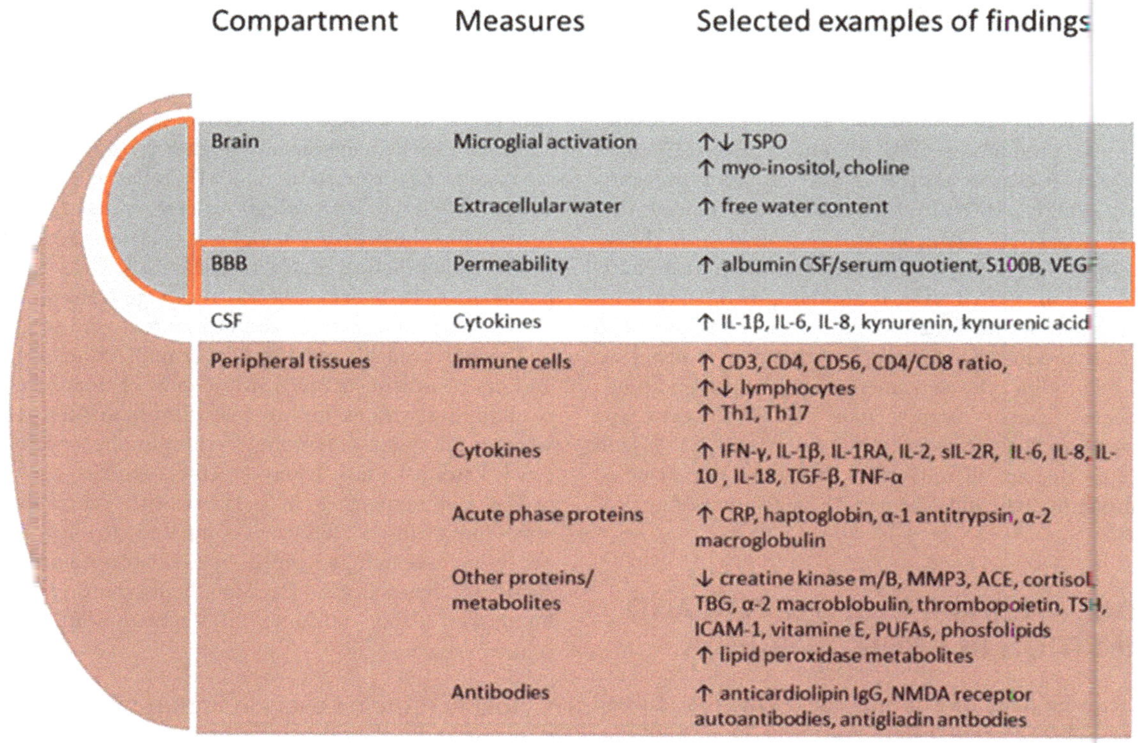

FIGURE 2 | Putative components comprising the immune signature in schizophrenia. BBB, blood-brain-barrier; CSF, cerebrospinal fluid; TSPO, translocator protein; VEGF, vascular endothelial growth factor; IL, interleukin; IFN, interferon; RA, receptor antibody; R, receptor; TGF, transforming growth factor; TNF, tumor necrosis factor; MMP, matrix metalloproteinase; ACE, angiotensine converting enzyme; TBG, thyroxine-binding globuline; TSH, thyrioidea stimulating hormone; ICAM, intercellular adhesion molecule; PUFAs, poly-unsaturated fatty acids; NMDA, N-methyl-D-aspartate.

subset of drug-naïve patients at the time of diagnosis is among the stronger underpinnings of the "inflammation hypothesis" in schizophrenia. However, as a general Th1/Th2 imbalance is not found the interpretation of the findings in terms of underlying immune disturbances is not clear (1).

Effects of antipsychotic treatment on cytokine levels

In a meta-analysis including 8 studies of drug-naïve patients with first-episode psychosis (FEP) a significant reduction after antipsychotic treatment for IL-2 and IL-6 was found. After excluding only one study IL-1β also declined significantly (50). The authors suggested that IL-1β, IL-2, and IL-6 could serve as markers for psychosis, while TNF-α, IL-17, and IFN-γ were still elevated after antipsychotic treatment. The analyses included in total between 69 (IL-2) and 253 (IL-6) subjects, and included studies with data available after 4 weeks of antipsychotic treatment. An earlier review of cytokine changes after antipsychotic treatment (4 to 52 weeks) including 39 studies with schizophrenia spectrum patients found that antipsychotic treatment was associated with reduced IL-2, increased sIL-2R and sTNF-R1/R2 and in some studies also an increase in IL-4 (51). Another meta analysis found that sIL-2R and IL-12 increased and IL-1β, IL-2, and IL-6 decreased with antipsychotic treatment after a mean period of 53 days with antipsychotic treatment (2) including studies with both first-episode and chronic patients. The most consistent finding is a reduction in IL-2 and/or increase in sIL-2R. IL-2 is primarily secreted from activated T-lymphocytes, and is an immunoregulator stimulating growth and development of immune cells in peripheral tissue early in the immune response, and the growth of oligodendrocytes in neural tissue (28). Accordingly, the reduction of IL-2 after antipsychotic treatment implies a decreased immune response.

Deficit syndrome—negative symptoms

A study in patients with the deficit syndrome of schizophrenia—a subgroup of patients with primary negative symptoms from the illness debut—found significantly elevated IL-6 and TNF-α in patients with deficit syndrome compared to in non-deficit schizophrenia and healthy controls (52). The association between negative symptoms and elevated specific cytokines is particularly interesting as antipsychotics are not effective treatment options for negative symptoms. Drug trials with immunomodulating agents targeting negative symptoms are specificly warranted.

A recent meta-analysis by Goldsmith et al. (53) summarized existing findings regarding cytokine alterations in schizophrenia, bipolar disorder and major depressive disorder (MDD), and also compared results from acute and chronic phases. IL-6, TNF-α, IL-1RA, and sIL-2R were all elevated in the acute phases of all three disorders. After treatment, IL-6 decreased both in schizophrenia and MDD, while TNF-α did not change. In chronic states, IL-6 was elevated in all three disorders, while IL-1β and sIL-2R were elevated in schizophrenia and bipolar disorder. The authors conclude that there is a distinct similarity between the acute phases across all three diagnoses and they highlight that the cytokines with elevated levels in the three disorders are all modulated by nuclear factor-κB, regularly found to be activated in autoimmune and inflammatory disorders (53).

Some of the pro-inflammatory cytokines can barely be measured in healthy persons, while in infection-associated inflammatory responses, the concentrations rise 10 to 100-fold In addition multiple confounders such as age, gender, smoking, body mass index (BMI), and diurnal variation may influence the results (2). Further, cytokine activity is interdependent with the hypothalamic pituitary adrenal axis. As a first psychotic episode generally induces high stress levels, it is unclear whether the observed cytokine rises are a general stress phenomenon, or a specific signature of psychosis. Finally, schizophrenia patients face a high burden of co-morbidity in terms of cardiometabolic disorders. As inflammation also plays a central role in the pathophysiology underlying these diseases, future research should address the nature of this relationship. Altered cytokine levels associated with schizophrenia could either be the result or cause of co-morbid disease, or there could be common immunopathogenetic mechanisms underlying both schizophrenia and for instance cardiovascular disease.

Having mentioned these problematic dimensions of cytokine measurement, the pro-inflammatory cytokines IL-1β, IL-6, and TNF-α seem to covariate with psychosis and could be useful tools for selecting participants to drug-studies with immune-modulating drugs targeting for example positive symptoms of schizophrenia.

Cytokine mRNA Levels

A study reporting differences in gene expression between 529 patients with schizophrenia and 660 healthy controls found 1,058 differentially expressed genes, of which 697 genes were upregulated (54). Gene set enrichment analysis showed that the upregulated genes were enriched in several processes involved in the response, activation and regulation of immunity. Differentially expressed immune genes included four complement genes: CR1, CR2, CD55, and C3, as well as TGFβ1 and TGM2. A study with combined measurement of mRNAs of cytokines and peripheral cytokines in plasma and serum aimed to define an inflammatory biotype of schizophrenia (20). This study used a recursive two-step cluster analysis to define subgroups of pro-inflammatory status on the basis of mRNAs of IL-18, IL-1β, IL-6, and IL-8. The cluster analysis included 68 controls and 82 patients. The results identified three clusters, cluster 1—low cytokine expression ($n = 89$), with below median expression of all measured cytokine mRNAs, cluster 2 ($n = 50$) was termed high cytokine expression and had above median for two and above third quartile for two cytokine mRNAs, while the very high cytokine expression group ($n = 11$) of cluster 3 were above the third quartile for all four cytokine mRNAs. 47.6% in the schizophrenia group was either cluster two or three compared to 32.4% in the healthy control group. The elevated/non-elevated subgroups of the schizophrenia participants did not differ with respect to gender, BMI, duration of illness or symptom severity as measured by the PANSS. Interestingly, the authors discussed the limited correlation between peripheral cytokine proteins and their mRNAs, and suggested that the main source of cytokine proteins may not be peripheral leucocytes. Furthermore, they suggested that mRNAs of pro-inflammatory cytokines could be used to select the patients who have an "elevated inflammation biotype" (20). In a study comparing 53 patients with schizophrenia and 53 healthy controls intracellular levels of IL-6 mRNA in the peripheral blood mononuclear cells (PBMC) analyzed with quantitative real-time polymerase chain reaction (RT-PCR) was found to be significantly elevated for patients with schizophrenia (55), and PBMC IL-6 mRNA was specifically suggested to be a candidate for a diagnostic marker for schizophrenia (55).

Acute Phase Proteins

CRP is an acute phase protein produced in the liver, stimulated by IL-1β, IL-6, and TNF (56) and released by macrophages and adipocytes. As demonstrated in the 2013 Guideline on the Assessment of Cardiovascular Risk from the American College of Cardiology and the American Heart Association (57) where CRP is now recommended as a supplementary test using a threshold of CRP ≥ 2 to indicate increased cardiovascular risk, CRP is widely used in clinical practice as a marker of inflammation. Another major advantage of CRP is that it can be measured reliably in most certified laboratories. A recent meta-analysis of 18 studies with 1,963 patients and 3,683 non-schizophrenia controls found that a diagnosis of schizophrenia was associated with a moderate increase in blood CRP (58), corroborating the results of a prior meta-analysis (4). Furthermore, patients from Asia or Africa and those who were younger than 30 years had higher CRP levels. The increase in CRP correlated with positive symptoms of schizophrenia but was unresponsive to initiation of antipsychotic treatment (4). A large and recent study ($n > 1{,}000$) reported elevated levels of CRP in patients with schizophrenia compared to controls, with levels of CRP correlating both to positive and negative symptoms (59). There is also evidence indicating a relationship between CRP and cognitive dysfunction in subjects with psychosis (60). In a recent systematic review by Orsolini et al. (61) elevated CRP levels were again identified in patients with schizophrenia and correlating with severity of symptoms. Interestingly, a large genome wide association study (GWAS) using mendelian randomization found that genetic factors that elevate CRP have a preventive effect with respect to developing schizophrenia (62), and the authors discussed that increased CRP in schizophrenia is more likely a result of developing and having the disease than being a predisposing factor. Various psychiatric disorders were investigated in a study assessing CRP in 599 admissions in a psychiatric catchment area. The prevalence of inflammation defined as CRP > 3 mg/L was 32% for psychotic disorders (ICD F 20–29), 21% for mood disorders (F30–39), 22% for neurotic disorders (F 40–48), and 42% for personality disorders (F60–69), indicating that low grade inflammation could be present in a whole range of psychiatric disorders (21). As obesity is more common among patients with a psychiatric diagnosis, the increase in adipose tissue and resulting higher risk for diabetes type 2 and cardiovascular illness could be an intermediating factor (63). Yet, even after adjusting for BMI CRP levels remain higher in patients (64). Furthermore in a study of patients with first admissions to hospital with diagnoses of schizophrenia, bipolar disorders or depression, survival-analyses showed that moderately elevated CRP (3–10 mg/L) was associated with an increase in all-cause mortality with adjusted hazard rate (HR) of 1.56 (95% CI: 1.02–2.38), and for levels above 10 mg/L the adjusted HR was 2.07 (95% CI: 1.30–3.29). To conclude, the acute phase protein CRP is elevated in a proportion of individuals with schizophrenia and other psychoses, the measure is reliable and widely available, and it has been found to correlate both with positive symptoms of schizophrenia and cognitive function. Expression profiles of the additional acute phase proteins—haptoglobin (HP), alpha-1 antitrypsin (A1T), and alpha-2 macroglobulin (A2M) were investigated with quantitative polymerase chain reaction (qPCR) in a sample with 43 FEP patients and 57 healthy controls followed up for 3 months (65). All three acute phase proteins were elevated during the study period, and correlated with PANSS positive, depressive, and excitement subscales. The results are in line with previous studies using proteomic techniques identifying changes in acute phase proteins in patients with schizophrenia supporting that inflammation is an important feature in schizophrenia (66, 67).

Additional Circulating Proteins and Metabolites Related to Inflammation

Several methods with the capacity to identify and quantify several hundreds to thousand molecules simultaneously have been used to analyse blood sera from patients with schizophrenia. These techniques are referred to as proteomics using multiplex immunoassay, two-dimensional gel electrophoresis and mass spectrometry for identifying proteins, and metabolomics using metabolomic mass spectrometry and ^{1}H-nuclear magnetic resonance spectroscopy (MRS) for identifying smaller circulating metabolites (68). Using proteomics, one interesting study comparing 17 drug-naïve FES to 17 healthy controls found that 9 proteins (creatine kinase m/B, MMP3, ACE, cortisol, TBG, α-2 macrobloblulin, thrombopoietin, TSH, and ICAM-1) displayed lower concentrations in the patients vs. the controls (69). The authors commented that most of these proteins are involved in endothelial cell function and inflammation. Another study recently reported results from a novel proteomic method on PBMC from 20 patients with schizophrenia assessed both while acutely ill and in the recovery phase and compared to healthy controls. Interestingly, the study found significant differences in α-defencins 1–3 between the acutely admitted patients and healthy controls (70). A systematic review of metabolite biomarkers of schizophrenia that included 63 studies discussed their findings of decreased levels of the antioxidant vitamin E, polyunsaturated fatty acids (PUFAs), and phospholipids together with high levels of lipid peroxidation metabolites to indicate an oxidative balance favoring pro-oxidants and thus also inflammation in patients with schizophrenia (71). Although proteomics or metabolomics have not yet been applied as tools in treatment guidance for individual patients with schizophrenia, some have suggested how the use of these methods could improve treatment (11, 72). As recently proposed for mood disorders, using immune-based biomarkers together with traditional clinical descriptions of the individual patients may potentially improve both drug studies and individual treatment (73). Schwarz et al. (74) used proteomics to divide patients with schizophrenia into three groups: those with immune signature, those with growth factor disturbances and those with hormonal abnormalities. Such subdivisions could help to identify patient groups for specific augmentation therapy, for example with components such as NSAIDs, metformin or selective estrogen receptor modulators. Future drug trials should implement the promising results from this rapidly developing field in order to enable and provide time-efficient and personalized treatment options approaches. By combining several proteomic/metabolomic markers indicating inflammation in patients with schizophrenia, these methods could offer specific and sensitive ways to select participants for drug trials and monitoring drug effects on the molecular level (72).

Antibodies

Elevation of some antibody-titers has been linked to schizophrenia. A systematic quantitative review including 81 studies, showed that increased anticardiolipin IgG and N-methyl-D-aspartate (NMDA) receptor autoantibody titers and several additional autoantibodies were more prevalent in patients with schizophrenia (75). In contrast, another study of three cohorts of patients with schizophrenia stated that peripheral NMDA receptor autoantibodies are very rare in patients with schizophrenia (76). Also antibodies to gliadin have been found elevated in studies comparing patients with schizophrenia to healthy controls, but this was not the case for antibodies more specific to coeliac disease (77). While the recognition and early treatment of auto-immune encephalitis is an important part in the differential diagnosis of schizophrenia, it is unclear if the presence of auto-antibodies in serum without specific symptoms of auto-immune encephalitis (convulsions, rapid progression, decreased consciousness, and stereotypic movements) warrant additional treatment (78). Although of considerable interest, the origin and effect of these findings in patients with schizophrenia are not yet clear, and their usefulness in the mapping of inflammation in schizophrenia is elusive.

Blood Brain Barrier Hyperpermeability

Evidence indicate increased permeability in the blood brain barrier (BBB) in a subset of patients with schizophrenia (79). One study found that 14 out of 39 patients with schizophrenia spectrum disorders displayed signs of BBB hyperpermeability including 9 patients with increased albumin cerebrospinal fluid (CSF)/serum concentration quotient (80). A recent meta-analysis by Orlovska-Waast et al. (81) with 32 studies concluded that patients with bipolar disorder and schizophrenia may display BBB abnormalities, but the authors also noted that the quality of available studies is rather low. Increased levels of S100B protein in blood and CSF that can be caused by BBB hyperpermeability

(82) and elevated vascular endothelial growth factor (VEGF), a protein known to increase BBB permeability, have been found in patients with schizophrenia (83). Also increased levels of vascular endothelial adhesion molecules and integrin receptor have been detected in schizophrenia (84). A PET study focusing on P-glycoprotein (P-gp), a major efflux pump in the BBB, found it to be more active in schizophrenia (85) but this finding needs to be replicated. Increased BBB permeability can have deleterious effects on the brain by pro-inflammatory cells and molecules entering in brain (79). Although, there is no concensus regarding the best way to monitor increased BBB permeability in patients with schizophrenia, several novel candidates including matrix metalloproteinase-9(MMP-9), ubiquitin carboxy-terminal hydrolase-L1(UCHL-L1), neurofilaments, brain derived neurotropic factor (BDNF), miRNA in addition to S100B and glial fibrillary acidic protein (GFAP) are available for future studies, and preferably aggregated and applied in panels of several biomarkers (86).

Assessments in the Brain

Neuroinflammation and Positron Emission Tomography (PET)

The concept of neuroinflammation indicates innate immune responses in the central nervous system (CNS) mainly produced by microglia and astrocytes (87), in contrast to the term neuroimmunology that denotes adaptive immunological changes within the CNS (88). However, the use of the term neuroinflammation to describe low-grade changes associated with depression and schizophrenia is controversial. One study that examined gene expression in brain in well-established inflammatory diseases (inflammatory bowel disease, juvenile dermatomyositis, MS, and ulcerative colitis) compared to the neurodevelopmental/neurodegenerative diseases Alzheimers disease, Parkinsons disease and schizophrenia reported a categorical difference between the neurodevelopmental/neurodegenerative diseases and the inflammatory diseases (89). The authors state that a distinction between classical neuroinflammatory conditions such as MS with typical mononuclear infiltrates and the smaller and ill-defined glial changes associated with secretion of various immune molecules must be established, and that missing this point may lead to unwarranted treatment trials (89). Nevertheless, classical neuroinflammation or more precisely microglial activation has been demonstrated to correlate with microglial expression of the translocator protein (TSPO) which is located at the outer mitochondrial membrane (90). While early studies with first generation TSPO PET tracers, for example [11C](R)-(1-[2-chrorophynyl]-N-methyl-N-[1-methylpropyl]-3 isoquinoline carboxamide (11C-(R)-PK11195) showed increased TSPO binding (91, 92), more recent studies did not find signs of microglial activation using the PK11195 tracer (93), and the specificity of TSPO binding to assess the inflammation associated with schizophrenia has been challenged (94). Second generation TSPO tracers have been developed, and in some studies increased microglial TSPO expression between patients with schizophrenia and healthy controls have been observed (95), while other did not find signs of increased TSPO expression (96). A recent meta-analysis that reviewed five studies with 75 patients and 77 healthy controls found that patients with schizophrenia had lower TSPO binding compared to controls, and concluded that this difference is caused either by lower density or altered function of brain immune cells (97). Hence, the advantage of measuring TSPO binding to assess low-grade inflammatory changes associated with schizophrenia seems to be in question, and the usefulness of the method to select patients with an "inflammatory" phenotype and monitoring effect of anti-inflammatory drugs appears to be low.

Magnetic Resonance Imaging (MRI) and Magnetic Resonance Spectroscopy (MRS)

MRI and MRS have also been proposed as potential means to measure the low-grade inflammatory changes associated with schizophrenia (98). MRS can measure concentrations of various molecules in defined volumes of the brain. Increased levels of glial markers as myo-inositol (MI), cholin (Cho) and total creatin, and reduced levels of neuronal markers as N-acetylaspartate and glutamate have been interpreted to indicate various dimensions of inflammation, such as increased density of glial cells and migration of glial cells into the inflamed area (98). MRS has so far been used in few studies to assess inflammation in schizophrenia. One study scanned 60 drug-naïve FES patients and 60 controls. The results showed elevated MI, Cho, and glutamate in the FES group (99) and were presented as evidence of inflammation in the early phase of schizophrenia. Also results from T1- and T2- weighted structural MRI and diffusion MRI free-water imaging may be used to assess low-scale brain inflammation (98, 100). The free-water imaging measures the amount of extracellular water in brain tissue and is postulated to correlate with oedema and possibly inflammation, and a few studies have identified increased free-water in samples of patients with schizophrenia compared to controls (101, 102). Taken together, MR based tecniques pose exciting opportunities to assess the subtle brain changes associated with schizophrenia. However, more research is needed to understand the relationship between these changes and other measures of inflammation, for example cytokine levels in CSF and the peripheral circulation, before they can be applied as markers of inflammation in the individual patient with schizophrenia. Prasad et al. found associations between diffusion tensor imaging measures and the levels of IL6 and CRP (103), but we have not identified studies exploring the relationship between more novel MRI methods and markers of inflammation in CSF or peripheral blood.

Cytokines in the Cerebrospinal Fluid

A meta-analysis including 16 studies comparing schizophrenia with healthy controls, found increased CSF levels of IL-1β, IL-6, IL-8, kynurenine, and kynurenic acid, while sIL-2R was decreased (104). With the exception of sIL-2R, increased levels of the same cytokines (IL-1β, IL-6, IL-8) have been reported in the periphery (2). A recent meta-analysis that included 32 studies also found that IL-6 and IL-8 were significantly elevated in schizophrenia (81). Presently it is not obvious that assessment of markers of inflammation in CSF to diagnose an inflammatory biotype in individual patients with schizophrenia will give additional gain vs. assessments in peripheral blood. With the exception of some countries, for example Germany and Denmark that investigate liquor in first episode patients to screen for Lyme's disease and other infectious causes, CSF assessment is not part of clinical practice for patients with psychosis. On the other hand, studies investigating CSF in schizophrenia are scarce and the number of participants are small compared to studies using peripheral measurements and future research might prove measuring inflammatory markers in CSF to be useful.

DRUG STUDIES TO TREAT IMMUNE DYSREGULATION OR INFLAMMATION IN SCHIZOPHRENIA

Non-steroidal Anti-inflammatory Drugs (NSAIDS)

Anti-inflammatory drugs have been used as add-on to antipsychotic treatment in patients with schizophrenia, with some success–see **Table 1**. The results are summarized in several meta-analyses: Sommer et al. included 4 studies with celecoxib, one with acetylsalicylic acid/aspirin (117), and reviewed 5 studies with celecoxib and 2 with aspirin in their broader meta-analysis of anti-inflammatory agents (16). A significant beneficial effect on PANSS total score of treatment with aspirin was found. As already mentioned, one randomized controlled trial (RCT) with aspirin showed stronger effects when stratifying participants on the basis of a marker of inflammation (27). Nitta et al. included 7 studies with celecoxib and 2 with aspirin (105). NSAIDS significantly reduced PANSS positive symptoms. The effects were moderated by aspirin treatment, in-patient treatment, first episode patients and lower PANSS negative scores. Zheng et al. conducted a meta-analysis including 8 studies with celecoxib conducted between 2002 and 2010, most of them were also included in the previously published meta-analyses (106). They concluded that treatment with celecoxib outperformed placebo in studies of first-episode patients, but not in patients with chronic schizophrenia. Effects were moderated by higher positive symptoms and lower negative symptoms at baseline. A few RCTs with anti-inflammatory drugs as add-on to antipsychotic treatment have been published after these overviews. Weiser et al. published a conference paper where they reanalyzed an RCT where patients with schizophrenia were randomized to treatment with either aspirine, minocycline, the dopamine-agonist pramipexole, or placebo (118). After subgrouping the participants according to CRP levels, they showed that in the upper third group with CRP above 3.8 mg/L, aspirine had a significant effect on PANSS positive symptoms. However, this was not found for other symptom measures, and not for participants treated with minocycline or pramipexole.

Steroidal Anti-inflammatory Drugs

Prednisolone, a synthetic corticosteroid, has been used for several decades in the treatment of various inflammatory and autoimmune disorders (119). The agent is more potent than NSAIDS as it targets several aspects of the immune system and interferes with almost all types of immune cells (120). Furthermore, prednisolone readily crosses the BBB. There are currently two recruiting randomized, placebo-controlled add-on trials investigating prednisolone in early phase schizophrena and related disorders (ClinicalTrials.gov Identifiers NCT03340909 and NCT02949232).

Novel Biological Drugs With Immune-Modulating Actions

The availability of monoclonal antibodies toward cytokines, cytokine receptors or other specific parts of the immune system, in combination with findings of elevated cytokine levels in schizophrenia imply that studies with these drugs would strongly enhance our knowledge about cytokine dysfunction in schizophrenia. Drawing upon the experience with targeted immune therapy in diseases such as rheumatoid arthritis, psoriasis, Chrohns disease, ulcerative colitis, spondyloarthritis, and systemic lupus erythematosus, it would have been interesting to try out this strategy in patients with schizophrenia. However, caution is warranted, as the cytokine antagonists have a range of adverse effects due to the multiple and pleiotropic functions of the cytokines (121). According to Baker and Isaacs (18), the novel biological drugs with immune-modulating properties can be described according to their target of action: (1) drugs directed toward activity in the T-helper 17 immune axis: drugs directed toward IL-23p19, IL-17, or IL-12/23p40, (2) drugs active against type I and II Interferons, (3) drugs interfering in the lymphocyte recruitment by intervening in the adhesion process either by sphingosine−1-phosphate receptor inhibition or by integrin blockade, (4) Janus kinase inhibitors—first generation and second generation selective inhibitors, (5) drugs targeting B cells, (6) drugs modulating T cell function, and (7) bispecific antibodies.

Two studies on the effect of novel biologicals in patients with schizophrenia have been published, both with tocilizumab which is a humanized IL-6 receptor monoclonal antibody. Tocilizumab was tried in an open label study (107), and 2017 an RCT of 36 patients with residual symptoms of schizophrenia was published (17). In the study by Miller et al. (107), 6 participants (4 with schizophrenia and 2 with schizoaffective disorder) entered and 5 completed an 8 week open trial of adjunctive injections with 4 mg/kg tocilizumab at baseline and after 4 weeks, with the aim of studying the effect on cognition. All subjects improved in a processing speed measure, and 5 out of 6 improved also on a global cognition measure. The authors state that the signal-to-noise ratio may be increased in future studies if only patients with baseline inflammation were included, which was not the case in this study. Girgis et al. (17) reported a study where 36 clinically stable individuals with schizophrenia and PANSS total scores >60 were randomized to treatment with 3 monthly injections with 8 mg/kg tocilizumab or placebo at baseline and after 4 weeks. The results showed no effect of tocilizumab on any behavioral outcome, while CRP decreased and IL-6 and IL-8 increased. No prediction of

TABLE 1 | Drug treatment of inflammation and immune dysregulation in schizophrenia.

Drugs	Level of evidence	Effect on primary outcome	Effect on secondary outcome
ANTI-INFLAMMATORY DRUGS			
NSAIDs			
Aspirin/acetyl-salicylic acid	Meta-analyses (16, 105)	↓PANSS total (16)	No effects in cognitive tests[c]
Celecoxib	Meta-analyses (16, 106)	↓PANSS total in subgroup first-episode patients (106)	↓Positive symptoms, negative symptoms, general psychopathology (106)
Steroids			
Prednisolone	Protocols for RCTs published[a]		
NOVEL BIOLOGICALS—MONOCLONAL ANTIBODIES AGAINST CYTOKINES/CYTOKINE RECEPTORS/CELL ADHESION MOLECULES			
Tocilizumab	One RCT in patients with residual symptoms (17)	No effect at week 12 on the PANSS total	No effects on the MATRICS, PANSS subscales, CGI, GAF, ↓CRP, ↑IL-6, and IL-8
	One open study (107)	↑BACS. No significant changes in psychopathology scores, cytokines or CRP	
	Protocol for RCT published[a]		
Siltuximab	Protocol for RCT published[a]		
Natalizumab	Protocol for RCT published[a]		
MISCELLANEOUS DRUGS WITH ANTI-INFLAMMATORY ACTION[b]			
N-acetylcysteine	Meta-analyses (16, 108)	↓Total psychopathology (SMD = −0.74). No effect on PANSS subscales (108)	No difference in any cause discontinuation rate or adverse drug reactions
Erythropoetin	One RCT[d] (109)	↑RBANS subtests delayed memory, language–semantic fluency, attention. ↓WCST-64–perseverative errors	No effect on other cognitive tests, psychopathology, or MRI brain volumes
Pioglitazone	One RCT (110)	↓PANSS negative	↓PANSS total. No difference in PANSS positive, HDRS
Simvastatin	One RCT (111)	↓PANSS negative	↓PANSS total. No difference PANSS positive or general psychopathology
Pravastatin	One RCT (112)	↓LDL cholesterol. No effect on CRP, PANSS total score, MATRICS over 12 weeks	↓PANSS positive at 6 weeks
Minocycline	Meta-analyses (113, 114)	↓PANSS total (113, 114)	↓PANSS positive (113), negative (113, 114), and general psychopathology (113, 114) subscales
	Two recent RCTs (115, 116)	No effect on PANSS total (115) or PANSS negative subscale (116)	No effects on secondary outcomes: PANSS subscales, general psychopathology measures, cognition

[a]At clinicaltrials.gov.
[b]Negative trials or drugs with negative findings in updated meta-analyses are not included.
[c]Assessed only in one study (27).
[d]The inclusion criteria included an RBANS score < 1 SD below mean.
NSAIDS, non-steroidal anti-inflammatory drugs; PANSS, Positive and Negative Syndrome Scale; RCT, randomized controlled trial; CGI, Clinical global impression; GAF, Global assessment of functioning; CRP, C-reactive protein; IL, interleukin; BACS, The Brief Assessment of Cognition in Schizophrenia; SMD, standardized mean difference; RBANS, Repeatable Battery for the Assessment of Neuropsychological Status; WCST, Wisconsin Card Sorting Test; MRI, Magnetic resonance imaging; LDL, low density lipoprotein.

outcome was seen by baseline CRP or the measured cytokines. No selection procedure based on elevated baseline inflammation measures was implemented, and the authors underlined the possibility that enriching the sample with inclusion of only individuals with an elevated CRP could have influenced the results.

We have not been able to identify other completed studies with novel biologicals targeting cytokines or cytokine receptors in schizophrenia. However, at the clinicaltrials.gov website three trials currently recruiting participants are listed, two from Augusta and one in London. One study conducted by the group of Brian Miller at Augusta University in Georgia, plans to randomize 30 stable outpatients with schizophrenia or schizoaffective disorder with CRP >5 mg/L to adjunct treatment with siltuximab which is a recombinant IL-6 monoclonal antibody, or placebo. In another study by the same group 20 stable outpatients with CRP >5 mg/L will be randomized to receive treatment with tocilizumab or placebo for 12 weeks. Lastly, a study conducted by Tiago Marques and Oliver Howes, Institute of Psychiatry at Kings college in London, plans to randomize 60 individuals with FES or other psychotic disorder to treatment with natalizumab, which is a humanized monoclonal antibody against the cell adhesion molecule α4-integrin, or placebo. The results are integrated in **Table 1**.

Miscellaneous Drugs With Anti-inflammatory Actions

N-acetylcysteine (NAC) is a drug with several established indications, including the treatment of paracetamol intoxication. NAC interacts with a wide range of physiological pathways, and has anti-oxidative and anti-inflammatory effects (122). A recent systematic review and meta-analysis summarizing the results from 3 RCTs with schizophrenia patients found that NAC improved total psychopathology (108). A recent RCT including 63 early psychosis patients found that NAC had no effects on positive and negative symptoms or functional outcome, but a significant effect on processing speed (123). Interestingly, patients with higher values of glutathione peroxidase activity in blood cells (GPx_{BC}), an indicator of oxidative stress and associated with brain glutathione levels, improved significantly on positive symptoms, leading the authors to suggest that GPx_{BC}, could be a theranostic marker for NAC treatment (123).

Erythropoetin (EPO) is a glycoprotein secreted by the kidney in response to hypoxia that stimulates bone-marrow erythropoiesis. EPO also has an anti-inflammatory effect in the brain by modulating microglia responses and decreasing BBB hyperpermeability (124), among a wide range of other pharmacological actions. Recombinant EPO is used as a drug to treat anemia associated with kidney failure and cancer therapy, and has also been tried to improve cognition in patients with schizophrenia. A systematic review with a quantitative synthesis included 78 animal and human studies (125), including only one double-blind RCT (109). The results of this 3 month study showed that the patients with schizophrenia improved on all cognitive tests but no improvement on the PANSS scores was found, and the authors suggest a role for EPO as an add-on treatment to antipsychotic drugs for patients with cognitive dysfunction. However, serious concerns regarding for example vascular side effects may limit the clinical use of EPO (125).

Statins have been tried in RCTs as add-ons to treatment with antipsychotics for patients with schizophrenia. Simvastatin showed effect on negative symptoms in an RCT with 66 patients randomized to simvastatin vs. placebo (111). According to the registrations on clinicaltrials (https://clinicaltrials.gov/), there are at least two on-going studies with simvastatin, one also with a published protocol (126). Vincenzi et al. randomized 60 patients with schizophrenia or schizoaffective disorder to pravastatine or placebo (112). Pravastatine significantly reduced PANSS total score from baseline to 6 weeks, but not at 12 weeks. Cholesterol and low density lipoprotein were reduced. In the subgroup with CRP above 2 mg/L cognitive measures were improved between baseline and 6 weeks.

Pioglitazone is an anti-diabetic drug also demonstrated to inhibit inflammatory pathways (127). Iranpour et al. randomized 40 patients with negative symptoms to pioglitazone vs. placebo as add-on to risperidone treatment and found significant decrease in negative symptoms after 8 weeks treatment (110).

Estrogens also have anti-inflammatory actions (128). The meta-analysis by Sommer et al. (16) included 8 studies, and concluded that treatment with estrogens have a significant effect on the PANSS total score. The same meta-analysis also included studies with davunetide ($n = 2$), fatty acids EPA/DHA($n = 7$), and minocycline($n = 4$). However, noen of these drugs showed a significant effect on the PANSS total score.

Minocycline is a second generation tetracycline with anti-inflammatory properties (129) and a potential for neuroprotective use for example after stroke (130). It has been tried for improving symptoms in schizophrenia in several studies, and the results summarized in meta-analyses (16, 113, 114). Solmi et al. (114) performed a systematic review and meta-analysis of studies published up to February 2016 and identified six RCTs with 215 participants randomized to minocycline and 198 to placebo. Minocyline was superior to placebo for PANSS total score, and the negative and general PANSS subscale, the conclusion was in contrast to the earlier meta-analysis by Sommer et al. (16) that included three studies with high heterogeneity. Xiang et al. (113) published a meta-analysis summarizing published RCTs upto January 2016 and included eight RCTs with 286 participants on minocycline and 262 on placebo. Also in this meta-analysis minocycline was superior to placebo in improving PANSS total, negative and general subscale, and here also for the positive subscale. However, two new RCTs do not find an effect of minocycline vs. placebo (115, 116). Deakin et al. (116) randomized 207 people with schizophrenia-spectrum disorder with an illness duration <5 years to minocycline or placebo, half and half. No effect on the primary outcome PANSS negative subscale or other symptoms of schizophrenia was identified after 12 months treatment. Weiser et al. (115) randomized 200 people with schizophrenia or schizoaffective disorder to 16 weeks treatment with minocycline or placebo as add-on to antipsychotic treatment. No effects on the primary outcome PANSS total or the secondary outcomes PANSS subscales, Clinical Global Impression Scale–Severity or–improvement scales, Brief Assessment of Cognition in Schizophrenia and drop out rates were identified. Thus, after these two negative, but rather large and well performed RCTs the status of minocycline as an agent to treat patients with schizophrenia is rather cloudy. However, and related to the main aim of this paper, the trials did not enrich their sample for patients with elevated measures of inflammation. It can not be ruled out that the negative and contrasting findings in the minocycline literature are caused by applying the minocycline to an unselected sample (131). Also the results for miscellaneous drugs are summarized in **Table 1**.

Theranostic Biomarkers in Studies With Anti-inflammatory/Immune-modulating Drugs for Patients With Schizophrenia

In summary, we did not find any completed studies on anti-inflammatory treatment or immune-modulating drugs that have selected patients based on elevated markers of inflammation. A few studies have analyzed subgroups of participants with for example elevated CRP, and indications of more beneficial effects of anti-inflammatory treatment in subgroups with raised CRP have been identified. However, this applies only to a minority of studies, and it is conceivable that the influence of anti-inflammatory treatment could have been stronger if the treatment were targeted to participants with elevated markers of inflammation. Several protocols for ongoing add-on trials have been published at clinicaltrials.gov/ and a few of these seem to plan selection of participants based on an elevated CRP level. If this strategy is successful, CRP could be regarded as a first theranostic biomarker for tailoring anti-inflammatory/immune-modulating treatment to patients with schizophrenia, which could pave a way for more sophisticated markers in the future. An interesting clustering of well-known and putative immune-modulating drugs based on the *in-vitro* influence on cytokine levels were done by Wallner et al. (132). They identified cyclosporine A and tacrolimus among other drugs as one group predominately influencing IFN-gamma, IL-2 and IL-17, while the JAK family of drugs inhibits IFN-γ and increases IL-2 and the chemokine MIP3-α. Consequently, if a specific immune/inflammation activation pattern can be repeatedly identified in patients with schizophrenia, a more specific and hopefully more effective immune-modulating drug therapy can be explored in future trials.

CONSTRUCTING THE INFLAMMATORY SIGNATURE OF SCHIZOPHRENIA FOR CLINICAL AND RESEARCH PURPOSE

The search for theranostic biomarkers for anti-inflammatory or immune-modulating treatment is still in its infancy. When selectively reviewing how inflammation and immunological dysregulation can be assessed in order to diagnose low-grade inflammation in patients with schizophrenia, two main issues need to be addressed. Firstly, the research conducted so far regarding immune dysregulation in schizophrenia has been focused to a large extent on finding differences on a group level comparing patients with schizophrenia and healthy controls, rather than determining the level of inflammation in the individual patient. Many advanced methods and bioinformatical tools are increasingly available and will doubtless be further developed to uncover cell populations or molecules that could serve as theranostic biomarkers and help assess the chances that anti-inflammatory or immune-modulating treatment will be of help to the individual patient. Secondly, although studies with proteomics, metabolomics and brain imaging offer exciting possibilities, presently the less sophisticated option of measuring the protein level of CRP and pro-inflammatory cytokines—IL-1β, IL-6, TNF-α, TGF-β–in serum is far more convenient for identifying patients with low-grade inflammation. Among the pro-inflammatory cytokines, IL-6 is found most often to be elevated in patients with schizophrenia (3), and has also been suggested as a possible state marker for acute relapse (2). However, as IL-6 seems to be both pro- and anti-inflammatory, more research is needed to establish the usefulness of IL-6 as a biomarker in schizophrenia (39). The general problem of assaying cytokines reliably and standardized remains and constrains further development of the field. Furthermore, and as discussed by Goldsmith et al. (53), it would be useful to agree internationally on a panel of cytokine network components to be studied in order to increase comparability between studies, and also to evaluate patterns of cytokines for example with cytokine ratios instead of focusing on individual cytokines.

There is some evidence indicating a link between peripheral levels of inflammation and symptom severity. For instance, CRP levels correlates with positive symptoms, negative symptoms, and cognitive dysfunction (60) and a level of CRP >3.8 mg/L increased the chance of therapeutic response to anti-inflammatory treatment with aspirin in one study (118). Besides this unique study, the literature offers little guidance as to the use of inflammatory parameters as theranostic biomarkers. In the current protocols for two ongoing studies with monoclonal antibodies conducted by dr. Brian Miller at Augusta University, the CRP level of 5 mg/L is chosen. In another study with add-on prednisolone, sponsored by Erik Johnsen at the Unversity of Bergen, a CRP level of >3.8 mg/L is chosen as an inclusion criterion (clinicaltrials.gov), based on the study by Weiser et al. (118). Adding to this, and based on the *in-vitro* findings of Wallner et al. (132), specific drugs could probably use specific measures to show response of treatment. We are certain that drug trials with anti-inflammatory or immune-modulating drugs would benefit from an concenting scientific community on how to select participants. This would increase comparability and also the possibility to show effect. Another important aspect calling for international collaborations is the need to increase the number of participants in drug trials in order to explore the fascinating possibility of disease-modifying treatment for schizophrenia posed by immune-modulating drugs.

Moreover, it seems clear that inflammation in this context should be regarded more as a dimension rather than a category. Thus, determining the degree of inflammation that causes or contributes to increased symptoms or deteriorating function is essential in the development of novel theranostic biomarkers (133). This can only be done in large longitudinal studies where multiple markers are monitored and predictors for increased symptoms, decreased function and other adverse developments are identified. Currently, biomarker panels are preferred to single markers (86), and individual differences must be accounted for (11).

SUMMARY

- The existing knowledge does not provide evidence to conclude that all patients with schizophrenia have increased inflammation, on the contrary; most studies report a low-grade inflammation in a subset of around 35–50% of patients with schizophrenia, and in the transition from descriptives on a group level to individual diagnosis the best way to diagnose inflammation in schizophrenia must be defined

- CRP and the pro-inflammatory cytokines are the proteins that at present should be further validated as biomarkers for inflammation in schizophrenia. Furthermore, they correlate at least in some studies with symptoms and phases of illness, and measurement is standardized and available from clinical laboratories
- More methods have the potential to develop biomarkers for inflammation in schizophrenia: immune cell characteristics measured by flow cytometry, proteins measured by proteomic methods, or other molecular elements mapped by metabolomics.
- The ultimal goal would be a panel of molecules with proven specificity and sensitivity as theranostic biomarkers which could be supported by brain imaging methods—to select patients for anti-inflammatory or immune-modulating treatment. Large longitudinal studies following standard development for biomarkers are needed to fulfill this goal.

AUTHOR CONTRIBUTIONS

RK, IS, VS, and EJ drafted the study. RK did the literature searches and wrote the first version. IS, VS, ID, and EJ commented, finalized the paper, and all approved the final version.

REFERENCES

1. Upthegrove R, Manzanares-Teson N, Barnes NM. Cytokine function in medication-naive first episode psychosis: a systematic review and meta-analysis. *Schizophr Res.* (2014) 155:101–8. doi: 10.1016/j.schres.2014.03.005
2. Miller B, Buckley P, Seabolt W, Mellor A, Kirkpatrick B. Meta-analysis of cytokine alterations in schizophrenia: clinical status and antipsychotic effects. *Biol Psychiatry* (2011) 70:663–71. doi: 10.1016/j.biopsych.2011.04.013
3. Rodrigues-Amorim D, Rivera-Baltanas T, Spuch C, Caruncho HJ, Gonzalez-Fernandez A, Olivares JM, et al. Cytokines dysregulation in schizophrenia: a systematic review of psychoneuroimmune relationship. *Schizophr Res.* (2017) S0920-9964(17)30718-1. doi: 10.1016/j.schres.2017.11.023
4. Fernandes BS, Steiner J, Bernstein HG, Dodd S, Pasco JA, Dean OM, et al. C-reactive protein is increased in schizophrenia but is not altered by antipsychotics: meta-analysis and implications. *Mol Psychiatry* (2016) 21:554–64. doi: 10.1038/mp.2015.87
5. Schizophrenia working group of the psychiatric genomics consortium. biological insights from 108 schizophrenia-associated genetic loci. *Nature* (2014) 511:421–7. doi: 10.1038/nature13595
6. Sekar A, Bialas AR, de Rivera H, Davis A, Hammond TR, Kamitaki N, et al. Schizophrenia risk from complex variation of complement component 4. *Nature* (2016) 530:177–83. doi: 10.1038/nature16549
7. Selten JP, Termorshuizen F. The serological evidence for maternal influenza as risk factor for psychosis in offspring is insufficient: critical review and meta-analysis. *Schizophr Res.* (2017) 183:2–9. doi: 10.1016/j.schres.2016.11.006
8. Sutterland AL, Fond G, Kuin A, Koeter MW, Lutter R, van Gool T, et al. Beyond the association. Toxoplasma gondii in schizophrenia, bipolar disorder, and addiction: systematic review and meta-analysis. *Acta Psychiatr Scand.* (2015) 132:161–79. doi: 10.1111/acps.12423
9. Flinkkila E, Keski-Rahkonen A, Marttunen M, Raevuori A. Prenatal inflammation, infections and mental disorders. *Psychopathology* (2016) 49:317–33. doi: 10.1159/000448054
10. Trepanier MO, Hopperton KE, Mizrahi R, Mechawar N, Bazinet RP. Postmortem evidence of cerebral inflammation in schizophrenia: a systematic review. *Mol Psychiatry* (2016) 21:1009–26. doi: 10.1038/mp.2016.90
11. Pickard BS. Schizophrenia biomarkers: translating the descriptive into the diagnostic. *J Psychopharmacol.* (2015) 29:138–43. doi: 10.1177/0269881114566631
12. Perkovic MN, Erjavec GN, Strac DS, Uzun S, Kozumplik O, Pivac N. Theranostic biomarkers for schizophrenia. *Int J Mol Sci.* (2017) 18:733. doi: 10.3390/ijms18040733
13. Delay J, Deniker P, Harl JM. Utilisation therapeutique psychiatrique d'une phenothiazine d'action centrale elective. *Ann Medico-Psychol.* (1952) 110:112–7.
14. Johnsen E, Kroken RA. Drug treatment developments in schizophrenia and bipolar mania: latest evidence and clinical usefulness. *Ther Adv Chronic Dis.* (2012) 3:287–300. doi: 10.1177/2040622312462275
15. Muller N, Riedel M, Scheppach C, Brandstatter B, Sokullu S, Krampe K, et al. Beneficial antipsychotic effects of celecoxib add-on therapy compared to risperidone alone in schizophrenia. *Am J Psychiatry* (2002) 159:1029–34. doi: 10.1176/appi.ajp.159.6.1029
16. Sommer IE, van Westrhenen R, Begemann MJH, de Witte LD, Leucht S, Kahn RS. Efficacy of anti-inflammatory agents to improve symptoms in patients with schizophrenia: an update. *Schizophrenia Bull.* (2014) 40:181–91. doi: 10.1093/schbul/sbt139
17. Girgis RR, Ciarleglio A, Choo T, Haynes G, Bathon JM, Cremers S, et al. A randomized, double-blind, placebo-controlled clinical trial of tocilizumab, an interleukin-6 receptor antibody, for residual symptoms in schizophrenia. *Neuropsychopharmacology* (2017) 43:1317–23. doi: 10.1038/npp.2017.258
18. Baker KF, Isaacs JD. Novel therapies for immune-mediated inflammatory diseases: what can we learn from their use in rheumatoid arthritis, spondyloarthritis, systemic lupus erythematosus, psoriasis, Crohn's disease and ulcerative colitis? *Ann Rheum Dis.* (2017) 77:175–87. doi: 10.1136/annrheumdis-2017-211555
19. Miller BJ, Buckley PF. The case for adjunctive monoclonal antibody immunotherapy in schizophrenia. *Psychiatr Clin North Am.* (2016) 39:187–98. doi: 10.1016/j.psc.2016.01.003
20. Boerrigter D, Weickert TW, Lenroot R, O'Donnell M, Galletly C, Liu D, et al. Using blood cytokine measures to define high inflammatory biotype of schizophrenia and schizoaffective disorder. *J. Neuroinflam.* (2017) 14:188. doi: 10.1186/s12974-017-0962-y
21. Osimo EF, Cardinal RN, Jones PB, Khandaker GM. Prevalence and correlates of low-grade systemic inflammation in adult psychiatric inpatients: an electronic health record-based study. *Psychoneuroendocrinology* (2018) 91:226–34. doi: 10.1016/j.psyneuen.2018.02.031
22. Fillman SG, Sinclair D, Fung SJ, Webster MJ, Shannon Weickert C. Markers of inflammation and stress distinguish subsets of individuals with schizophrenia and bipolar disorder. *Trans Psychiatry* (2014) 4:e365. doi: 10.1038/tp.2014.8
23. Carpenter WT Jr. Schizophrenia: disease, syndrome, or dimensions? *Fam Process.* (2007) 46:199–206. doi: 10.1111/j.1545-5300.2007.00204.x
24. Keshavan MS, Nasrallah HA, Tandon R. Schizophrenia, "Just the Facts" 6. Moving ahead with the schizophrenia concept: from the elephant to the mouse. *Schizophr Res.* (2011) 127:3–13. doi: 10.1016/j.schres.2011.01.011
25. Weinberger JF, Raison CL, Rye DB, Montague AR, Woolwine BJ, Felger JC, et al. Inhibition of tumor necrosis factor improves sleep continuity in patients with treatment resistant depression and high inflammation. *Brain Behav Immun.* (2015) 47:193–200. doi: 10.1016/j.bbi.2014.12.016
26. Raison CL, Rutherford RE, Woolwine BJ, Shuo C, Schettler P, Drake DF, et al. A randomized controlled trial of the tumor necrosis factor antagonist infliximab for treatment-resistant depression: the role of baseline inflammatory biomarkers. *JAMA Psychiatry* (2013) 70:31–41. doi: 10.1001/2013.jamapsychiatry.4
27. Laan W, Grobbee DE, Selten JP, Heijnen CJ, Kahn RS, Burger H. Adjuvant aspirin therapy reduces symptoms of schizophrenia spectrum disorders:

results from a randomized, double-blind, placebo-controlled trial. *J Clin Psychiatry* (2010) 71:520–7. doi: 10.4088/JCP.09m05117yel
28. Dembic Z. *The Cytokines of the Immune System - The Role of Cytokines in Disease Related to Immune Response*. Oxford: Academic Press (2015).
29. Dean B. Understanding the role of inflammatory-related pathways in the pathophysiology and treatment of psychiatric disorders: evidence from human peripheral studies and CNS studies. *Int. J. Neuropsychopharmacol.* (2011) 14:997–1012. doi: 10.1017/S1461145710001410
30. Debnath M, Berk M. Functional implications of the IL-23/IL-17 immune axis in schizophrenia. *Mol Neurobiol.* (2017) 54:8170–8. doi: 10.1007/s12035-016-0309-1
31. Korn T, Bettelli E, Oukka M, Kuchroo VK. IL-17 and Th17 Cells. *Ann Rev Immunol.* (2009) 27:485–517. doi: 10.1146/annurev.immunol.021908.132710
32. Garlanda C, Dinarello CA, Mantovani A. The interleukin-1 family: back to the future. *Immunity* (2013) 39:1003–18. doi: 10.1016/j.immuni.2013.11.010
33. Dinarello CA. Immunological and inflammatory functions of the interleukin-1 family. *Annu Rev Immunol.* (2009) 27:519–50. doi: 10.1146/annurev.immunol.021908.132612
34. Maggio M, Guralnik JM, Longo DL, Ferrucci L. Interleukin-6 in aging and chronic disease: a magnificent pathway. *J Gerontol Ser A.* (2006) 61:575–84. doi: 10.1093/gerona/61.6.575
35. Kimura A, Kishimoto T. IL-6: Regulator of Treg/Th17 balance. *Eur J Immunol.* (2010) 40:1830–5. doi: 10.1002/eji.201040391
36. Gabay C, Kushner I. Acute-phase proteins and other systemic responses to inflammation. *N Engl J Med.* (1999) 340:448–54.
37. Schindler R, Mancilla J, Endres S, Ghorbani R, Clark SC, Dinarello CA. Correlations and interactions in the production of interleukin-6 (IL-6), IL-1, and tumor necrosis factor (TNF) in human blood mononuclear cells: IL-6 suppresses IL-1 and TNF. *Blood* (1990) 75:40–7.
38. Tilg H, Trehu E, Atkins MB, Dinarello CA, Mier JW. Interleukin-6 (IL-6) as an anti-inflammatory cytokine: induction of circulating IL-1 receptor antagonist and soluble tumor necrosis factor receptor p55. *Blood* (1994) 83:113–8.
39. Raison CL, Knight JM, Pariante C. Interleukin (IL)-6: a good kid hanging out with bad friends (and why sauna is good for health). *Brain Behav Immun.* (2018) 73:1–2. doi: 10.1016/j.bbi.2018.06.008
40. Popa C, Netea MG, van Riel PL, van der Meer JW, Stalenhoef AF. The role of TNF-alpha in chronic inflammatory conditions, intermediary metabolism, and cardiovascular risk. *J Lipid Res.* (2007) 48:751–62. doi: 10.1194/jlr.R600021-JLR200
41. Miller BJ, Gassama B, Sebastian D, Buckley P, Mellor A. Meta-analysis of lymphocytes in schizophrenia: clinical status and antipsychotic effects. *Biol Psychiatry* (2013) 73:993–9. doi: 10.1016/j.biopsych.2012.09.007
42. Fernandez-Egea E, Vertes PE, Flint SM, Turner L, Mustafa S, Hatton A, et al. Peripheral immune cell populations associated with cognitive deficits and negative symptoms of treatment-resistant schizophrenia. *PLoS ONE* (2016) 11:e0155631. doi: 10.1371/journal.pone.0155631
43. Bergink V, Gibney SM, Drexhage HA. Autoimmunity, inflammation and psychosis: a search for peripheral markers. *Biol Psychiatry* (2014) 75:324–31. doi: 10.1016/j.biopsych.2013.09.037
44. Drexhage RC, Hoogenboezem TA, Cohen D, Versnel MA, Nolen WA, van Beveren NJ, et al. An activated set point of T-cell and monocyte inflammatory networks in recent-onset schizophrenia patients involves both pro- and anti-inflammatory forces. *Int J Neuropsychopharmacol.* (2011) 14:746–55. doi: 10.1017/S1461145710001653
45. Ding M, Song X, Zhao J, Gao J, Li X, Yang G, et al. Activation of Th17 cells in drug naïve, first episode schizophrenia. *Prog Neuropsychopharmacol Biol Psychiatry* (2014) 19:78–82. doi: 10.1016/j.pnpbp.2014.01.001
46. Finckley AG, Foulds GA, Oughton JA, Kerkvliet NI, Multhoff G. Immune cell phenotyping using flow cytometry. *Curr Protoc Toxicol.* (2015) 66:18.8.1–34. doi: 10.1002/0471140856.tx1808s66
47. Frydecka D, Krzystek-Korpacka M, Lubeiro A, Stramecki F, Stanczykiewicz B, Beszlej JA, et al. Profiling inflammatory signatures of schizophrenia: a cross-sectional and meta-analysis study. *Brain Behav Immun.* (2018) 71:28–36. doi: 10.1016/j.bbi.2018.05.002
48. Antonelli M, Kushner I. It's time to redefine inflammation. *FASEB J.* (2017) 31:1787–91. doi: 10.1096/fj.201601326R
49. Zeni-Graiff M, Rizzo LB, Mansur RB, Maurya PK, Sethi S, Cunha GR, et al. Peripheral immuno-inflammatory abnormalities in ultra-high risk of developing psychosis. *Schizophr Res.* (2016) 176:191–5. doi: 10.1016/j.schres.2016.06.031
50. Capuzzi E, Bartoli F, Crocamo C, Clerici M, Carra G. Acute variations of cytokine levels after antipsychotic treatment in drug-naive subjects with a first-episode psychosis: a meta-analysis. *Neurosci Biobehav Rev.* (2017) 77:122–8. doi: 10.1016/j.neubiorev.2017.03.003
51. Tourjman V, Kouassi É, Koué M-È, Rocchetti M, Fortin-Fournier S, Fusar-Poli P, et al. Antipsychotics' effects on blood levels of cytokines in schizophrenia: a meta-analysis. *Schizophrenia Res.* (2013) 151:43–7. doi: 10.1016/j.schres.2013.10.011
52. Goldsmith DR, Haroon E, Miller AH, Strauss GP, Buckley PF, Miller BJ. TNF-alpha and IL-6 are associated with the deficit syndrome and negative symptoms in patients with chronic schizophrenia. *Schizophr Res.* (2018) 199:281–4. doi: 10.1016/j.schres.2018.02.048
53. Goldsmith DR, Rapaport MH, Miller BJ. A meta-analysis of blood cytokine network alterations in psychiatric patients: comparisons between schizophrenia, bipolar disorder and depression. *Mol Psychiatry* (2016) 21:1696–709. doi: 10.1038/mp.2016.3
54. Sanders AR, Drigalenko EI, Duan J, Moy W, Freda J, Goring HHH, et al. Transcriptome sequencing study implicates immune-related genes differentially expressed in schizophrenia: new data and a meta-analysis. *Transl Psychiatry* (2017) 7:e1093. doi: 10.1038/tp.2017.47
55. Chase KA, Cone JJ, Rosen C, Sharma RP. The value of interleukin 6 as a peripheral diagnostic marker in schizophrenia. *BMC Psychiatry* (2016) 16:152. doi: 10.1186/s12888-016-0866-x
56. Wu Y, Potempa LA, El Kebir D, Filep JG. C-reactive protein and inflammation: conformational changes affect function. *Biol Chem.* (2015) 396:1181–97. doi: 10.1515/hsz-2015-0149
57. Goff DC Jr, Lloyd-Jones DM, Bennett G, Coady S, D'Agostino RB, Sr, Gibbons R, et al. 2013 ACC/AHA guideline on the assessment of cardiovascular risk: a report of the American College of Cardiology/American Heart Association Task Force on Practice Guidelines. *J Am College Cardiol.* (2014) 63(25 Pt B):2935–59. doi: 10.1016/j.jacc.2013.11.005
58. Wang Z, Li P, Chi D, Wu T, Mei Z, Cui G. Association between C-reactive protein and risk of schizophrenia: an updated meta-analysis. *Oncotarget* (2017) 8:75445–54. doi: 10.18632/oncotarget.17995
59. Liemburg EJ, Nolte IM, Klein HC, Knegtering H. Relation of inflammatory markers with symptoms of psychotic disorders: a large cohort study. *Prog Neuropsychopharmacol Biol Psychiatry* (2018) 86:89–94. doi: 10.1016/j.pnpbp.2018.04.006
60. Johnsen E, Fathian F, Kroken RA, Steen VM, Jorgensen HA, Gjestad R, et al. The serum level of C-reactive protein (CRP) is associated with cognitive performance in acute phase psychosis. *BMC Psychiatry* (2016) 16:60. doi: 10.1186/s12888-016-0769-x
61. Orsolini L, Sarchione F, Vellante F, Fornaro M, Matarazzo I, Martinotti G, et al. Protein-C reactive as biomarker predictor of schizophrenia phases of illness? A systematic review. *Curr Neuropharmacol.* (2018) 16:583–606. doi: 10.2174/1570159X16666180119144538
62. Prins BP, Abbasi A, Wong A, Vaez A, Nolte I, Franceschini N, et al. Investigating the causal relationship of C-reactive protein with 32 complex somatic and psychiatric outcomes: a large-scale cross-consortium mendelian randomization study. *PLoS Med.* (2016) 13:e1001976. doi: 10.1371/journal.pmed.1001976
63. Asztalos BF, Horan MS, Horvath KV, McDermott AY, Chalasani NP, Schaefer EJ. Obesity associated molecular forms of C-reactive protein in human. *PLoS ONE* (2014) 9:e109238. doi: 10.1371/journal.pone.0109238
64. Rethorst CD, Bernstein I, Trivedi MH. Inflammation, obesity, and metabolic syndrome in depression: analysis of the 2009-2010 National Health and Nutrition Examination Survey (NHANES). *J Clin Psychiatry* (2014) 75:e1428–32. doi: 10.4088/JCP.14m09009
65. Yee JY, Nurjono M, Ng WY, Teo SR, Lee TS, Lee J. Peripheral blood gene expression of acute phase proteins in people with first episode psychosis. *Brain Behav Immun.* (2017) 65:337–41. doi: 10.1016/j.bbi.2017.06.006

66. Yang Y, Wan C, Li H, Zhu H, La Y, Xi Z, et al. Altered levels of acute phase proteins in the plasma of patients with schizophrenia. *Anal Chem.* (2006) 78:3571–6. doi: 10.1021/ac051916x
67. Wan C, La Y, Zhu H, Yang Y, Jiang L, Chen Y, et al. Abnormal changes of plasma acute phase proteins in schizophrenia and the relation between schizophrenia and haptoglobin (Hp) gene. *Amino Acids* (2007) 32:101–8. doi: 10.1007/s00726-005-0292-8
68. Guest PC, Guest FL, Martins-de Souza D. Making sense of blood-based proteomics and metabolomics in psychiatric research. *Int J Neuropsychopharmacol.* (2016) 19. doi: 10.1093/ijnp/pyv138
69. Herberth M, Rahmoune H, Schwarz E, Koethe D, Harris LW, Kranaster L, et al. Identification of a molecular profile associated with immune status in first-onset schizophrenia patients. *Clin Schizophr Relat Psychoses* (2014) 7:207–15. doi: 10.3371/CSRP.HERA.020113
70. Huang TL, Lo LH, Shiea J, Su H. Rapid and simple analysis of disease-associated biomarkers of Taiwanese patients with schizophrenia using matrix-assisted laser desorption ionization mass spectrometry. *Clin Chim Acta* (2017) 473:75–81. doi: 10.1016/j.cca.2017.08.011
71. Davison J, O'Gorman A, Brennan L, Cotter DR. A systematic review of metabolite biomarkers of schizophrenia. *Schizophr Res.* (2018) 195:32–50. doi: 10.1016/j.schres.2017.09.021
72. Steiner J, Guest PC, Martins-de-Souza D. Application of proteomic techniques for improved stratification and treatment of schizophrenia patients. *Adv Exp Med Biol.* (2017) 974:3–19. doi: 10.1007/978-3-319-52479-5_1
73. Amare AT, Schubert KO, Baune BT. Pharmacogenomics in the treatment of mood disorders: strategies and opportunities for personalized psychiatry. *EPMA J* (2017) 8:211–27. doi: 10.1007/s13167-017-0112-8
74. Schwarz E, van Beveren NJ, Ramsey J, Leweke FM, Rothermundt M, Bogerts B, et al. Identification of subgroups of schizophrenia patients with changes in either immune or growth factor and hormonal pathways. *Schizophr Bull.* (2014) 40:787–95. doi: 10.1093/schbul/sbt105
75. Ezeoke A, Mellor A, Buckley P, Miller B. A systematic, quantitative review of blood autoantibodies in schizophrenia. *Schizophrenia Res.* (2013) 150:245–51. doi: 10.1016/j.schres.2013.07.029
76. de Witte LD, Hoffmann C, van Mierlo HC, Titulaer MJ, Kahn RS, Martinez-Martinez P. Absence of N-methyl-D-aspartate receptor IgG autoantibodies in schizophrenia: the importance of cross-validation studies. *JAMA Psychiatry* (2015) 72:731–3. doi: 10.1001/jamapsychiatry.2015.0526
77. Ergun C, Urhan M, Ayer A. A review on the relationship between gluten and schizophrenia: is gluten the cause? *Nutr Neurosci.* (2017) 21:455–66. doi: 10.1080/1028415X.2017.1313569
78. Titulaer MJ, Dalmau J. Antibodies to NMDA receptor, blood-brain barrier disruption and schizophrenia: a theory with unproven links. *Mol Psychiatry* (2014) 19:1054. doi: 10.1038/mp.2014.25
79. Najjar S, Pahlajani S, De Sanctis V, Stern JNH, Najjar A, Chong D. Neurovascular unit dysfunction and blood-brain barrier hyperpermeability contribute to schizophrenia neurobiology: a theoretical integration of clinical and experimental evidence. *Front Psychiatry* (2017) 8:83. doi: 10.3389/fpsyt.2017.00083
80. Bechter K, Reiber H, Herzog S, Fuchs D, Tumani H, Maxeiner HG. Cerebrospinal fluid analysis in affective and schizophrenic spectrum disorders: identification of subgroups with immune responses and blood-CSF barrier dysfunction. *J Psychiatr Res.* (2010) 44:321–30. doi: 10.1016/j.jpsychires.2009.08.008
81. Orlovska-Waast S, Kohler-Forsberg O, Brix SW, Nordentoft M, Kondziella D, Krogh J, et al. Cerebrospinal fluid markers of inflammation and infections in schizophrenia and affective disorders: a systematic review and meta-analysis. *Mol Psychiatry* (2018). doi: 10.1038/s41380-018-0220-4. [Epub ahead of print].
82. Najjar S, Pearlman D, Alper K, Najjar A, Devinsky O. Neuroinflammation and psychiatric illness. *J Neuroinflammation* (2013) 10:43. doi: 10.1186/1742-2094-10-43
83. Pillai A, Howell KR, Ahmed AO, Weinberg D, Allen KM, Bruggemann J, et al. Association of serum VEGF levels with prefrontal cortex volume in schizophrenia. *Mol Psychiatry* (2016) 21:686–92. doi: 10.1038/mp.2015.96
84. Masopust J, Maly R, Andrys C, Valis M, Bazant J, Hosak L. Markers of thrombogenesis are activated in unmedicated patients with acute psychosis: a matched case control study. *BMC Psychiatry* (2011) 11:2. doi: 10.1186/1471-244X-11-2
85. de Klerk OL, Willemsen AT, Bosker FJ, Bartels AL, Hendrikse NH, den Boer JA, et al. Regional increase in P-glycoprotein function in the blood-brain barrier of patients with chronic schizophrenia: a PET study with [(11)C]verapamil as a probe for P-glycoprotein function. *Psychiatry Res.* (2010) 183:151–6. doi: 10.1016/j.pscychresns.2010.05.002
86. Chmielewska N, Szyndler J, Makowska K, Wojtyna D, Maciejak P, Plaznik A. Looking for novel, brain-derived, peripheral biomarkers of neurological disorders. *Neurol Neurochirurgia Polska* (2018) 52:318–25. doi: 10.1016/j.pjnns.2018.02.002
87. Streit WJ, Mrak RE, Griffin WS. Microglia and neuroinflammation: a pathological perspective. *J Neuroinflamm.* (2004) 1:14. doi: 10.1186/1742-2094-1-14
88. Khansari P, Sperlagh B. Inflammation in neurological and psychiatric diseases. *Inflammopharmacology* (2012) 20:103–7. doi: 10.1007/s10787-012-0124-x
89. Filiou MD, Arefin AS, Moscato P, Graeber MB. 'Neuroinflammation' differs categorically from inflammation: transcriptomes of Alzheimer's disease, Parkinson's disease, schizophrenia and inflammatory diseases compared. *Neurogenetics* (2014) 15:201–12. doi: 10.1007/s10048-014-0409-x
90. Winkeler A, Boisgard R, Awde AR, Dubois A, Theze B, Zheng J, et al. The translocator protein ligand [(1)(8)F]DPA-714 images glioma and activated microglia *in vivo*. *Eur J Nuclear Med Mol Imaging* (2012) 39:811–23. doi: 10.1007/s00259-011-2041-4
91. Doorduin J, de Vries EFJ, Willemsen ATM, de Groot JC, Dierckx RA, Klein HC. Neuroinflammation in schizophrenia-related psychosis: a PET study. *J Nuclear Med.* (2009) 50:1801–7. doi: 10.2967/jnumed.109.066647
92. van Berckel BN, Bossong MG, Boellaard R, Kloet R, Schuitemaker A, Caspers E, et al. Microglia activation in recent-onset schizophrenia: a quantitative (R)-[11C]PK11195 positron emission tomography study. *Biol Psychiatry* (2008) 64:820–2. doi: 10.1016/j.biopsych.2008.04.025
93. Di Biase MA, Zalesky A, O'Keefe G, Laskaris L, Baune BT, Weickert CS, et al. PET imaging of putative microglial activation in individuals at ultra-high risk for psychosis, recently diagnosed and chronically ill with schizophrenia. *Transl Psychiatry* (2017) 7:e1225. doi: 10.1038/tp.2017.193
94. Notter T, Coughlin JM, Gschwind T, Weber-Stadlbauer U, Wang Y, Kassiou M, et al. Translational evaluation of translocator protein as a marker of neuroinflammation in schizophrenia. *Mol Psychiatry* (2018) 23:323–34. doi: 10.1038/mp.2016.248
95. Bloomfield PS, Selvaraj S, Veronese M, Rizzo G, Bertoldo A, Owen DR, et al. Microglial activity in people at ultra high risk of psychosis and in schizophrenia: an [(11)C]PBR28 PET brain imaging study. *Am J Psychiatry* (2016) 173:44–52. doi: 10.1176/appi.ajp.2015.14101358
96. Coughlin JM, Wang Y, Ambinder EB, Ward RE, Minn I, Vranesic M, et al. *In vivo* markers of inflammatory response in recent-onset schizophrenia: a combined study using [(11)C]DPA-713 PET and analysis of CSF and plasma. *Transl Psychiatry* (2016) 6:e777. doi: 10.1038/tp.2016.40
97. Plaven-Sigray P, Matheson GJ, Collste K, Ashok AH, Coughlin JM, Howes OD, et al. Positron emission tomography studies of the glial cell marker translocator protein in patients with psychosis: a meta-analysis using individual participant data. *Biol Psychiatry* (2018) 84:433–42. doi: 10.1016/j.biopsych.2018.02.1171
98. Pasternak O, Kubicki M, Shenton ME. *In vivo* imaging of neuroinflammation in schizophrenia. *Schizophr Res.* (2016) 173:200–12. doi: 10.1016/j.schres.2015.05.034
99. Plitman E, de la Fuente-Sandoval C, Reyes-Madrigal F, Chavez S, Gomez-Cruz G, Leon-Ortiz P, et al. Elevated myo-inositol, choline, and glutamate levels in the associative striatum of antipsychotic-naive patients with first-episode psychosis: a proton magnetic resonance spectroscopy study with implications for glial dysfunction. *Schizophr Bull.* (2016) 42:415–24. doi: 10.1093/schbul/sbv118
100. Pasternak O, Kelly S, Sydnor VJ, Shenton ME. Advances in microstructural diffusion neuroimaging for psychiatric disorders. *Neuroimage* (2018) 182:259–82. doi: 10.1016/j.neuroimage.2018.04.051

101. Pasternak O, Westin C, Bouix S, Seidman L, Goldstein J, Woo T, et al. Excessive extracellular volume reveals a neurodegenerative pattern in schizophrenia onset. *J Neurosci.* (2012) 32:17365–72. doi: 10.1523/JNEUROSCI.2904-12.2012
102. Oestreich LK, Pasternak O, Shenton ME, Kubicki M, Gong X, McCarthy-Jones S, et al. Abnormal white matter microstructure and increased extracellular free-water in the cingulum bundle associated with delusions in chronic schizophrenia. *NeuroImage Clin.* (2016) 12:405–14. doi: 10.1016/j.nicl.2016.08.004
103. Prasad KM, Upton CH, Nimgaonkar VL, Keshavan MS. Differential susceptibility of white matter tracts to inflammatory mediators in schizophrenia: an integrated DTI study. *Schizophr Res.* (2015) 161:119–25. doi: 10.1016/j.schres.2014.09.043
104. Wang AK, Miller BJ. Meta-analysis of cerebrospinal fluid cytokine and tryptophan catabolite alterations in psychiatric patients: comparisons between schizophrenia, bipolar disorder, and depression. *Schizophr Bull.* (2018) 44:75–83. doi: 10.1093/schbul/sbx035
105. Nitta M, Kishimoto T, Müller N, Weiser M, Davidson M, Kane JM, et al. Adjunctive use of nonsteroidal anti-inflammatory drugs for schizophrenia: a meta-analytic investigation of randomized controlled trials. *Schizophrenia Bull.* (2013) 39:1230–41. doi: 10.1093/schbul/sbt070
106. Zheng W, Cai DB, Yang XH, Ungvari GS, Ng CH, Muller N, et al. Adjunctive celecoxib for schizophrenia: a meta-analysis of randomized, double-blind, placebo-controlled trials. *J Psychiatr Res.* (2017) 92:139–46. doi: 10.1016/j.jpsychires.2017.04.004
107. Miller BJ, Dias JK, Lemos HP, Buckley PF. An open-label, pilot trial of adjunctive tocilizumab in schizophrenia. *J Clin Psychiatry* (2016) 77:275–6. doi: 10.4088/JCP.15l09920
108. Zheng W, Zhang QE, Cai DB, Yang XH, Qiu Y, Ungvari GS, et al. N-acetylcysteine for major mental disorders: a systematic review and meta-analysis of randomized controlled trials. *Acta Psychiatr Scand.* (2018) 137:391–400. doi: 10.1111/acps.12862
109. Ehrenreich H, Hinze-Selch D, Stawicki S, Aust C, Knolle-Veentjer S, Wilms S, et al. Improvement of cognitive functions in chronic schizophrenic patients by recombinant human erythropoietin. *Mol Psychiatry* (2007) 12:206–20. doi: 10.1038/sj.mp.4001907
110. Iranpour N, Zandifar A, Farokhnia M, Goguol A, Yekehtaz H, Khodaie-Ardakani MR, et al. The effects of pioglitazone adjuvant therapy on negative symptoms of patients with chronic schizophrenia: a double-blind and placebo-controlled trial. *Hum Psychopharmacol.* (2016) 31:103–12. doi: 10.1002/hup.2517
111. Tajik-Esmaeeli S, Moazen-Zadeh E, Abbasi N, Shariat SV, Rezaei F, Salehi B, et al. Simvastatin adjunct therapy for negative symptoms of schizophrenia: a randomized double-blind placebo-controlled trial. *Int Clin Psychopharmacol.* (2017) 32:87–94. doi: 10.1097/YIC.0000000000000159
112. Vincenzi B, Stock S, Borba CP, Cleary SM, Oppenheim CE, Petruzzi LJ, et al. A randomized placebo-controlled pilot study of pravastatin as an adjunctive therapy in schizophrenia patients: effect on inflammation, psychopathology, cognition and lipid metabolism. *Schizophr Res.* (2014) 159:395–403. doi: 10.1016/j.schres.2014.08.021
113. Xiang YQ, Zheng W, Wang SB, Yang XH, Cai DB, Ng CH, et al. Adjunctive minocycline for schizophrenia: a meta-analysis of randomized controlled trials. *Eur Neuropsychopharmacol.* (2017) 27:8–18. doi: 10.1016/j.euroneuro.2016.11.012
114. Solmi M, Veronese N, Thapa N, Facchini S, Stubbs B, Fornaro M, et al. Systematic review and meta-analysis of the efficacy and safety of minocycline in schizophrenia. *CNS Spectr.* (2017) 22:415–26. doi: 10.1017/S1092852916000638
115. Weiser M, Levi L, Burshtein S, Chirita R, Cirjaliu D, Gonen I, et al. The effect of minocycline on symptoms in schizophrenia: Results from a randomized controlled trial. *Schizophr Res.* (2018). doi: 10.1016/j.schres.2018.10.023. [Epub ahead of print].
116. Deakin B, Suckling J, Barnes TRE, Byrne K, Chaudhry IB, Dazzan P, et al. The benefit of minocycline on negative symptoms of schizophrenia in patients with recent-onset psychosis (BeneMin): a randomised, double-blind, placebo-controlled trial. *Lancet Psychiatry* (2018) 5:885–94. doi: 10.1016/S2215-0366(18)30345-6
117. Sommer I, de Witte L, Begemann M, Kahn R. Nonsteroidal anti-inflammatory drugs in schizophrenia: ready for practice or a good start? a meta-analysis. *J Clin Psychiatry* (2011) 73:414–9. doi: 10.4088/JCP.10r06823
118. Weiser M, Burstein S, Fodoreanu L, Shirita R, Talau G, Cirjaliu D, et al. Positive symptoms respond to add-on aspirin in schizophrenia patients with high sera CRP levels: a post-hoc analysis of an RCT. *Schizophr Res* (2014) 153(Suppl. 1):S79. doi: 10.1016/S0920-9964(14)70256-7
119. Lowenberg M, Stahn C, Hommes DW, Buttgereit F. Novel insights into mechanisms of glucocorticoid action and the development of new glucocorticoid receptor ligands. *Steroids* (2008) 73:1025–9. doi: 10.1016/j.steroids.2007.12.002
120. Spies CM, Bijlsma JW, Burmester GR, Buttgereit F. Pharmacology of glucocorticoids in rheumatoid arthritis. *Curr Opin Pharmacol.* (2010) 10:302–7. doi: 10.1016/j.coph.2010.02.001
121. Baldo BA. Side effects of cytokines approved for therapy. *Drug Saf.* (2014) 37:921–43. doi: 10.1007/s40264-014-0226-z
122. Berk M, Malhi GS, Gray LJ, Dean OM. The promise of N-acetylcysteine in neuropsychiatry. *Trends Pharmacol Sci.* (2013) 34:167–77. doi: 10.1016/j.tips.2013.01.001
123. Conus P, Seidman LJ, Fournier M, Xin L, Cleusix M, Baumann PS, et al. N-acetylcysteine in a double-blind randomized placebo-controlled trial: toward biomarker-guided treatment in early psychosis. *Schizophr Bull.* (2018) 44:317–27. doi: 10.1093/schbul/sbx093
124. Maiese K, Li F, Chong ZZ. Erythropoietin in the brain: can the promise to protect be fulfilled? *Trends Pharmacol Sci.* (2004) 25:577–83. doi: 10.1016/j.tips.2004.09.006
125. Fond G, Macgregor A, Attal J, Larue A, Brittner M, Ducasse D, et al. Treating patients with schizophrenia deficit with erythropoietin? *Psychiatry Clin Neurosci.* (2012) 66:375–82. doi: 10.1111/j.1440-1819.2012.02359.x
126. Chaudhry IB, Husain N, Husain MO, Hallak J, Drake R, Kazmi A, et al. Ondansetron and simvastatin added to treatment as usual in patients with schizophrenia: study protocol for a randomized controlled trial. *Trials* (2013) 14:101. doi: 10.1186/1745-6215-14-101
127. Munhoz CD, Garcia-Bueno B, Madrigal JL, Lepsch LB, Scavone C, Leza JC. Stress-induced neuroinflammation: mechanisms and new pharmacological targets. *Braz J Med Biol Res.* (2008) 41:1037–46. doi: 10.1590/S0100-879X2008001200001
128. Uchoa MF, Moser VA, Pike CJ. Interactions between inflammation, sex steroids, and Alzheimer's disease risk factors. *Front Neuroendocrinol.* (2016) 43:60–82. doi: 10.1016/j.yfrne.2016.09.001
129. Garrido-Mesa N, Zarzuelo A, Galvez J. Minocycline: far beyond an antibiotic. *Br J Pharmacol.* (2013) 169:337–52. doi: 10.1111/bph.12139
130. Malhotra K, Chang JJ, Khunger A, Blacker D, Switzer JA, Goyal N, et al. Minocycline for acute stroke treatment: a systematic review and meta-analysis of randomized clinical trials. *J Neurol.* (2018) 265:1871–9. doi: 10.1007/s00415-018-8935-3
131. Kishimoto T, Horigome T, Takamiya A. Minocycline as a treatment for schizophrenia: is the discussion truly finished? *Lancet Psychiatry* (2018) 5:856–7. doi: 10.1016/S2215-0366(18)30389-4
132. Wallner FK, Hultquist Hopkins M, Woodworth N, Lindvall Bark T, Olofsson P, Tilevik A. Correlation and cluster analysis of immunomodulatory drugs based on cytokine profiles. *Pharmacol Res.* (2018) 128:244–51. doi: 10.1016/j.phrs.2017.10.012
133. Rodrigues-Amorim D, Rivera-Baltanas T, Lopez M, Spuch C, Olivares JM, Agis-Balboa RC. Schizophrenia: a review of potential biomarkers. *J Psychiatr Res.* (2017) 93:37–49. doi: 10.1016/j.jpsychires.2017.05.009

3

Blood-Based Lipidomics Approach to Evaluate Biomarkers Associated with Response to Olanzapine, Risperidone and Quetiapine Treatment in Schizophrenia Patients

Adriano Aquino[1†], *Guilherme L. Alexandrino*[2†], *Paul C. Guest*[1], *Fabio Augusto*[2], *Alexandre F. Gomes*[3], *Michael Murgu*[3], *Johann Steiner*[4,5] and *Daniel Martins-de-Souza*[1,6,7*]

[1] Laboratory of Neuroproteomics, Department of Biochemistry and Tissue Biology, Institute of Biology, University of Campinas, Campinas, Brazil, [2] Gas Chromatography Laboratory, Chemistry Institute, University of Campinas, Campinas, Brazil, [3] Mass Spectrometry Applications & Development Laboratory, Waters Corporation, São Paulo, Brazil, [4] Department of Psychiatry and Psychotherapy, University of Magdeburg, Magdeburg, Germany, [5] Center for Behavioral Brain Sciences, Magdeburg, Germany, [6] UNICAMP's Neurobiology Center, Campinas, Brazil, [7] Instituto Nacional de Biomarcadores em Neuropsiquiatria (INBION), Conselho Nacional de Desenvolvimento Científico e Tecnológico, São Paulo, Brazil

***Correspondence:**
Daniel Martins-de-Souza
dmsouza@unicamp.br

† These authors have contributed equally to this work.

This is the first study to identify lipidomic markers in plasma associated with response of acutely ill schizophrenia patients in response to specific antipsychotic treatments. The study population included 54 schizophrenia patients treated with antipsychotics for 6 weeks. Treatment led to significant improvement in positive and negative symptoms for 34 patients with little or no improvement for 20 patients. In addition, 37 patients showed an increase in body mass index after the 6 week treatment period, consistent with effects on metabolism and the association of such effects with symptom improvement. Profiling of plasma samples taken prior to therapy using liquid chromatography tandem mass spectrometry (LC-MS/MS) resulted in identification of 38, 10, and 52 compounds associated with the olanzapine, risperidone, and quetiapine treatment groups, which could be used to distinguish responders from non-responders. Limitations include the retroactive active nature of the study and the small sample size. Further investigations with larger sample sets could lead to the development of a molecular test that could be used to help psychiatrists determine the best treatment options for each patient.

Keywords: schizophrenia, drug response, antipsychotics, lipidomics, biomarkers

INTRODUCTION

Disease management of acute schizophrenia is achieved by administration of antipyschotics. However, ~40% of patients do not respond adequately to these medications and around 60% end up abandoning treatment due to intolerable side effects (1). As a consequence, the mood-related and cognitive functions of the patients may not improve, making these individuals less capable of functioning adequately in society. The side effects of second-generation (atypical) antipsychotics like olanzapine, risperidone, and quetiapine include metabolic-related responses such as hyperglycaemia, insulin resistance, and weight gain (2). Interestingly, some researchers have suggested that weight gain and other metabolic effects may be linked to the improvement of symptoms (3). These side effects are most likely related to the high affinity of these compounds for other receptor systems in the brain, which are involved in regulation of appetite and food intake (4–6). Such effects can have a deleterious impact on the overall health of patients and can potentially lead to conditions such as insulin resistance, type 2 diabetes, obesity, and cardiovascular complications (7, 8). These issues have led to recommendations for clinicians to closely monitor antipsychotic-treated psychiatric patients for early signs of such side effects (9–11). This has included concerted efforts by researchers from academia and the pharmaceutical industry to identify biomarkers that can be used to predict or monitor treatment responses (8, 12).

These issues have led academic and pharmaceutical industry researchers to embark on biomarker discovery initiatives to help guide treatment decisions and potentially pave the way toward novel therapeutic approaches. A number of molecular studies have already been carried out using multiplex immunoassay profiling of serum/plasma proteins to identify potential relationships between antipsychotic treatment responses and biomarker levels (12–14). However, none of these studies attempted to identify biomarker profiles that are predictive of response in cohorts treated separately with different antipsychotics. This is critical since different patients may show a better response to a distinct drug. In a recent publication, we reported on the analysis of plasma samples from a cohort of 58 schizophrenia patients using shotgun mass spectrometry proteomic profiling (15). Our objective was to identify proteins and protein pathways involved with an effective response to atypical antipsychotics, although, as with the above studies, no attempt was made to identify treatment-specific signatures.

Given the effects on metabolic functions mentioned above, we have carried out a lipidomic profiling study of plasmasamples obtained from the same schizophrenia patients prior to their treatment with the different antipsychotics. The analysis consisted of ultra-performance liquid-chromatography tandem mass spectrometry (UPLC-MS/MS) followed by the multivariate data analysis of the overall lipidomic profiles from all patients simultaneously (16). The main objective was to identify lipid profiles that could be used to predict response to treatment with either olanzapine, risperidone, or quetiapine. This is the first study which has attempted to assign specific biomarker profiles for predicting response to distinct antipsychotics. This study provides the groundwork for development of objective clinical tests that can be used to help psychiatrists in the choice of treatments for individuals presenting with acute schizophrenia in line with personalized medicine objectives.

METHODS

Samples

The samples had already been obtained from a cohort comprised of 54 acute schizophrenia patients who were treated with either olanzapine (n = 17), risperidone (n = 23), or quetiapine (n = 14) (**Supplementary Table 1**), as described previously (15). Diagnoses were performed using DSM-IV criteria and the Structured Clinical Interview (SCID-I) (17). Blood samples had been collected by venous puncture in the psychiatric clinic at the University of Magdeburg, Germany, as part of naturalistic study of acutely ill in-patients who were un-medicated for at least 6 weeks prior to inclusion. Citrate plasma samples were prepared and analyzed at a time when the patients were suffering from acute illness [designated time zero (T0)]. Individuals with other medical diseases were not included in the study. After the 6-week treatment period, all samples were grouped according to whether (n = 34) or not (n = 20) the patients responded favorably to the treatment. A favorable response was defined as a 50% reduction of total Positive and Negative Syndrome Scale (PANSS) scores. These scores were corrected by subtraction of the minimum the scores which represented no symptoms (7, 7, and 16 for PANSS positive, negative and general scores, respectively) (15). Exclusion criteria included substance abuse disorder or symptoms induced by a non-psychiatric medical illness or treatment, including immune diseases, immunomodulatory treatment, cancer, chronic terminal disease, cardiovascular disorders, dyslipidemia, diabetes, and severe trauma. The institutional review board (ethics commission of the University of Magdeburg) approved the study, (process 110/07, from November 26th, 2007 amended on February 11th, 2013). Written informed consent was obtained from all participants.

Sample Preparation

Lipids from 25 µL plasma samples taken at T0 were extracted by addition of 100 µL isopropanol. Samples were vortexed for 1 min and then incubated 10 min at room temperature. The samples were kept at −20°C for 18 h and centrifuged at 14,000g for 20 min. The pellet was discarded and the supernatant dried in a vacuum centrifuge and reconstituted in 100 µL isopropanol (IPA)/acetonitrile (ACN)/water (2:1:1 v:v:v) (18). Ten quality control (QCs) injections were run along with the clinical samples. These were composed by equal aliquots of each of the plasma sample to monitor the preparation and LC-MS/MS performance.

Liquid Chromatography

All chemicals were purchased from Sigma-Aldrich (Seelze, Germany) and were of high performance liquid chromatography (HPLC) grade, or higher, purity. An Acquity H-Class UPLC (Waters Corporation, Milford, MA, USA) was used as the inlet for mass spectrometry. The column used was an ACQUITY UPLC® CSH C18, 2.1 × 100 mm, 1.7 µm particle size (Waters Corporation), operating at a flow rate of 0.4 mL/min and at 55°C. The chromatographic separation was performed in gradient mode using a mobile phase system consisted by two solvents, A and B. Solvent A was ACN/water (60:40, v:v) with 10 mM ammonium formate and 0.1% formic acid, and phase B was IPA/ACN (90:10, v:v) with 10 mM ammonium formate and 0.1% formic acid. The gradient steps started with 60% A and 40% B, changing linearly to 57% A and 43% B in 2.0 min, to 50% A and 50% B in 2.1 min, to 46% A and 54% B in 12.0 min, to 30% A and 70% B in 12.1 min, to reach 1% A and 99% B in 18.0 min and then returning to the initial composition (60% A and 40% B) in 18.1 min. The buffer remained at this composition until 20 min prior to preparing the system for the next injection. The injection volume was 1.0 µL.

Mass Spectrometry

The inlet system was coupled to a hybrid quadrupole orthogonal time-of-flight mass spectrometer, Xevo G-2 XS QT of (Waters

Corporation, Manchester, UK), controlled by MassLynx 4.1 software. Data were acquired in positive electrospray ionization (ESI+) with the capillary voltage set to 2.0 kV, cone voltage to 30 eV and source temperature to 150°C. The desolvation gas was nitrogen, with flow of 900 L/h and temperature of 550°C. Data were acquired from m/z 100 to 2,000 in MS^E mode during which the collision energy was alternated between low (2 eV) and high (ramped from 20 to 30 eV). Leucine-enkephalin (Waters Corporation, Milford, MA, USA), $C_{28}H_{37}N_5O_7$, ([M+H]+ = 556.2771 m/z) was used as lock mass reference at concentration of 0.2 ng/L with flow rate of 10 μL/min.

Data Processing and Statistical Analyses

Progenesis QI 2.2 (Nonlinear Dynamics, Indianapolis, IN, USA) software was used to process data for peak detection, multivariate analysis and identification. All samples were normalized using the total ionic current. After that, data filtering was performed by removing ions present in blank samples. The ion abundance threshold filtering was also applied, which evaluated the minimal ion abundance that could provide a good precursor ion signal with a consistent isotopic pattern. A final filtering step was made based on retention time by checking sample chromatograms to define the retention time window over which the lipids eluted. After the data filtering steps, the normalization option was changed from total ion current to the summed ion abundance of all compounds. For compound identification, the Lipidmaps database was used, with searching parameters as follows: precursor mass error ≤ 10 ppm, fragment tolerance ≤ 10 ppm. Other parameters such as fragmentation score were also considered for disambiguation.

Data Analysis

The output variables were the ion abundance of the chromatographic signals from the lipids according to their corresponding mass/charge (m/z) obtained from the mass spectrometer. Approximately 1,600 m/z signals with different elution times were detected in total. To identify the appropriate adducts for data processing, a spectral evaluation of different lipid classes and ion abundances were carried out. The selected adducts were [M+H-H2O]+, [M+H]+, [M+Na]+, [M+K]+, [2M+H]+ and [2M+Na]+. The normalized m/z signals were imported into Matlab® R2013b (The Matworks, Natick, MA, USA) as single data matrices Xi(I × J) for each treatment, with i = 1 (risperidone), 2 (olanzapine), or 3 (quetiapine), I = number of samples in the corresponding treatment, and J = number of m/z signals: risperidone = 1,610; olanzapine = 1,632; and quetiapine = 1,628. Multivariate analyses were performed with the autoscaled data using Partial Least Squares-Discriminant Analysis (PLS-DA) and Principal Component Analysis (PCA), employing the Pls Toolbox 8.1 (Eigenvector Research Inc., Wenatchee, WA, USA). One-way ANOVA *F*-Test analyses were performed in Matlab using in-house scripts.

PLS-DA

The most relevant m/z signals from baseline samples used to distinguish the patients who did or did not respond to the treatments were extracted from each Xi data matrix using a variable selection approach based on double cross-validation (CV2) PLS-DA (19). For CV2, Xi matrices were randomly split into 2 submatrices Xical (A, J) and Xitest (B, J), with A = 17, 12, or 9, and B = 5, 4, or 2, for either risperidone, olanzapine, and quetiapine, respectively. This approach helped to keep the proportion of the overall m/z signals between responders and non-responders in the submatrices similar to the corresponding Xi matrices. PLS-DA was performed only for Xical, using 4-fold Venetian blind cross-validation for model optimization. Xical submatrices were also arranged to allow simultaneous extraction of rows from both responder and non-responder groups of patients during the inner cross-validation process, and the correct number of latent variables (LVs) for the models was obtained in the lowest root mean squares error of cross-validation (RMSECV). After model optimization, only the Variable Importance for Projection (VIP) scores upon a threshold were selected while extracting the most informative m/z signals for the classification from Xical submatrices. This threshold was defined iteratively based on reaching the point below which the PLS-DA models did not increase their RMSECV. This was computed for new models each time a new threshold was established. The overall CV2 procedure was performed 500 times, and only those m/z signals that were selected in at least 80% (risperidone and olanzapine) and 95% (quetiapine) of the iterations were considered relevant for distinguishing between responders and non-responders. The remaining m/z signals were discarded, since the contrary approach resulted in an overall increase of the RMSECV and misclassification of predictions from the Xitest. No additional variable selection step was performed once the Xi matrix contained only the most frequent m/z signals selected previously from the histograms. This approach of combining variable selection into double cross-validated PLS-DA models provided the most important m/z signals from the pooled data without fitting overly-optimistic PLS-DA models. This is due to the fact that the final m/z signals were selected based on non-biased histograms of random iterations and because model performances were strictly evaluated, given that they were computed for independent samples. A similar approach using PLS-DA for analyte selection has been published elsewhere (20). Here we intended to apply a high stringency model, so that only the most robust data are selected. The drawback is that some valid signals may be filtered out.

One-Way ANOVA *F*-Test and PCA

The final m/z signals selected from the PLS-DA modeling were ranked individually according to their ability to distinguish between responder and non-responder patients, using one-way ANOVA *F*-test analysis. False discovery rates (FDR) were also estimated for the respective m/z signals according to a null distribution ANOVA *F*-test approach, as described previously in metabolomics studies (21, 22). Next, PCA was performed to highlight the separation between responders and non-responders to each antipsychotic treatment when considering only the selected compounds in which FDR ≤ 0.05 (i.e., probability of type-I error ≤ 5%).

Data Sharing

The ethics committee approval for this project does not include sharing the mass spectrometry raw files obtained here, as these are pertinent information to the participants of the study. Interested researchers should look for us in order to sign a non-disclosure agreement to be submitted to the ethics committee.

RESULTS

Patient Response to Treatment

According to the criteria set in the Methods section, 34 out of 54 total patients showed a good response to treatment (see **Supplementary Table 1**). There were no significant differences observed for age, illness duration, BMI, gender, smoking, PANSS negative, or PANSS general scores at baseline between the responders and non-responders (**Table 1**). However, significantly higher PANSS positive scores ($P = 0.005$) were observed at baseline for the responders compared to the non-responders. In addition, 38 out of the 54 patients showed an increase in BMI following the treatment. In the responder group, 27 out of the 34 patients showed an increase in BMI with an average increase of 1.22 ± 1.42 kg/m^2 (mean $\pm$ sd; $n = 34$). In the non-responder group, 11 out of the 20 patients had an increased BMI ($0.22 + 1.43$; $n = 20$). There difference in the BMI gain across the responders and non-responders was significant ($p = 0.033$; Mann–Whitney test).

Selection of m/z Peaks for Best Separation of Responders and Non-responders for Each Treatment Group

PLS-DA models were used to extract the most relevant m/z signals from the pooled data for the best separation of responders and non-responders in each treatment group. This resulted in selection of 134, 36, and 119 m/z signals for the olanzapine, risperidone, and quetiapine treatment groups, respectively out of more than 1,600 compounds in total (**Table 2**). Due to the fact that the PLS-DA extracts linear correlations in the multivariate data to maximize discrimination of the samples in a supervised manner, some false positive signals might be included. For this reason, the ability of each m/z signal to distinguish between responders and non-responders was tested using one-way ANOVA *F*-test analysis combined with FDR estimations. The F-ratio thresholds for estimating the FDR (confidence level $\geq$ 99%), obtained from the null-distribution ANOVA F-ratio approach, considered all possible null class comparisons in both groups (i.e., response or non-response) of patients, for each antipsychotic treatment group. The compounds for which the FDR was <5% are more likely to be associated to the medication effectiveness. Therefore, these compounds were tentatively identified for the selected olanzapine, risperidone, and quetiapine signals (**Supplementary Tables 2–4**; non-identified m/z signals are provided in **Supplementary Table 5**). The PCA plots considering only those m/z signals for which the FDR $\leq$ 5% resulted in clear discrimination between responders and non-responders for the olanzapine (**Figure 1A**), risperidone (**Figure 1B**), and quetiapine (**Figure 1C**) treatments. These separations were associated with a total (i.e., identified and non-identified) of 66 compounds for olanzapine (**Figure 1A**), 24 compounds for risperidone (**Figure 1B**) and 52 compounds for quetiapine (**Figure 1C**).

TABLE 1 | Assessment of baseline variables, comparing patients in the responder (R, $n = 34$) and non-responder (NR, $n = 20$) groups.

		Median (Q1, Q3)	*P*-value
Age (years)	R	36.0 (30.3, 47.3)	0.199[a]
	NR	31.5 (25.0, 43.3)	
Illness duration (years)	R	1.5 (0.0, 9.3)	0.689[a]
	NR	1.5 (0.0, 9.3)	
BMI (kg/m^2)	R	23.8 (21.6, 29.8)	0.484[a]
	NR	23.5 (22.0, 26.8)	
PANSS positive scores	R	26.0 (16.3, 21.0)	**0.005**[a]
	NR	21.0 (16.8, 24.5)	
PANSS negative scores	R	9.5 (5.0, 18.0)	0.429[a]
	NR	11.5 (6.0, 22.3)	
PANSS general scores	R	27.0 (22.0, 32.8)	0.255[a]
	NR	30.0 (21.0, 39.8)	
Gender (male/female)	R	19/15	0.821[b]
	NR	13/7	
Smoking (yes/no)	R	23/11	0.807[b]
	NR	15/5	

As the data were unevenly distributed, Shapiro-Wilk tests were use to determine significance values for continuous variables (median and quartiles 1 and 3 shown) and Fisher's exact test was applied for contingency variables. Values which were significantly different are indicated using bold font.
a, H-test; b, Fisher's exact test.

DISCUSSION

This is the first study to use a lipidomic profiling approach in an attempt to detect lipid-based molecules in plasma samples taken from patients prior to treatment that could be used for prediction of response to specific antipsychotic treatments. The PLS-DA models resulting in low root mean squares error of cross-validation and misclassifications infers robustness (non-biased) of the final selected lipid signals, given that the models correctly classified most of the patients independently throughout the random cross validation iterations. These results, along with the ranking of the signals according to their respective ability to distinguish between responder and non-responder patients, was provided by the one-way ANOVA *F*-test analysis combined with the corresponding false-positive probability estimations. This guided the biological

TABLE 2 | Performance of double cross-validated PLS-DA models after $N = 500$ random iteration (average values and standard deviations in the brackets) to select the main m/z signals while classifying between responders and non-responders for each treatment group.

	Risperidone	Olanzapine	Quetiapine
# of latent variables	1.06 (0.40)	1.23 (0.46)	1.12 (0.33)
RMSECV	0.005 (0.024)	0.04 (0.06)	0.03 (0.05)
Misclassified	0.4 (4.5) %	0.3 (2.3) %	0
M/Z selected	36	134	119

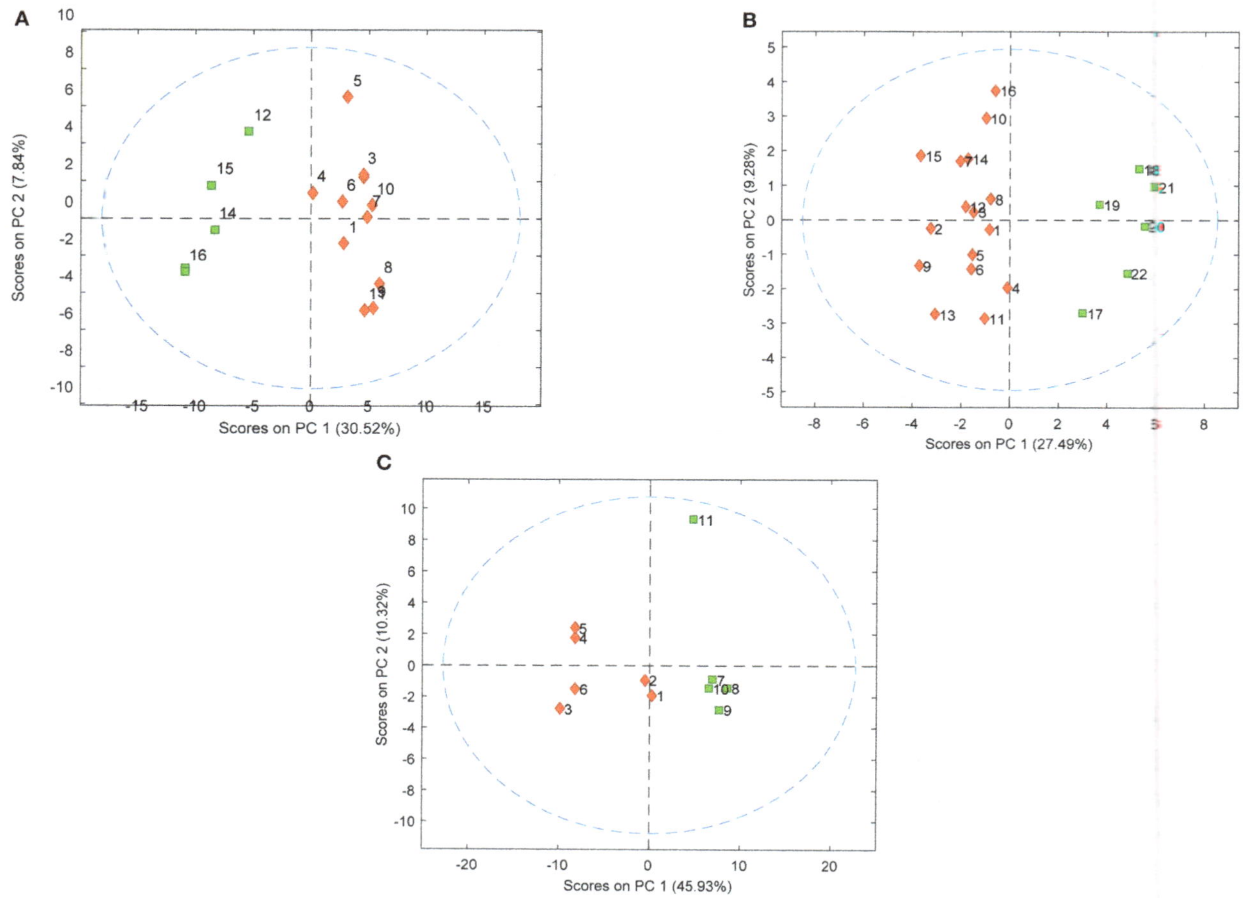

FIGURE 1 | PCA plots showing separation of patients who either responded or did not respond to **(A)** olanzapine, **(B)** risperidone, and **(C)** quetiapine treatment using baseline plasma lipid levels (each symbol represents a patient sample). Responders and non-responders are represented in red and green, respectively.

investigation toward only those potential hits closely related to the responses of patients to treatment with the specific antipsychotics. The m/z signals that were not designated as potential hits do not necessarily infer non-relevance to the study. Instead, they have a higher probability (>5%) of being false-positives in these datasets, according to the adopted statistical metric.

The brain is rich in lipids, which act within specific brain regions to regulate processes that can impact complex processes such as behavior, emotions, cognition, and learning (23). Evidence has accrued that phospholipids play an important role in the structure and function of membranes and the associated pathways appear to be impaired in schizophrenia (24). Therefore, counter changes in phospholipids may be associated with the therapeutic response to antipsychotics in schizophrenia patients. Recent developments in the field of lipidomics have allowed characterization of hundreds of individual lipid species in human blood which may be altered in disease states (25). For example, deregulation of cholesterol has been associated with altered levels of some steroid hormones and development psychiatric disorders including autism (26), altered metabolism of sphingolipids such as ceramide has been observed in some cases of depression (27) and patients with psychosis often show subclinical dyslipidemia (28).

Most antipsychotics in current use act as dopamine and serotonin blockers and. the circulating levels of drugs such as risperidone and quetiapine are metabolized in the liver to produce the active metabolites (29) and some classes of lipids can inhibit the activity of the metabolizing enzymes. Altered phospholipid content in the membrane can affect metabolism through the cytochrome P450 family of metabolic enzymes by altering protein conformation and interactions essential for activity (30). Cirulating nutritional factors including lipids can also affect the efficiency of these metabolizing enzymes (31). This may be important as response of schizophrenia patients to antipsychotics may be related to metabolism of these drugs in the liver. For example, olanzapine is normally metabolized to its 10-and 4′-N-glucuronides, 4′-N-desmethylolanzapine [cytochrome P450 (CYP)1A2] and olanzapine N-oxide (flavin mono-oxygenase 3) (32), risperidone is metabolized primarily by CYP2D6 and to a lesser extent by CYP3A4, and quetiapine is known to undergo an N-dealkylation catalyzed by CYP3A4/5 (33). Furthermore, olanzapine is metabolized by direct glucuronidationby CYP1A2 and by CYP2D6 and CYP3A4, although the later two enzymes play a smaller role in this conversion. In addition, quetiapineis metabolized by CYP3A4 although aldehyde oxidase is the enzyme responsible for most of its metabolism (34). Thus, an altered composition of lipid in blood could lead to changes in the levels of some of these metabolites and thereby affect treatment response. Further studies should investigate the effect of specific lipids on metabolism of each of these antipsychotics, given the potential link to treatment response. This study has provided a list of lipids associated with treatment response to olanzapine, risperidone, and quetiapine which could be used as potential starting point in such an investigation.

LIMITATIONS

There are a number of limitations of this study. Firstly, this was a retroactive analysis of samples provided from a previous naturalistic study and there was only a limited sample size for determining effects of each separate drug treatments. Thus, replication is required using a different sample set with larger numbers for each treatment group. Also, patients who showed a good response to the treatment also had the most severe symptoms at baseline, as assessed by the PANSS positive scoring system. Although the small sample size was a limitation of this study from a statistical point of view, the data treatment strategy comprising variable selection and statistical double cross-validation presented here assured the non-biased selection of only the most robust m/z signals that distinguish responders and non-responders groups of patients in the dataset. Finally, the natural heterogeneity of schizophrenia makes identification of biomarkers challenging (35). Further studies should be carried out using patient populations that have been stratified strictly using either clinical or molecular biomarkers. Finally, although the results give high confidence on identification of the lipid class, size of carbon chains and number of double bonds, it was not possible to distinguish between isomer candidates. Specifically, the observed fragmentation helped to define the size and number of double bonds of each carbon chain for many compounds, considering the sn-1 and sn-1-H_2O (and sn-2 and sn-2-H_2O for lipids with more than one carbon chain). However, the position of the double bonds could not be determined using the current mass spectrometry approach as this would require comparison with analytical standards. Finally, it is important to highlight that our aim here is to look for a molecular signature to predict antipsychotic responsiveness. As it can be seen in the Supplementary Tables, among the compounds we analyzed, a number of them are unidentified. We are not focusing here in their identification. If these are consistently present in the samples analyzed and are able to separate responders from non-responders, we reached our objective. We are currently working on their identification, in order to describe which of these compounds are triggering molecular pathways associated to an effective antipsychotic response and which are involved with poor response. This data will provide, in the future, biological leads that may be useful for the development of new treatments.

CONCLUSIONS

Previous studies have demonstrated that first onset schizophrenia patients may also show signs of metabolic syndrome (7, 36). This includes elevated levels of insulin-related peptides (37, 38), increased insulin resistance (39, 40) and altered lipid profiles (28) in the blood. This is the first study to identify specific lipidomic signatures for prediction of response to specific antipsychotics. Given further validation of these findings, the signatures could be developed into a rapid assay using a platform such as selective reaction monitoring (SRM) mass spectrometry to aid the process of antipsychotic selection in the treatment of patients with acute psychosis. This fits in with ongoing strategies of translational and personalized medicine for improved treatment outcomes of patients suffering from this debilitating psychiatric disease.

AUTHOR CONTRIBUTIONS

DM-d-S conceived, organized, and supervised all steps of the study. DM-d-S and PG wrote the paper together with PG. JS collected and provided blood plasma samples and contributed with paper writing. AA prepared plasma samples and ran the mass spectrometry experiments helped by AG and MM. GA performed all statistical analyses supervised by FA. PG helped in data analyses. All authors had access to the final version of the manuscript.

FUNDING

AA, DM-d-S, and GA are supported by São Paulo Research Foundation (FAPESP), grants 2015/09159-8, 2015/08201-0, 2013/08711-3, 2014/10068-4 and 2017/25588-1. DM-d-S is also supported by Serrapilheira Institute (grant number Serra-1709-16349) and by the Brazilian National Council for Scientific and Technological Development (CNPq, 302453/2017-2).

ACKNOWLEDGMENTS

The authors sincerely thank sample donors for their willingness to contribute to our study, which is dedicated to patients. We also thank Anke Dudeck, Daniela Fenker, Gabriela Meyer-Lotz, and Jeanette Schadow who participated in the sample characterization and collection.

SUPPLEMENTARY MATERIAL

Supplementary Table 1 | Patients demographics.

Supplementary Tables 2-4 | List of compounds (FDR was <5%) associated to the medication effectiveness. Non-identified m/z signals are provided in Supplementary Table 5.

Supplementary Table 5 | List of non-identified compounds for each of the medication evaluated.

REFERENCES

1. Tandon R, Nasrallah HA, Keshavan MS. Schizophrenia, "Just the Facts" 5. Treatment and prevention past, present, and future. *Schizophr Res.* (2010) **122**:1–23. doi: 10.1016/j.schres.2010.05.025
2. Newcomer JW. Second-generation (atypical) antipsychotics and metabolic effects: a comprehensive literature review. *CNS Drugs* (2005) **19**:1–93. doi: 10.2165/00023210-200519001-00001
3. Jones B, Basson BR, Walker DJ, Crawford AM, Kinon BJ. Weight change and atypical antipsychotic treatment in patients with schizophrenia. *J Clin Psychiatry* (2001) **62**(Suppl. 2):41–4. doi: 10.1177/0269881105058378
4. Kim SF, Huang AS, Snowman AM, Teuscher C, Snyder SH. From the cover: antipsychotic drug-induced weight gain mediated by histamine H1 receptor-linked activation of hypothalamic AMP-kinase. *Proc Natl Acad Sci USA.* (2007) **104**:3456–9. doi: 10.1073/pnas.0611417104
5. Benarroch L, Kowalchuk C, Wilson V, Teo C, Guenette M, Chintoh A, et al. Atypical antipsychotics and effects on feeding: from mice to men. *Psychopharmacology* (2016) **233**:2629–53. doi: 10.1007/s00213-016-4324-8
6. Huang XF, Weston-Green K, Yu Y. Decreased 5-HT2cR and GHSR1a interaction in antipsychotic drug-induced obesity. *Obes. Rev.* (2017) **19**:396–405. doi: 10.1111/obr.12638
7. Harris LW, Guest PC, Wayland MT, Umrania Y, Krishnamurthy D, Rahmoune H, et al. Schizophrenia: metabolic aspects of aetiology, diagnosis and future treatment strategies. *Psychoneuroendocrinology* (2013) **38**:752–66. doi: 10.1016/j.psyneuen.2012.09.009
8. Zhang JP, Lencz T, Zhang RX, Nitta M, Maayan L, John M, et al. Pharmacogenetic associations of antipsychotic drug-related weight gain: a systematic review and meta-analysis. *Schizophr Bull.* (2016) **42**:1418–37. doi: 10.1093/schbul/sbw058
9. Correll CU, Lencz T, Malhotra AK. Antipsychotic drugs and obesity. *Trends Mol Med.* (2011) **17**:97–107. doi: 10.1016/j.molmed.2010.10.010
10. Himmerich H, Minkwitz J, Kirkby KC. Weight gain and metabolic changes during treatment with antipsychotics and antidepressants. *Endocr Metab Immune Disord Drug Targets* (2015) **15**:252–60. doi: 10.2174/1871530315666150623092031
11. Musil R, Obermeier M, Russ P, Hamerle M. Weight gain and antipsychotics: a drug safety review. *Expert Opin Drug Saf.* (2015) **14**:73–96. doi: 10.1517/14740338.2015.974549
12. Schwarz E, Steiner J, Guest PC, Bogerts B, Bahn S. Investigation of molecular serum profiles associated with predisposition to antipsychotic-induced weight gain. *World J Biol Psychiatry* (2015) **16**:22–30. doi: 10.3109/15622975.2013.817685
13. Schwarz E, Guest PC, Steiner J, Bogerts B, Bahn S. Identification of blood-based molecular signatures for prediction of response and relapse in schizophrenia patients. *Transl Psychiatry* (2012) **2**:e82. doi: 10.1038/tp.2012.3
14. Tomasik J, Schwarz E, Lago SG, Rothermundt M, Leweke FM, van Beveren NJM, et al. Pretreatment levels of the fatty acid handling proteins H-FABP and CD36 predict response to olanzapine in recent-onset schizophrenia patients. *Brain Behav Immun.* (2016) **52**:178–86. doi: 10.1016/j.bbi.2015.10.019
15. Martins-de-Souza D, Solari FA, Guest PC, Zahedi RP, Steiner J. Biological pathways modulated by antipsychotics in the blood plasma of schizophrenia patients and their association to a clinical response. *NPJ Schizophrenia* (2015) **1**:15050. doi: 10.1038/npjschz.2015.50
16. Prata PS, Alexandrino GL, Mogollón NG, Augusto F. Discriminating Brazilian crude oils using comprehensive two-dimensional gas chromatography-mass spectrometry and multiway principal component analysis. *J Chromatogr A* (2016) **1472**:99–106. doi: 10.1016/j.chroma.2016.10.044
17. First MB, Spitzer RL, Gibbon M, Williams JBW. *Structured Clinical Interview for DSM-IV-TR Axis I disorders, Research Version, Patient Edition (SCID-I/P).* New York, NY: Biometrics Research, New York State Psychiatric Institute (2002).
18. Sarafian MH, Gaudin M, Lewis MR, Martin FP, Holmes E, Nicholson JK, et al. Objective set of criteria for optimization of sample preparation procedures for ultra-high throughput untargeted blood plasma lipid profiling by UPLC-MS. *Anal Chem.* (2014) **86**:5766–74. doi: 10.1021/ac500317c
19. Szymanska E, Saccenti E, Smilde AK, Westerhuis JA. Double-check: validation of diagnostic statistics for PLS-DA models in metabolomics studies. *Metabolomics* (2012) **8**(Suppl. 1):3–16. doi: 10.1007/s11306-011-0330-3
20. Khakimov B, Poulsen SK, Savorani F, Acar E, Gürdeniz G, Larsen TM, et al. New nordic diet versus average danish diet: a randomized controlled trial revealed healthy long-term effects of the New Nordic Diet by GC–MS blood plasma metabolomics. *J Proteome Res.* (2016) **15**:1939–54. doi: 10.1021/acs.jproteome.6b00109
21. Parsons BA, Marney LC, Siegler WCS, Hoggard JC, Wright BW, Synovec RE. Tile-Based fisher ratio analysis of comprehensive two-dimensional gas chromatography time-of-flight mass spectrometry (GC × GC-TOFMS) data using a null distribution approach. *Anal Chem.* (2015) **87**:3812–9. doi: 10.1021/ac504472s
22. Watson NE, Parsons BA, Synovec RE. Performance evaluation of tile-based Fisher Ratio analysis using a benchmark yeast metabolome dataset. *J Chromatogr A* (2016) **1459**:101–11. doi: 10.1016/j.chroma.2016.06.067
23. Fernandes MF, Mutch DM, Leri F. The Relationship between fatty acids and different depression-related brain regions, and their potential role as biomarkers of response to antidepressants. *Nutrients* (2017) **9**:E298. doi: 10.3390/nu9030298
24. Kaddurah-Daouk R, McEvoy J, Baillie RA, Lee D, Yao JK, Doraiswamy PM, et al. Metabolomic mapping of atypical antipsychotic effects in schizophrenia. *Mol Psychiatry* (2007) **12**:934–945. doi: 10.1038/sj.mp.4002000
25. Huynh K, Martins RN, Meikle PJ. Lipidomic profiles in diabetes and dementia. *J Alzheimers Dis.* (2017) **59**:433–44. doi: 10.3233/JAD-161215
26. Gillberg C, Fernell E, Kočovská E, Minnis H, Bourgeron T, Thompson L, et al. The role of cholesterol metabolism and various steroid abnormalities in autism spectrum disorders: A hypothesis paper. *Autism Res.* (2017) **10**:1022–44. doi: 10.1002/aur.1777
27. Dinoff A, Herrmann N, Lanctôt KL. Ceramides and depression: a systematic review. *J Affect Disord.* (2017) **213**:35–43. doi: 10.1016/j.jad.2017.02.008
28. Misiak B, Stanczykiewicz B, Łaczmanski Ł, Frydecka D. Lipid profile disturbances in antipsychotic-naive patients with first-episode non-affective psychosis: A systematic review and meta-analysis. *Schizophr Res.* (2017) **190**:18–27. doi: 10.1016/j.schres.2017.03.031
29. Maier W, Zobel A. Contribution of allelic variations to the phenotype of response to antidepressants and antipsychotics. *Eur. Arch Psychiatry Clin Neurosci.* (2008) **258**(Suppl. 1):12–20. doi: 10.1007/s00406-007-1004-z
30. Brignac-Huber LM, Park JW, Reed JR, Backes WL. Cytochrome P450 organization and function are modulated by endoplasmic reticulum phospholipid heterogeneity. *Drug Metab Dispos.* (2016) **44**:1859–66. doi: 10.1124/dmd.115.068981
31. Bidlack WR, Brown RC, Mohan C. Nutritional parameters that alter hepatic drug metabolism, conjugation, and toxicity. *Fed Proc.* (1986) **45**:142–8.
32. Callaghan JT, Bergstrom RF, Ptak LR, Beasley CM. Olanzapine. Pharmacokinetic and pharmacodynamic profile. *Clin Pharmacokinet.* (1999) **37**:177–93. doi: 10.2165/00003088-199937030-00001
33. Zanger UM, Schwab M. Cytochrome P450 enzymes in drug metabolism: Regulation of gene expression, enzyme activities, and impact of genetic variation. *Pharmacol Ther.* (2013) **138**:103–41. doi: 10.1016/j.pharmthera.2012.12.007
34. Urichuk L, Prior TI, Dursun S, Baker G. Metabolism of atypical antipsychotics: involvement of cytochrome p450 enzymes and relevance for drug-drug interactions. *Curr Drug Metab.* (2008) **9**:410–18. doi: 10.2174/138920008784746373
35. Fond G, d'Albis MA, Jamain S, Tamouza R, Arango C, Fleischhacker WW, et al. The promise of biological markers for treatment response in first-episode psychosis: a systematic review. *Schizophr Bull.* (2015) **41**:559–73. doi: 10.1093/schbul/sbv002
36. Meyer J, Koro CE, L'Italien GJ. The metabolic syndrome and schizophrenia: a review. *Int Rev Psychiatry* (2005) **17**:173–80. doi: 10.1080/09540260500071798

37. Guest PC, Wang L, Harris LW, Burling K, Levin Y, Ernst A, et al. Increased levels of circulating insulin-related peptides in first-onset, antipsychotic naïve schizophrenia patients. *Mol Psychiatry* (2010) **15**:118–9. doi: 10.1038/mp.2009.81
38. Guest PC, Schwarz E, Krishnamurthy D, Harris LW, Leweke FM, Rothermundt M, et al. Altered levels of circulating insulin and other neuroendocrine hormones associated with the onset of schizophrenia. *Psychoneuroendocrinology* (2011) **36**:1092–6. doi: 10.1016/j.psyneuen.2010.12.018
39. Ryan MC, Collins P, Thakore JH. Impaired fasting glucose tolerance in first-episode, drug-naive patients with schizophrenia. *Am J Psychiatry* (2003) **160**:284–9. doi: 10.1176/appi.ajp.160.2.284
40. Spelman LM, Walsh PI, Sharifi N, Collins P, Thakore JH. Impaired glucose tolerance in first-episode drug-naive patients with schizophrenia. *Diabet Med.* (2007) **24**:481–5. doi: 10.1111/j.1464-5491.2007.02092.x

4

Cognitive and Neurophysiological Recovery Following Electroconvulsive Therapy: A Study Protocol

Ben J. A. Palanca[1,2], Hannah R. Maybrier[1], Angela M. Mickle[1], Nuri B. Farber[3], R. Edward Hogan[4], Emma R. Trammel[1], J. Wylie Spencer[1], Donald D. Bohnenkamp[3], Troy S. Wildes[1], ShiNung Ching[2,5], Eric Lenze[3], Mathias Basner[6], Max B. Kelz[7] and Michael S. Avidan[1,8]*

[1] Department of Anesthesiology, Washington University School of Medicine in St. Louis, St Louis, MO, United States, [2] Division of Biology and Biomedical Sciences, Washington University School of Medicine in St. Louis, St Louis, MO, United States, [3] Department of Psychiatry, Washington University School of Medicine in St. Louis, St Louis, MO, United States, [4] Department of Neurology, Washington University School of Medicine in St. Louis, St Louis, MO, United States, [5] Department of Electrical Systems and Engineering, Washington University, St Louis, MO, United States, [6] Department of Psychiatry, University of Pennsylvania Perelman School of Medicine, Philadelphia, PA, United States, [7] Department of Anesthesiology, University of Pennsylvania Perelman School of Medicine, Philadelphia, PA, United States, [8] Department of Surgery, Washington University School of Medicine in St. Louis, St Louis, MO, United States

***Correspondence:**
Ben J. A. Palanca
palancab@wustl.edu

Electroconvulsive therapy (ECT) employs the elective induction of generalizes seizures as a potent treatment for severe psychiatric illness. As such, ECT provides an opportunity to rigorously study the recovery of consciousness, reconstitution of cognition, and electroencephalographic (EEG) activity following seizures. Fifteen patients with major depressive disorder refractory to pharmacologic therapy will be enrolled (Clinicaltrials.gov, NCT02761330). Adequate seizure duration will be confirmed following right unilateral ECT under etomidate anesthesia. Patients will then undergo randomization for the order in which they will receive three sequential treatments: etomidate + ECT, ketamine + ECT, and ketamine + sham ECT. Sessions will be repeated in the same sequence for a total of six treatments. Before each session, sensorimotor speed, working memory, and executive function will be assessed through a standardized cognitive test battery. After each treatment, the return of purposeful responsiveness to verbal command will be determined. At this point, serial cognitive assessments will begin using the same standardized test battery. The presence of delirium and changes in depression severity will also be ascertained. Sixty-four channel EEG will be acquired throughout baseline, ictal, and postictal epochs. Mixed-effects models will correlate the trajectories of cognitive recovery, clinical outcomes, and EEG metrics over time. This innovative research design will answer whether: (1) time to return of responsiveness will be prolonged with ketamine + ECT compared with ketamine + sham ECT; (2) time of restoration to baseline function in each cognitive domain will take longer after ketamine + ECT than after ketamine + sham ECT; (3) postictal delirium is associated with delayed restoration of baseline function in all cognitive domains; and (4) the sequence of reconstitution of cognitive domains following the three treatments in this study is similar to that occurring after an isoflurane general anesthetic (NCT01911195). Sub-studies will assess the relationships of cognitive recovery to the EEG preceding, concurrent, and following individual ECT sessions. Overall, this study will lead the development of biomarkers for tailoring the cogno-affective recovery of patients undergoing ECT.

Keywords: electroconvulsive therapy, electroencephalography, major depressive disorder, ketamine, anesthesia, seizures, neurocognitive disorders, consciousness

INTRODUCTION

Seizures—Unique States for Probing the Return Consciousness and Cognition

The return of consciousness following reversible states of unresponsiveness is relevant to neuroscience and clinical practice. Neural mechanisms underlying these processes appear to be distinct, with implications for anesthetic practice (1) and sleep/wake disorders (2). While states incurred by general anesthesia (3–5) and sleep (6, 7) have suggested neural substrates necessary for sustaining consciousness (8), the recovery from these depressed states of neural activity remains poorly characterized. Comparatively less is known regarding the recovery from states of highly synchronized neural activity incurred through generalized seizures (9, 10). Characterizing the recovery of neural activity and cognitive function following these states may provide a system to complement states of brain suppression given that: (1) action potential synchronization is a fundamental mode of information processing in the cerebral cortex distinct from neuronal firing rates and (2) seizures arise from changes in the excitatory and inhibitory synaptic balance in different brain regions.

The relationships of underlying electroencephalographic (EEG) activity and the recovery from generalized seizures is currently limited and challenging to investigate (11). Generalized seizures are characterized by the loss of consciousness coincident with ictal EEG spike-and-wave complexes, polyspike-and-wave complexes, and spikes (12). External phenotypes, ranging from convulsions to immobile staring, likely depend on the precise disruption in subcortical arousal systems, cortical-subcortical interactions, or neocortical connectivity (9, 10, 13). Inter-individual heterogeneity among clinical seizures may arise from diverse structural or metabolic derangements. Moreover, seizures are typically sporadic, unpredictable in occurrence, and may vary in intensity and character, making them difficult to study systematically. Following the disappearance of epileptiform EEG signatures, the postictal period begins and culminates in a return of consciousness and cognitive function. There is little standardization of postictal clinical and behavioral testing to facilitate objective comparison to EEG changes during the postictal period. Critical barriers to generating inferences from reproducible seizures may be addressed in the context of electroconvulsive therapy (ECT) (14), where seizures are electrically induced under safely controlled conditions.

EEG Activity and Cognitive Dysfunction Following ECT

The potential of EEG to inform clinicians on the future efficacy and side effects of ECT has not been fully realized. EEG is commonly monitored during ECT, a proven treatment for depression, bipolar illness, and psychosis (15). Following the delivery of the ECT stimulus charge, epileptiform activity in the bilateral fronto-mastoid EEG can complement the assessment of peripheral tonic-clonic muscle activity (16). Clinically relevant EEG measures beyond the length of seizure duration (17) have unclear clinical utility (18). Optimally, EEG markers would be available for predicting and refining ECT administration to balance efficacy and side effects that accrue over the course of therapy. EEG measurements acquired on the day of treatment would inform clinicians prior to stimulus delivery. The spatial, temporal, and spectral properties of such markers remain unknown. Once ascertained, translation to clinical practice would require a sparse montage of EEG sensors that can generalize across patient gender, age, and recovery from general anesthesia. Similar advances in the field have not occurred since prior work establishing a relationship between cognitive performance and ECT stimulation parameters (19, 20). This void may be due to the paucity of studies that have characterized EEG across widely distributed brain regions using either 10–20 montages (21–24) or high-density EEG. The spatial resolution offered by high-density EEG is likely needed to associate cognitive and affective perturbations to specific EEG patterns. High-density scalp EEG has shown superiority over standard 10–20 montage recordings in guiding surgical treatment for epileptic seizures (25). Extension of this paradigm to the ECT setting may yield clinically relevant EEG markers for tailoring treatment at an individual patient level.

During the ictal period, seemingly stereotyped EEG patterns develop and resolve (26), with proposed phases of activity (21). Brief periods of EEG suppression or rhythmic bilateral 14-22 Hz oscillations may first emerge (21). Induction of bilateral polyspike activity occurs, often with greater power on the side of the stimulation electrode in unilateral ECT (21, 27). Spike/spike-and-wave complexes then arise, followed by termination within 3 min (21, 26). This ictal activity may be followed by postictal generalized EEG suppression, a marker associated with ECT therapeutic efficacy (17, 28, 29) and with potential implications for understanding sudden unexpected death in epilepsy (30, 31). Delta waves (<4 Hz) (26) emerge that are gradually replaced by theta (4–8 Hz), alpha (8–13 Hz), and beta (13–30 Hz) rhythms (26). The dynamics of these EEG changes may aid in our understanding of seizures in general and help to reveal the efficacy/side effects of ECT in the postictal period following future large-scale investigations.

The continued resolution of postictal EEG changes may also correlate with the cognitive impairments incurred immediately after individual sessions and progress over the course of ECT treatments. Perturbations in processed EEG measures persist even when individuals appear to be awake in the postictal period (32–34). Patients with greater suppression in processed EEG measures following ECT are more likely to experience prolonged memory impairment (35). Specific EEG markers that can be linked to both underlying neurobiology and cognitive function have not been developed for the acute period after ECT. Beyond individual sessions, persistent slow theta and delta oscillations have been observed in the EEG (36) and may resolve only weeks following the last session (37, 38). These markers that remain weeks after ECT sessions may be linked to either therapeutic efficacy (38) or the extent of disorientation and retrograde amnesia (39). Definitive relationships remain speculative.

The recovery of cognitive function following individual ECT sessions has not been fully characterized. Recent analyses have shed light on the incidence and persistence of cognitive side effects related to this procedure (40). Approximately 5–12% of patients experience postictal agitation and disorientation after ECT (41, 42) that may last 1–2 h after ECT. Postictal agitation does not occur reproducibly in the same patients following subsequent treatments (43). Disorientation during the early postictal recovery from ECT appears to decrease with number of sessions (44). In contrast, interictal confusion accumulates with successive ECT sessions (44). Cognitive side effects may persist for 90 min following seizure termination (45). The temporal development and progression over the course of ECT remain unclear, but deficits in verbal memory, executive function (46), and visuospatial memory (47) have been identified. Cognitive impairments during the course of ECT can delay treatment (48), contribute to missed work, burden caregivers. Given that each session of ECT requires the administration of general anesthesia during seizure induction, systematic study requires accounting for these potent neuromodulatory agents.

Control for Anesthetic Exposure

Elucidating cognitive recovery following seizures in the context of ECT requires a control to account for the effects of general anesthesia. This is because modern ECT is conducted under general anesthesia and pharmacologic neuromuscular paralysis. Anesthetics with mechanisms invoking γ-aminobutyric acid (GABA) A-type receptor agonism (e.g., etomidate) or NMDA-receptor antagonism (ketamine) are commonly used. Ketamine has received greater attention recently since subanesthetic doses of ketamine have shown efficacy in treating refractory depression (49–52). Relative to other anesthetics in use for ECT, ketamine may provide faster recovery from cognitive impairment on the day of treatment (53, 54) or offer additive benefits on ECT efficacy (54). Thus, ketamine may be useful in a sham ECT condition to control for anesthetic exposure while offering potential therapeutic effects even in the absence of electrical stimulation.

Hypotheses and Aims

This is a randomized crossover trial to investigate the recovery of cognitive and neurophysiological function following right-unilateral ECT in individuals with treatment-resistant depression. We hypothesize that the reconstitution among different cognitive domains will markedly vary in rate and order, depending on the presence of seizures induced by electrical brain stimulation. Our specific aims include: (1) assess whether the time to return of responsiveness will be prolonged with ketamine + ECT compared with ketamine + sham ECT; (2) ascertain whether the time of restoration to baseline function in each cognitive domain will take longer after ketamine + ECT than after ketamine + sham ECT; (3) determine if postictal delirium is associated with delayed restoration of baseline function in all cognitive domains; and (4) determine whether the sequence of reconstitution across cognitive domains is similar to that occurring after an isoflurane general anesthetic; we also anticipate these cognitive disturbances to mirror recovery in EEG power spectral measures, despite substantial variability across our sample.

METHODS AND ANALYSIS

This protocol includes elements elaborated in the Standard Protocol Items: Recommendations for Interventional Trials (SPIRIT) checklist (55, 56).

Participants

Ethics Approval

The HRPO at Washington University School in St. Louis has approved the study. The study will be conducted with strict adherence to Washington University Institutional Review Board protocol. American Board of Anesthesiology board-certified anesthesiologists with experience in conducting clinical studies will lead the study. Safety and privacy of study participants will be safeguarded in compliance with the Health Insurance Portability and Accountability Act.

Inclusion and Exclusion Criteria

Inclusion criteria include: (1) Referral for ECT via right unilateral stimulation for treatment-resistant non-psychotic unipolar depression or bipolar disorder, (2) Fluency in English, (3) Age greater than 18 years, and (4) Ability to provide written informed consent. Exclusion criteria are: (1) Known brain lesions or neurological illness with sufficient cognitive impairment to prevent cognitive testing prior to ECT initiation, (2) Schizophrenia, (3) Schizoaffective disorder, (4) Blindness or deafness that may impair performance on cognitive testing, or (5) Inadequate seizure duration with etomidate general anesthesia, defined at our institution as bilateral spike-and-wave complexes present for less than 10 s. Past suicidality or substance use disorder will not exclude patients from enrollment.

Design and Procedure

Recruitment

Given the sample size used in our prior study (57), 15 patients will be recruited over a span of three years. Psychiatrists will brief prospective patients on the study to determine eligibility and interest. Trained study team members will formally screen and enroll interested patients during a preoperative clinic visit or in the hospital ward. All enrolled patients will provide written informed consent, with adherence to the Declaration of Helsinki. Patients will not be charged for participating and will receive remuneration of $100 per completed treatment session, up to $600.

Interventions

Each patient will be scheduled for an initial dose-charge titration and six treatment sessions over the initial 2 weeks of the ECT treatment cycle (**Figure 1**) at Barnes-Jewish Hospital, St. Louis, MO, USA. Patients will receive three sequential treatments: etomidate + ECT, ketamine + ECT, and ketamine + sham ECT. These treatments will be repeated in the same sequence over the subsequent week. The study focuses on changes in in cognoaffective function over the initial period of the ECT index course prior to maintenance therapy. A 2-week duration of involvement was chosen to maximize patient tolerance of study procedures and minimize repetition of stimuli.

Randomization and Blinding

A trained team member will use a computer-generated randomization algorithm among 18 potential combinations of initial cognitive task and order of study interventions. Random assignments will account for investigator-physician availability for ketamine + sham ECT sessions. The patient will be blind to the order of treatment condition. Study and clinician teams will be aware of the treatment arm at each session and maintain routine checks and monitoring before and after anesthetic induction. In order to maximize adherence to the intervention protocol, a study coordinator will inform research and clinical teams of the treatment condition prior to the study session day, and brief these teams on study procedures immediately before the subject's scheduled treatment session. To maintain sufficient blinding of the subject to the treatment condition, patients will not be able to view the syringe during anesthetic induction during any treatment session. Furthermore, stimulation electrode and conducting gel will also be placed on the scalp following loss and prior to return of responsiveness during sham-ECT sessions. Post-anesthetic evaluation by anesthesiology, psychiatry, and nursing staff will be consistent across sessions.

To maximize study rigor and reproducibility, investigators evaluating study measurements for data quality and development of analytical tools will be blinded to the details of the treatment intervention, whenever possible (58).

Timeline of Treatment Visits

Dose-Charge Titration

As part of standard care, the patient will be admitted for an initial dose-charge titration to induce a generalized seizure of adequate duration under etomidate general anesthesia. This session will serve to determine the seizure threshold and tolerance for the study procedures (**Figure 2A**). During this visit, the study team will assess baseline cognitive function and EEG prior to ECT, tolerability of cognitive testing and EEG recording, and feasibility of etomidate as the anesthetic for study and subsequent treatments. ECT charge will be delivered via a Thymatron System IV (Somatics, LLC, Venice, FL, USA). Per ECT laboratory procedures, stimulation parameters include a current of 0.9 amperes, pulse width of 0.3 ms, with escalating dosage: (5% total charge: 24.9 millicoulombs, 10 Hz stimulation, 4.6 s duration; 10% total charge: 50.8 millicoulombs,

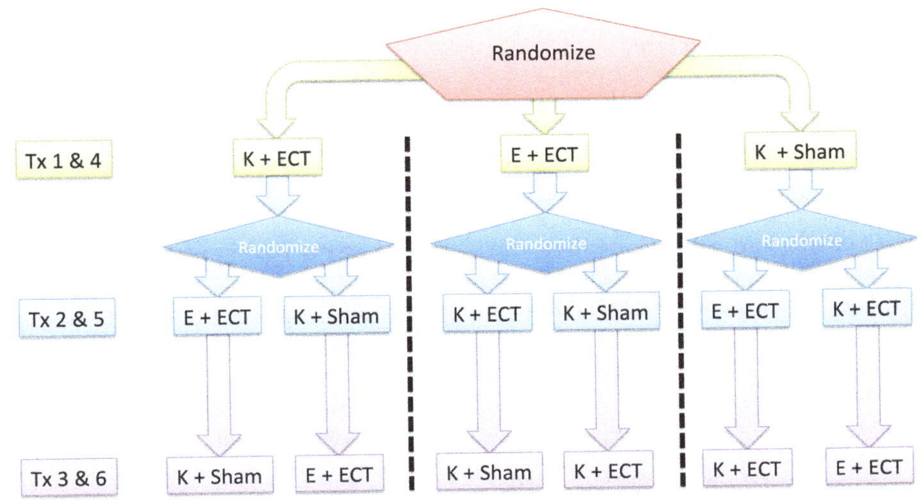

FIGURE 1 | Overall study design. Patients are randomized to repeated testing on three different treatment (Tx) interventions: Etomidate + ECT (E + ECT), ketamine + ECT (K + ECT), and ketamine + sham ECT (K + Sham). These interventions occur over a 2-week period following a dose-charge titration session that determines the adequate ECT charge for treatment-resistant depression.

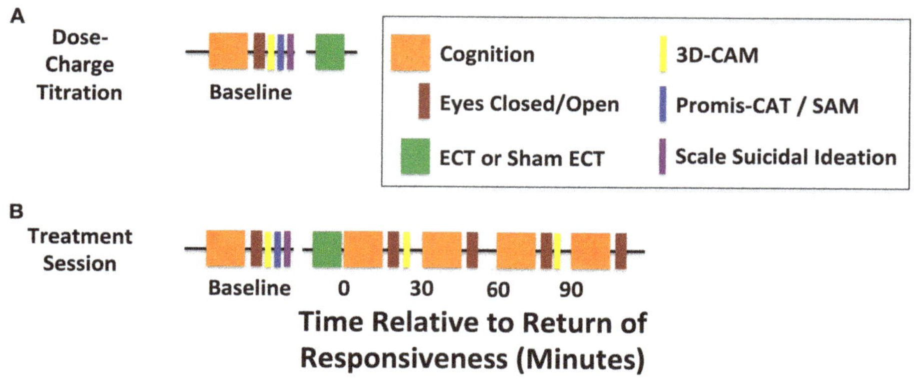

FIGURE 2 | Timelines for dose-charge titration and treatment sessions. (A) Baseline cognitive assessments are acquired before the dose-charge titration session with etomidate general anesthesia. **(B)** Baseline cognitive assessments are acquired before each treatment session and serially from the return of responsiveness to verbal command (T = 0) and up to 90 min afterwards (T = 90). Continuous high-density EEG is acquired during baseline assessments and treatment sessions.

20 Hz stimulation, 4.65 s duration, 15% total charge: 75.6 millicoulombs, 20 Hz stimulation, 6.98 s duration). Subsequent planned ECT treatment is based on a six-fold increase in charge delivery. Thus, individuals without suitable seizure duration at a projected 100% charge will be withdrawn from the study if subsequently scheduled for bilateral ECT. Participants will not be withdrawn if their standard-of-care anesthetic is changed from etomidate to another anesthetic, such as ketamine.

Study Intervention Treatment Sessions 1–6

Following randomization, each patient will initiate a complete course of therapy with participation in six treatment sessions (**Figure 2B**). During four of these six sessions, the patients will receive care within standard practice for ECT: general anesthesia (etomidate or ketamine), muscle paralysis (succinylcholine), and electrical stimulation. For the remaining two sessions, patients will undergo a ketamine general anesthetic without muscle paralysis or ECT stimulation.

High-density EEG, bilateral fronto-mastoid clinical EEG, and full American Society of Anesthesiologists (ASA) monitoring will commence prior to the induction of general anesthesia. Additionally, audible squeeze toys will be placed in each hand of the patient, who will be instructed to follow serial commands to either "Squeeze your left hand twice" or "Squeeze your right hand twice." Every 30 s, one of these recorded audio commands will be played at random, to monitor loss and return of responsiveness to verbal command. Patients will be pre-oxygenated by mask and anesthesia will be induced with ketamine, approximately 2 mg/kg, or etomidate, approximately 0.2 mg/kg. Following bolus of the induction agent, loss of responsiveness and eyelash reflex will be confirmed. Loss of responsiveness to verbal command will be recorded as the first time when a subject fails to correctly respond to the standardized auditory commands. Care adherent to the ASA guidelines will be performed regardless of treatment session. For sessions with ECT, pre-stimulation hyperventilation and assisted ventilation will also be performed. Central seizure duration will be assessed from bilateral fronto-mastoid EEG by the psychiatry team. Peripheral seizure duration will be determined through monitoring of tonic-clonic activity (16). During all sessions other drugs will also be administered according to current practice and as clinically indicated (e.g. for nausea or headache).

During the recovery from the study intervention, the study team will note spontaneous eye opening and compliance to commands to ascertain the timing for return of responsiveness. The ability to extend the thumb to verbal command ("thumbs up") will be assayed every 30 s. Timing for opening of eyes to command will be noted. These requests will be preceded with the patient's name to increase emotional valence. Return of responsiveness will be defined as the first time at which the patient squeezes the correct hand precisely as instructed via the standardized auditory commands. At this time, defined as t = 0 min, the subject will begin a series of cognitive and behavioral assessments, which are repeated every 30 min up to 90 min after return of responsiveness. Patients will be permitted to take brief breaks to use the restroom and eat or drink, as necessary. They will be discharged according to standard post-anesthesia care unit discharge criteria upon completing the last neurocognitive test battery. A study site coordinator will contact each subject within 24 h of the study day to assess and document any adverse events, as well as confirm the subject's continued involvement in the study.

DATA COLLECTION

The overall design of data collection for the dose-charge titration session and the experimental treatment sessions differ in the emergence period after ECT or sham ECT (**Figure 2**). Primary study measurements and outcomes are listed in **Table 1**. Patient demographics and clinical measures will be maintained using the Research Electronic Data Capture (REDCap) application (59).

Primary and Secondary Outcomes

Primary outcomes include: the temporal recovery profiles for cognitive task performance, as measured using the Cognition assessment battery (60); times for the return of responsiveness

TABLE 1 | Summary of study measurements and outcomes for primary analyses.

Type	Measure/Outcome	Purpose
Responsiveness	Spontaneous eye opening	Spontaneous return of arousal
	Eye opening to verbal command	Verbal probe
	Mimicking "thumbs up" gesture	Probe with visual cues
	Squeezing of hand to verbal command	Standardized auditory probe
Cognitive Task Performance	Motor Praxis Test	Sensorimotor speed
	Psychomotor Vigilance Test	Reaction time
	Digit Symbol Substitution	Visual scanning
	Fractal-2-Back	Working memory
	Visual Object Learning Test	Memory for complex shapes
	Abstract Matching Test	Executive function
Clinical Outcomes	Scale of Suicidal Ideation	Suicidal Ideation
	PROMIS-CAT	Depression: Computer-based
	Self-Assessment Manikin	Depression: Visual-analog
	3D-CAM	Delirium Assessment
	QIDS-SR16	Depression: Self-report
Seizure Markers	Frequency	Rate of ictal complexes
	Scalp Topology	Spatial characteristics
	Morphology	Temporal characteristics
	Postictal Generalized EEG Suppression	Efficacy marker
Power Spectral Measures	Delta Band (1–4 Hz)	
	Theta Band (4–8 Hz)	
	Alpha Band (8–13 Hz)	Spectral content
	Beta Band (13–30 Hz)	
	Gamma Band (30–70 Hz)	

to auditory command; and the presence of delirium, evaluated through the 3-minute Diagnostic Assessment for CAM-defined delirium (3D-CAM) (61).

Secondary outcome measures based on the EEG will include characterization of the seizures by both expert reader interpretation and quantitative techniques (62). Central seizure duration will be visually determined by clinician evaluation of the frontal-mastoid bipolar EEG ictal complexes. Additional measures will be calculated from windowed analyses of the high-density EEG: power spectral measures of the interval between anesthetic induction to delivery of ECT stimulus charge; the seizure envelope for 1–12 Hz EEG power; peak-to-peak amplitude, calculated from the difference in maximum and minimum voltages within 200 ms time; periodicity of epileptiform discharges; inter-hemispheric symmetry of seizure discharges; intra- and inter-hemispheric coherence. When possible, these measures and power spectral estimates will be derived from different phases of the ictal waveforms (27). The following postictal EEG measures will be assessed: duration and signal amplitude of postictal EEG suppression; power spectral parameters flanking the return of responsiveness to verbal command; and power spectral parameters from eyes open and closed epochs, including assessments of the posterior dominant rhythm. Spatiotemporal analyses will also focus on the propagation of EEG signatures during the ictal and early postictal period.

Additional secondary outcomes include: suicidality, mood, depression severity, delirium, and treatment course outcome.

Cognition Test Battery

Cognitive assessments will be administered on a Dell Latitude E5430 Laptop with a 14-inch liquid crystal display (Round Rock, TX, USA) using Cognition test battery software (60). Cognition consists of 10 brief neuropsychological tests with known cerebral representation that cover a wide range of cognitive domains (60). Patients will watch a standardized instructional video for baseline testing prior to the dose-charge titration session. Additional pre-intervention baseline assessments will also be performed on each treatment session prior to induction of general anesthesia. Post-treatment testing will occur at return of responsiveness to auditory command ($t = 0$) and at $t = 30$, 60, and 90 min. Each testing bout will take approximately 15–20 min to complete wherein the first cognitive test will be repeated as the last test at each time point. The order in which the tests are administered will be randomized between subjects but will be held constant across treatment sessions for a given patient. These tests have been previously employed in probing cognitive function during the recovery from isoflurane general anesthesia (57).

Motor Praxis Test (MPT)

This test assesses sensorimotor speed (63). Participants use a touchpad to click on squares that appear at random locations on the screen. The difficulty of tracking increases as successive squares become smaller.

Psychomotor Vigilance Test (PVT)

The PVT evaluates reaction time for detecting visual stimuli at random inter-stimulus intervals (64). During this 3-min test, subjects are instructed to monitor for a counter on the screen and to hit the space bar as quickly as possible once the counter appears.

Digit Symbol Substitution Test (DSST)

This test assesses memory, complex scanning, and visual tracking based on a paradigm used in the Wechsler Adult Intelligence Scale (65). Subjects are presented with a legend that pairs unique symbols to digits (1 through 9). Symbols are then sequentially presented on the screen in random order over a 90 s testing period. Participants are instructed to press the corresponding number key as soon as possible.

Fractal-2-Back (F2B)

As a variant of the Letter 2-Back task (66), the F2B assesses working memory through sequential presentation of fractal patterns that fill the screen. During the testing bout, each pattern may have multiple presentations. Subjects are asked to press the space bar when the current stimulus matches the pattern displayed two fractals previously.

Visual Object Learning Test (VOLT)

Memory for complex visual figures is evaluated by the VOLT (67). Ten complex three-dimensional figures are presented on the screen for participants to memorize. Participants are then asked to select these ten objects from a set that also contains ten decoys, with each of the 20 objects presented individually in random order.

Abstract Matching Test (AMT)

This test assesses components of executive function, including the development of implicit abstract rules (68). During the AMT, two pairs of objects are shown, one at the bottom left, and one at the bottom right of the screen. A target object appearing in the middle of the screen must be classified as fitting better with one of the two groups based on shape or fill pattern.

MPT, PVT, and DSST use stimuli that are randomly generated prior to each test administration. For F2B, VOLT, and AMT, 15 unique versions exist, and up to 14 versions will be used for this protocol. The same stimuli will be repeated after the 14 versions of these tests have been exhausted. Due to the number of stimuli and the time between ECT sessions, it is unlikely that subjects will remember specific stimulus sequences or stimuli across ECT sessions.

Median reaction time and accuracy will be computed for each of the multiple testing bouts within each session, including pre-treatment baseline and during recovery. For each treatment session, parameters obtained after the return of responsiveness to verbal command will be subtracted from baseline to arrive at repeated measures that account for the recovery in task performance over time.

Suicidal Ideation, Depression Severity, and Delirium Assessment

At the beginning of each study session, the first two questions of the Scale of Suicidal Ideation (69) will be used to assess the patient's subjective desire to hurt him- or herself. These two questions, "Wish to live?" and "Wish to die?", have been used previously for assessing changes in suicidal ideation before and after a brief ketamine infusion for major depressive disorder (70).

Depression severity will be assessed using the Patient-Reported Outcomes Measures Information System-Computer Adaptive Testing (PROMIS®-CAT) survey for depression. Mood will be quantified via the Self-Assessment Manikin (SAM, Supplementary Material 1) (71), a brief scale appropriate for patients with transient cognitive impairment following ECT. Baseline assessments will be performed prior to the dose-charge titration. To determination improvement on the day of treatment, the PROMIS®-CAT and the SAM will be administered prior to anesthetic induction on all study sessions and after the last cognitive battery of each treatment session. As part of standard care for tracking depression symptoms during an ECT course, treating psychiatry teams will administer the Quick Inventory of Depressive Symptomatology, Self-Report (16-Item), QIDS-SR16 (72).

Delirium will be assessed with the 3-min Diagnostic Assessment for CAM-defined delirium (3D-CAM) (61). The 3D-CAM will be administered at baseline, prior to the dose-charge titration visit, prior to each treatment visit, and post-treatment at $t = 0$, and 60. However, if the patient is negative for the 3D-CAM assessment at any time during the recovery, subsequent assessments will not be performed during the remainder of the session.

To assess quality of treatment blinding, the patient will be asked their impression of whether they received ECT at the last testing point on each treatment session. The patient will be asked, "Do you feel that you received ECT today? Was ECT painful?"

EEG and Video Acquisition

EEG will be collected during the dose-charge titration session and during all treatment sessions to assess pre-ECT and pre-anesthetic baseline EEG recordings. An appropriately fitted 64-channel EEG Geodesics Sensor Net (Electrical Geodesics, Inc. Eugene, OR, USA) will be affixed to the scalp and face. Elefix electrode paste (Nihon Kohden America, Inc., Irvine, CA, USA) will be injected to maintain conductivity to the silver/silver-chloride electrodes. Electrode impedances on each channel will be optimized to be less than 100 kOhms/channel, per manufacturer's suggestions. EEG signals (500 Hz sampling rate) will be acquired with a Net Amps 400 amplifier and Net Station version 5.0 and above (Electrical Geodesics, Inc. Eugene, OR, USA) via a Late 2012 Mac Pro Workstation (Apple Cupertino, CA, USA). Whenever possible, video synchronized to EEG will be acquired using an Axis P3364LV network camera (Axis Communications, Lund, Sweden).

EEG Preprocessing and Analysis

Netstation Tools and EEGLab will be used to assess for quality and to reduce artifact related to motion and eye movements (73). Bad channels will be identified by visual inspection. Signals will be filtered from 1 to 100 Hz and subsequently downsampled to 250 Hz. Modules of the PREP pipeline (74) will be used to reduce artifact related to line noise and movement. Reduction of eye movement artifacts will employ independent component analysis. For ictal recordings, preprocessing will be tailored to minimize distortion of seizure complexes. The following analysis time epochs will be evaluated for secondary outcomes related to EEG activity: pre-ECT and post-ECT periods with either eyes open or eyes closed, the interval between anesthetic induction and ECT stimulation, the period between stimulus delivery and cessation of ictal waveforms/spike-and-wave complexes, postictal period of EEG suppression and slowing, and both 5-min epochs flanking the return of responsiveness to verbal command.

Spectral analysis will be performed using the Chronux Toolbox (75), including five tapers, time frequency bandwidth of 3, and 6-s non-overlapping time windows. Total power and peak amplitude will be computed within the delta (1–4 Hz), theta (4–8 Hz), alpha (8–13 Hz), and beta (13–30 Hz) bands. Sub-studies will focus on coherence and phase lag indices, as computed using the Chronux toolbox. Global coherence (76) and permutation entropy will also be computed (77).

In parallel to power spectral analyses, we will track the time-varying connectivity between the measured brain regions. Data will be windowed into 5–10 s epochs within which several cross-channel connectivity metrics will be computed. These measures will include the Pearson correlation, directed entropy, and Shannon mutual information. Thus, windows will manifest different "networks," each describing the association between channels (regions) according to its respective metric. These networks will be clustered into a set of distinct motifs, or microstates, by using a k-means algorithm with least-squares error criterion. Other methods to characterize the time-varying dynamics of the observed brain activity, including those based on network control theory, will also be considered.

Visualization and analyses of epileptiform EEG activity will be performed using Net Station and Persyst software (Persyst, Solana Beach, CA, USA), following interpolation of bad channels and re-referencing to the average signal. EEG dipole localization, inter-hemispheric generalization, and phase-reversals will be assessed by epilepsy board-certified neurologists. Seizures will be staged according to the previously described phases that follow ECT stimulation (phase I with initial 14–22 Hz rhythmic beta activity, phase II with arrhythmic polyspike activity, and phase III with rhythmic 2.5–3.5 Hz. spike/polyspike activity (27)) The duration and amplitude of post-ictal generalized EEG suppression (PGES) will also be determined. Additionally, expanding on previous analyses of stationarity in epileptiform activity induced by ECT (24), we will use high-density EEG to topographically map rhythmic sharp-wave discharges. To maintain rigor, evaluators will be blinded to the study intervention. Quantitative metrics will be derived from spectral and time-based analyses of the ictal EEG. These measures will evaluate seizure energy, periodicity, and symmetry, as well as propagation, and termination.

Sample Size

We based our targeted enrollment on safety consideration for a ketamine general anesthetic, expected differences in the recovery patterns of different domains assessed by the Cognition test battery, and prior volunteer data with isoflurane emergence (57). Sample size calculations were based on 1-way pairwise of ANOVA (Analysis of Variance) comparisons of 5 means ($t = 0$, 30, 60, 90, and 120 min). Expected effect sizes for differences in the modeled trajectories of cognitive function ranged from 20 to 40 min. Standard deviations were expected to range between 20 and 40 min. Using conservative assumptions, we calculated a sample size of 24 subjects (effect size, μ_A-μ_B, of 20 min; standard deviation, σ, of 20 min; two-sided alpha of 0.05; power of 80%). With liberal assumptions, we estimated a sample size of 12 participants (μ_A-μ_B of 40 min; σ of 20 min; two-sided alpha of 0.05; power of 99%). With this range of estimates and expected attrition of participants, we targeted for data collection from 15 to 20 participants.

Statistical Analyses

We will employ mixed-effects models to quantify trajectories of cognitive recovery over time while addressing inter-subject variance and missing data. Linear models with appropriate transformations will be used preferentially over non-linear models. Time and treatment intervention group will be included as fixed effects while random effects will account for repeated measures provided by each participant. Day of treatment relative to the dose-charge titration session will allow consideration of cumulative effects of treatment order that may remain biased despite randomization. To address differences in ECT-stimulation responsiveness, regression approaches will account for dose charge, central seizure duration, and age. Models will assess for the effects of treatment on the timing for the return of responsiveness to verbal command and the presence of delirium. Separate mixed-effects models will be generated to assess task performance in a group of young healthy volunteers during the recovery from isoflurane general anesthesia (57). For example, the following damped-exponential equations will be used for mixed-effects models of cognitive task performance over time t, for an individual k.

$$\text{Reaction Time}\,(t,k) = \Phi_1(t,k) - \Phi_2(t,k) \times \exp(-\Phi_3(t,k)) \quad (1)$$

$$\text{Accuracy}\,(t,k) = \Phi_1(t,k) + \Phi_2(t,k) \times \exp(-\Phi_3(t,k)) \quad (2)$$

Where parameters $\Phi_1(t,k)$, $\Phi_2(t,k)$, $\Phi_3(t,k)$ are optimized at an individual and group level based on changes in these measures relative to pre-intervention baseline within a treatment session. A change in performance at time 0 (return of responsiveness) would be accounted by $\Phi_1(k)$, the asymptotic value on recovery by $\Phi_2(t,k)$, and the rate of recovery modeled by Φ_3.

Primary Pre-specified Analyses

Recovery of Responsiveness

Given that the induction of generalized seizures by electrical stimulation may compound the recovery from general anesthesia, we expect that interval from loss to return of responsiveness following ketamine + ECT will be longer compared to the period for ketamine + sham ECT. We will determine the median and 95% confidence intervals for this measure in relation to the treatment intervention.

Recovery of Cognition

Given that postictal suppression may be prolonged with ketamine than with etomidate (78), we hypothesize that the time needed for the return of cognition to baseline on individual sessions will be greatest for ketamine + ECT, followed by etomidate + ECT, and ketamine + sham ECT. Separate mixed-effects models will be generated based on reaction time and accuracy. We will determine the time of convergence for 95% confidence intervals for the marginal responses related to the three treatment groups. To determine the timing for the recovery to baseline, we will determine the time when the same 95% confidence intervals include 0.

Postictal Delirium and Cognitive Recovery

We expect the incidence of delirium (3D-CAM) to be associated with delayed restoration of baseline function in all cognitive domains. The magnitude and significance of this relationship will be determined from the mixed-effects models for each cognitive test.

Comparison of Cognitive Recovery After ECT and Isoflurane General Anesthesia

We hypothesize that the time for recovery to baseline will be quicker for treatments involving ECT compared to that for the recovery from isoflurane general anesthesia. Convergence for 95% confidence intervals will be compared between treatment groups.

Secondary Pre-specified Analyses

Recovery of Cognition

Principal measures of performance are based on preliminary data (60) of the Cognition test battery. Additional measures include: PVT response speed, DSST throughput, PVT lapses, VOLT duration and accuracy, AM duration and accuracy, and DSST errors. Cognition performance measures associated with lower effect sizes will also be assessed. These include AM accuracy, VOLT accuracy, F2B reaction time, MPT accuracy, MPT duration, and F2B accuracy. Overall, we expect F2B, VOLT, and AMT to recover the slowest due to taxing of short-term memory after ketamine + ECT compared to ketamine + sham ECT.

Recovery in the Spontaneous EEG

We will evaluate mixed-effects models to test the hypotheses that the predominance of frontal delta or theta power during passive eyes opening or occipital alpha power during eyes closure predict cognitive performance (Cognition scores) or delirium (3D-CAM scores). We will also compare these EEG spectral measures across treatment sessions to evaluate the impact of anesthetic and ECT.

Relationship of ECT Seizure Duration to Return of Responsiveness to Verbal Command

We expect that the length of ECT-induced seizures will correlate with the intervals from the loss of responsiveness to the return of responsiveness.

Mood and Depression Severity

We expect improvement in these clinical outcomes to be greatest with ketamine + ECT, followed by etomidate + ECT, and then ketamine + sham ECT.

Treatment Satisfaction

We expect satisfaction to be greatest for ketamine + ECT, followed by ketamine + sham ECT, and then by etomidate + ECT.

RISKS AND JUSTIFICATION

Candidates for ECT are refractory to multiple medical modalities. These patients may benefit from a greater understanding of the impact of anesthetics and ECT on the severity of the underlying psychiatric illness and the recovery of cognitive function. Ketamine may improve the efficacy of ECT and recovery of cognitive function following ECT. Patients may benefit from the additional EEG monitoring in the postictal period during which non-convulsive status epilepticus is rarely manifested. Risks from exposure to ketamine include self-limited tachycardia, hypertension, hallucinations, agitation, and delusions.

RESEARCH CONDUCT

Treatment sessions will be conducted at Washington University School of Medicine under the general supervision of a board-certified anesthesiologist who is familiar with post-anesthetic and post-intervention care. Patients will be monitored during emergence and recovery from anesthesia by the anesthetic and nursing staff in the ECT suite as per standard care. Additionally, research personnel trained in good clinical practices will be present during the acquisition of data. Monitoring and safety will be according to the current clinical standard. Patient confidentiality will be maintained through de-identification of personal health information. Identity and linking information will be stored in a locked cabinet within the principal investigator's office, which is locked outside of business hours. Electronic data will be password-encrypted on secure servers.

Patient satisfaction will be monitored throughout the study (Supplementary Material 2). Discontinuation of study procedures will be proposed if withdrawal is in the best interest of the patient or if removal of treatment blinding is requested. In the event that different interventions are needed from those allocated, the patient will be withdrawn from the study. Participants will be given a satisfaction survey to be returned by mail following the last study session (79).

ADVERSE EVENTS AND PREMATURE DISCONTINUATION

The Washington University in St. Louis Human Research Protection Office (HRPO) and the Data and Safety Monitoring Committee (DSMC) will oversee the study's progression and adherence to protocol. The study was approved by HRPO on March 24, 2016. Following each intervention, the principal investigators will affirm continued involvement or withdrawal based on patient tolerance and data quality. All adverse events will be reviewed by the DSMC and reported to HRPO, following the reporting policies and procedures, and followed until satisfactory resolution. The description of the adverse experience will include the time of onset, duration, intensity, known etiology, relationship to the study, and any treatment required. The trial steering committee will be responsible for all major decisions regarding changes to the protocol. The committee will communicate these changes to HRPO and appropriate parties.

DISSEMINATION

The final trial dataset will be the property of the investigative team and shall not be shared without permission from the principal investigators. Dissemination plans include presentations at local, national and international scientific conferences. Every effort will be made to publish results of this trial in peer-reviewed journals. Dissemination of results to study participants and their family members will be available upon request. Updates and results of the study will be available to the public at www.clinicaltrials.gov. The trial was first registered on April 30, 2016 as NCT02761330. The first participant was enrolled on May 3, 2016.

DISCUSSION

This study will be the first to elaborate the time course and sequence whereby consciousness, cognition, and EEG activity recover following seizures induced for ECT. The randomized, repeated methods design of the study is powerful, as it will allow several within-patient comparisons. Specifically, the design will allow us to distinguish between the effect of ketamine anesthesia alone versus the combined effect of ketamine and ECT. Recovery of consciousness after etomidate is expected to be rapid, on the order of minutes. Therefore, the etomidate + ECT arm should provide an additional comparator condition to the ketamine + ECT arm. Intra-patient repetition of each of the three exposures over 2 weeks will help to establish the reproducible effect of each exposure on the outcomes of interest.

Past EEG studies during and after ECT show interesting correlates with clinical outcomes, including degree of increased post-ECT slowing (theta and delta activity) during the course of treatment for depression (80). However, EEG acquisition techniques have varied widely in past studies, with some studies using limited EEG electrode coverage of the bifrontal regions (45) and others using more conventional standard clinical EEG montages (38). Techniques with broad head coverage and high sensor density, such as magnetoencephalography, have already shown promise in further characterizing post-ECT changes such as increases in slow delta and theta rhythms, and decreases in faster alpha and beta rhythms (81). The use of high-density EEG in the current study offers an extension of current clinical monitoring with extensive electrode coverage over the scalp. This approach may expand the possibility of detecting meaningful EEG changes that correlate with post-ECT changes in consciousness and treatment effects.

Limitations of the study include an inability of our sample size to account for variability across medical treatment regimens. Despite our efforts to minimize subjective bias across treatment arms, patient unblinding is possible due to psychoactive effects of ketamine that are not associated with etomidate. Furthermore, the lack of pharmacologic muscle paralysis during sham ECT treatments may also contribute if muscle aches are encountered during the study. Without drug levels of ketamine, we will be unable to rule out the possibility that any prolongation in depressed cognition or consciousness is related to changes in hepatic blood flow or function during ECT compared to sham treatments. Finally, the effects of timing between treatments and of successive treatments over time may not be fully addressed by our study design.

The cognitive domains assessed through the study test battery are components of complex cognoaffective processes that may be more closely linked to activities of daily living. Further investigation will be able to address measures that integrate cognitive domains and emotional valence or account for cognitive distortions (82). While potentially more difficult to assess, these meaningful outcomes will yield a greater understanding of how patients perceive and interact with their environment.

An underlying motivation for this work is that cognitive impairments incurred over the ECT index course limit patient functionality and adherence to this important treatment modality. Comparisons of task performance before and after an index course have identified deficits in orientation (83, 84) and different forms of memory (47, 85–90). Cumulative treatments of ECT are associated with anterograde (91) and retrograde amnesia (92), primarily following the entire course regimen (40). Cognitive deficits resolve within days (40) to weeks after the index course of therapy (87, 88, 90, 93). The links between these longer-term deficits and the perturbations incurred over the shorter time scales of the proposed investigation constitute future avenues of inquiry.

We anticipate our findings to lay the groundwork for larger mechanistic studies for generating markers that reflect the efficacy and side effects of ECT across an array of psychiatric illnesses. These insights could impact our understanding of other neuromodulatory therapies. Overall, ECT remains an established and effective modality for treating refractory mental illness. Future neural markers for aiding decision-making of patients and clinicians could demystify ECT, thereby improving access, adoption, and adherence.

AUTHOR CONTRIBUTIONS

BP, HM, AM, NF, ET, EL, MB, and MA contributed to study design; BP, HM, AM, NF, RH, ET, JS, TW, SC, EL, MB, MK, and MA contributed to the writing of the manuscript.

FUNDING

This study has been awarded funding for 3 years by the James S. McDonnell Foundation (PI: Michael Avidan): The James S. McDonnell Foundation 1034 S. Brentwood Blvd. Ste 1850 St. Louis, MO 63117.

ACKNOWLEDGMENTS

We appreciate the initial contributions by George Mashour, MD, PhD for the design and manuscript. We also acknowledge the feedback and suggestions of Warren Ugalde, RN, and Michael Jarvis, MD, PhD to improve the workflow, safety, and comfort for our study patients. Kristopher Bakos, Pharm D provided valuable logistical contributions for the administration of study medications. We also thank members of the Reconstructing

Consciousness and Cognition Phase 2 (RCC2) Research Collaborative at Washington University School of Medicine: Jamila Burton; Jordan Oberhaus; Shelly Gupta; Amil Patel; Chloe Stallion; Ying Jiang; Ravi Upadhyayula; Changwei Wei; Alaira Lourido.

REFERENCES

1. Kelz MB, Sun Y, Chen J, Cheng Meng Q, Moore JT, Veasey SC, et al. An essential role for orexins in emergence from general anesthesia. *Proc Natl Acad Sci USA.* (2008) **105**:1309–14. doi: 10.1073/pnas.0707146105
2. Trotti LM. Waking up is the hardest thing I do all day: sleep inertia and sleep drunkenness. *Sleep Med Rev.* (2016) **35**:76–84. doi: 10.1016/j.smrv.2016.08.005
3. Boveroux P, Vanhaudenhuyse A, Bruno MA, Noirhomme Q, Lauwick S, Luxen A, et al. Breakdown of within- and between-network resting state functional magnetic resonance imaging connectivity during propofol-induced loss of consciousness. *Anesthesiology* (2010) **113**:1038–53. doi: 10.1097/ALN.0b013e3181f697f5
4. Palanca BJ, Mitra A, Larson-Prior L, Snyder AZ, Avidan MS, Raichle ME. Resting-state functional magnetic resonance imaging correlates of sevoflurane-induced unconsciousness. *Anesthesiology* (2015) **122**:346–56. doi: 10.1097/ALN.0000000000000731
5. Ranft A, Golkowski D, Kiel T, Riedl V, Kohl P, Rohrer G, et al. Neural correlates of sevoflurane-induced unconsciousness identified by simultaneous functional magnetic resonance imaging and electroencephalography. *Anesthesiology* (2016) **125**:861–72. doi: 10.1097/ALN.0000000000001322
6. Massimini M, Ferrarelli F, Esser SK, Riedner BA, Huber R, Murphy M, et al. Triggering sleep slow waves by transcranial magnetic stimulation. *Proc Natl Acad Sci USA.* (2007) **104**:8496–501. doi: 10.1073/pnas.0702495104
7. Landsness EC, Crupi D, Hulse BK, Peterson MJ, Huber R, Ansari H, et al. Sleep-dependent improvement in visuomotor learning: a causal role for slow waves. *Sleep* (2009) **32**:1273–84. doi: 10.1093/sleep/32.10.1273
8. Koch C, Massimini M, Boly M, Tononi G. Neural correlates of consciousness: progress and problems. *Nat Rev Neurosci.* (2016) **17**:307–21. doi: 10.1038/nrn.2016.22
9. Yu L, Blumenfeld H. Theories of impaired consciousness in epilepsy. *Ann N Y Acad Sci.* (2009) **1157**:48–60. doi: 10.1111/j.1749-6632.2009.04472.x
10. Englot DJ, Yang L, Hamid H, Danielson N, Bai X, Marfeo A, et al. Impaired consciousness in temporal lobe seizures: role of cortical slow activity. *Brain* (2010) 133(Pt 12):3764–77. doi: 10.1093/brain/awq316
11. So NK, Blume WT. The postictal EEG. *Epilepsy Behav.* (2010) **19**:121–6. doi: 10.1016/j.yebeh.2010.06.033
12. Hrachovy RA, Frost JDJr. The EEG in selected generalized seizures. *J Clin Neurophysiol.* (2006) **23**:312–32. doi: 10.1097/01.wnp.0000228496.66246.e0
13. Blumenfeld H. Impaired consciousness in epilepsy. *Lancet Neurol.* (2012) **11**:814–26. doi: 10.1016/S1474-4422(12)70188-6
14. Fink M. *Convulsive Therapy: Theory and Practice.* New York, NY: Rave Press. (1979).
15. Lisanby SH. Electroconvulsive therapy for depression. *N Engl J Med.* (2007) **357**:1939–45. doi: 10.1056/NEJMct075234
16. Fink M, Johnson L. Monitoring the duration of electroconvulsive therapy seizures: 'cuff' and EEG methods compared. *Arch Gen Psychiatry* (1982) **39**:1189–91. doi: 10.1001/archpsyc.1982.04290100055009
17. Mayur P. Ictal electroencephalographic characteristics during electroconvulsive therapy: a review of determination and clinical relevance. *J ECT* (2006) **22**:213–7. doi: 10.1097/01.yct.0000235922.14623.39
18. Dinwiddie SH, Glick DB, Goldman MB. The effect of propofol-remifentanil anesthesia on selected seizure quality indices in electroconvulsive therapy. *Brain Stimul.* (2012) **5**:402–7. doi: 10.1016/j.brs.2011.06.008
19. Weiner RD, Rogers HJ, Davidson JR, Kahn EM. Effects of electroconvulsive therapy upon brain electrical activity. *Ann N Y Acad Sci.* (1986) **462**:270–81. doi: 10.1111/j.1749-6632.1986.tb51261.x
20. Abrams R. *Electroconvulsive Therapy.* New York, NY: Oxford University Press. (2002).
21. Brumback RA, Staton RD. The electroencephalographic pattern during electroconvulsive therapy *Clin Electroencephalogr.* (1982) **13**:148–53.
22. Luber B, Nobler MS, Moeller JR, Katzman GP, Prudic J, Devanand DP, et al. Quantitative EEG during seizures induced by electroconvulsive therapy: relations to treatment modality and clinical features. II. Topographic analyses. *J ECT* (2000) **16**:229–43. doi: 10.1097/00124509-200009000-00003
23. Nobler MS, Luber B, Moeller JR, Katzman GP, Prudic J, Devanand DP, et al. Quantitative EEG during seizures induced by electroconvulsive therapy: relations to treatment modality and clinical features. I. Global analyses. *J ECT* (2000) **16**:211–28. doi: 10.1097/00124509-200009000-00002
24. Zoldi SM, Krystal A, Greenside HS. Stationarity and redundancy of multichannel EEG data recorded during generalized tonic-clonic seizures. *Brain Topogr.* (2000) **12**:187–200. doi: 10.1023/A:1023489807177
25. Brodbeck V, Spinelli L, Lascano AM, Wissmeier M, Vargas MI, Vulliemoz S, et al. Electroencephalographic source imaging: a prospective study of 152 operated epileptic patients. *Brain* (2011) 134(Pt 10):2887–97. doi: 10.1093/brain/awr243
26. Weiner RD. Electroencephalographic correlates of ECT. *Psychopharmacol Bull.* (1982) **18**:78–81.
27. Gerst JW, Enderie JD, Staton RD, Barr CE, Brumback RA. The electroencephalographic pattern during electroconvulsive therapy II. Preliminary analysis of spectral energy. *Clin Electroencephalogr.* (1982) **13**:251–6.
28. Krystal AD, Weiner RD. EEG correlates of the response to ECT: a possible antidepressant role of brain-derived neurotrophic factor. *J ECT* (1999) **15**:27–38. doi: 10.1097/00124509-199903000-00004
29. Azuma H, Fujita A, Sato K, Arahata K, Otsuki K, Hori M, et al. Postictal suppression correlates with therapeutic efficacy for depression in bilateral sine and pulse wave electroconvulsive therapy. *Psychiatry Clin Neurosci.* (2007) **61**:168–73. doi: 10.1111/j.1440-1819.2007.01632.x
30. Ryvlin P, Nashef L, Lhatoo SD, Bateman LM, Bird J, Bleasel A, et al. Incidence and mechanisms of cardiorespiratory arrests in epilepsy monitoring units (MORTEMUS): a retrospective study. *Lancet Neurol.* (2013) **12**:966–77. doi: 10.1016/S1474-4422(13)70214-X
31. Bauer PR, Thijs RD, Lamberts RJ, Velis DN, Visser GH, Tolner EA, et al. Dynamics of convulsive seizure termination and postictal generalized EEG suppression. *Brain* (2017) **140**:655–68. doi: 10.1093/brain/aww322
32. Gunawardane PO, Murphy PA, Sleigh JW. Bispectral index monitoring during electroconvulsive therapy under propofol anaesthesia. *Br J Anaesth.* (2002) **88**:184–7. doi: 10.1093/bja/88.2.184
33. Thimmaiah R, Thirthalli J, Ramesh VJ, Radhakrishnan MC, Muralidharan K, Mahadevaiah M, et al. Effect of a course of electroconvulsive therapy on interictal bispectral index values: a prospective study. *J ECT* (2012) **28**:20–3. doi: 10.1097/YCT.0b013e318235b658
34. Soehle M, Kayser S, Ellerkmann RK, Schlaepfer TE. Bilateral bispectral index monitoring during and after electroconvulsive therapy compared with magnetic seizure therapy for treatment-resistant depression. *Br J Anaesth.* (2014) **112**:695–702. doi: 10.1093/bja/aet410
35. Koitabashi T, Oyaizu T, Ouchi T. Low bispectral index values following electroconvulsive therapy associated with memory impairment. *J Anesth.* (2009) **23**:182–7. doi: 10.1007/s00540-008-0722-3
36. Volavka J, Feldstein S, Abrams R, Dornbush R, Fink M. EEG and clinical change after bilateral and unilateral electroconvulsive therapy. *Electroencephalogr Clin Neurophysiol.* (1972) **32**:631–9. doi: 10.1016/0013-4694(72)90100-9
37. Kolbeinsson H, Petursson H. Electroencephalographic correlates of electroconvulsive therapy. *Acta Psychiatr Scand.* (1988) **78**:162–8. doi: 10.1111/j.1600-0447.1988.tb06316.x
38. Sackeim HA, Luber B, Katzman GP, Moeller JR, Prudic J, Devanand DP, et al. The effects of electroconvulsive therapy on quantitative electroencephalograms. Relationship to clinical outcome. *Arch Gen Psychiatry* (1996) **53**:814–24. doi: 10.1001/archpsyc.1996.01830090060009
39. Sackeim HA, Luber B, Moeller JR, Prudic J, Devanand DP, Nobler MS. Electrophysiological correlates of the adverse cognitive effects of electroconvulsive therapy. *J ECT* (2000) **16**:110–20. doi: 10.1097/00124509-200006000-00003
40. Semkovska M, McLoughlin DM. Objective cognitive performance associated with electroconvulsive therapy for depression: a systematic

review and meta-analysis. *Biol Psychiatry* (2010) **68**:568–77. doi: 10.1016/j.biopsych.2010.06.009
41. Kranaster L, Janke C, Hoyer C, Sartorius A. Management of severe postictal agitation after electroconvulsive therapy with bispectrum electroencephalogram index monitoring: a case report. *J ECT* (2012) **28**:e9–e10. doi: 10.1097/YCT.0b013e31823d2fef
42. Tzabazis A, Schmitt HJ, Ihmsen H, Schmidtlein M, Zimmermann R, Wielopolski J, et al. Postictal agitation after electroconvulsive therapy: incidence, severity, and propofol as a treatment option. *J ECT* (2013) **29**:189–95 doi: 10.1097/YCT.0b013e3182887b5b
43. Fink M. Post-ECT Delirium. *Convuls Ther.* (1993) **9**:326–30.
44. Calev A, Cohen R, Tubi N, Nigal D, Shapira B, Kugelmass S, et al. Disorientation and bilateral moderately suprathreshold titrated, E. C. T. *Convuls Ther.* (1991a) **7**:99–110.
45. Perera TD, Luber B, Nobler MS, Prudic J, Anderson C, Sackeim HA. Seizure expression during electroconvulsive therapy: relationships with clinical outcome and cognitive side effects. *Neuropsychopharmacology* (2004) **29**:813–25. doi: 10.1038/sj.npp.1300377
46. Vasavada MM, Leaver AM, Njau S, Joshi SH, Ercoli L, Hellemann G, et al. Short- and long-term cognitive outcomes in patients with major depression treated with electroconvulsive therapy. *J ECT* (2017) **33**:278–85. doi: 10.1097/YCT.0000000000000426
47. Falconer DW, Cleland J, Fielding S, Reid IC. Using the Cambridge Neuropsychological Test Automated Battery (CANTAB) to assess the cognitive impact of electroconvulsive therapy on visual and visuospatial memory. *Psychol Med.* (2010) **40**:1017–25. doi: 10.1017/S0033291709991243
48. Miller ME, Siris SG, Gabriel AN. Treatment delays in the course of electroconvulsive therapy. *Hosp Commun Psychiatry* (1986) **37**:825–7. doi: 10.1176/ps.37.8.825
49. Mathew SJ, Shah A, Lapidus K, Clark C, Jarun N, Ostermeyer B, et al. Ketamine for treatment-resistant unipolar depression: current evidence. *CNS Drugs* (2012) **26**:189–204. doi: 10.2165/11599770-000000000-00000
50. Mathews DC, Zarate CAJr. Current status of ketamine and related compounds for depression. *J Clin Psychiatry* (2013) **74**:516–7. doi: 10.4088/JCP.13ac08382
51. Murrough JW, Iosifescu DV, Chang LC, Al Jurdi RK, Green CE, Perez AM, et al. Antidepressant efficacy of ketamine in treatment-resistant major depression: a two-site randomized controlled trial. *Am J Psychiatry* (2013a) **170**:1134–42. doi: 10.1176/appi.ajp.2013.13030392
52. Murrough JW, Perez AM, Pillemer S, Stern J, Parides MK, aan het Rot M, et al. Rapid and longer-term antidepressant effects of repeated ketamine infusions in treatment-resistant major depression. *Biol Psychiatry* (2013b) **74**:250–6. doi: 10.1016/j.biopsych.2012.06.022
53. McDaniel WW, Sahota AK, Vyas BV, Laguerta N, Hategan L, Oswald J. Ketamine appears associated with better word recall than etomidate after a course of 6 electroconvulsive therapies. *J ECT* (2006) **22**:103–6. doi: 10.1097/00124509-200606000-00005
54. MacPherson RD, Loo CK. Cognitive impairment following electroconvulsive therapy–does the choice of anesthetic agent make a difference? *J ECT* (2008) **24**:52–6. doi: 10.1097/YCT.0b013e31815ef25b
55. Chan AW, Tetzlaff JM, Altman DG, Laupacis A, Gotzsche PC, Krleza-Jeric K, et al. SPIRIT 2013 statement: defining standard protocol items for clinical trials. *Ann Intern Med.* (2013a) **158**:200–7. doi: 10.7326/0003-4819-158-3-201302050-00583
56. Chan AW, Tetzlaff JM, Gotzsche PC, Altman DG, Mann H, Berlin JA, et al. SPIRIT 2013 explanation and elaboration: guidance for protocols of clinical trials. *BMJ* (2013b) **346**:e7586. doi: 10.1136/bmj.e7586
57. Maier KL, McKinstry-Wu AR, Palanca BJ, Tamal V, Blain-Moraes S, Basner M, et al. Protocol for the reconstructing human consciousness and cognition study. *Front Hum Neurosci.* (2017) **11**:284. doi: 10.3389/fnhum.2017.00284
58. Nuzzo R. How scientists fool themselves - and how they can stop. *Nature* (2015) **526**:182–5. doi: 10.1038/526182a
59. Harris PA, Taylor R, Thielke R, Payne J, Gonzalez N, Conde JG. Research electronic data capture (REDCap)–a metadata-driven methodology and workflow process for providing translational research informatics support. *J Biomed Inform.* (2009) **42**:377–81. doi: 10.1016/j.jbi.2008.08.010
60. Basner M, Savitt A, Moore TM, Port AM, McGuire S, Ecker AJ, et al. Development and validation of the cognition test battery for spaceflight. *Aerosp Med Hum Perform.* (2015) **86**:942–52. doi: 10.3357/AMHP.4343.2015
61. Marcantonio ER, Ngo LH, O'Connor M, Jones RN, Crane PK, Metzger ED, et al. 3D-CAM: derivation and validation of a 3-minute diagnostic interview for CAM-defined delirium: a cross-sectional diagnostic test study. *Ann Intern Med.* (2014) **161**:554–61. doi: 10.7326/M14-0865
62. Haider HA, Esteller R, Hahn CD, Westover MB, Halford JJ, Lee JW, et al. Sensitivity of quantitative EEG for seizure identification in the intensive care unit. *Neurology* (2016) **87**:935–44. doi: 10.1212/WNL.0000000000003034
63. Gur RC, Ragland JD, Moberg PJ, Turner TH, Bilker WB, Kohler C, et al. Computerized neurocognitive scanning: I. Methodology and validation in healthy people. *Neuropsychopharmacology* (2001) **25**:766–76. doi: 10.1016/S0893-133X(01)00278-0
64. Basner M, Mollicone D, Dinges DF. Validity and sensitivity of a brief psychomotor vigilance test (PVT-B) to total and partial sleep deprivation. *Acta Astronaut.* (2011) **69**:949–59. doi: 10.1016/j.actaastro.2011.07.015
65. McLeod DR, Griffiths RR, Bigelow GE, Yingling J. An automated version of the digit symbol substitution test (DSST). *Behav Res Methods Instrum.* (1982) **14**:463–6. doi: 10.3758/BF03203313
66. Ragland JD, Turetsky BI, Gur RC, Gunning-Dixon F, Turner T, Schroeder L, et al. Working memory for complex figures: an fMRI comparison of letter and fractal n-back tasks. *Neuropsychology* (2002) **16**:370–9. doi: 10.1037/0894-4105.16.3.370
67. Glahn DC, Gur RC, Ragland JD, Censits DM, Gur RE. Reliability, performance characteristics, construct validity, and an initial clinical application of a visual object learning test (VOLT). *Neuropsychology* (1997) **11**:602–12. doi: 10.1037/0894-4105.11.4.602
68. Glahn DC, Cannon TD, Gur RE, Ragland JD, Gur RC. Working memory constrains abstraction in schizophrenia. *Biol Psychiatry* (2000) **47**:34–42. doi: 10.1016/S0006-3223(99)00187-0
69. Beck AT, Kovacs M, Weissman A. Assessment of suicidal intention: the Scale for Suicide Ideation. *J Consult Clin Psychol.* (1979) **47**:343–52. doi: 10.1037/0022-006X.47.2.343
70. Ballard ED, Ionescu DF, Vande Voort JL, Niciu MJ, Richards EM, Luckenbaugh DA, et al. Improvement in suicidal ideation after ketamine infusion: relationship to reductions in depression and anxiety. *J Psychiatr Res.* (2014) **58**:161–6. doi: 10.1016/j.jpsychires.2014.07.027
71. Bradley MM, Lang PJ. Measuring emotion: the self-assessment manikin and the semantic differential. *J Behav Ther Exp Psychiatry* (1994) **25**:49–59. doi: 10.1016/0005-7916(94)90063-9
72. Rush AJ, Trivedi MH, Ibrahim HM, Carmody TJ, Arnow B, Klein DN, et al. The 16-Item Quick Inventory of Depressive Symptomatology (QIDS), clinician rating (QIDS-C), and self-report (QIDS-SR): a psychometric evaluation in patients with chronic major depression. *Biol Psychiatry* (2003) **54**:573–83. doi: 10.1016/S0006-3223(02)01866-8
73. Delorme A, Makeig S. EEGLAB: an open source toolbox for analysis of single-trial EEG dynamics including independent component analysis. *J Neurosci Methods* (2004) **134**:9–21. doi: 10.1016/j.jneumeth.2003.10.009
74. Bigdely-Shamlo N, Mullen T, Kothe C, Su KM, Robbins KA. The PREP pipeline: standardized preprocessing for large-scale EEG analysis. *Front Neuroinform.* (2015) **9**:16. doi: 10.3389/fninf.2015.00016
75. Mitra PP, Bokil H. *Observed Brain Dynamics.* New York, NY: Oxford University Press (2008).
76. Cimenser A, Purdon PL, Pierce ET, Walsh JL, Salazar-Gomez AF, Harrell PG, et al. Tracking brain states under general anesthesia by using global coherence analysis. *Proc Natl Acad Sci USA.* (2011) **108**:8832–7. doi: 10.1073/pnas.1017041108
77. Bandt C, Pompe B. Permutation entropy: a natural complexity measure for time series. *Phys Rev Lett.* (2002) **88**:174102. doi: 10.1103/PhysRevLett.88.174102
78. Hoyer C, Kranaster L, Janke C, Sartorius A. Impact of the anesthetic agents ketamine, etomidate, thiopental, and propofol on seizure parameters and seizure quality in electroconvulsive therapy: a retrospective study. *Eur Arch Psychiatry Clin Neurosci.* (2014) **264**:255–61. doi: 10.1007/s00406-013-0420-5
79. Sienaert P, De Becker T, Vansteelandt K, Demyttenaere K, Peuskens J. Patient satisfaction after electroconvulsive therapy. *J ECT* (2005) **21**:227–31. doi: 10.1097/01.yct.0000183268.62735.c0
80. Farzan F, Boutros NN, Blumberger DM, Daskalakis ZJ. What does the electroencephalogram tell us about the mechanisms of action

of ECT in major depressive disorders? *J ECT* (2014) **30**:98–106. doi: 10.1097/YCT.0000000000000144

81. Sperling W, Martus P, Alschbach M. Evaluation of neuronal effects of electroconvulsive therapy by magnetoencephalography (MEG). *Prog Neuropsychopharmacol Biol Psychiatry* (2000) **24**:1339–54. doi: 10.1016/S0278-5846(00)00145-7
82. Gonda X, Pompili M, Serafini G, Carvalho AF, Rihmer Z, Dome P. The role of cognitive dysfunction in the symptoms and remission from depression. *Ann Gen Psychiatry* (2015) **14**:27. doi: 10.1186/s12991-015-0068-9
83. Summers WK, Robins E, Reich T. The natural history of acute organic mental syndrome after bilateral electroconvulsive therapy. *Biol Psychiatry* (1979) **14**:905–12.
84. Daniel WF, Crovitz HF. Disorientation during electroconvulsive therapy. Technical, theoretical, and neuropsychological issues. *Ann N Y Acad Sci.* (1986) **462**:293–306. doi: 10.1111/j.1749-6632.1986.tb51264.x
85. Daniel WF, Crovitz HF. Acute memory impairment following electroconvulsive therapy [2]. Effects of electrode placement. *Acta Psychiatr Scand.* (1983b) **67**:57–68.
86. Daniel WF, Crovitz HF. Acute memory impairment following electroconvulsive therapy [1]. Effects of electrical stimulus waveform and number of treatments. *Acta Psychiatr Scand.* (1983a) **67**:1–7.
87. Calev A, Nigal D, Shapira B, Tubi N, Chazan S, Ben-Yehuda Y, et al. Early and long-term effects of electroconvulsive therapy and depression on memory and other cognitive functions. *J Nerv Ment Dis.* (1991b) **179**:526–33.
88. Lisanby SH, Maddox JH, Prudic J, Devanand DP, Sackeim HA. The effects of electroconvulsive therapy on memory of autobiographical and public events. *Arch Gen Psychiatry* (2000) **57**:581–90. doi: 10.1001/archpsyc.57.6.581
89. Schat A, van den Broek WW, Mulder PG, Birkenhager TK, van Tuijl R, Murre JM. Changes in everyday and semantic memory function after electroconvulsive therapy for unipolar depression. *J ECT* (2007) **23**:153–7. doi: 10.1097/yct.0b013e318065aa0c
90. Fernie G, Bennett DM, Currie J, Perrin JS, Reid IC. Detecting objective and subjective cognitive effects of electroconvulsive therapy: intensity, duration and test utility in a large clinical sample. *Psychol Med.* (2014) **44**:2985–94. doi: 10.1017/S0033291714000658
91. Sobin C, Sackeim HA, Prudic J, Devanand DP, Moody BJ, McElhiney MC. Predictors of retrograde amnesia following ECT. *Am J Psychiatry* (1995) **152**:995–1001. doi: 10.1176/ajp.152.7.995
92. Nobler MS, Sackeim HA. Neurobiological correlates of the cognitive side effects of electroconvulsive therapy. *J ECT* (2008) **24**:40–5. doi: 10.1097/YCT.0b013e31815d6957
93. Bodnar A, Krzywotulski M, Lewandowska A, Chlopocka-Wozniak M, Bartkowska-Sniatkowska A, Michalak M, et al. Electroconvulsive therapy and cognitive functions in treatment-resistant depression. *World J Biol Psychiatry* (2016) **17**:159–64. doi: 10.3109/15622975.2015.1091501

5

Psychopathology—A Precision Tool in Need of Re-Sharpening

Frauke Schultze-Lutter[1], Stefanie J. Schmidt[2] and Anastasia Theodoridou[3]*

[1] Department of Psychiatry and Psychotherapy, Medical Faculty, Heinrich-Heine University, Düsseldorf, Germany,
[2] Department of Clinical Psychology and Psychotherapy, University of Bern, Bern, Switzerland, [3] Department of Psychiatry, Psychotherapy and Psychosomatics, Psychiatric Hospital, University of Zürich, Zürich, Switzerland

***Correspondence:**
Frauke Schultze-Lutter
frauke.schultze-lutter@lvr.de

Psychopathology is the scientific exploration of abnormal mental states that, for more than a century, has provided a *Gestalt* for psychiatric disorders and guided clinical as well as scientific progress in modern psychiatry. In the wake of the immense technical advances, however, psychopathology has been increasingly marginalized by neurobiological, genetic, and neuropsychological research. This ongoing erosion of psychiatric phenomenology is further fostered by clinical casualness as well as pressured health care and research systems. The skill to precisely and carefully assess psychopathology in a qualified manner used to be a core attribute of mental health professionals, but today's curricula pay increasingly less attention to its training, thus blurring the border between pathology and variants of the "normal" further. Despite all prophecies that psychopathology was doomed, and with neurobiological parameters having yet to show their differential-diagnostic superiority and value for differential indication, psychiatric diagnosis continues to rely exclusively on psychopathology in DSM-5 and ICD-11. Their categorical systematic, however, is equally challenged, and, supported by advances in machine learning, a personalized symptom-based approach to precision psychiatry is increasingly advocated. The current paper reviews the objectives of psychopathology and the recent debate on the role of psychopathology in future precision psychiatry—from guiding neurobiological research by relating neurobiological changes to patients' experiences to giving a framework to the psychiatric encounter. It concludes that contemporary research and clinic in psychiatry do not need less but rather more differentiated psychopathologic approaches in order to develop approaches that integrate professional knowledge and patients' experience.

Keywords: descriptive psychopathology, clinical psychopathology, theoretical psychopathology, neuroscience, self-experiences, mind, brain, machine-learning

The term "psychopathology," from the Greek ψυχή (psyche) for "soul" or "spirit," πάθος (pathos) for "suffering," and λογότυπα (logos) for "reason," "discourse" or "opinion," roughly translates into "teachings of the sufferings of the soul" and was coined in 1878 by the German psychiatrist Hermann Emminghaus (1). Yet, as a scientific discipline, psychopathology is commonly agreed to have started only 35 years later, in 1913 with the publication of Karl Japers' book "Allgemeine Psychopathologie" [(2), English: "General Psychopathology"] (3–10). To Jaspers, the subject of psychopathology was broadly "the individual as a whole in his illness, as far as it is a mental and psychogenic illness" and "the soul of the individual," respectively [(8), p. 845]. With it, psychopathology had become the core science in psychiatry that, over the past century, has provided a "Gestalt" for psychiatric disorders and successfully guided clinical as well as scientific progress in psychiatry and clinical psychology (5, 6, 11). Yet, in the wake of tremendous technological advances, within recent decades, psychopathology has been increasingly eclipsed by neurobiological approaches in both research and teaching (6, 8, 11, 12). In the following, we will therefore revisit the objectives of psychopathology and discuss their current state and their potential future role.

OBJECTIVES OF PSYCHOPATHOLOGY

In line with Jaspers' general definition, psychopathology is currently broadly defined, e.g., as "the scientific exploration of abnormal mental states" [(6), p. S147], "the subject matter of psychiatry, that is, pathologies of the psyche" [(9), p. 559], or "the discipline that assesses and makes sense of abnormal human subjectivity" [(10), p. 169]. Yet, despite this seeming agreement, the specific objectives of psychopathology and—consequently—its role in current and future psychiatric work and research still lack common understanding in psychiatry (6, 8). In 2010, the Task Force on Nosology and Psychopathology of the World Federation of Societies of Biological Psychiatry (WFSBP) thus reviewed approaches, theories, tasks, and tools of psychopathology in order to identify the main objectives of psychopathology in order to evaluate its role in the twenty-first century (8). It identified three main objectives of interrelated and partly interdependent tasks—descriptive, clinical and theoretical psychopathology (8). Illustrated by examples from (early) psychosis research, these are outlined and discussed in the following.

DESCRIPTIVE PSYCHOPATHOLOGY

The main tasks of descriptive or general psychopathology are two-fold (8). The first task is to describe and to denominate persons' subjective experiences and behaviors in a way that allows objective communication about them that is free of personal, cultural and school-specific interpretations (8–10). In doing so, ideally, psychopathology would provide a shared language (10). Yet, some of the critique on general psychopathology might in fact stem from the failure of the psychopathological community to provide, maintain, and impart an unambiguous nomenclature, i.e., from the lack of "a common language in the "Tower of Babel" that science has become" [(8), p. 848].

The early detection and intervention in psychoses is one such recent field of research in psychiatry in that such a persistent Babylonian speech confusion and its effects can be observed (13, 14). For example, in a recent critique of the ultra-high risk (UHR) approach (15), the majority of arguments were based on the assumed equality of UHR-relevant attenuated psychotic symptoms (APS) assessed by clinicians in patient samples using specific semi-standardized instruments and "psychotic-like experiences" assessed in the community by lay-persons using fully standardized instruments or by self-rating instruments (13, 14). In the critique (15), positive results in both assessment modes were equally regarded as "slightly-but-not quite psychotic," "low-grade psychotic symptoms," or "psychotic experiences," albeit studies showing that such community measures commonly overestimate the presence of clinician-assessed APS to a degree that casts serious doubts on their comparability (14, 16–18). This lack of psychopathological understanding and the resulting falsely assumed equality of phenomena of similar names (13, 14) then paved the way to unfounded—if not, from a clinical point of view, absurd—conclusions (14) such as "psychotic experiences" merely being "a marker for the severity of non-psychotic states" [(15), p.201].

However, Babylonian speech confusion is not restricted to wrongly assuming phenomenological equality by using similar terms interchangeably (13) but also includes using different terms for equal phenomena—often in the context of different schools. An example of this in psychosis literature is the current nomenclature of patients' self-descriptions of deviations in their mental processes. While these, within a biomedical theoretical framework, are known as "basic symptoms" (19–23), within the framework of the phenomenological tradition in philosophy, they are called "self-disturbances," "anomalous self- or subjective experiences" and "self-disorders" or "anomalous world experiences" (21, 22, 24–26). Thus, already in light of such imponderability of nomenclature, it might not be all surprising that, in psychiatry and related fields, researchers and clinicians alike increasingly seek rescue in neuroscience and its more definite terms and palpable constructs.

The second task of general psychopathology, including "special" and "functional" psychopathology, is to distinguish "abnormal" from "normal" experiences and behaviors and to describe the nature and developments of these "symptoms" (8). In special psychopathology, the focus has been on patients' self-experiences and self-reports of their mental states rather than on their observable expressions and behaviors that are regarded as important but less specific than personal experiences in terms of first-person perspective narratives (5, 6, 9). Functional psychopathology adopted a different strategy by defining deviant mental functions by clinicians' or third-persons' observations either of persons' expressions and behaviors or by their test performances, e.g., in neuropsychological tasks (8). With regard to test performances, functional psychopathology commonly defines the "abnormal" by standard deviations from the mean or similar measures, e.g., in case of the construct "intelligence" or of the 6th dimension, "cognitive impairment" of the severity assessment of symptoms of psychosis introduced in DSM-5 (27).

Traditionally, focus in psychiatry has been on special psychopathology. Yet, in the development of criteria-based operational diagnoses in DSM and ICD, emphasis was laid on interrater reliability rather than validity. Therefore, functional psychopathology was given a more prominent role along with the use of fully structured and sometimes even fully standardized instruments in special psychopathology (5, 6, 8, 12). In special psychopathology, however, empathy has been the main clinical tool to recreate and understand the patients' self-experience and to shape the psychiatric encounter. Thereby, the clinician systematically explores patients' self-experiences and translates these and certain accompanying aspects of their expression and behavior into specific predefined symptoms (5, 6, 9). Such an empathetic, understanding approach does not rule out the biomedical approach of seeing abnormal phenomena as symptoms whose underlying dysfunctions are to be cured but rather compliments it by exploring patients' meaning of their symptoms (9, 10). Besides, it does not rule out the use of semi-structured interviews to ensure addressing all relevant symptoms, including interviews specifically addressing self-experienced "abnormalities" (25, 26, 28, 29). Yet, this should be done in a conversational, context-sensitive way that supports giving a *Gestalt* to the patient's complaints (5, 9, 10, 12). The *Gestalt* arising from a careful, detailed and thorough exploration is more than simply an aggregation of symptoms—just as the picture arising from a jigsaw puzzle is more than the sum of its pieces; it is a coherent picture of the patient's mind and the foundation of a valid clinical and diagnostic appraisal.

The skill to precisely and carefully assess special psychopathology in a qualified manner used to be a core attribute of mental health professionals, but today's curricula pay increasingly less attention to its time-consuming training (5, 9, 12, 30). As a consequence, the border between pathology and variants of the "normal," whose supposed lack of clear definition is often held against special psychopathology, is further blurred. This ongoing erosion of the core skill of psychiatry is further fostered by clinical casualness as well as (economically) pressured health care and research systems (9) and endeavors such as the Research Domain Criteria (RDoC) project, whose aim is to classify "mental disorders based on dimensions of observable behavior and neurobiological measures" using big data approaches [(31), p.1205].

CLINICAL PSYCHOPATHOLOGY

Based on the descriptive psychopathology, nosological, or clinical psychopathology identifies symptoms that are significant to supposed nosographical distinctions and groups them together in nosographical systems, i.e., syndromes and diagnostic entities (8–10)—nowadays, increasingly with help of some kind of statistical modeling (8). In doing so, it has laid the grounds for studies into the causes of mental disorders, i.e., etiological psychopathology, and to the development of evidence-based treatment guidelines (8). Yet, mental disorders neither exist per se nor are they distinct diagnostic entities, but commonly share features. In mental health research, however, shared features are not only problem of clinical psychopathology but also of genetics (32) and neurobiology (33, 34).

Furthermore, these diagnostic entities in terms of mental disorders are not merely defined by a selected group of symptoms. In addition, they generally make objective requirements on symptoms' course, such as their minimum time of persistence (thus including some consideration of the crucial dimension of time (6)), their presentation (such as current frequency of occurrence or association–or lack of it–with certain situations or life events) and their non-functionality. Thus, a certain self-experience might only become a "symptom" in a pathological sense of meaning under certain circumstances, and symptoms and syndromes or disorders should not be equaled in discussions, such as in the exemplary critique of the UHR approach (14, 15). The presence of a clinician-assessed APS does not constitute presence of a UHR criterion that, in addition, makes requirements on its frequency and course as well as consideration of the context in that it occurs (14, 35–37). For this reason, roughly only one of ten persons of the community who had reported APS in a clinician-conducted interview actually met UHR criteria (35). Thus, some of the problems of distinguishing "normal" mental states from "abnormal" mental disorder might not pertain to the definition of phenomena but rather to their frequency and persistence allowances in diagnostic criteria, which are often not decided based on data but expert consensus.

Furthermore, current diagnostic manuals–and recent approaches toward a dimensional nosology such as the Hierarchical Taxonomy Of Psychopathology (HiTOP) initiative (38, 39)–only rely on a fraction of possible symptoms that merely convey a fragmented picture of a patient's mind and whose selection was mainly driven by reliability rather than validity aspects (5, 12). Today's psychiatric training, however, is focusing on only diagnosis-relevant symptoms (9, 10, 12, 30) that are frequently observable epiphenomena arising from patient's coping (incl. the search for meaning and explanation) with different, often distressing self-experiences (5, 30). These symptoms, however, had been initially intended only as gatekeepers in terms of the minimum symptoms needed to make a diagnosis rather than perceived as a conclusive description of symptoms associated with the respective diagnosis (12). Thus, in the wake of the introduction of DSM and ICD, "classics of psychopathology are now largely ignored" and "research in psychopathology is a dying (or dead) enterprise" [(12), p. 111]; and clinicians are discouraged from getting to know the individual patient and from understanding the *Gestalt* of his or her state of mind (5, 9, 10, 12, 30). Yet, as one commonly only finds what one is looking for, findings of a study examining case notes for descriptions of basic symptoms (40) are not surprising. Basic symptoms, which represent a prototype of patients' self-experiences but are completely unconsidered in diagnostic criteria of DSM and ICD, were 16 times more likely reported by patients with psychotic disorder in a special interview (28) than they were recorded in their case notes (40).

THEORETICAL PSYCHOPATHOLOGY

Exceeding, yet depending on and interacting with both descriptive and clinical psychopathology, theoretical psychopathology is the study of etiology or pathogenesis and, thus, strongly links psychopathology to neuroscience ((8); see also 'psychopathology in neuroscience and precision psychiatry' below). It lends some validity to mental syndromes but also provides the foundations for etiological and pathogenetic research (8). However, with sacrificing validity to reliability in DSM, the research targets provided by its diagnoses might be the wrong ones (12), thus gradually weakening the cause of psychopathology. Furthermore, while theoretical psychopathology borrowed methods from other science that were subordinated to the needs of psychopathological research in the past, with immense advances in neuroscience and genetics, these increasingly took a life on their own, thereby losing their already weakened psychopathological foundation (8). Thus, with increasing separation of neuroscience and genetics from the very subject of psychiatry—i.e., the mind, the "dehumanizing impact" of DSM on the practice of psychiatry [(12), p. 111] will be multiplied.

PSYCHOPATHOLOGY IN NEUROSCIENCE AND PRECISION PSYCHIATRY

Psychiatry and psychopathological research, in particular theoretical psychopathology, has always been positioned on a continuum between (natural) facts and (human) constructs (8, 10). This is a unique, yet often forgotten feature of psychiatry within biomedical science; and it is the mind rather than "brain events by themselves" that is of interest in psychiatry (5, 8, 10). Yet, this intermediate position has always fueled discussions on the role and value of psychopathology between advocates of different positions on this continuum, e.g., between neuroscientists located on the pole of natural facts and philosophers located on the pole of human constructs, who often lack a common language (8). Thus, with the two positions drifting further and further apart in the process of increasing specialization in science, psychopathology will have to make their re-integration, i.e., the reintegration of "mind" and "brain," its explicit objective (8, 10).

In order to reach these aims, the still widely accepted limited range of symptoms currently considered in diagnostic criteria and the structures of diagnosis need to be broadened again to the full range of patients' self-experiences in descriptive psychopathology and reassessed in clinical psychopathology (5, 10–12). The same applies to specific concepts of properties of the "psyche" or symptoms that often have been established decades ago without subsequent examination of their nowadays' social, historical and philosophical appropriateness and that are often used without sufficient knowledge of their origin and historical development (11, 13). Thus, today, neuroscientists and geneticists who try to find the neurobiological or genetic correlates of mental disorders or properties are faced with likely inadequate concepts of mental disorders. Additionally, they often lack understanding of the conceptual basis of their target (disorder or property) and the validity of its assessment methods; and rarely have a team member, e.g., a psychopathologist, able to expertly address these matters (11).

In the last few years, machine learning has made huge progress as a statistical method to classify and predict human experiences and behavior, incl. mental disorders, based on interpreting different kinds of information (41–44). Compared to more traditional prediction methods (such as regression analyses), predictive accuracy with machine learning methods (such as Support Vector Machines, Random Forests, and Deep Learning) increases from 30 to 40% to frequently over 90% in individualized prediction that is the basis of precision psychiatry (45). The use of these methods, however, is not restricted to neuroscience—in that it is currently mainly used—but can well be applied in psychopathology. In fact, it was recently shown that clinical variables can perform as well as neurobiological ones (46). Furthermore, other next generation statistical approaches such as joint modeling, time series analyses or network models might help identifying valid syndromes of little overlap if not based only on the "small world" of symptoms currently included in the definition of mental disorders (47, 48). Promising to this aim are patients' self-experiences in terms of basic symptoms and anomalous self- or world experiences, respectively (5, 20–23, 28, 29). These, in particular basic symptoms, have the unbeatable advantage to clearly distinguish "normal" from "abnormal" experiences as, by definition, they differ from what patients consider to be their normal mental self and functions. These subtle disturbances in any kind of mental process (e.g., stress tolerance, drive, affect, thinking, speech, perception, motor action, and central-vegetative functions) are self-experienced with immediate and full insight into their abnormal nature, and reported by patients as "abnormalities" (20–23, 28, 29).

For all these different aspects to be considered, the different specialties involved in this endeavor (incl. psychiatry, psychology, neuroscience, philosophy, genetics, epidemiology, computer science, and mathematics) will have to closely work together on equal footing in order to succeed in understanding the underpinnings and mechanisms of mental disorders. Developing a clear common language and bringing together their particular skills and expertise, multidisciplinary projects are needed:

- to validly define on a basic, fine-grained level what is "abnormal" and "normal" both in human experience and in brain function (10),
- to develop valid, reliable, broadly applicable, and sufficiently economic instruments for the assessment of such "abnormalities" whose assessment time should be fully covered by health insurances—this bringing in health politics (11),
- to detect if and how these "abnormalities" and "normalities" relate to each other over time (6, 10, 11),
- to newly define valid and reliable nosological constructs, i.e., syndromes or mental disorders, based on these "abnormalities" (5, 6, 8, 10, 12, 49),
    - that are also in terms with and perceptive about the full range of complaints with that patients will present themselves (5, 6, 10, 12, 49),
    - allow precise personalized diagnosis and prognosis (6),
    - for that efficient benign treatments exist or can be developed, likely as modular therapies (49),
- to include the dimension of time, i.e., the likely course of symptoms, in order to not only classify and treat the current mental state ("Zustandsbild") but the underlying illness ("Krankheit") and its psychosocial functional consequences (6).

CONCLUSION

Psychopathology is currently a neglected, if not dying science—not least, because current concepts of mental disorders failed to produce adequate neurobiological and genetic targets. Yet, as we demonstrated, problems within the field of psychopathology and the resulting neglect of psychopathology have brought about this failure. Thus, contemporary research and clinic in psychiatry do not need less but rather more differentiated psychopathologic approaches in order to develop approaches that integrate professional knowledge and patients' self-experience and offer more appropriate valid targets for neurobiological and genetic research than the broad, rather ill-defined constructs that definitions of mental disorders currently represent, i.e., as Nancy Andreasen has pointed out repeatedly over more than 20 years [(11), p. 112]:

> "We need to make a serious investment in training a new generation of real experts in the science and art of psychopathology. Otherwise, we high-tech scientists may wake up in 10 years [that is, now; comment by authors] and discover that we face a silent spring. Applying technology without the companionship of wise clinicians with specific expertise in psychopathology will be a lonely, sterile, and perhaps fruitless enterprise."

AUTHOR CONTRIBUTIONS

FS-L was responsible for the conception of the work and drafted the first version of this work. SS and AT revised it critically for important intellectual contents. All authors provided approval for publication of the content.

REFERENCES

1. Emminghaus H. *Allgemeine Psychopathologie zur Einführung in das Studium der Geistesstörungen*. Leipzig: F.C.W. Vogel (1878). 492.
2. Jaspers K. *Allgemeine Psychopathologie. Ein Leitfaden für Studierende, Ärzte und Psychologen*. Berlin: Springer (1913). 338.
3. Berrios GE. Phenomenology and psychopathology: was there ever a relationshhip? *Compr Psychiatry* (1993) 34:213–20. doi: 10.1016/0010-440X(93)90001-K
4. Beumont PJ. Phenomenology and the history of psychiatry. *Aust N Z J Psychiatry* (1992) 26:532–45. doi: 10.3109/00048679209072085
5. Parnas J, Sass LA, Zahavi D. Rediscovering psychopathology: the epistemology and phenomenology of the psychiatric object. *Schizophr Bull.* (2012) 39:270–7. doi: 10.1093/schbul/sbs153
6. Heckers S. Future in psychopathology research. *Schizophr Bull.* (2014) 40(Suppl. 2):S147–51. doi: 10.1093/schbul/sbt159
7. Huber G. The psychopathology of K. Jaspers and K. Schneider as a fundamental method for psychiatry. *World J Biol Psychiatry* (2002) 3:50–7. doi: 10.3109/15622970209150601
8. Musalek M, Larach-Walters V, Lepine JP, Millet B, Gaebel W on behalf of the WSFSBP Task Force on Nosology and Psychopathology. Psychopathology in the 21st century. *World J Biol Psychiatry* (2010) 11:844–51. doi: 10.3109/15622975.2010.510207
9. Stanghelli G. The meanings of psychopathology. *Curr Opin Psychiatry* (2009) 22 559–64. doi: 10.1097/YCO.0b013e3283318e36
10. Stanghelli G, Broome MR. Psychopathology as the basic science of psychiatry. *Br J Psychiatry* (2014) 205:169–70. doi: 10.1192/bjp.bp.113.138974
11. Torres-Correia D, Sampaio D. Historical roots of psychopathology. *Front Psychol.* (2016) 7:905. doi: 10.3389/fpsyg.2016.00905
12. Andreasen NC. DSM and the death of phenomenology in America: an example of unintended consequences. *Schizophr Bull.* (2006) 33:108–12. doi: 10.1093/schbul/sbl054
13. Schultze-Lutter F, Schimmelmann BG, Ruhrmann S. The near Babylonian speech confusion in early detection of psychosis. *Schizophr Bull.* (2011) 37:653–5. doi: 10.1093/schbul/sbr039
14. Schultze-Lutter F, Klosterkötter J, Gaebel W, Schmidt SJ. Psychosis-risk criteria in the general population: frequent misinterpretations and current evidence. *World Psychiatry* (2018) 17:109–10. doi: 10.1002/wps.20498
15. van Os J, Guloksuz S. A critique of the "ultra-high risk" and "transition" paradigm. *World Psychiatry* (2017) 16:200–6. doi: 10.1002/wps.20423
16. Schultze-Lutter F, Renner F, Paruch J, Julkowski D, Klosterkötter J, Ruhrmann S. Self-reported psychotic-like experiences are a poor estimate of clinician-rated attenuated and frank delusions and hallucination. *Psychopathology* (2014) 47:194–201. doi: 10.1159/000355554
17. Linscott RJ, van Os J. An updated and conservative systematic review and meta-analysis of epidemiological evidence on psychotic experiences in children and adults: on the pathway from proneness to persistence to dimensional expression across mental disorders. *Psychol Med.* (2013) 43:1133–49. doi: 10.1017/S0033291712001626
18. Spitz A, Studerus E, Koranyi S, Rapp C, Ramyead A, Ittig S, et al. Correlations between self-rating and observer-rating od psychopathology in at-risk mental state and first-episode psychosis patients: influence of disease stage and gender. *Early Interv Psychiatry* (2017) 11:461–70. doi: 10.1111/eip.12270
19. Huber G. Reine defektsyndrome und basisstadien endogener psychose. *Fortschr Neurol Psychiatr.* (1966) 34:409–26.
20. Schultze-Lutter F. Subjective symptoms of schizophrenia in research and the clinic: the basic symptom concept. *Schizophr Bull.* (2009) 35:5–8. doi: 10.1093/schbul/sbn139
21. Schultze-Lutter F, Debbané M, Theodoridou A, Wood SJ, Raballo A, Michel C, et al. Revisiting the basic symptom concept: towards translating risk symptoms for psychosis into neurobiological targets. *Front Psychiatry* (2016) 7:9. doi: 10.3389/fpsyt.2016.00009
22. Schultze-Lutter F, Theodoridou A. The concept of basic symptoms: its relevance in research and the clinic. *World Psychiatry* (2017) 16:104–5. doi: 10.1002/wps.20404
23. Schultze-Lutter F, Ruhrmann S, Fusar-Poli P, Bechdolf A, Schimmelmann BG, Klosterkötter J. Basic symptoms and the prediction of first-episode psychosis. *Curr Pharm Des.* (2012) 18:351–7. doi: 10.2174/138161212799316064
24. Parnas J, Raballo A, Handest P, Jansson L, Vollmer-Larsen A, Sæbye D. Self-experience in the early phases of schizophrenia: 5-year follow-up of the Copenhagen Prodromal Study. *World Psychiatry* (2011) 10:200–4. doi: 10.1002/j.2051-5545.2011.tb00057.x
25. Parnas J, Møller P, Kircher T, Thalbitzer J, Jansson L, Handest P, et al. EASE: Examination of Anomalous Self-Experience. *Psychopathology* (2005) 38:236–58. doi: 10.1159/000088441
26. Sass L, Pienkos E, Skodlar B, Stanghellini G, Fuchs T, Parnas J, et al. EAWE: Examination of Anomalous World Experience. *Psychopathology* (2017) 50:10–54. doi: 10.1159/000454928
27. American Psychiatric Association (APA). *Diagnostic and Statistical Manual of Mental Disorders.* 5th ed (DSM-5). Arlington, VA: APA (2013). 991.
28. Schultze-Lutter F, Addington J, Ruhrmann S, Klosterkötter J. *Schizophrenia Proneness Instrument, Adult Version (SPI-A)*. Rome: Giovanni Fioriti Editore s.r.l (2007). 97.
29. Schultze-Lutter F, Marshall M, Koch E. *Schizophrenia Proneness Instrument, Child and Youth Version; Extended English Translation (SPI-CY EET)*. Rome: Giovanni Fioriti Editore s.r.l (2012). 167.
30. Huber G. Psychopathologie – eine versiegende Quelle? Ein kritischer Kommentar. *Fortschr Neurol Psychiatr.* (2002) 70:393–402. doi: 10.1055/s-2002-33058
31. Cuthbert BN. Translating intermediate phenotypes into psychopathology: the NIMH research domain criteria. *Psychophysiology* (2014) 51:1205–6. doi: 10.1111/psyp.12342

32. Brainstorm Consortium, Anttila V, Bulik-Sullivan B, Finucane HK, Walters RK, Bras J, et al. Analysis of shared heritability in common disorders of the brain. *Science* (2018) 360:eaap8757. doi: 10.1126/science.aap8757
33. Pasternak O, Kelly S, Sydnor VJ, Shenton ME. Advances in microstructural diffusion neuroimaging for psychiatric disorders. *Neuroimage* (2018). doi: 10.1016/j.neuroimage.2018.04.051. [Epub ahead of print].
34. Power BD, Nguyen T, Hayhow B, Looi J. Neuroimaging in psychiatry: an update on neuroimaging in the clinical setting. *Australas Psychiatry* (2016) 24:157–63. doi: 10.1177/1039856215618525
35. Schultze-Lutter F, Michel C, Ruhrmann S, Schimmelmann BG. Prevalence and clinical relevance of interview-assessed psychosis risk symptoms in the young adult community. *Psychol Med.* (2018) 48:1167–78. doi: 10.1017/S0033291717002586
36. Schultze-Lutter F, Ruhrmann S, Schimmelmann BG, Michel C. 'A rose is a rose is a rose', but at-risk criteria differ. *Psychopathology* (2013) 46:75–87. doi: 10.1159/000339208
37. Schultze-Lutter F, Hubl D, Schimmelmann BG, Michel C. Age effect on prevalence of ultra-high risk for psychosis symptoms: replication in a clinical sample of an early detection of psychosis service. *Eur Child Adolesc Psychiatry* (2017) 26:1401–5. doi: 10.1007/s00787-017-0994-y
38. Kotov R, Krueger RF, Watson D, Achenbach TM, Althoff RR, Bagby RM, et al. The Hierarchical Taxonomy of Psychopathology (HiTOP): a dimensional alternative to traditional nosologies. *J Abnorm Psychol.* (2017) 126:454–77. doi: 10.1037/abn0000258
39. Kotov R, Krueger RF, Watson D. A paradigm shift in psychiatric classification: the Hierarchical Taxonomy Of Psychopathology (HiTOP). *World Psychiatry* (2018) 17:24–5. doi: 10.1002/wps.20478
40. Eisener E, Drake R, Lobban F, Bucci S, Emsley R, Barrowclough C. Comparing early signs and basic symptoms as methods for predicting psychotic relapse in clinical practice. *Schizophr Res.* (2018) 192:124–30. doi: 10.1016/j.schres.2017.04.050
41. Basili R, Bellomaria V, Bugge NJ, Croce D, De Michele F, Federico FN, et al. Monitoring adolescents' distress using social web data as a Source: the insideout project. In: Basili R, Nissim M, Satta G, editors. *Proceedings of the Fourth Italian Conference on Computational Linguistics CLiC-it 2017.* Torino: Academia University Press (2017), 24–9.
42. Howes C, Purver M, McCabe R. Linguistic indicators of severity and progress in online text-based therapy for depression. In: Association for Computational Linguistics, editor. *ACL Workshop on Computational Linguistics and Clinical Psychology: From Linguistic Signal to Clinical Reality.* Baltimore, MA: Association for Computational Linguistics (2014). 7–16.
43. McManus K, Mallory EK, Goldfeder RL, Haynes WA, Tatum JD. Mining Twitter Data to improve detection of schizophrenia. *AMIA Jt Summits Transl Sci Proc.* (2015) 2015:122–6.
44. Park M, McDonald DW, Cha M. Perception differences between the depressed and non-depressed users in twitter. In: Kiciman E, Ellison NB, Hogan B, Resnick P, Soboroff I, editors. *Proceedings of the Seventh International Conference on Weblogs and Social Media.* Cambridge, MA: AAAAI Press (2013). 476–85.
45. Goodfellow I, Bengio Y, Courville A. *Deep Learning.* Vol. 1. Cambridge, MA: MIT Press (2016). 864.
46. Koutsouleris N, Kambeitz-Ilankovic L, Ruhrmann S, Rosen M, Ruef A, Dwyer DB, et al. Individualized prediction of functional outcomes in mental healthcare: a multi-modal, multi-site machine learning analysis in the clinical high-risk state for psychosis and recent-onset depression. *JAMA Psychiatry* (2018).
47. Borsboom D, Cramer AO, Schmittmann VD, Epskamp S, Waldorp LJ. The small world of psychopathology. *PLoS ONE* (2011) 6:e27407. doi: 10.1371/journal.pone.0027407
48. Nelson B, McGorry PD, Wichers M, Wigman JTW, Hartmann JA. Moving from static to dynamic models of the onset of mental disorder: a review. *JAMA Psychiatry* (2017) 74:528–34. doi: 10.1001/jamapsychiatry.2017.0001
49. Goldberg D. Psychopathology and classification in psychiatry. *Soc Psychiatry Psychiatr Epidemiol.* (2015) 50:1–5. doi: 10.1007/s00127-014-0924-y

6

Neural and Behavioral Predictors of Treatment Efficacy on Mood Symptoms and Cognition in Mood Disorders

Ida Seeberg[1,2], *Hanne L. Kjaerstad*[1] *and Kamilla W. Miskowiak*[1,2*]

[1] *Neurocognition and Emotion in Affective Disorders Group, Copenhagen Affective Disorder Research Centre, Psychiatric Centre Copenhagen, Rigshospitalet, Copenhagen University Hospital, Copenhagen, Denmark,* [2] *Department of Psychology, University of Copenhagen, Copenhagen, Denmark*

Correspondence:
Kamilla W. Miskowiak
Kamilla@miskowiak.dk

Background: The clinical and etiological heterogeneity of mood disorders impede identification of effective treatments for the individual patient. This highlights a need for early neuronal and behavioral biomarkers for treatment efficacy, which can provide a basis for more personalized treatments. The present systematic review aimed to identify the most consistent neuronal and behavioral predictors of treatment efficacy on mood symptoms and cognitive impairment in mood disorders.

Methods: We identified and included 60 original peer-reviewed studies investigating neuroimaging and behavioral predictors of treatment efficacy within the domains of emotional and non-emotional cognition, structural neuroimaging, and resting state functional connectivity in patients with unipolar or bipolar disorder.

Results: Lower baseline responsivity in limbic regions coupled with heightened medial and dorsal prefrontal responses to emotional stimuli were the most consistent predictors of response to pharmacotherapy for depression. In contrast, heightened limbic and ventral prefrontal reactivity to emotional stimuli seemed to predict efficacy of psychological interventions. Early modulation of fronto-limbic activity and reduction in negative bias were also associated with treatment response. Better performance on non-emotional tests at baseline was relatively consistently associated with efficacy on mood symptoms, whereas the association between neural activity during non-emotional tests and treatment response was less clear. Other baseline factors associated with treatment response were greater white matter integrity, resting state functional connectivity, more prefrontal gray matter volume as well as an early increase following short administered treatment. Finally, emerging evidence indicates that baseline cognitive deficits are associated with greater chances of achieving treatment efficacy on cognition.

Conclusions: Patients' profile of emotional and non-emotional cognition and neural activity—and the early treatment-associated changes in neural and cognitive function—may be useful for guiding treatments for depression. While cognitive deficits at baseline seem to improve chances of treatment efficacy on cognition, more studies of this association are urgently needed.

Keywords: mood disorders, treatment, biomarker, cognition, neuroimaging, treatment efficacy, personalized medicine, precision medicine

INTRODUCTION

Unipolar depression (UD) and bipolar disorder (BD) are among top contributors to the global burden of disease, with UD being the single largest contributor to global disability worldwide (1). At a global level, more than 300 million people suffer from UD and 60 million from BD (1) and the economic cost of these affective disorders is estimated to be €113 billion in Europe and $128 billion in the United States per year (2, 3). Despite the major economic imperatives to optimize treatment for these disorders, current treatment options are limited by insufficient efficacy on depressive symptoms for 30–40% of patients, general time lag of several months before an effective treatment can be identified for the individual patient, and frequent residual cognitive impairments (4–6). Specifically, cognitive impairment has emerged as a new treatment target based on evidence for persistent mild to moderate cognitive impairments beyond the acute illness episodes in both UD and BD that impede patients' functional recovery and quality of life (7, 8).

Presently, first-line treatments for mood disorders include pharmacological treatment with selective serotonin reuptake inhibitors (SSRI) and/or evidence-based psychotherapy, such as cognitive-behavioral therapy (CBT) (9). However, it is often unclear which treatment is optimal for the individual patient until after several weeks of treatment given the delay in the onset of response to pharmacotherapy and psychotherapy of 4–6 weeks (10). Therefore present clinical practice and guidelines for best treatment strategy relies on a trial and error approach and a pragmatic advice on switching to a different treatment after 4–6 weeks of continued treatment with a therapeutic dose. As most patients do not respond to their first prescribed treatment, this leads to a substantial time lag of several months before an effective treatment can be identified for the individual patient. In this time, patients' ability to work and function in everyday life is severely affected, resulting in great personal and socioeconomic costs. Notwithstanding, there is no clinically useful guideline as to which specific treatment would be the most optimal for the individual patient based on their particular symptom presentation (9–11).

The clinical and etiological heterogeneity of patients with mood disorders implicates distinct pathophysiological profiles for each individual patient (12, 13). This highlights a pressing need for identification of biomarkers of treatment efficacy that can serve as a platform for personalized treatments. A major focus of recent research has therefore been to identify associations between biological or psychological measures and treatment response. Clinical predictors of treatment efficacy, such as severity or depressive clinical subtypes, have so far shown disappointing predictive value of improvement on mood symptoms. Genetic testing, neuroimaging, psychological and psychophysiological approaches have therefore been employed (9, 14). In particular, identification of early predictors of antidepressant response at neural and cognitive level seems an essential step to more effectively personalized treatment options (10). However, the findings from the large number of neuroimaging and behavioral studies of efficacy markers vary, and there is no clear understanding of what are the most robust neurocognitive biomarkers of treatment efficacy on mood symptoms.

More recently, studies have begun to investigate treatments that directly target residual cognitive impairments in mood disorders. Specifically, recent studies have found global or selective cognitive difficulties in 50–70% remitted patients with mood disorders, and poorer quality of life, more stress and impaired work capacity in cognitively impaired patients relatively to those who are "cognitively intact" (8). While there is currently no clinically available treatment for cognitive impairment in mood disorders, there is strong preliminary evidence for several candidate treatments including, modafinil, vortioxetine, erythropoietin, lurasidone and cognitive remediation (15–20). Nevertheless, treatment development targeting cognition is hampered by the lack of insight into the neurobiological underpinnings of cognitive improvement and lack insight into baseline predictors of efficacy on cognition.

Taken together, there is a need for insight into what are the most robust biomarkers of treatment efficacy on mood symptoms and cognition to aid more effective, personalized treatments. The aim of the present systematic review is therefore to provide a "landscape" view of putative functional and structural neuroimaging and behavioral predictors of treatment efficacy on depressive symptoms and cognition in mood disorders. Based on this, a discussion will be formed on the identified putative biomarkers and how they may be integrated in the clinical assessments of patients to aid speed and efficacy of future treatment strategies.

METHODS

Selection Criteria

The initial search criteria were defined in accordance to PICO framework (Population, Intervention, Comparison, Outcome). We included original peer-reviewed articles involving predictive intervention studies on patients with a mood disorder (unipolar or bipolar disorder) and no comorbid schizophrenia/schizoaffective disorder. The primary criterion was a focus on prediction of treatment response or remission using either neuroimaging (fMRI or MRI) or objective neurocognitive testing as a measure. We excluded articles that were naturalistic in design with no control of treatment; involved pediatric, adolescent or geriatric participants; only assessed cognitive measures with subjectively informed ratings; only looked at single drug administrations (with no follow-up of treatment efficacy following longer term treatment). Other reasons for exclusion were: other languages than English; meeting abstract, case report or study protocol; animal studies; comorbid schizoaffective disorder.

Search Strategy

A systematic computerized search was performed on PubMed/MEDLINE, EMBASE and PsychInfo databases from inception up until October 2017. The search profile included three elements: "biomarker," "neuroimaging OR cognition" and "mood disorder AND therapy/treatment" with each their combinations in the respective databases (see supplementary material for more details).

Two of the authors (IS and HLK) independently performed a primary title/abstract screening for potentially eligible articles and, following this, a secondary full-text screening was conducted. In both primary and secondary screening, we considered each of the unique references according to inclusion/exclusion criteria, but only provided information on the specific reasons for exclusion of papers in the secondary screening. Finally, a hand search was performed by tracking and screening the citations of the included articles for possible extra inclusions. Agreement between the two authors who performed the screening (IS and HK) was good (primary: 94%, secondary: 87%), and any disagreements were discussed and consensus was reached in all cases. This systematic review has followed the procedures of the *Preferred reporting items for systematic reviews and meta-analysis* (PRISMA) statement (21), and a PRISMA flowchart can be seen in **Figure 1**.

RESULTS

The initial screening identified 2030 articles (duplicate hits excluded). Out of these, 158 articles were included for titles/abstracts screening, resulting in 89 full-text articles evaluated for eligibility. Of these, 60 met inclusion criteria and were included in this review. In total, 58 studies explored different predictors of treatment efficacy on *mood symptoms*: 26 investigated "hot" (emotional) cognition with behavioral and functional neuroimaging measures, 15 investigated neuroimaging and behavioral measures of "cold" (non-emotional) cognition as predictors of treatment response on mood symptoms, ten investigated resting-state functional neuroimaging measures, and eight investigated structural neuroimaging measures. Only two studies investigated predictors of treatment efficacy on *cognition* using demographic variables and behavioral measures of cognition.

Emotional Cognition to Predict Treatment Response on Mood Symptoms

The 26 studies of "hot" cognition as a putative biomarker of treatment response examined behavioral and neuroimaging measures of facial emotion processing and regulation, implicit processing of emotion pictures, emotional self-referential processing, and reward processing (see Supplementary Table 1 for study details).

Behavioral Measures of Emotion Processing

Only one published study to date examined early change in behavioral assays of emotion processing as a predictor of subsequent treatment response (22). The study revealed that early increase in the recognition of happy facial expressions in the first 2 weeks of treatment with the SSRI citalopram or the SNRI reboxetine predicted clinical improvement indicated by reduction in total score on Clinical Outcome in Routine Evaluation (CORE). In contrast, early treatment-associated improvements in the recognition of disgust and surprise were not associated with treatment response.

Neuroimaging Data on Emotion Processing

Neural response to emotional faces

Fourteen studies explored whether treatment response was associated with baseline neural activity to emotional faces or with the early effects of treatment on neural response to emotional faces in UD or BD (23–36).

Overall, the studies found that those patients who went on to respond to antidepressant treatment (i.e., treatment responders) exhibited amygdala *hypo*-activity to negative facial expressions at baseline compared to healthy controls (32, 34). Further, one study compared responders to healthy controls and specified that the association between baseline amygdala *hypo*-activity to facial emotions signaling reward and threat and treatment response was independent of medication type (SSRIs escitalopram or sertraline vs. SNRI venlafaxine). In keeping with this, the study reported an association between amygdala *hyper*-activity to sad facial expression and non-response to venlafaxine compared to healthy controls (32). One study found that this association between amygdala *hypo*-activity to sad faces and subsequent treatment response to the anticholinergic antidepressant scopalomine could only be observed when patients were required to attend to the faces (i.e., instructed to focus explicitly on the faces' portion of the picture) in the presence of meaningful distractor stimuli (34). Consistent with this, one study reported that lowered baseline activity in middle occipital cortex (i.e., visual processing area) during encoding and recognition of faces with (task-irrelevant) emotional expressions was associated with better treatment response to scopalomine (29). Notably, Redlich et al. (36) did not find any significant predictors of treatment response to electroconvulsive therapy (ECT), though reported that both treatment groups (ECT and pharmacotherapy) showed increased amygdala reactivity to sad faces at baseline compared to healthy controls.

Studies have also found consistent associations between responses to either drug treatment or chronotherapy (combinations of repeated total sleep deprivation and light therapy) and baseline prefrontal activity in UD and BD (23, 27, 31). Specifically, UD responders to SSRIs fluoxetine or sertraline exhibited *greater* anterior cingulate cortex (ACC) response to fearful, angry and sad faces compared to non-responders (23, 30, 31). In keeping with this, BD-I responders to chronotherapy showed greater ACC and medial prefrontal cortex (MPFC) response during implicit processing of fearful and angry facial expressions compared to non-responders (31). Further, greater dorsomedial PFC (DMPFC) and posterior cingulate cortex (PCC) response to sad faces in UD was associated with better response to treatment with the noradrenergic and specific serotonergic antidepressant (NaSSA) mirtazapine or venlafaxine (27).

Finally, three studies reported an association between greater functional connectivity (FC) (i.e., closer to healthy controls) and treatment response to chronotherapy or pharmacotherapy (26, 31, 35). In particular, two studies found that responders to either chronotherapy or SSRI showed greater baseline activity and FC within fronto-limbic networks during implicit processing of fearful and angry faces (31, 35). In accordance with this, responders to either venlafaxine or mirtazapine had increased

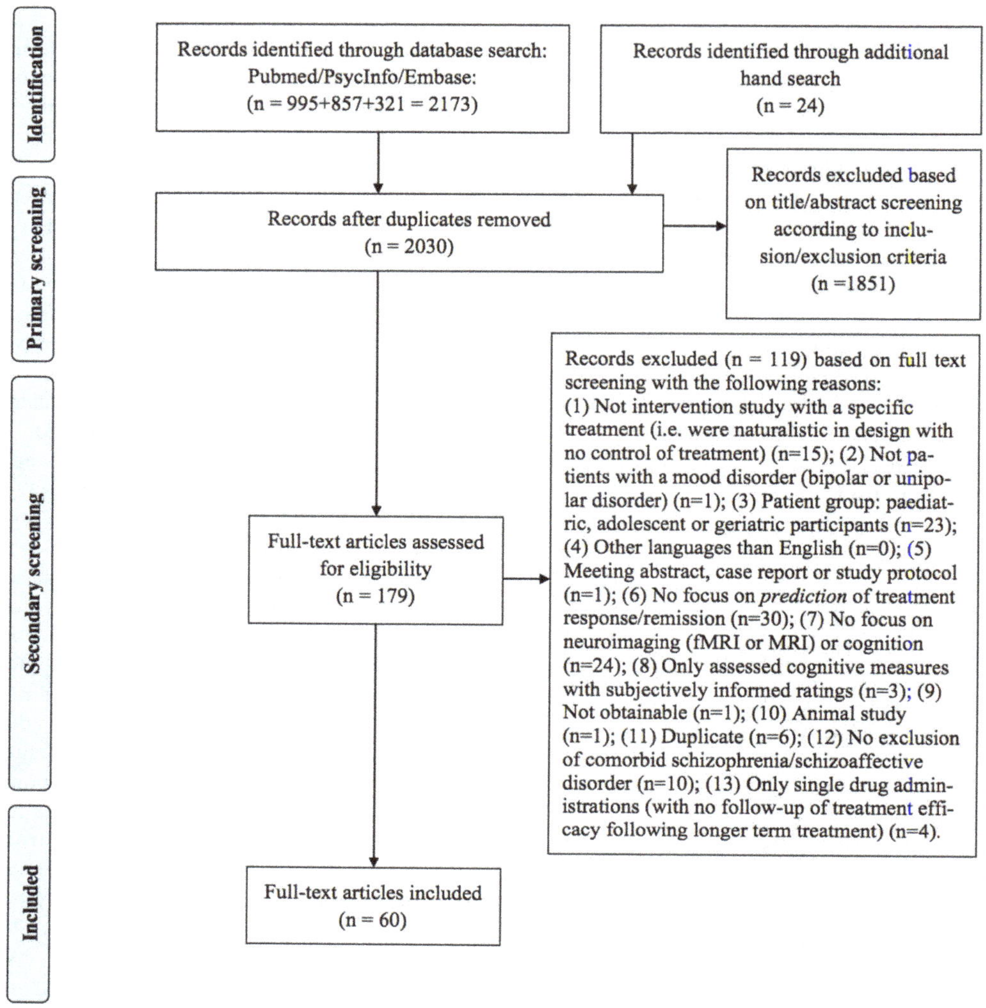

FIGURE 1 | PRISMA flow-chart.

FC of the orbitofrontal cortex (OFC) in the left precentral gyrus and internally within the right middle OFC during an emotional face-matching task at baseline (26).

Notably, two studies of CBT revealed the opposite association between baseline neural activity and treatment response (24, 25). Specifically, responders to CBT displayed *lower* dorsal ACC (DACC) activity to sad faces at baseline compared to non-responders (24). In fact, responders' DACC response to sad faces was more "normal" (i.e., more similar to the activity in healthy controls) than non-responders'. Moreover, one study reported that the FC during processing of sad faces at the lowest and highest intensities identified patients who had a full clinical response to CBT (25).

Only a few studies (all conducted on patients with UD) explored whether *early changes* in neural response to emotional faces can predict subsequent treatment efficacy (28, 29, 33). Nevertheless, these studies provide consistent evidence for early modulation of limbic-subcortical-prefrontal brain networks being predictive of subsequent treatment efficacy. One study found that early treatment-related *decrease* (toward normal levels) in ACC, insula, amygdala, and thalamus reactivity to fearful faces after 1 week characterized responders vs. non-responders to escitalopram (33). In contrast, responders to the SSRI paroxetine showed an early treatment-related *decrease* in amygdala response to negative faces (relative to baseline) compared to non-responders, as well as an *increase* in lower dorsal regions (DLPFC and DMPFC) to negative faces (toward "normal" levels) after six weeks of treatment relative to non-responders (28). This suggests that paroxetine exposure over time improves dorsal prefrontal regulation of abnormal limbic activity. Another study found that following short-term (1 week) scopalomine administration, responders exhibited *increased* response (closer to "normal") in bilateral middle occipital cortex (relative to baseline) during encoding and recognition of faces with (task-irrelevant) emotional expressions (29).

Neural response to emotional pictures

Five fMRI studies investigated the predictive value of baseline neural activity during emotional reactivity and emotional regulation using emotion-laden picture stimuli for efficacy of pharmacotherapy in UD (37–41). Responders to a combination treatment with fluoxetine and antipsychotic olanzapine or to venlafaxine were characterized by *greater* baseline activity to *negative* images in the ACC and premotor cortex and to *positive* images in the posterior cingulate gyrus and precuneus than non-responders (37, 40). Further, *lower* ventrolateral PFC (VLPFC) activity at baseline during attempts to suppress positive emotions elicited by pleasant pictures was associated with greater reduction in anhedonia after venlafaxine or fluoxetine treatment (38). Finally, a study of CBT found that *greater* pre-treatment activity in the DLPFC and anterior temporal lobe (ATL) to negative images and to pictures in general (emotional and neutral) predicted symptom improvement after CBT (39).

Only one study investigated the predictive value of early changes in neural activity in response to the mood-stabilizer lithium or the atypical antipsychotic quetiapine for subsequent treatment efficacy (41). Patients with BD-I who later achieved remission exhibited an early *increase* in MPFC, temporal, and posterior cortical areas to emotional (unpleasant) pictures after 1 week of either lithium or quetiapine treatment. Also, while amygdala activity at baseline and after short-term treatment administration did not predict treatment remission, non-remission was associated with baseline *hypo*-activity in the amygdala in comparison to healthy controls and remitted subjects (41).

Neural response during emotional self-referential processing

Four fMRI studies explored the predictive value of neural response during emotional self-referential processing at baseline (i.e., in which patients were instructed to judge the personal relevance of a picture or word) (42–45). Delaveau et al. (45) found that UD remitters to treatment with the atypical antidepressant agomelatine (melatonin and serotonin receptor antagonist) displayed lower baseline activation in the rostral DMPFC, PCC, and DLPFC during self-referential processing of emotional and neutral pictures compared to non-remitters. Consistent with this, Miller et al. (44) found that UD responders to escitalopram displayed lower baseline responses to negative self-referent words in midbrain, DLPFC, paracingulate, ACC, thalamus and caudate nuclei compared to non-responders.

Two studies of baseline neural activity predictors for response to CBT revealed a somewhat different pattern (42, 43). Specifically, patients with amygdala *hyper*-activity and low subgenual ACC (sgACC) reactivity during self-referent processing of negative emotional words displayed the most improvement after CBT (42, 43). In addition sgACC activity remained low for patients in remission after treatment, suggesting that successful treatment did not operate by normalizing this mechanism but rather by remaining more like healthy individuals from pretreatment to posttreatment measurements (43). Notably, no studies of self-referent processing explored the association between early neural activity changes and subsequent clinical improvement in response to pharmacological or psychological interventions.

Neuroimaging and behavioral measures of reward processing

Two studies of reward processing as a putative biomarker for response to behavioral activation therapy for depression (BATD) (46, 47) found that neural response to monetary awards at baseline was predictive of treatment efficacy. Specifically, increased frontostriatal connectivity during reward anticipation and increased capacity to sustain ACC activity when receiving rewards, were found to be associated with greater treatment response (46, 47). Consistent with this, Carl et al. (46) reported that greater change in reaction time during reward trials (i.e., faster response at run 2) at baseline predicted treatment response.

Interim Summary

In sum, responders to pharmacotherapy tend to be characterized by heightened PFC top-down control as well as *greater* recruitment of ACC and/or lowered limbic and visual cortical reactivity during the processing of emotional stimuli than non-responders. Accordingly, particularly *less* limbic and occipital reactivity to task-irrelevant emotional aspects of faces in preference for cognitively demanding tasks was associated with better antidepressant efficacy. In contrast, responders to psychological interventions seem to be characterized by a pattern of *greater* baseline limbic reactivity, *less* PFC response to emotional stimuli and *greater* neural response to reward stimuli.

Additionally, the small number of studies investigating *change* in neural activity after 1–6 weeks of pharmacological treatment consistently indicate that treatment-related reduction in limbic activity and increase in DPFC top-down control to negative valence emotional stimuli are putative early predictors of response to distinct biological interventions.

Non-emotional Cognition to Predict Treatment Response on Mood Symptoms

A total of 13 studies investigated "cold" cognition as a putative biomarker for treatment response on mood symptoms (see Supplementary Table 2 for study details). Five studies assessed neuroimaging measures, while eight studies examined purely behavioral assays of non-emotional cognition as biomarkers of treatment efficacy (7, 15, 48–58).

Combined Neuroimaging and Behavioral Measures of Non-emotional Cognition

Five studies used a combination of neuroimaging and neurocognitive assessment to investigate baseline predictors for treatment response on mood symptoms in patients with UD (51, 52, 55, 57, 58). Two studies of inhibitory control found that aberrant neural activity within prefrontal regions during a parametric Go/No-go task predicted subsequent treatment efficacy. In one study, patients who responded well to duloxetine, escitalopram or citalopram treatment showed more *unsuccessful* inhibition (i.e., more performance errors) at baseline as well as less recruitment (i.e., *lower activation)* of brain areas important for cognitive control and/or interference resolution, including the ACC, left VMPFC and right VLPFC (58). In contrast, the other study found that *greater* rostral ACC activation during *unsuccessful* inhibition was associated with subsequent treatment response (51).

Two studies of patients with UD found an association between aberrant neural activity during verbal working memory and clinical response to fluoxetine and rTMS, respectively (52, 57). Specifically, the fluoxetine study reported *lower* DACC during verbal n-back working memory at baseline in responders vs. non-responders (52). In contrast, the rTMS study found that responders displayed a *combination* of lower activity in perigenual, medial OFC, and middle frontal cortices, and a greater activation in the ventral-caudal putamen during a word-generation task at baseline compared to non-responders (57). Notably, a third study (55) found no significant associations between treatment response to rTMS and structural or behavioral measures at baseline.

Behavioral Measures of Non-emotional Cognition

Seven studies explored purely *behavioral* assays of non-emotional baseline cognition (i.e., performance accuracy and speed) as potential predictors of treatment response on depression symptoms in patients with UD and BD (7, 15, 48–50, 53, 54).

Four studies reported that *better* cognitive performance across several domains predicted response to antidepressant treatment (7, 48, 50, 53). In particular, two studies of UD patients found that responders to fluoxetine displayed better baseline performance in executive functioning and mental processing speed than non-responders (48, 50). The third study showed that greater attention performance at baseline was associated with better clinical outcome in UD patients treated with agomelatine (7). Finally, the fourth study found that UD and BD patients with less over-general memory (i.e., lack of memory for specific episodes, which is a key feature of depression) recovered faster from depression and were at lower risk for relapse after ECT (53).

In contrast, one study found that *poor* cognitive performance predicted subsequent clinical response. Specifically, UD responders to the new norepinephrine–dopamine reuptake inhibitor bupropion displayed visual memory deficits and slowed mental processing speed at baseline (15).

Finally, two studies showed that a *combination* of high and low performance within different cognitive domains predicted treatment response to SSRIs (49, 54). In particular, one study found that a combination of good sustained attention performance and poor psychomotor speed and planning performance predicted response to fluoxetine (54). A similar pattern of good cognitive performance on "simple" tasks and poor performance in "complex" tasks (requiring more demanding effort and maintenance) was observed in responders vs. non-responders to SSRI (drug not specified) (49).

Only one study investigated *early change* in cognition as a biomarker for treatment response in patients with UD and BD (56). This study revealed that early improvement in visuospatial memory after 2–3 weeks of rTMS treatment predicted eventual treatment response. Interestingly, the initial cognitive changes appeared to be independent of antidepressant efficacy, since patients' cognitive improvement occurred *before* any mood changes. In contrast, early treatment-related improvements in verbal learning and memory and attention span were not related to subsequent treatment response (56).

Interim Summary

Taken together, findings from functional neuroimaging studies highlight aberrant neural activity during non-emotional cognition tasks as a putative prognostic biomarker. The most consistent marker of treatment response seems to be less recruitment of dorsal PFC during cognitive performance. Studies of *behavioral* performance measures on non-emotional cognitive tests in UD and BD patients provided more consistent findings. Specifically, it was demonstrated in several studies that *high* performance across attention, executive function, and memory tests was a predictor of response to pharmacological interventions (SSRI and SNRI), rTMS, and ECT for depression (7, 48, 50, 53). Additionally, a couple of other studies found that a combination of good performance on simple tests and poor performance on complex tests might predict treatment efficacy (49, 54).

Combined Emotional and Non-emotional Cognition to Predict Mood Improvement

Two studies investigated whether a pattern of emotional and non-emotional cognitive performance could be used to identify the individual patients who would achieve clinical remission in response to escitalopram, sertraline, or venlafaxine (11, 59) (see Supplementary Table 3 for study details). Using a novel pattern classification analysis, Etkin et al. (59) and colleagues showed poorer treatment outcomes for a subgroup of depressed participants (approximately one-quarter of patients) with impairment across most cognitive and emotional capacities. High task performance predicted remission after escitalopram treatment (but not other medications) with 72% accuracy. The other study investigated whether predictions of remission could be made with a larger cognitive assessment battery, including eight non-emotional tests tapping into several cognitive domains and one emotional identification test (11). The study reported that the test battery thresholds established a negative predictive value of ≥80%, which identified 41% of participants not remitting on escitalopram, 77% of participants not remitting on sertraline, and 39% of participants not remitting on venlafaxine (all including 20% false negatives). These findings provide promising ways to predict treatment efficacy with a high sensitivity and specificity for each individual patient, although replication is needed to establish an applicable tool for clinical use.

Resting State Functional Connectivity to Predict Treatment Response on Mood Symptoms

Ten studies investigated the association between resting state and FC at baseline and treatment response in UD and BD (9, 10, 60–67) (see Supplementary Table 4 for study details).

Four of these found that greater baseline resting-state FC in the PFC predicted response to treatment with rTMS applied to either DLPFC or DMPFC (60–62, 67). Specifically, Ge et al. (67) found that both UD and BD patients who responded well to treatment displayed enhanced contributions to functional connectivity, namely hyper-connectivity in ACC/VMPFC within the anterior default mode network (DMN) and DACC/insula within the salience network. Downar et al. (60) found that at baseline, UD and BD responders showed increased connectivity within reward pathways, including left VMPFC, the ventral tegmental area, and striatum compared with non-responders. Liston et al. (61) found that baseline hyperconnectivity between the sgACC and multiple areas of the DMN and central executive network independently predicted greater clinical improvements after TMS. Finally, Salomons et al. (62) found that higher baseline FC between DLPFC and a medial prefrontal cluster spanning the subgenual cingulate gyrus and DMPFC was associated with better response to treatment in UD and BD. In addition, patients with low baseline cortico-thalamic (DMPFC-medial dorsal thalamus), cortico-striatal (DMPFC-putamen), and cortico-limbic (sgACC-amygdala and sgACC-hippocampus) connectivity also experienced a greater response to the treatment (62).

Among UD patients treated with BATD, responders were characterized by greater baseline connectivity between the right insula and right middle temporal gyrus (63). For UD patients given CBT, remission was predicted by greater positive FC at baseline with the subcallosal cingulate cortex and three regions: the dorsal midbrain, VLPFC/insula, and VMPFC (9). The latter study also compared patients receiving CBT with those treated with antidepressant medications (escitalopram or duloxetine). This revealed that *negative* FC (i.e., anti-correlations of activity over time) between the same regions was associated with remission in medication-treated patients (9). The study thus suggests that the direction of baseline FC can be used to predict whether an individual is more likely to benefit from psychotherapy or pharmacotherapy. Finally, assessment of UD patients with treatment-resistant depression (TRD) receiving ECT (64) revealed that the brain areas in which resting-state activity provided the largest contribution in predicting subsequent remission were the cingulate cortex, medial- and orbitofrontal cortices, although the direction of connectivity (increased vs. decreased) was not specified.

Four studies of both UD and BD patients found evidence of *early change* in neural activity during resting state that predicted subsequent response to various biological treatments (10, 62, 65, 66). Specifically, efficacy of rTMS and ECT was associated with early *increase* in positive/negative fronto-limbic connectivity, respectively (62, 65). Also, another study using transcutaneous vagus nerve stimulation (tVNS) for treatment of UD found that treatment responders exhibited early increase in left anterior insula activity after the first treatment session (66). In contrast, Cheng et al. (10) found that responders to escitalopram were characterized by early decrease in occipital cortex activity and increase in DLPFC, DMPFC, and middle cingulate cortex activity only 5 h after initial treatment administration. However, the best predictor of clinical remission was increased activity in ACC, midcingulate cortex, and right superior temporal gyrus (STG) 5 h after administration of escitalopram to endpoint. Moreover, aberrant (increased and decreased, respectively) FC between cingulate and limbic areas was predictive of response in patients who were treated with either ECT or rTMS (62, 65).

Interim Summary

Taken together, the findings support the idea that greater positive fronto-limbic connectivity during resting state at baseline is predictive of treatment response to a psychotherapeutic intervention. In contrast, decreased fronto-limbic connectivity is predictive of response for antidepressant medication treatment. Additionally, response to antidepressant treatment was associated with early *increase* (positive and negative) in fronto-limbic connectivity during resting state.

Structural Abnormalities to Predict Treatment Response on Mood Symptoms

Grey Matter

Four studies investigated the association between gray matter (GM) and treatment response in UD (23, 68–70) (see Supplementary Table 5 for study details). Two studies found that at baseline, decreased hippocampal volume and increased subgenual cingulate gyrus volume, respectively, were associated with better clinical response to electroconvulsive therapy (ECT) (69, 70). In addition a study of patients undergoing pharmacotherapy with fluoxetine found that greater GM volume at baseline in the ACC, insula, and right temporo-parietal cortex predicted faster and better symptom improvement (23). In keeping with this, one study of patients undergoing either pharmacotherapy with fluoxetine or CBT found that clinical remission to pharmacotherapy was predicted by greater GM volume density in the right rostral ACC, left PCC, whereas no prediction was found for CBT (68). Two studies have investigated the association between early change in GM and treatment efficacy to ECT (69, 70). These revealed early increase in hippocampal and amygdala volume (as well as in clinical symptoms) that is observable already after two ECT sessions and that this increase in volume (and the improved symptoms) predicted subsequent response to ECT (69, 70). Redlich et al. (70) also found increased GM volume in left hippocampus in patients receiving ECT over time (mean 6 weeks), pointing to a reversal of hippocampal volume loss in these patients.

White Matter

Four studies investigated whether white matter (WM) integrity is predictive of treatment efficacy (71–74) (see Supplementary Table 5 for study details). A study of WM integrity in BD patients undergoing treatment with the atypical antipsychotic lurasidone showed that greater baseline fractional anisotropy (FA) in multiple regions, including tracts in the frontal and parietal lobes, predicted greater reduction in depressive symptoms (74). The other two studies investigated WM integrity in UD undergoing treatment with escitalopram (71, 72). One study found that remission was predicted by a pattern of higher FA in the cingulum cingulate tract (that connects the cingulate gyrus to the hippocampus) and lower FA in the stria terminalis tract (that connects the hippocampus to the hypothalamus and the rest of the limbic system) (72). The other study (71) found that lower baseline FA in the right amygdala tracts originating from the mid-brain could distinguish non-remitters from remitters. The study also showed a correlation between average FA in tracts to the right amygdala and SSRI treatment response. One final study examining WM integrity in BD undergoing chronotherapy (a combination of total sleep deprivation and morning light therapy) observed how the degree of reduction of WM integrity also biases the efficacy of treatment, so that clinical improvement negatively correlated with WM integrity (73).

Interim Summary

Overall, findings from structural neuroimaging studies point to lower hippocampal GM volume and greater ACC volume at baseline being predictors of response to pharmacotherapy and ECT in UD.

Non-emotional Cognition to Predict Clinically Relevant Cognitive Improvements

Only two studies to date have explored the impact of cognitive performance at baseline on treatment efficacy on cognition (18, 19) (see Supplementary Table 6 for study details). Both were based on a randomized controlled study of erythropoietin (EPO) treatment of patients with BD in partial remission or with treatment-resistant UD patients. The reports revealed that patients with cognitive dysfunction at baseline—as reflected by cognitive performance levels that were ≥1 SD below the norm on the targeted memory domain (18) or ≥1 on two or more domains (19) were substantially more likely to achieve treatment efficacy on cognition than those who were less impaired. This was not related to simple regression toward the mean with repeated cognitive testing since no such effect of baseline deficits was observed in the placebo group (18). In contrast, subjectively self-reported cognitive difficulties were only weakly (albeit statistically significantly) associated with better chances of achieving treatment efficacy on cognition in one (18) but not the other study (19). Taken together these two studies highlight the importance of baseline deficits in cognition for treatment efficacy on cognition. However, further studies with different interventions are necessary before any firm conclusions can be drawn regarding the impact of baseline cognition on the chances of treatment efficacy on cognitive impairment.

DISCUSSION

Overall Findings

There is a pressing need for insight into how we can most effectively adapt treatments for mood disorders to the individual patient. This systematic review identified sixty functional or structural neuroimaging and/or behavioral studies of *baseline* and *early change* biomarkers that were predictive of subsequent clinical efficacy on either depressive symptoms or cognitive impairments. An overview of the results is presented in **Figure 2**. The vast majority of studies (58 of 60) focused on delineating predictors of treatment response on depressive symptoms. The most consistent predictors of mood improvement were heightened PFC top-down control and greater recruitment of ACC and/or lowered limbic reactivity to negative emotional stimuli as well as high behavioral performance on non-emotional cognitive tests at baseline. Specifically, lower baseline reactivity in limbic and occipital regions coupled with greater recruitment of dorsal and medial PFC regions seems to predict better response to *pharmacotherapy*. Further, early treatment-related increase in happiness recognition and modulation of neural activity to negative stimuli in the cortico-limbic circuitry were found in several studies to predict response to several biological treatments. In contrast, *greater* baseline reactivity in limbic regions and *lower* PFC response to negative information, greater fronto-striatal connectivity as well as sustained ACC activity to reward stimuli were the most consistent predictors of response to *psychological* interventions. In addition, resting state fMRI studies showed some evidence for *lower* fronto-limbic connectivity at baseline and for an early increase in fronto-limbic connectivity predicting response to pharmacological interventions. In contrast, more positive fronto-limbic connectivity was found in resting state fMRI studies to predict response to psychotherapeutic interventions. Finally, lower baseline hippocampal GM volume, greater ACC volume and greater FA were found in structural neuroimaging studies to predict response to pharmacotherapy and ECT, while one study found that increased volume in hippocampus and amygdala after only two ECT sessions predicted later clinical response. In contrast to the large number of studies investigating predictors of mood improvement, only two studies investigated baseline predictors of treatment efficacy on cognition. These randomized, controlled studies revealed preliminary evidence for a strong association between objectively measured cognitive deficits at baseline and subsequent clinically relevant cognitive improvement. Notably, no published studies explored whether improvement in cognition could be predicted by neuronal response during cognitive testing, resting state functional connectivity or structural neuroimaging measures.

Emotional Cognition and Resting State Neural Activity as Biomarkers of Efficacy on Mood

Neural responses to emotional stimuli as well as functional connectivity during resting state seem to differentially predict treatment response to pharmacotherapy vs. psychological interventions and thereby aid treatment selection. For pharmacotherapy, the studies showed the best treatment response for patients exhibiting close to "normal" neural responses (i.e., low limbic reactivity and high PFC top-down control). Pharmacotherapy is hypothesized to normalize aberrant fronto-limbic activity to emotional stimuli by reducing the overwhelming influx of automatic negative cues early in treatment (75). This may explain why pharmacotherapy is more effective for patients with less aberrant neural network dysfunction. Regarding psychotherapy, the findings support the notion that heightened neural and cognitive reactivity (i.e., enhanced functional connectivity between limbic and prefrontal regions) are predictors of treatment response. It is tempting to speculate that patients with such greater limbic reactivity

BASELINE PREDICTORS OF TREATMENT RESPONSE	EARLY CHANGE PREDICTORS OF TREATMENT RESPONSE
Behavioural measures • ↑ Cognition predicts response on mood symptoms • ↓ Cognition may predict treatment efficacy on cognition	**Behavioural measures** • Early ↓ in cognitive response to negative stimuli seems to predict subsequent efficacy on mood symptoms
Activation-based fMRI measures • ↓ Limbic and ↑ medial and dorsal prefrontal response to emotional stimuli predict response to *pharmacotherapy* • ↑ Limbic and ventral prefrontal reactivity to emotional stimuli seems to predict efficacy of *psychological* interventions	**Activation-based fMRI measures** • Early modulation of fronto-limbic reactivity to emotional stimuli seems to be associated with subsequent response on mood symptoms
Resting state fMRI measures • ↓ Fronto-limbic connectivity predicts response to *pharmacotherapy* • ↑ Fronto-limbic connectivity seems to predict response to *psychological* interventions	**Resting state fMRI measures** • Early ↑ in fronto-limbic connectivity predicts subsequent response to *pharmacotherapy*
Structural MRI measures • ↑ Prefrontal grey matter volume seems to predict response on mood symptoms • ↑ White matter integrity seems to predict response on mood symptoms	**Structural MRI measures** • Early ↑ in hippocampal volume may predict subsequent response to electroconvulsive therapy

No studies investigated whether treatment-related improvement in cognition could be predicted by early change in neural response during non-emotional cognitive testing, resting state functional connectivity or structural neuroimaging measures.

FIGURE 2 | An overview of identified main predictors of treatment response.

to emotional stimuli may also engage more emotionally in psychotherapy and thereby benefit more from this type of intervention. Further, therapy can help patients restore the network dysfunction by strengthening their conscious PFC top-down control through cognitive reappraisal and cognitive restructuring of negative automatic thoughts (42, 76). This is interesting as functional neuroimaging studies of PTSD patients treated with CBT show that excessive fear processing of emotional stimuli in the limbic system is associated with poor clinical improvement (77). This is opposite to our findings on mood disorders and therefor underlines the importance of differentiating the profiles of the patients with affective disorders including anxiety disorders.

Non-emotional Cognition, Neural Activity and Structural Measures as Biomarkers of Efficacy on Mood

Overall, the included studies reported highly consistent evidence for better performance on non-emotional cognitive tests as a predictor of antidepressant treatment efficacy on mood symptoms. In addition, greater ACC volume and FA at baseline, as well as early volume increase in limbic regions, were predictors of response to biological treatments. Taken together, the greater cognitive performance and PFC volume in treatment responders may reflect greater capacity for neuroplasticity and is consistent with evidence for a link between good treatment prognosis and a cognitive reserve (i.e., the brain's capacity to compensate for neuropsychological damage and ability to maximize performance through recruitment of different brain networks and cognitive strategies) (8). Notably, lower hippocampal volume at baseline was also a predictor of treatment response (69, 70). This is interesting since longer duration and greater severity of depression are associated with more hippocampal volume reduction (78, 79). In light of these findings, the association between lower hippocampal volume and better treatment response could suggest that enhancement of hippocampal plasticity and neurogenesis may be key mechanisms of antidepressant drug treatment (80).

The findings from fMRI investigations on neural activity during non-emotional tests were generally unclear. Specifically, some studies found that *lower* task-related PFC activity during unsuccessful inhibition as well as a verbal working memory tasks at baseline predicted treatment response (52, 58), while other studies found that *greater* task-related PFC activity predicted treatment response (51), or that a combination of lower and higher task-related activity at baseline were predictors (i.e., lower activity in perigenual, medial OFC, and middle frontal cortices with greater activation in ventral-caudal putamen) (57). However, the overall most consistent predictor of treatment response seems to be lower response in prefrontal regions (in the absence of differences in cognitive performance) suggesting that those patients with the *most efficient* brain functioning (i.e., closer to normal with less recruitment of prefrontal resources during cognitive testing) responded better to pharmacological treatment. This adds to the notion that better brain function at baseline is a predictor of treatment response. Considering this, the discrepancies in results are likely due to the features of the different cognitive tasks employed (e.g., tests of psychomotor speed vs. executive functioning), as well as task difficulty, which have considerable effects on the strength and extent of the neural response (52). Other possible reasons for the discrepancies are patient selection (e.g., the severity of the depressive illness, illness course, inpatients vs. outpatients) and treatment modalities (different medications and clinical trial methodologies), as different pharmacological interventions might have subtle differences in mechanisms and therefore also different neuropsychological profiles for the responders.

Non-emotional Cognition as an Emerging Biomarker of Efficacy on Cognition

The emerging evidence for an association between cognitive dysfunction at baseline and patients' chances of achieving treatment efficacy on cognition has potential significance for future trials targeting cognition and for future clinical treatment of patients' cognitive deficits. Specifically, this association suggests that future intervention studies may improve their chances of demonstrating treatment efficacy by pre-screening patients for cognitive impairments before trial entry (18, 19). In addition, the use of a brief objective cognitive screener seems feasible for clinical decisions regarding which patients should be given a treatment for neurocognitive impairments rather than mood symptoms. However, notably this evidence comes from only two studies, and there is a remarkable absence of research into functional and structural neuroimaging predictors of treatment efficacy on cognition. This is a major impediment for development of better treatment strategies to target cognition. This issue and other major methodological challenges in cognition trials in mood disorders were recently addressed by a global task force of international experts in the field under the International Society for Bipolar Disorders (ISBD) (8, 16). The absence of insight into neuroimaging biomarkers for efficacy on cognition impedes insight into neurobiological targets of pro-cognitive interventions (8). Future cognition trials are therefore encouraged to implement neuroimaging assessments to increase our insight into the neurobiological predictors of cognitive improvements.

Limitations

A limitation of this systematic review was that the included studies did not consistently report on patient demographics (e.g., the severity of the depressive illness, illness course, inpatients vs. outpatients), and hence these factors were not controlled for. Also, the inclusion criterion for study design was non-specific and did not only include randomized controlled studies, adding to a question of study quality. Adding to this, another methodological limitation to the present systematic review is that only original peer-reviewed articles were included, and a current matter in neuroimaging literature is that studies with small sample sizes or negative results may be prone to publication bias (81, 82). However, the present systematic review followed the PRISMA guidelines including multiple procedures for identification of articles, thus limiting risk of bias (21). Nevertheless this review provides a landscape overview of prediction biomarkers for treatment efficacy on depressive symptoms and cognition in both unipolar and bipolar depression by combining neuroimaging and behavioral findings. This integrated understanding of pre-treatment and early change biomarkers are only preliminary, though very promising and may have a great impact in the clinical assessments of patients to aid in efficient treatment strategies.

CONCLUSION

In conclusion, this systematic review revealed several promising baseline biomarkers for prediction of treatment efficacy on mood symptoms including behavioral and neural measures of emotional and non-emotional cognition as well as cortico-limbic functional connectivity. The review also highlights a need for more studies of early treatment-related changes in these measures, since recent emerging evidence points to informative early change in emotional and non-emotional cognition before any clinical response in symptom reduction. While cognition is a new important treatment target in mood disorders, only two studies assessed the predictors of treatment response on cognition. These two reports found greater chances of treatment efficacy on cognition in patients presenting objective cognitive deficits at baseline. Nevertheless, there is a paucity of studies examining predictors of treatment-associated cognitive improvement. This highlights a pressing need for further investigation of cognitive measures and associated neuronal networks that can guide in the development of new treatment strategies targeting cognition.

AUTHOR CONTRIBUTIONS

KM as principal investigator had the overall responsibility of the systematic review. IS conducted the literature searches, under supervision of KM. IS and HK conducted the primary and secondary screening of articles for inclusion. IS and HK wrote the initial draft of the manuscript in collaboration with KM. All authors contributed to and approved the final report.

REFERENCES

1. WHO. *Depression and Other Common Mental DIsorders, Global Health Estimates.*(2017). Available online at: http://www.who.int/mental_health/management/depression/prevalence_global_health_estimates/en/: WHO
2. Wyatt RJ, Henter I. An economic evaluation of manic-depressive illness–1991. *Soc Psychiatry Psychiatr Epidemiol.* (1995) 30:213–9.
3. Olesen J, Gustavsson A, Svensson M, Wittchen HU, Jonsson B. The economic cost of brain disorders in Europe. *Eur J Neurol.* (2012) 19:155–62. doi: 10.1111/j.1468-1331.2011.03590.x
4. Hansen R, Gaynes B, Thieda P, Gartlehner G, Deveaugh-Geiss A, Krebs E, et al. Meta-analysis of major depressive disorder relapse and recurrence with second-generation antidepressants. *Psychiatr Serv.* (2008) 59:1121–30. doi: 10.1176/ps.2008.59.10.1121
5. Bourne C, Aydemir O, Balanza-Martinez V, Bora E, Brissos S, Cavanagh JT, et al. Neuropsychological testing of cognitive impairment in euthymic bipolar disorder: an individual patient data meta-analysis. *Acta Psychiatr Scand.* (2013) 128:149–62. doi: 10.1111/acps.12133
6. Bora E, Murray RM. Meta-analysis of cognitive deficits in ultra-high risk to psychosis and first-episode psychosis: do the cognitive deficits progress over, or after, the onset of psychosis? *Schizophr Bull.* (2014) 40:744–55. doi: 10.1093/schbul/sbt085
7. Clery-Melin ML, Gorwood P. A simple attention test in the acute phase of a major depressive episode is predictive of later functional remission. *Depress Anxiety* (2017) 34:159–70. doi: 10.1002/da.22575
8. Miskowiak KW, Burdick KE, Martinez-Aran A, Bonnin CM, Bowie CR, Carvalho AF, et al. Methodological recommendations for cognition trials in bipolar disorder by the International Society for Bipolar Disorders Targeting Cognition Task Force. *Bipolar Disord.* (2017) 19:614–26. doi: 10.1111/bdi.12534

9. Dunlop BW, Rajendra JK, Craighead WE, Kelley ME, Mcgrath CL, Choi KS, et al. Functional connectivity of the subcallosal cingulate cortex and differential outcomes to treatment with cognitive-behavioral therapy or antidepressant medication for major depressive disorder. *Am J Psychiatry* (2017) 174:533–45. doi: 10.1176/appi.ajp.2016.16050518
10. Cheng Y, Xu J, Arnone D, Nie B, Yu H, Jiang H, et al. Resting-state brain alteration after a single dose of SSRI administration predicts 8-week remission of patients with major depressive disorder. *Psychol Med.* (2017) 47:438–50. doi: 10.1017/S0033291716002440
11. Gordon E, Rush AJ, Palmer DM, Braund TA, Rekshan W. Toward an online cognitive and emotional battery to predict treatment remission in depression. *Neuropsychiatr Dis Treat.* (2015) 11:517–31.
12. Krishnan V, Nestler EJ. Linking molecules to mood: new insight into the biology of depression. *Am J Psychiatry* (2010) 167:1305–20. doi: 10.1176/appi.ajp.2009.10030434
13. Miskowiak KW, Kjaerstad HL, Meluken I, Petersen JZ, Maciel BR, Kohler CA, et al. The search for neuroimaging and cognitive endophenotypes: a critical systematic review of studies involving unaffected first-degree relatives of individuals with bipolar disorder. *Neurosci Biobehav Rev.* (2017) 73:1–22. doi: 10.1016/j.neubiorev.2016.12.011
14. Dunlop BW. Prediction of treatment outcomes in major depressive disorder. *Expert Rev Clin Pharmacol.* (2015) 8:669–72. doi: 10.1586/17512433.2015.1075390
15. Herrera-Guzman I, Gudayol-Ferre E, Lira-Mandujano J, Herrera-Abarca J, Herrera-Guzman D, Montoya-Perez K, et al. Cognitive predictors of treatment response to bupropion and cognitive effects of bupropion in patients with major depressive disorder. *Psychiatry Res.* (2008) 160:72–82. doi: 10.1016/j.psychres.2007.04.012
16. Miskowiak KW, Carvalho AF, Vieta E, Kessing LV. Cognitive enhancement treatments for bipolar disorder: a systematic review and methodological recommendations. *European Neuropsychopharmacology* (2016) 26:1541–61. doi: 10.1016/j.euroneuro.2016.08.011
17. Miskowiak KW, Petersen JZ, Ott CV, Knorr U, Kessing LV, Gallagher P, et al. Predictors of the discrepancy between objective and subjective cognition in bipolar disorder: a novel methodology. *Acta Psychiatr Scand.* (2016) 134:511–21. doi: 10.1111/acps.12649
18. Miskowiak KW, Rush AJJr, Gerds TA, Vinberg M, Kessing LV. Targeting treatments to improve cognitive function in mood disorder: suggestions from trials using erythropoietin. *J Clin Psychiatry* (2016) 77:e1639–e1646. doi: 10.4088/JCP.15m10480
19. Ott CV, Vinberg M, Kessing LV, Miskowiak KW. The effect of erythropoietin on cognition in affective disorders–Associations with baseline deficits and change in subjective cognitive complaints. *Eur Neuropsychopharmacol.* (2016) 26:1264–73. doi: 10.1016/j.euroneuro.2016.05.009
20. Vinberg M, Weikop P, Olsen NV, Kessing LV, Miskowiak K. Effect of recombinant erythropoietin on inflammatory markers in patients with affective disorders: A randomised controlled study. *Brain Behav Immun.* (2016) 57:53–7. doi: 10.1016/j.bbi.2016.05.006
21. Moher D, Liberati A, Tetzlaff J, Altman DG. Preferred reporting items for systematic reviews and meta-analyses: the PRISMA statement. *J Clin Epidemiol.* (2009) 62:1006–12. doi: 10.1016/j.jclinepi.2009.06.005
22. Tranter R, Bell D, Gutting P, Harmer C, Healy D, Anderson IM. The effect of serotonergic and noradrenergic antidepressants on face emotion processing in depressed patients. *J Affect Disord.* (2009) 118:87–93. doi: 10.1016/j.jad.2009.01.028
23. Chen CH, Ridler K, Suckling J, Williams S, Fu CH, Merlo-Pich E, et al. Brain imaging correlates of depressive symptom severity and predictors of symptom improvement after antidepressant treatment. *Biol Psychiatry* (2007) 62:407–14. doi: 10.1016/j.biopsych.2006.09.018
24. Fu CH, Williams SC, Cleare AJ, Scott J, Mitterschiffthaler MT, Walsh ND, et al. Neural responses to sad facial expressions in major depression following cognitive behavioral therapy. *Biol Psychiatry* (2008) 64:505–12. doi: 10.1016/j.biopsych.2008.04.033
25. Costafreda SG, Khanna A, Mourao-Miranda J, Fu CH. Neural correlates of sad faces predict clinical remission to cognitive behavioural therapy in depression. *Neuroreport* (2009) 20:637–41. doi: 10.1097/WNR.0b013e3283294159
26. Lisiecka D, Meisenzahl E, Scheuerecker J, Schoepf V, Whitty P, Chaney A, et al. Neural correlates of treatment outcome in major depression. *Int J Neuropsychopharmacol.* (2011) 14:521–34. doi: 10.1017/S1461145710001513
27. Samson AC, Meisenzahl E, Scheuerecker J, Rose E, Schoepf V, Wiesmann M, et al. Brain activation predicts treatment improvement in patients with major depressive disorder. *J Psychiatr Res.* (2011) 45:1214–22. doi: 10.1016/j.jpsychires.2011.03.009
28. Ruhe HG, Booij J, Veltman DJ, Michel MC, Schene AH. Successful pharmacologic treatment of major depressive disorder attenuates amygdala activation to negative facial expressions: a functional magnetic resonance imaging study. *J Clin Psychiatry* (2012) 73:451–9. doi: 10.4088/JCP.10m06584
29. Furey ML, Drevets WC, Hoffman EM, Frankel E, Speer AM, Zarate CAJr. Potential of pretreatment neural activity in the visual cortex during emotional processing to predict treatment response to scopolamine in major depressive disorder. *JAMA Psychiatry* (2013) 70:280–90. doi: 10.1001/2013.jamapsychiatry.60
30. Victor TA, Furey ML, Fromm SJ, Ohman A, Drevets WC. Changes in the neural correlates of implicit emotional face processing during antidepressant treatment in major depressive disorder. *Int J Neuropsychopharmacol.* (2013) 16:2195–208. doi: 10.1017/S146114571300062X
31. Vai B, Poletti S, Radaelli D, Dallaspezia S, Bulgarelli C, Locatelli C, et al. Successful antidepressant chronotherapeutics enhance fronto-limbic neural responses and connectivity in bipolar depression. *Psychiatry Res.* (2015) 233:243–53. doi: 10.1016/j.pscychresns.2015.07.015
32. Williams LM, Korgaonkar MS, Song YC, Paton R, Eagles S, Goldstein-Piekarski A, et al. Amygdala reactivity to emotional faces in the prediction of general and medication-specific responses to antidepressant treatment in the randomized iSPOT-D trial. *Neuropsychopharmacology* (2015) 40:2398–408. doi: 10.1038/npp.2015.89
33. Godlewska BR, Browning M, Norbury R, Cowen PJ, Harmer CJ. Early changes in emotional processing as a marker of clinical response to SSRI treatment in depression. *Transl Psychiatry* (2016) 6:e957. doi: 10.1038/tp.2016.130
34. Szczepanik J, Nugent AC, Drevets WC, Khanna A, Zarate CAJr, Furey ML. Amygdala response to explicit sad face stimuli at baseline predicts antidepressant treatment response to scopolamine in major depressive disorder. *Psychiatry Res.* (2016) 254:67–73. doi: 10.1016/j.pscychresns.2016.06.005
35. Vai B, Bulgarelli C, Godlewska BR, Cowen PJ, Benedetti F, Harmer CJ. Fronto-limbic effective connectivity as possible predictor of antidepressant response to SSRI administration. *Eur Neuropsychopharmacol.* (2016) 26:2000–10. doi: 10.1016/j.euroneuro.2016.09.640
36. Redlich R, Burger C, Dohm K, Grotegerd D, Opel N, Zaremba D, et al. Effects of electroconvulsive therapy on amygdala function in major depression - a longitudinal functional magnetic resonance imaging study. *Psychol Med.* (2017) 47:2166–76. doi: 10.1017/S0033291717000605
37. Davidson RJ, Irwin W, Anderle MJ, Kalin NH. The neural substrates of affective processing in depressed patients treated with venlafaxine. *Am J Psychiatry* (2003) 160:64–75. doi: 10.1176/appi.ajp.160.1.64
38. Light SN, Heller AS, Johnstone T, Kolden GG, Peterson MJ, Kalin NH, et al. Reduced right ventrolateral prefrontal cortex activity while inhibiting positive affect is associated with improvement in hedonic capacity after 8 weeks of antidepressant treatment in major depressive disorder. *Biol Psychiatry* (2011) 70:962–8. doi: 10.1016/j.biopsych.2011.06.031
39. Ritchey M, Dolcos F, Eddington KM, Strauman TJ, Cabeza R. Neural correlates of emotional processing in depression: changes with cognitive behavioral therapy and predictors of treatment response. *J Psychiatr Res.* (2011) 45:577–87. doi: 10.1016/j.jpsychires.2010.09.007
40. Rizvi SJ, Salomons TV, Konarski JZ, Downar J, Giacobbe P, Mcintyre RS, et al. Neural response to emotional stimuli associated with successful antidepressant treatment and behavioral activation. *J Affect Disord.* (2013) 151:573–81. doi: 10.1016/j.jad.2013.06.050
41. Strakowski SM, Fleck DE, Welge J, Eliassen JC, Norris M, Durling M, et al. fMRI brain activation changes following treatment of a first bipolar manic episode. *Bipolar Disord.* (2016) 18:490–501. doi: 10.1111/bdi.12426
42. Siegle GJ, Carter CS, Thase ME. Use of FMRI to predict recovery from unipolar depression with cognitive behavior therapy. *Am J Psychiatry* (2006) 163:735–8. doi: 10.1176/ajp.2006.163.4.735
43. Siegle GJ, Thompson WK, Collier A, Berman SR, Feldmiller J, Thase ME, et al. Toward clinically useful neuroimaging in depression treatment: prognostic

utility of subgenual cingulate activity for determining depression outcome in cognitive therapy across studies, scanners, and patient characteristics. *JAMA Psychiatry* (2012) 69:913–24. doi: 10.1001/archgenpsychiatry.2012.65

44. Miller JM, Schneck N, Siegle GJ, Chen Y, Ogden RT, Kikuchi T, et al. FMRI response to negative words and SSRI treatment outcome in major depressive disorder: a preliminary study. *Psychiatry Res.* (2013) 214:296–305. doi: 10.1016/j.pscychresns.2013.08.001
45. Delaveau P, Jabourian M, Lemogne C, Allaili N, Choucha W, Girault N, et al. Antidepressant short-term and long-term brain effects during self-referential processing in major depression. *Psychiatry Res.* (2016) 247:17–24. doi: 10.1016/j.pscychresns.2015.11.007
46. Carl H, Walsh E, Eisenlohr-Moul T, Minkel J, Crowther A, Moore T, et al. Sustained anterior cingulate cortex activation during reward processing predicts response to psychotherapy in major depressive disorder. *J Affect Disord.* (2016) 203:204–12. doi: 10.1016/j.jad.2016.06.005
47. Walsh E, Carl H, Eisenlohr-Moul T, Minkel J, Crowther A, Moore T, et al. Attenuation of frontostriatal connectivity during reward processing predicts response to psychotherapy in major depressive disorder. *Neuropsychopharmacology* (2017) 42:831–43. doi: 10.1038/npp.2016.179
48. Dunkin JJ, Leuchter AF, Cook IA, Kasl-Godley JE, Abrams M, Rosenberg-Thompson S. Executive dysfunction predicts nonresponse to fluoxetine in major depression. *J Affect Disord.* (2000) 60:13–23. doi: 10.1016/S0165-0327(99)00157-3
49. Kampf-Sherf O, Zlotogorski Z, Gilboa A, Speedie L, Lereya J, Rosca P, et al. Neuropsychological functioning in major depression and responsiveness to selective serotonin reuptake inhibitors antidepressants. *J Affect Disord.* (2004) 82:453–9. doi: 10.1016/j.jad.2004.02.006
50. Taylor BP, Bruder GE, Stewart JW, Mcgrath PJ, Halperin J, Ehrlichman H, et al. Psychomotor slowing as a predictor of fluoxetine nonresponse in depressed outpatients. *Am J Psychiatry* (2006) 163:73–8. doi: 10.1176/appi.ajp.163.1.73
51. Langenecker SA, Kennedy SE, Guidotti LM, Briceno EM, Own LS, Hooven T, et al. Frontal and limbic activation during inhibitory control predicts treatment response in major depressive disorder. *Biol Psychiatry* (2007) 62:1272–80. doi: 10.1016/j.biopsych.2007.02.019
52. Walsh ND, Williams SC, Brammer MJ, Bullmore ET, Kim J, Suckling J, et al. A longitudinal functional magnetic resonance imaging study of verbal working memory in depression after antidepressant therapy. *Biol Psychiatry* (2007) 62:1236–43. doi: 10.1016/j.biopsych.2006.12.022
53. Raes F, Sienaert P, Demyttenaere K, Peuskens J, Williams JM, Hermans D. Overgeneral memory predicts stability of short-term outcome of electroconvulsive therapy for depression. *J Ect.* (2008) 24:81–3. doi: 10.1097/YCT.0b013e31814da995
54. Gudayol-Ferre E, Herrera-Guzman I, Camarena B, Cortes-Penagos C, Herrera-Abarca JE, Martinez-Medina P, et al. The role of clinical variables, neuropsychological performance and SLC6A4 and COMT gene polymorphisms on the prediction of early response to fluoxetine in major depressive disorder. *J Affect Disord.* (2010) 127:343–51. doi: 10.1016/j.jad.2010.06.002
55. Furtado CP, Hoy KE, Maller JJ, Savage G, Daskalakis ZJ, Fitzgerald PB. Cognitive and volumetric predictors of response to repetitive transcranial magnetic stimulation (rTMS) - a prospective follow-up study. *Psychiatry Res.* (2012) 202:12–9. doi: 10.1016/j.pscychresns.2012.02.004
56. Hoy KE, Segrave RA, Daskalakis ZJ, Fitzgerald PB. Investigating the relationship between cognitive change and antidepressant response following rTMS: a large scale retrospective study. *Brain Stimul.* (2012) 5:539–46. doi: 10.1016/j.brs.2011.08.010
57. Hernández-Ribas R, Deus J, Pujol J, Segalàs C, Vallejo J, Menchón JM, et al. Identifying brain imaging correlates of clinical response to repetitive transcranial magnetic stimulation (rTMS) in major depression. *Brain Stimul.* (2013) 6:5[illegible]–61. doi: 10.1016/j.brs.2012.01.001
58. Crane NA, Jenkins LM, Bhaumik R, Dion C, Gowins JR, Mickey BJ, et al. Multidimensional prediction of treatment response to antidepressants with cognitive control and functional MRI. *Brain* (2017) 140:472–86. doi: 10.1093/brain/aww326
59. Etkin A, Patenaude B, Song YJ, Usherwood T, Rekshan W, Schatzberg AF, et al. A cognitive-emotional biomarker for predicting remission with antidepressant medications: a report from the iSPOT-D trial. *Neuropsychopharmacology* (2015) 40:1332–42. doi: 10.1038/npp.2014.333
60. Downar J, Geraci J, Salomons TV, Dunlop K, Wheeler S, Mcandrews MP, et al. Anhedonia and reward-circuit connectivity distinguish nonresponders from responders to dorsomedial prefrontal repetitive transcranial magnetic stimulation in major depression. *Biol Psychiatry* (2014) 76:176–85. doi: 10.1016/j.biopsych.2013.10.026
61. Liston C, Chen AC, Zebley BD, Drysdale AT, Gordon R, Leuchter B, et al. Default mode network mechanisms of transcranial magnetic stimulation in depression. *Biol Psychiatry* (2014) 76:517–26. doi: 10.1016/j.biopsych.2014.01.023
62. Salomons TV, Dunlop K, Kennedy SH, Flint A, Geraci J, Giacobbe P, et al. Resting-state cortico-thalamic-striatal connectivity predicts response to dorsomedial prefrontal rTMS in major depressive disorder. *Neuropsychopharmacology* (2014) 39:488–98. doi: 10.1038/npp.2013.222
63. Crowther A, Smoski MJ, Minkel J, Moore T, Gibbs D, Petty C, et al. Resting-state connectivity predictors of response to psychotherapy in major depressive disorder. *Neuropsychopharmacology* (2015) 40:1659–73. doi: 10.1038/npp.2015.12
64. Van Waarde JA, Scholte HS, Van Oudheusden LJ, Verwey B, Denys D, Van Wingen GA. A functional MRI marker may predict the outcome of electroconvulsive therapy in severe and treatment-resistant depression. *Mol Psychiatry* (2015) 20:609–14. doi: 10.1038/mp.2014.78
65. Cano M, Cardoner N, Urretavizcaya M, Martínez-Zalacaín I, Goldberg X, Via E, et al. Modulation of limbic and prefrontal connectivity by electroconvulsive therapy in treatment-resistant depression: a preliminary study. *Brain Stimul.* (2016) 9:65–71. doi: 10.1016/j.brs.2015.08.016
66. Fang J, Egorova N, Rong P, Liu J, Hong Y, Fan Y, et al. Early cortical biomarkers of longitudinal transcutaneous vagus nerve stimulation treatment success in depression. *NeuroImage Clin.* (2017) 14:105–11. doi: 10.1016/j.nicl.2016.12.016
67. Ge R, Blumberger DM, Downar J, Daskalakis ZJ, Dipinto AA, Tham JCW, et al. Abnormal functional connectivity within resting-state networks is related to rTMS-based therapy effects of treatment resistant depression: a pilot study. *J Affect Disord.* (2017) 218:75–81. doi: 10.1016/j.jad.2017.04.060
68. Costafreda SG, Chu C, Ashburner J, Fu CH. Prognostic and diagnostic potential of the structural neuroanatomy of depression. *PLoS ONE* (2009) 4:e6353. doi: 10.1371/journal.pone.0006353
69. Joshi SH, Espinoza RT, Pirnia T, Shi J, Wang Y, Ayers B, et al. Structural plasticity of the hippocampus and amygdala induced by electroconvulsive therapy in major depression. *Biol Psychiatry* (2016) 79:282–92. doi: 10.1016/j.biopsych.2015.02.029
70. Redlich R, Opel N, Grotegerd D, Dohm K, Zaremba D, Burger C, et al. Prediction of Individual Response to Electroconvulsive Therapy via Machine Learning on Structural Magnetic Resonance Imaging Data. *JAMA Psychiatry* (2016) 73:557–64. doi: 10.1001/jamapsychiatry.2016.0316
71. Delorenzo C, Delaparte L, Thapa-Chhetry B, Miller JM, Mann JJ, Parsey RV. Prediction of selective serotonin reuptake inhibitor response using diffusion-weighted MRI. *Front Psychiatry* (2013) 4:5. doi: 10.3389/fpsyt.2013.00005
72. Korgaonkar MS, Williams LM, Song YJ, Usherwood T, Grieve SM. Diffusion tensor imaging predictors of treatment outcomes in major depressive disorder. *Br J Psychiatry* (2014) 205:321–8. doi: 10.1192/bjp.bp.113.140376
73. Bollettini I, Poletti S, Locatelli C, Vai B, Smeraldi E, Colombo C, et al. Disruption of white matter integrity marks poor antidepressant response in bipolar disorder. *J Affect Disord.* (2015) 174:233–40. doi: 10.1016/j.jad.2014.11.010
74. Lan MJ, Rubin-Falcone H, Motiwala F, Chen Y, Stewart JW, Hellerstein DJ, et al. White matter tract integrity is associated with antidepressant response to lurasidone in bipolar depression. *Bipolar Disord.* (2017) 19:444–9. doi: 10.1111/bdi.12509
75. Harmer CJ, Duman RS, Cowen PJ. How do antidepressants work? New perspectives for refining future treatment approaches *Lancet Psychiatry* (2017) 4:409–18. doi: 10.1016/S2215-0366(17)30015-9
76. Franklin G, Carson AJ, Welch KA. Cognitive behavioural therapy for depression: systematic review of imaging studies. *Acta Neuropsychiatr.* (2016) 28:61–74. doi: 10.1017/neu.2015.41

77. Bryant RA, Felmingham K, Whitford TJ, Kemp A, Hughes G, Peduto A, et al. Rostral anterior cingulate volume predicts treatment response to cognitive-behavioural therapy for posttraumatic stress disorder. *J Psychiatry Neurosci.* (2008) 33:142–6.
78. Sheline YI, Gado MH, Kraemer HC. Untreated depression and hippocampal volume loss. *Am J Psychiatry* (2003) 160:1516–8. doi: 10.1176/appi.ajp.160.8.1516
79. Bearden CE, Thompson PM, Avedissian C, Klunder AD, Nicoletti M, Dierschke N, et al. Altered hippocampal morphology in unmedicated patients with major depressive illness. *ASN Neuro.* (2009) 1: e00020. doi: 10.1042/AN20090026
80. Santarelli L, Saxe M, Gross C, Surget A, Battaglia F, Dulawa S, et al. Requirement of hippocampal neurogenesis for the behavioral effects of antidepressants. *Science* (2003) 301:805–9. doi: 10.1126/science.1083328
81. Sandercock P. Negative results: why do they need to be published? *Int J Stroke* (2012) 7:32–3. doi: 10.1111/j.1747-4949.2011.00723.x
82. Button KS, Ioannidis JP, Mokrysz C, Nosek BA, Flint J, Robinson ES, et al. Power failure: why small sample size undermines the reliability of neuroscience. *Nat Rev Neurosci.* (2013) 14:365–76. doi: 10.1038/nrn3475

7

Encephalitis, Mild Encephalitis, Neuroprogression, or Encephalopathy—Not Merely a Question of Terminology

Karl Bechter*

Department Psychiatry and Psychotherapy II, Bezirkskrankenhaus Günzburg, Ulm University, Ulm, Germany

***Correspondence:**
Karl Bechter
karl.bechter@bkh-guenzburg.de

Background: Psychoneuroimmunology research has presented emerging evidence of the involvement of inflammatory and immune mechanisms in the pathogenesis of severe mental disorders. In this context, new terms with increasing clinical relevance have been proposed, challenging the existing terms, and requiring consensus definitions of the new ones.

Method: From a perspective of longstanding personal involvement in clinical settings and research in psychoneuroimmunology, the new and the existing terms are critically reconsidered.

Results: Meningoencephalitis and encephalitis are comparably well defined clinical terms in neuropsychiatry, although in the individual case approach diagnosis can be difficult, for example in some cases of encephalitis that are described with normal cerebrospinal fluid findings, or often in chronic encephalitis. Encephalopathy is also a widely accepted term, however, with a surprisingly broad meaning with regard to the assigned underlying pathophysiology, ranging from one-hit traumatic encephalopathy to inflammatory encephalopathy, the latter term addressing a type of brain dysfunction secondary to acute systemic inflammation without proven brain autochthonus inflammation (neuroinflammation). However, this latter assumption and term may be wrong as neuroinflammation is difficult to prove *in vivo*. With emerging insights into prevailing inflammatory and neuroinflammatory mechanisms that are involved in the pathogenesis of severe mental disorders, the interdependent aspects of sensitive assessment and potential clinical relevance of mild neuroinflammation are becoming more apparent and of increasing clinical interest. The new terms "mild encephalitis," "parainflammation," and "neuroprogression" show considerable overlap in addition to gaps and hardly defined borders. However, details are hard to discuss as available studies use many biomarkers, but most of these are done without an established categorical attribution to exclusive terms. Most important, the three new concepts (neruoprogression, parainflammation, and mild encephalitis) are not mutually exclusive, even at the individual case level, and therefore will require state-related individual assessment approaches beyond large confirmatory studies.

Conclusion: The newly proposed terms of mild encephalitis, parainflammation, and neuroprogression have an emerging clinical relevance, but respective borders, gaps and overlap in between them remain unclear, and these concepts may even be seen as complementary. Categorical delineation of the new and reconsideration of the existing terms with respect to individualized psychiatric treatment is required for better clinical use, eventually requiring a consensus approach. Here, a critique based on available data and a focus on clinical perspective was outlined, which may help to enhance fruitful discussion. The idea followed here is in line with pillar number six as proposed for the Research Diagnostic Domains, i.e., to provide and follow new concepts in psychiatric research.

Keywords: meningoencephalitis, encephalitis, neuroinflammation, inflammation, parainflammation

INTRODUCTION

Neuroinflammation, like inflammation in general, represents a dimensional or graded response embedded in time and space. Such a principle is even true in neurodevelopmental perspectives, recently exemplified for microglia (1). For clinical purposes, such a dynamic is split into separate categories, because categorization is helpful and needed to guide diagnostic management and especially appropriate treatment decisions. Inherent to such an approach is not only a partial loss of the dynamic perspective, but it poses also the new problem to define borders between neighboring categories as exactly as possible. However, categorical definition is based on actual theories and evidence and not least diagnostic methods available in the clinical approach. The paradigm of clinically relevant neuroinflammation represents infectious (meningo-)encephalitis, representing an acute, strong type of neuroinflammation, thus up to now also dominating the definition of terms beyond states of classical acute neuroinflammation. Suggestive or possible clinically relevant states of (mild) neuroinflammation not fulfilling the definition of meningoencephalitis, were not well classified or might sometimes even have been assigned as "non-inflammatory" diseases in clinical use and research (see below definition of neuroinflammation), with the terms mild neuroinflammation or parainflammation not in use. However, lower grades of neuroinflammation as compared to classical defined neuroinflammation might also be clinically relevant, especially when lasting over longer periods of time, but apparently are *a priori* more difficult to diagnose in individual cases and to categorize within a theoretical framework. The idea that mild encephalitis (ME) may be under-recognized though clinically relevant for severe mental disorders (SMI) (2), was not well accepted when first published in 2001 (3), but is gaining more support now (3–5). The discovery of NMDAR autoantibodies in 2007/8 by Josep Dalmau and his group and the since-emerging recognition and definition of Autoimmune Encephalitis (AE) for a widening spectrum of neurological disorders (4, 5) have especially moved the field, because AE can be well diagnosed as a result of presenting with severe neurologic symptoms. Most important, the early stages of AE are associated with various and varying, initially pure psychiatric syndromes, with neurological symptoms appearing only later in more severe stages, in addition to psychiatric syndromes (4, 5). Thus, mild neuroinflammation, or ME, can retrospectively be assumed to have been present during early stages of AE, as is evidenced from clinical course and by the later, more severe findings and symptoms categorized as AE. The emerging insight that some cases of psychosis may even represent previously undetected cases of AE (6, 7), led to an enhanced interest in improved and new diagnostic approaches to ME and a search for appropriate treatments in new-onset and therapy-resistant SMI. This was strongly reinforced by single case reports of successful immune modulatory treatments of cases of Autoimmune Psychosis (AP), with AP cases not fulfilling the diagnostic criteria of AE (8–13). Given the widely unexplained causality of SMI, one should recognize that ME in theory and practice appears sufficient and even prone to cause a spectrum of psychiatric symptoms even though it presents without neurological symptoms (at least without so-called neurological hard signs), and is thus within a spectrum of SMI (2). Therefore, the question of potentially prevailing but under-diagnosed ME in SMI is of great interest and relevance for improved treatments, including those with potentially rapid therapeutic success. Such a situation requires also a critical reconsideration of existing clinical terms in use, because more refined categorical classification is then required for research and clinical approaches. This is attempted here from a clinical and research.

CRITICAL OUTLINE OF TERMS IN CLINICAL USE AROUND NEUROINFLAMMATION

(Meningo-)Encephalitis

Encephalitis is used to term meningoencephalitis when involvement of meninges is apparent with respect to clinical symptoms and/or by findings (14). The most important diagnostic measure is CSF examination plus neuroimaging. Most diagnosed cases represent a type of acute severe encephalitis, with the disease sometimes being life-threatening.

Chronic encephalitis is overall rare. A clear definition of chronicity is difficult and a time frame of 4 weeks and beyond appears to be used by some in the clinical field, but a generally accepted sound definition of the term "chronic" was not to be found. Chronic encephalitis presents—with regard to the clinical picture—similarly to acute encephalitis, with the course just being protracted *a priori*, possibly with dominating or exclusive psychiatric symptoms in extended early stages of the disease. Respective psychiatric syndromes are typically unspecific, i.e., various and variant, though some symptom characteristics may be found, especially when including systemic signs and findings (14, 15).

Acute encephalitis is usually represented by severe acute brain inflammation possibly involving the brain and the meninges. Nevertheless, a theoretically sound definition is difficult (for example, exact delineation of encephalitis vs. with or without meningitis? Or is there always some co-occurrence?), whereas consensus on clinical case definition and diagnostic approach is well established (16). Of note is that in rare cases even CSF examination, the most sensitive diagnostic procedure followed by neuroimaging, may present with normal findings [Benninger and Steiner in Deisenhammer et al. (14), Venkatesan et al. (16)].

Encephalopathy

The term encephalopathy appears to be broadly used, with a long tradition but with an apparent weakness of precision in its meaning. Encephalopathy was mainly used for lasting consequences of various insults to the brain, for example traumatic encephalopathy, vascular encephalopathy or epileptic encephalopathy. A recent case definition differentiates encephalitis from inflammatory encephalopathy, the latter addressing the case of brain dysfunction from severe systemic inflammation [compare with (16)]. In the context of the new developments in the field of psychoneuroimmunology the weakness of the existing term becomes clear; for example, the term "inflammatory encephalopathy" left open the question of possibly prevailing mild neuroinflammation beyond mere signaling effects in the brain from circulating cytokines and inflammatory markers, the latter mechanism assumed to underlie the "encephalopathy." Also, with epileptic encephalopathy the problem becomes apparent; it is established that repeated epileptic seizures can lead to subtle damage of the brain, which can be prevented with good control of seizures, and such pathology would match, like traumatic encephalopathy, with the traded use of the term, typically addressing cases of lasting brain pathology from single or multiple hits. From a pathogenetic point of view, a completely different scenario represents a subgroup of epileptic disorders, which is consistent with rather new findings, which is caused by a subtype of AE and can be successfully treated with immune modulatory treatments (17, 18). The pathogenetic scenarios behind these two types of epileptic "encephalopathy" (when using the term encephalopathy in the broad sense as often found yet in actual literature) apparently differ strongly. The first one represents a state of defect, the second one a state of active neuroinflammation though clinically presenting nearly identically and appearing seemingly "non-inflammatory," if not differentiated by the new diagnostic methods available for AE, and creating a new case group of AE presenting as epilepsy. To use the term encephalopathy for such differing pathogenetic scenarios is hardly acceptable, because such broad meaning of terminology is inappropriate to guide clinical decisions.

Autoimmune Encephalitis (AE)

The only recently described subtype—AE—of encephalitis was mainly related to the discovery of CNS autoantibodies, found in blood and more sensitively in CSF, with cases presenting various neurological signs of encephalitis as established in clinical neurology (19–22). Most interestingly, the spectrum of neurological disorders associated with the prevalence of CNS autoantibodies is emerging since the discovery of NMDAR-autoantibodies, much beyond the previously-known cases of limbic encephalitis and tumor-associated paraneoplastic encephalitis, and emerging as well is the number of CNS autoantibodies discovered (23–30). However, many questions remain to be solved, especially with regard to the role of CNS autoantibodies in psychiatric disorders (27, 31–37).

Mild Encephalitis (ME)

ME was proposed as a term in 2001 (3), placed categorically in between encephalopathy and encephalitis. Mild forms of encephalitis (or minor neuroinflammation) have been detected with careful histopathological investigation in certain disease phases of experimental Borna disease virus infection, a strongly neurotropic virus that causes classical-type meningoencephalitis in some species and in others presents just mild neuroinflammation paralleled by behavioral syndromes. Most important, the observed symptoms and course aspects over years (in animals) remembered variant symptomatology and courses of major psychiatric disorders in humans (3). Indeed, many findings including epidemiological and course aspects in affective and schizophrenic spectrum disorders would match with an ME scenario subgroup, just the limited sensitivity of available clinical methods may explain that diagnosis of ME cases failed in clinical reality (2, 3). Meanwhile, evidence is increasing that an ME subgroup indeed prevails in broadly defined affective and schizophrenic spectrum disorders [compare (8, 9, 38–43)]. In only very rare cases of subacute psychoses, performance of a brain biopsy was indicated for apparent ethical reasons; these rare though important studies demonstrated not only mild neuroinflammation in the cortex, but even more importantly, demonstrated good response to immune modulatory treatments (13, 38, 44). Given the rather high prevalence of minor CSF abnormalities in SMI groups (45–48), the size of an apparent prevailing ME subgroup in SMI patients remains to be carefully investigated.

Autoimmune Psychosis (AP)

The term autoimmune psychosis was proposed recently (49) and taken up by other groups (8, 9). The term AP could well make sense, despite a yet-limited precision of its definition in a pathogenetic perspective. Primarily addressing the presence of CNS autoantibodies [compare with (49)] or, in an extended definition of AP, some apparent clinical plausibility of a prevailing autoimmune process [compare (9)], does not convincingly demonstrate the assumed neuroinflammatory mechanisms behind psychosis, except in cases with respective findings in brain biopsy or CSF or neuroimaging. Nevertheless, respective criteria of a consensus diagnosis of AP are just being developed. It seems that the problem of diagnosis/definition of AP (dependent on the methods used and available, see above) is rather similar to the problem with the term and definition/diagnosis of "inflammatory encephalopathy," leaving major open questions about the categorical borders between parainflammation (see below) vs. mild neuroinflammation vs. classical neuroinflammation.

Parainflammation

The term parainflammation represents a new definition for low-grade inflammation (50), recently adapted for mental health disorders and exemplified for "stress-induced parainflammation" by Wohleb (51): Wohleb proposed a situation similar to general parainflammation as proposed by Medzhitov to represent the underlying pathophysiological mechanism in some mental health disorders, a mild form of inflammation assigned as parainflammation of the brain when being inducible and induced by systemic inflammatory activation, especially stress. Parainflammation would be characterized by evolving neuroimmune processes and microglial changes, with the altered microglia-neuron interactions eventually leading to neuroplasticity deficits and neuronal dystrophy. The (para-)inflammatory changes from homeostasis were considered modest in quality and degree as compared to changes which defined neuroinflammation. CNS-related parainflammation was discussed to play a role in mental health disorders like anxiety and depressive-like behavior in aging and in neurodegenerative disorders. Criteria to define stress-induced parainflammation of the CNS appeared however difficult to establish and reliably reproduce, if not in the stress paradigm. The respective claimed borders to neuroinflammation appear rather unclear or arbitrary and must be worked out. The relation of CNS parainflammation to neuroprogression remained open, but conceptual overlap apparently exists. Nevertheless, the concept of CNS parainflammation appears to represent another valuable attempt to tackle the problem of a refined grading of immune-inflammatory responses in the CNS in clinically useful categories.

Neuroinflammation (NI)

The definition of NI differs in details between different fields (virology, histopathology, clinical field, others) due to the differing assessment methods used in respective fields. Therefore, a simple translation of the definition of NI from one field to the other is complicated and, for evident reasons, the case of mild chronic NI is more problematic as compared to severe acute NI. A general problem of the clinical definition of NI relates to the limited approach to the brain in clinical patients; even the diagnosis of severe acute NI requires the use of a combination of various methods, each with an overall limited sensitivity to detect NI at the individual patient level. The most relevant diagnostic methods herein are represented by CSF examination followed by neuroimaging. The most sensitive method in principle represented brain biopsy, but its application is strongly limited due to apparent ethical reasons and, even when indicated, from the difficulty of choosing the appropriate brain site for taking the biopsy, the latter aspect reducing its *a priori* high sensitivity. A critical review of the theoretical and practical gaps in defining NI in the various fields dealing with NI is hardly found in the literature.

An indirect example to critically review the clinical definition of NI can be found with actual recommendations for the use of CSF in biomarker studies (52): definitions and names of control groups (overall 6 groups) are as follows: Healthy Controls, Spinal Anesthesia Subjects, Central Inflammatory Neurologic Disease Controls, Peripheral Inflammatory Neurologic Disease Controls, Noninflammatory Neurologic Disease Controls, Symptomatic Controls. The defining criteria of each group are based on multilevel clinical findings, including exclusion criteria by CSF findings. The use of CSF findings to define controls apparently represents in some way a circular argument for definition, but to find better options for definition is difficult, at least not available, because completely healthy controls are not only hard to find as controls in studies requiring invasive methods, but is also hardly justified to use controls in all studies. The compromises needed to deal with the problem of controls in studies may, however, posit a major problem for studies about mild neuroinflammation, although less so with classical severe acute neuroinflamamtion. Herein, the most apparent weak aspect in defining categories/subgroups of controls was the CSF criteria for non-inflammatory neurologic disorders (cell count must be normal, QAlb can be normal or elevated). The idea of mild neuroinflammation appears, at least to me, still poorly understood, given the high frequency of minor CSF abnormalities in SMI groups (see also above). One should consider that normal values for CSF parameters were established in clinical neurology, which from apparent circumstantial factors may cause a preference for observing severe neurological disorders only and, in the case of NI, a preference for observing only cases with severe neuroinflammation. This may lead to missing milder forms of NI or even missing cases of severe meningoencephalitis, which can be observed with normal CSF numbers (see above). Therefore, a justified conclusion is that available methods, including even the major pillars of NI diagnostics in the clinic, CSF examination and neuroimaging, are likely, and by many experts admittedly, insensitive for an individualized diagnosis of mild NI.

Neuroprogression

The term neuroprogression, proposed by Berk et al. (53), refers to a combination of treatment non-responsiveness, relapsing and declining course of illness, and progressive neuropathological changes commonly seen in several psychiatric disorders (54). The concept of neuroprogression is emerging and well supported (55–58). To establish defining criteria of neuroprogression in an individualized approach appears, however, presently unsolved, because neuroprogression involves many pathogenic mechanisms including microglial activation, inflammation and systemic toxicity (59). Nevertheless, for clinical use, eventually a categorical definition will be required to guide appropriate therapeutic approaches at the individual case level (60). The theory appears yet fully informative for select testing of respective treatment approaches in study design, which does not appear to be the case for individual treatment approaches like with the ME hypothesis (see above). The problems of overlap and unclear categorical differences between neuroprogression, parainflammation, and mild neuroinflammation, also discussed in context with AP and inflammatory encephalopathy, are apparent, but all these concepts have innovative power. A crucial question herein is whether, how and when, which one of the three newly introduced concepts (meaning in principle more or less strong active states of neuro-immuno-inflammation) may be relevant at an individual case level and in the course of the disease.

Relation to Research Domain Criteria (RDoC) Research

The development of RDoCs under the guidance of the National Institutes of Health to improve the basics of available diagnostic systems in psychiatry is driven by limited progress in psychiatric therapies from psychiatric research; to overcome this frustrating situation new approaches are claimed to be grounded on seven new pillars (61). Along this new line of orientation of psychiatric research, the sixth pillar is approached here; that is, a new conceptualization, respectively constructs with immediate relevance for new individualized treatments. An emerging collection of single cases demonstrates the utility of the ME concept in severe SMI at the individual case approach of selected cases. The new concepts of parainflammation and of neuroprogression may be of more general relevance. Parainflammation may act as a contributive or triggering factor in severe mental disorders and as a causative factor for minor psychiatric disorders as presented with the still theoretical concept, which is able to explain a number of established findings as at least one possible interpretation; neuroprogression appears to be relevant to understand the long-term aspects and consequences from lasting neuroinflammatory dysregulation in rather large subgroups of SMI, a conclusion that is backed by a number of emerging studies to support the concept with good theoretical plausibility. Nevertheless, this evaluation of these two concepts does not disregard the possibility that the concept of ME is appropriate even in a larger subgroup of SMI. The three new concepts may be relevant in a complementary perspective in general and over time during the course of SMI illness.

Arguments for the relevance of the ME concept are as follows: observed single cases of therapy-resistant schizophrenia-like syndromes (but diagnosed before as schizophrenia) or of severe major depression of rapid and often full remission (conclusion: cases were seemingly chronic, but in retrospect better considered subacute or mild NI) under various immune modulatory treatments including CSF filtration (62, 63); brain biopsy-proven ME in major depression (13); cortisone or antiepileptics (64–66); complex immune treatment with refined diagnosis of systemic autoimmune disorder underlying the psychiatric syndrome (seeming to be of a chronic-inactive character but in retrospect rather representing a subacute or waxing-waning immune-inflammatory pathology) (12); or a differential diagnosis of a difficult-to-detect agent related autoimmunity—that is, persistent infection-related autoimmunity, treatable by antibiotics and/or immune modulatory measures (11, 67–69).

CONCLUSION

The traded clinical terms dealing with neuroinflammatory and other brain damaging disease states like neuroinflammation, (meningo-)encephalitis and encephalopathy should be reconsidered in light of recent developments in neuropsychoimmunology and completed by new terms. With new insights into the frequent prevalence of milder forms of neuroinflammation in severe mental disorders and in a variety of neurodegenerative disorders including dementia, parkinsonism and others not discussed in this review, a detailed categorical terminology of neuroinflammatory and neuroimmune mechanisms with respective clinical relevance would be helpful. Establishing refined new terms is however difficult due to many problems inherent to the diagnostic approach to the individual patient and the slowly emerging insights about the possible pathogenic relevance of new findings indicating some neuroinflammatory or neuroimmune aberrances. The key question about any potential relevance of identified factors in the pathogenesis of the respective disorder (causal or contributive factor, relative weight of single factor), is difficult to evaluate *a priori*. However, this is complicated by uncertainties about the sensitivity and limits of diagnostic methods available, the latter aspect directly influencing the validity of clinical definitions, which becomes a circular problem. For example, although prevalence of some neuroinflammatory activation was well established in the pathogenesis of dementia, the respective inflammatory CSF markers appear to be less important compared to metabolic biomarkers (70), thus raising the question of the weight of neuroinflammatory changes in respective disease pathogenesis. The newly proposed terms Mild Encephalitis, Neuroprogression, Stress-induced Parainflammation and Autoimmune Psychosis appear of special relevance for research on severe mental disorders, although they may yet remain difficult or impossible to assess with available clinical methods in an individual patient approach. However, also in theoretical framework and with respect to categorical borders of one term to another, overlap and gaps of knowledge have to be recognized and solved, but the new terms may set the stage for further research and development. With regard to existing terminology, the new terms can bridge the most apparent gaps in the clinical approach to the dimensional and quality aspects of (neuro-)inflammation by addressing potentially relevant though overall mild forms of neuroinflammation in the pathogenesis of severe mental disorders and in minor stress-induced mental disorders, thus they might importantly contribute to progress in psychiatric research and clinical settings. Teaching examples like the psychosomatics of gastric/duodenal ulcers vs. the bacterial triggered dysfunction/inflammation might be kept in mind. The term encephalopathy appears to be rather weakly defined, often used to assign various seemingly brain-diseased states in general medicine, neurology, and psychiatry. A most appropriate use of the term encephalopathy might represent disease states "after" some insult to the brain, like post-traumatic or post-encephalitic states, or in the case of preliminary diagnosis or of a scientifically unclear weight of identified single pathogenic factors within a complex brain disease pathogenesis. The term inflammatory encephalopathy appears rather questionable and should represent a focus of further research regarding the underlying brain pathology and detailed pathogenesis behind it [compare (16)]. A rather important step in such a direction was to perform CSF examination more frequently than presently done in the psychiatric field (59) and by advanced and newly developed diagnostic methods (71, 72). Such an approach follows the RDoC initiative assumed to bring psychiatric individualized treatments forward into a new, more successful level.

AUTHOR CONTRIBUTIONS

The author confirms being the sole contributor of this work and has approved it for publication.

REFERENCES

1. Matcovitch-Natan O, Winter DR, Giladi A, Vargas Aguilar S, Spinrad A, Sarrazin S, et al. Microglia development follows a stepwise program to regulate brain homeostasis. *Science* (2016) 353:aad8670. doi: 10.1126/science.aad8670
2. Bechter K. Updating the mild encephalitis hypothesis of schizophrenia. *Prog Neuropsychopharmacol Biol Psychiatry* (2013) 42:71–91. doi: 10.1016/j.pnpbp.2012.06.019
3. Bechter K. Mild encephalitis underlying psychiatric disorders-a reconsideration and hypothesis exemplified on Borna disease. *Neurol Psychiatry Brain Res.* (2001) 9:55–70.
4. Graus F, Titulaer MJ, Balu R, Benseler S, Bien CG, Cellucci T, et al. A clinical approach to diagnosis of autoimmune encephalitis. *Lancet Neurol.* (2016) 15:391–404. doi: 10.1016/S1474-4422(15)00401-9
5. Herken J, Prüss H. Red flags: clinical signs for identifying autoimmune encephalitis in psychiatric patients. *Front Psychiatry* (2017) 8:25. doi: 10.3389/fpsyt.2017.00025
6. Steiner J, Walter M, Glanz W, Sarnyai Z, Bernstein HG, Vielhaber S, et al. Increased prevalence of diverse N-methyl-D-aspartate glutamate receptor antibodies in patients with an initial diagnosis of schizophrenia: specific relevance of IgG NR1a antibodies for distinction from N-methyl-D-aspartate glutamate receptor encephalitis. *JAMA Psychiatry* (2013) 70:271–8. doi: 10.1001/2013.jamapsychiatry.86
7. Lennox BR, Coles AJ, Vincent A. Antibody-mediated encephalitis: a treatable cause of schizophrenia. *Br J Psychiatry* (2012) 200:92–4. doi: 10.1192/bjp.bp.111.095042
8. Al-Diwani A, Pollak TA, Langford AE, Lennox BR. Synaptic and neuronal autoantibody-associated psychiatric syndromes: controversies and hypotheses. *Front Psychiatry* (2017) 8:13. doi: 10.3389/fpsyt.2017.00013
9. Najjar S, Steiner J, Najjar A, Bechter K. A clinical approach to new-onset psychosis associated with immune dysregulation: The concept of autoimmune psychosis. *J Neuroinflammation* (2018) 15:40. doi: 10.1186/s12974-018-1067-y
10. Bechter K, Herzog S, Schreiner V, Wollinsky KH, Schuettlert R. Cerebrospinal fluid filtration in Borna-disease-virus-encephalitis-related schizophrenia A new therapeutic perspective in psychiatry NPBR. *Acad.* (1998) 6:85–86.
11. Bechter K, Bindl A, Horn M, Schreiner V. Therapieresistente depression mit fatigue. Fall einer vermutlichen streptokokkenassoziierten Autoimmunkrankheit. *Der Nervenarzt.* (2007) 78:338–340. doi: 10.1007/s00115-006-2178-8
12. Mack A, Pfeiffer C, Schneider EM, Bechter K. Schizophrenia or atypical lupus erythematosus with predominant psychiatric manifestations over 25 years: case analysis and review. *Front Psychiatry* (2017) 8:131. doi: 10.3389/fpsyt.2017.00131
13. Najjar S, Pearlman DM, Hirsch S, Friedman K, Strange J, Reidy J, et al. Brain biopsy findings link major depressive disorder to neuroinflammation, oxidative stress, and neurovascular dysfunction: a case report. *Biol Psychiatry* (2014) 75:e23–6. doi: 10.1016/j.biopsych.2013.07.041
14. Deisenhammer F, Teunissen CE, Tumani H, editors. *Cerebrospinal Fluid in Neurologic Disorders.* Amsterdam; Kidlington; Cambridge, MA: Elsevier (2017).
15. Bechter K. Diagnosis of infectious or inflammatory psychosyndromes. *Open Neurol J.* (2012) 6:113–8. doi: 10.2174/1874205X01206010113
16. Venkatesan A, Tunkel AR, Bloch KC, Lauring AS, Sejvar J, Bitnun A, et al. Case definitions, diagnostic algorithms, and priorities in encephalitis: consensus statement of the international encephalitis consortium. *Clin Infect Dis.* (2013) 57:1114–28. doi: 10.1093/cid/cit458
17. Al-Ajlan FS, Althobiti A, Baz S, Al-Attas A. Autoimmune encephalopathy and drug refractory seizures with the presence of two autoantibodies specific for the neuronal cell surface. *Epilepsy Behav Case Rep.* (2014) 2:199–202. doi: 10.1016/j.ebcr.2014.06.002
18. Al-Diwani A, Butterworth RJ, Nibber A, Lang B, Vincent A, Irani SR. Acute onset of focal seizures, psychiatric features and confusion: A case of autoimmune encephalitis? *BMJ Case Rep.* (2012) 2012:bcr2012006881. doi: 10.1136/bcr-2012-006881
19. Gresa-Arribas N, Titulaer MJ, Torrents A, Aguilar E, McCracken L, Leypoldt F, et al. Diagnosis and significance of antibody titers in anti-NMDA receptor encephalitis, a retrospective study. *Lancet Neurol.* (2014) 13:167–77. doi: 10.1016/S1474-4422(13)70282-5
20. Dalmau J. The case for autoimmune neurology. *Neurol Neuroimmunol Neuroinflamm.* (2017) 4:373. doi: 10.1212/NXI.0000000000000373
21. Dalmau J. Identifying targets for diagnosis, prognosis, and treatment. *Neurol Neuroimmunol Neuroinflamm.* (2015) 2:87. doi: 10.1212/NXI.0000000000000087
22. Armangue T, Leypoldt F, Dalmau J. Autoimmune encephalitis as differential diagnosis of infectious encephalitis. *Curr Opin Neurol.* (2014) 27:361–8. doi: 10.1097/WCO.0000000000000087
23. Bien CG, Holtkamp M. "Autoimmune epilepsy": encephalitis with autoantibodies for epileptologists. *Epilepsy Curr.* (2017) 17:134–41. doi: 10.5698/1535-7511.17.3.134
24. Chefdeville A, Honnorat J, Hampe CS, Desestret V. Neuronal central nervous system syndromes probably mediated by autoantibodies. *Eur J Neurosci.* (2016) 43:1535–52. doi: 10.1111/ejn.13212
25. Chiba Y, Katsuse O, Takahashi Y, Yoneda M, Kunii M, Ihata A, et al. Anti-glutamate receptor $\varepsilon 2$ antibodies in psychiatric patients with anti-thyroid autoantibodies–a prevalence study in Japan. *Neurosci Lett.* (2013) 534:217–22. doi: 10.1016/j.neulet.2012.10.060
26. Cornelius DC, Lamarca B. TH17- and IL-17- mediated autoantibodies and placental oxidative stress play a role in the pathophysiology of pre-eclampsia. *Minerva Ginecol.* (2014) 66:243–9.
27. Coutinho E, Harrison P, Vincent A. Do neuronal autoantibodies cause psychosis? A neuroimmunological perspective. *Biol Psychiatry* (2014) 75:269–75. doi: 10.1016/j.biopsych.2013.07.040
28. Faust TW, Chang EH, Kowal C, Berlin R, Gazaryan IG, Bertini E, et al. Neurotoxic lupus autoantibodies alter brain function through two distinct mechanisms. *Proc Natl Acad Sci USA.* (2010) 107:18569–74. doi: 10.1073/pnas.1006980107
29. Geis C, Ritter C, Ruschil C, Weishaupt A, Grünewald B, Stoll G, et al. The intrinsic pathogenic role of autoantibodies to aquaporin 4 mediating spinal cord disease in a rat passive-transfer model. *Exp Neurol.* (2015) 265:8–21. doi: 10.1016/j.expneurol.2014.12.015
30. Bowes E, Levy F, Lawson J, Mandalis A, Mohan A, Shannon Weickert C. Anti-N-methyl-D-aspartate encephalitis - a case study of symptomatic progression. *Australas Psychiatry* (2015) 23:422–5. doi: 10.1177/1039856215588229
31. Ilias I, Karagiorga V, Paraskevas G, Bougea A, Bourbouli M, Pappa A, et al. Thyroid autoantibodies in the cerebrospinal fluid of subjects with and without thyroid disease: implications for Hashimoto's encephalopathy. *J Thyroid Res.* (2015) 2015:819072. doi: 10.1155/2015/819072

32. Hammer C, Stepniak B, Schneider A, Papiol S, Tantra M, Begemann M, et al. Neuropsychiatric disease relevance of circulating anti-NMDA receptor autoantibodies depends on blood-brain barrier integrity. *Mol Psychiatry* (2014) 19:1143–9. doi: 10.1038/mp.2013.110
33. Kimura A, Sakurai T, Koumura A, Yamada M, Hayashi Y, Tanaka Y, et al. High prevalence of autoantibodies against phosphoglycerate mutase 1 in patients with autoimmune central nervous system diseases. *J Neuroimmunol.* (2010) 219:105–8. doi: 10.1016/j.jneuroim.2009.11.014
34. Kreye J, Wenke NK, Chayka M, Leubner J, Murugan R, Maier N, et al. Human cerebrospinal fluid monoclonal N-methyl-D-aspartate receptor autoantibodies are sufficient for encephalitis pathogenesis. *Brain* (2016) 139(Pt 10):2641–52. doi: 10.1093/brain/aww208
35. Lang K, Prüss H. Frequencies of neuronal autoantibodies in healthy controls: estimation of disease specificity. *Neurol Neuroimmunol Neuroinflamm.* (2017) 4:386. doi: 10.1212/NXI.0000000000000386
36. Mader S, Brimberg L, Diamond B. The role of brain-reactive autoantibodies in brain pathology and cognitive impairment. *Front Immunol.* (2017) 8:1101. doi: 10.3389/fimmu.2017.01101
37. Pathmanandavel K, Starling J, Dale RC, Brilot F. Autoantibodies and the immune hypothesis in psychotic brain diseases: challenges and perspectives. *Clin Dev Immunol.* (2013) 2013:257184. doi: 10.1155/2013/257184
38. Najjar S, Pahlajani S, Sanctis V de, Stern JNH, Najjar A, Chong D. Neurovascular unit dysfunction and blood–brain barrier hyperpermeability contribute to schizophrenia neurobiology: a theoretical integration of clinical and experimental evidence. *Front Psychiatry* (2017) 8:83. doi: 10.3389/fpsyt.2017.00083
39. Bernstein H-G, Steiner J, Guest PC, Dobrowolny H, Bogerts B. Glial cells as key players in schizophrenia pathology: recent insights and concepts of therapy. *Schizophr Res.* (2015) 161:4–18. doi: 10.1016/j.schres.2014.03.035
40. Bogerts B, Winopal D, Schwarz S, Schlaaff K, Dobrowolny H, Mawrin C, et al. Evidence of neuroinflammation in subgroups of schizophrenia and mood disorder patients: a semiquantitative postmortem study of CD3 and CD20 immunoreactive lymphocytes in several brain regions. *Neurol Psychiatry Brain Res.* (2017) 23:2–9. doi: 10.1016/j.npbr.2016.11.001
41. Schubert KO, Clark SR, Baune BT. The use of clinical and biological characteristics to predict outcome following First Episode Psychosis. *Aust N Z J Psychiatry* (2015) 49:24–35. doi: 10.1177/0004867414560650
42. Singhal G, Jaehne EJ, Corrigan F, Toben C, Baune BT. Inflammasomes in neuroinflammation and changes in brain function: a focused review. *Front Neurosci.* (2014) 8:315. doi: 10.3389/fnins.2014.00315
43. Fillman SG, Sinclair D, Fung SJ, Webster MJ, Shannon Weickert C. Markers of inflammation and stress distinguish subsets of individuals with schizophrenia and bipolar disorder. *Transl Psychiatry* (2014) 4:e365. doi: 10.1038/tp.2014.8
44. Najjar S, Pearlman DM. Neuroinflammation and white matter pathology in schizophrenia: Systematic review. *Schizophr Res.* (2015) 161:102–12. doi: 10.1016/j.schres.2014.04.041
45. Bechter K, Reiber H, Herzog S, Fuchs D, Tumani H, Maxeiner HG. Cerebrospinal fluid analysis in affective and schizophrenic spectrum disorders: Identification of subgroups with immune responses and blood-CSF barrier dysfunction. *J Psychiatr Res.* (2010) 44:321–30. doi: 10.1016/j.jpsychires.2009.08.008
46. Kuehne LK, Reiber H, Bechter K, Hagberg L, Fuchs D. Cerebrospinal fluid neopterin is brain-derived and not associated with blood-CSF barrier dysfunction in non-inflammatory affective and schizophrenic spectrum disorders. *J Psychiatr Res.* (2013) 47:1417–22. doi: 10.1016/j.jpsychires.2013.05.027
47. Maxeiner H-G, Marion Schneider E, Kurfiss S-T, Brettschneider J, Tumani H, Bechter K. Cerebrospinal fluid and serum cytokine profiling to detect immune control of infectious and inflammatory neurological and psychiatric diseases. *Cytokine* (2014) 69:62–7. doi: 10.1016/j.cyto.2014.05.008
48. Maxeiner H-G, Rojewski MT, Schmitt A, Tumani H, Bechter K, Schmitt M. Flow cytometric analysis of T cell subsets in paired samples of cerebrospinal fluid and peripheral blood from patients with neurological and psychiatric disorders. *Brain Behav Immun.* (2009) 23:134–42. doi: 10.1016/j.bbi.2008.08.003
49. Ellul P, Groc L, Tamouza R, Leboyer M. The clinical challenge of autoimmune psychosis: learning from anti-NMDA receptor autoantibodies. *Front Psychiatry* (2017) 8:54. doi: 10.3389/fpsyt.2017.00054
50. Medzhitov R. Origin and physiological roles of inflammation. *Nature* (2008) 454:428–35. doi: 10.1038/nature07201
51. Wohleb ES. Neuron-microglia interactions in mental health disorders: "For Better, and For Worse". *Front Immunol.* (2016) 7:544. doi: 10.3389/fimmu.2016.00544
52. Teunissen CE, Verheul C, Willemse EAJ. The use of cerebrospinal fluid in biomarker studies. *Handb Clin Neurol.* (2017) 146:3–20. doi: 10.1016/b978-0-12-804279-3.00001-0
53. Berk M, Conus P, Kapczinski F, Andreazza AC, Yücel M, Wood SJ, et al. From neuroprogression to neuroprotection: implications for clinical care. *Med J Aust.* (2010) 193(4 Suppl): S36-40.
54. Haroon E, Miller AH. Inflammation effects on glutamate as a pathway to neuroprogression in mood disorders. *Mod Trends Pharmacopsychiatry* (2017) 31:37–55. doi: 10.1159/000470805
55. Maes M, Leonard B, Fernandez A, Kubera M, Nowak G, Veerhuis R, et al. (Neuro)inflammation and neuroprogression as new pathways and drug targets in depression: from antioxidants to kinase inhibitors. *Prog Neuropsychopharmacol Biol Psychiatry* (2011) 35:659–63. doi: 10.1016/j.pnpbp.2011.02.019
56. Berk M, Williams LJ, Jacka FN, O'Neil A, Pasco JA, Moylan S, et al. So depression is an inflammatory disease, but where does the inflammation come from? *BMC Med.* (2013) 11:200. doi: 10.1186/1741-7015-11-200
57. Maes M, Anderson G, Kubera M, Berk M. Targeting classical IL-6 signalling or IL-6 trans-signalling in depression? *Expert Opin Ther Targets* (2014) 18:495–512. doi: 10.1517/14728222.2014.888417
58. Davis J, Moylan S, Harvey BH, Maes M, Berk M. Neuroprogression in schizophrenia: Pathways underpinning clinical staging and therapeutic corollaries. *Aust N Z J Psychiatry* (2014) 48:512–29. doi: 10.1177/0004867414533012
59. Müller N. Neuroprogression in schizophrenia and psychotic disorders: the possible role of inflammation. *Mod Trends Pharmacopsychiatry* (2017) 31:1–9. doi: 10.1159/000470802
60. Tang SW, Helmeste DM, Leonard BE. Neurodegeneration, neuroregeneration, and neuroprotection in psychiatric disorders. *Mod Trends Pharmacopsychiatry* (2017) 31:107–23. doi: 10.1159/000470811
61. Cuthbert BN, Insel TR. Toward the future of psychiatric diagnosis: the seven pillars of RDoC. *BMC Med.* (2013) 11:126. doi: 10.1186/1741-7015-11-126
62. Bechter K, Herzog S, Schreiner V, Wollinsky KH, Schüttler R. Cerebrospinal fluid filtration in a case of schizophrenia related to 'subclinical' Borna disease virus encephalitis. In: Müller N. editor. *Psychiatry, Psychoneuroimmunology and Viruses, Key Top Brain Research.* Wien: Springer (1999). p. 19–35
63. Bechter K, Schreiner V, Herzog S, Breitinger N, Wollinsky KH, Brinkmeier H, et al. Liquorfiltration als experimentelle Therapie bei therapieresistenten Psychosen Borna-Disease-Virus-seropositiver Patienten—Therapeutische Effekte, Befunde. *Psychiatr Prax* (2003) 30(Suppl 2):216–20. doi: 10.1055/s-2003-39747
64. Endres D, Perlov E, Riering AN, Maier V, Stich O, Dersch R, et al. Steroid-responsive chronic schizophreniform syndrome in the context of mildly increased antithyroid peroxidase antibodies. *Front Psychiatry* (2017) 8:64. doi: 10.3389/fpsyt.2017.00064
65. Endres D, Perlov E, Feige B, Altenmüller D-M, Venhoff N, van Tebartz Elst L. Schizophrenia associated with epileptiform discharges without seizures successfully treated with levetiracetam. *Front Psychiatry* (2017) 8:12. doi: 10.3389/fpsyt.2017.00012
66. Endres D, Perlov E, Stich O, Meyer PT, Lützen N, van Tebartz Elst L. Case report: low-titre anti-Yo reactivity in a female patient with psychotic syndrome and frontoparieto-cerebellar atrophy. *BMC Psychiatry* (2015) 15:122. doi: 10.1186/s12888-015-0486-x
67. Thienemann M, Murphy T, Leckman J, Shaw R, Williams K, Kapphahn C, et al. Management of pediatric acute-onset neuropsychiatric syndrome: part I-psychiatric and behavioral interventions. *J Child Adolesc Psychopharmacol.* (2017) 27:566–73. doi: 10.1089/cap.2016.0145
68. Ong LTC, Galambos G, Brown DA. Primary Sjogren's syndrome associated with treatment-resistant obsessive-compulsive disorder. *Front Psychiatry* (2017) 8:124. doi: 10.3389/fpsyt.2017.00124
69. Swedo SE, Frankovich J, Murphy TK. Overview of treatment of pediatric acute-onset neuropsychiatric syndrome. *J Child Adolesc Psychopharmacol.* (2017) 27:562–5. doi: 10.1089/cap.2017.0042

70. Zetterberg H, Rohrer JD, Schott JM. Cerebrospinal fluid in the dementias. *Handb Clin Neurol.* (2017) 146:85–97. doi: 10.1016/B978-0-12-804279-3.00006-X
71. Engelborghs S, Niemantsverdriet E, Struyfs H, Blennow K, Brouns R, Comabella M, et al. Consensus guidelines for lumbar puncture in patients with neurological diseases. *Alzheimers Dement.* (2017) 8:111–26. doi: 10.1016/j.dadm.2017.04.007
72. Nath S, Koziarz A, Badhiwala JH, Alhazzani W, Jaeschke R, Sharma S, et al. Atraumatic versus conventional lumbar puncture needles: a systematic review and meta-analysis. *The Lancet* (2018) 391:1197–204. doi: 10.1016/S0140-6736(17)32451-0

8

Bright Light as a Personalized Precision Treatment of Mood Disorders

Julia Maruani [1,2,3,4] and Pierre Alexis Geoffroy [1,2,3,4]*

[1] Inserm, U1144, Paris, France, [2] Université Paris Descartes, UMR-S 1144, Paris, France, [3] Université Paris Diderot, Sorbonne Paris Cité, UMR-S 1144, Paris, France, [4] AP-HP, GH Saint-Louis–Lariboisière–F. Widal, Pôle de Psychiatrie et de Médecine Addictologique, Paris, France

Correspondence:
Pierre Alexis Geoffroy
pierre.a.geoffroy@gmail.com

Background: The use of light for its antidepressant action dates back to the beginnings of civilization. Three decades ago, the use of bright-light therapy (BLT) for treating Seasonal Affective Disorder (SAD) was officially proposed. Since then, a growing scientific literature reports its antidepressant efficacy in both unipolar and bipolar disorders (BD), with or without seasonal patterns. This review aims to examine the management of BLT as a personalized and precision treatment in SAD, unipolar, and BD.

Methods: We conducted a narrative review using Medline and Google Scholar databases up to June 2018.

Results: BLT has physiological effects by resynchronizing the biological clock (circadian system), enhancing alertness, increasing sleep pressure (homeostatic system), and acting on serotonin, and other monoaminergic pathways. Effects of BLT on mood depend on several factors such as light intensity, wavelength spectrum, illumination duration, time of the day, and individual circadian rhythms. A growing body of evidence has been generated over the last decade about BLT evolving as an effective depression treatment not only to be used in SAD, but also in non-seasonal depression, with efficiency comparable to fluoxetine, and possibly more robust in patients with BD. The antidepressant action of BLT is fast (within 1-week) and safe, with the need in BD to protect against manic switch with mood stabilizers. Side effects might be nausea, diarrhea, headache, and eye irritation, and are generally mild and rare. This good safety profile may be of particular interest, especially in women during the perinatal period or for the elderly. The management of BLT needs to be clarified across mood disorders and future studies are expected to compare different dose-titration protocols, to validate its use as a maintenance treatment, and also to identify predictive biomarkers of response and tolerability. We propose clinical guidelines for BLT use in SAD, non-seasonal depression, and BD.

Conclusions : BLT is an efficient antidepressant strategy in mono- or adjunct-therapy, that should be personalized according the unipolar or bipolar subtype, the presence or absence of seasonal patterns, and also regarding its efficacy and tolerability.

Keywords: bright light therapy, circadian rhythms, sleep, seasonal affective disorder, non-seasonal depression, bipolar disorder

INTRODUCTION

The use of light for its antidepressant action dates back to the beginnings of civilization (1). Three decades ago, the use of bright-light therapy (BLT) for treating Seasonal Affective Disorder (SAD) was officially proposed. It is now acknowledged as an antidepressant strategy for mood disorders (2–4). In the 1980s, BLT was developed in SAD to extend daytime photoperiod and counteract winter darkness (5). BLT is now considered to be the first line treatment for SAD in therapeutic guidelines (2). Since then, a growing scientific literature reports its antidepressant efficacy in both unipolar and bipolar disorders (BD), without such seasonal patterns. Indeed, the sustained antidepressant efficacy of BLT, used alone or in combination with antidepressant drugs–but also with some mood stabilizers and sleep deprivation, has been evidenced in numerous clinical studies (2, 6, 7). This antidepressant effect may be both due to light's effect on the biological clock -by phase advance and alignment of circadian rhythms- and/or actions on non-circadian pathways (8). Indeed, light modulates the activation of efferent serotonergic neurons, decreases the serotonin reuptake transporter (5-HTT) levels, and increases serotonin (5-HT) levels in mood regulatory areas such as the anterior cingulate and prefrontal Cortex (1, 9). Recent reviews discuss how light may influence mood, and emphasize recent finding of light's direct effects on enhancing alertness and the sleep homeostasis (10). Thus, light exerts strong effects on mood thanks to many circadian and non-circadian actions that may combine: phase shifting of circadian rhythms, enhancement alertness, sleep homeostasis by increasing EEG delta activity and sleep pressure, and modulation of the serotonin and other monoaminergic pathways. These effects of BLT on mood depend on several factors such as light intensity, wavelength spectrum, illumination duration, time of the day, and individual circadian rhythms (3).

However, the management of BLT continues to be a point of debate in mood disorders, with no evidence-based guidelines for implementing BLT in patients across mood disorders (2, 11, 12). This review aims to examine the management of BLT as a personalized and precision mood disorders treatment, encompassing both unipolar and bipolar disorders, and seasonal and non-seasonal characteristics.

MATERIALS AND METHODS

Search Strategy

We aimed to consider papers examining efficacy of BLT in mood disorder including SAD, unipolar and bipolar disorders, with or without seasonal characteristics. Only data published in English and French were included in this review. We conducted a narrative review using Medline and Google Scholar databases up to June 2018, using the following keywords combination: ("depression" or "bipolar disorder" or "unipolar disorder," or "seasonal affective disorder") and ("light therapy" or "phototherapy").

Study Selection

Two authors (JM, PAG) reviewed the title and abstract of identified publications in order to identify eligible studies. The two resulting article lists were compared and, in case of disagreement, the final decision as to inclusion was made by consensus. JM and PG independently and then jointly selected studies for detailed extraction of information, mostly based on the full text. In cases where full text was not available, corresponding authors were contacted. If a reply was not obtained following a 6-month waiting period, abstracts were then considered in the review only if the appropriate information was included. The exclusion criteria included reviews, meta-analyses, commentaries, case reports, and studies where bright light therapy on patients with BD or SAD or unipolar depression was not investigated. Finally, we decided to divide literature results in four main sections: (1) BLT in SAD; (2) BLT in non-seasonal depression; (3) BLT in BD depression; (4) BLT for sleep and circadian rhythms abnormalities associated in chronic mood disorders.

RESULTS

The literature search returned 234 records pertaining to BLT, SAD, and unipolar and bipolar disorders, with or without seasonal characteristics. Following preliminary screening of the titles and abstracts, 125 records were excluded (reviews, meta-analyses, commentaries, case reports, and studies where bright light therapy on patients with BD or SAD or unipolar depression was not investigated). With 41 studies identified from the related articles function of the PubMed database and the reference list of retained studies, 84 independent studies were retained in the qualitative analysis. These investigations were classified according to their studied parameters: (1) 17 Studies explored BLT in SAD; (2) 40 studies explored BLT in non-seasonal depression; (3) 12 studies explored BLT in BD depression; (4) 15 studies explored BLT for sleep and circadian rhythms abnormalities associated in chronic mood disorders.

Bright Light Therapy in Seasonal Affective Disorders (SAD)

BLT as an Effective Curative Treatment in SAD

Among mood disorders, seasonal affective disorder (SAD) corresponds to the seasonal pattern of recurrent major depressive episodes occurring during the same time of the year, usually in autumn or winter with spontaneous remission in the spring or summer (5). This disorder is frequent, with prevalence varying between 0.4 and 16% in the general population according to latitude, age, sex, and the method of measurement used (13). SAD is a severe transdiagnostic disorder that may affect patients with both unipolar and bipolar disorders (5, 14). Over the past two decades, researchers, and clinicians have mainly focused on the pathophysiological mechanisms involved in SAD. Studies support the existence of interactions between a genetic vulnerability and chronobiological factors, and brain process alterations including noradrenergic and serotoninergic neurotransmissions (8). Several international therapeutic guidelines and many studies suggest that BLT is a non-pharmacological antidepressant that has proved to be effective in SAD and is now used as the first line treatment for individuals with SAD because of its low side effects profile and high response rate about 67% in patients with milder SAD and 40% in severe SAD patients (2–4, 15–17).

Usage in SAD

BLT is classically delivered through a light box that is equipped with fluorescent tubes and a reflector or diffusing screen. Patients sit in front of the light box mounted on a table with their eyes open. BLT may be also administered thanks to light glasses or visors (18, 19).

Treatment in SAD may begin with exposition duration of 30 min, using a light intensity of 10,000 lux. Early morning administration offers greater chances for remission (20, 21). Measured at eye level, a therapeutic distance of 60–80 cm from the light box can be seen as standard requirements (some other devices recommend a distance of 30 cm, so we advise to follow the device recommendations that take into account light parameters and distance). Lower intensities also appear to be effective, but need longer exposure durations: 2,500 Lux for 2 h/day, 5,000 Lux for 1 h/day. Significant effects appear only at 2–3 weeks of treatment. Treatment is usually continued until the time of usual spontaneous remission in the spring or summer because the effects of LT do not persist after discontinuation of BLT. In addition, it has been observed that low-intensity blue-enriched light has a therapeutic effect comparable to standard bright light (10,000 lux) in treating SAD (22). Finally, BLT is well-tolerated by patients; adverse effects such as headache, eyestrain, nausea and agitation, are usually transient and mild (23, 24). Main contraindications are ophthalmic disorders (cataract, macular degeneration, glaucoma, retinitis pigmentosa) and disorders affecting the retina (retinopathy, diabetes, herpes, etc.); and patients at risk (or if there is a doubt) should have pretreatment ophthalmological examinations (3).

BLT as a Preventive Device for Seasonal Affective Disorder

Patients with SAD might benefit from prophylactic use of BLT (25, 26). A recent Cochrane review assessed the efficacy of BLT in preventing SAD (27). Both forms of preventive light therapy (light boxes and visor) reduced the incidence of SAD compared with no light therapy. Although not statistically significant, they observed that BLT reduced the risk of SAD incidence of 36% (27). However, given methodological limitations (small sample sizes of available RCTs, and lack of power for some analyses), authors concluded that the decision for or against initiating preventive treatment of SAD and the treatment selected should be strongly based on patient preferences.

Bright Light Therapy for Non-seasonal Depression

BLT as an Effective Treatment in Non-seasonal Depression

In the last two decades, the interest in BLT has expanded far beyond SAD. Indeed, several studies investigated the efficacy of BLT in treating non-seasonal depression disorders as alternative or adjunctive treatment. This is of major interest because depression affects an estimated 350 million people worldwide and is projected to become the second global leading cause of disability by the year 2020 (28). Moreover, only 50–60% of patients respond to first line antidepressants and only 35–40% experience remission of symptoms (29). Last but not least, pharmacological antidepressant strategies as first line treatments take at least 4 weeks to build up its effect and work fully (11).

Recent systematic reviews and meta-analyses confirmed this extent of antidepressant efficacy in non-seasonal depressions. Indeed the APA Committee on Research on Psychiatric treatment (2) and a Cochrane review (12) observed significant effect sizes equivalent to those in most antidepressant pharmacotherapy trials that were about 0.84. Reports and double blind placebo controlled studies suggest that the efficacy of BLT as an adjunct therapy in treating non-seasonal depression in its initial phase is faster and is perceived during the first week of treatment (7, 30, 31). These studies also confirmed the efficacy of the combination of BLT and selective serotonin reuptake inhibitors (SSRIs) with benefit after 1 month of treatment. BLT combined with SSRI lead to a faster (within a week) and better remission of patients (by reducing 30% of symptoms) in patients with non-seasonal depression than SSRIs alone (7, 31). In line with this, results are confirmed in a recent meta-analysis that also conclude that BLT are effective for patients with non-seasonal depression with clinical significant effect (SMD $= -0.62$, $P < 0.001$, $I^2 = 37\%$) and can be a helpful additional treatment for depression (32). This meta-analysis included 419 patients with non-seasonal depression (unipolar or bipolar depression) from 9 trials: 211 receiving BLT and 208-placebo controls. Most participants received BLT as a monotherapy except in two trials where they had BLT in addition to antidepressant. First, their results reported significant effects in the first week when administered in the early morning (2, 12). They found the largest antidepressant effect of BLT for an exposure duration of 2–5 weeks, and unfortunately were not able to propose an optimal intensity of BLT given the heterogeneity of the trials. Another recent meta-analysis of randomized controlled trials (11), including 881 participants from 20 RCTs used BLT as monotherapy compared to an inactive placebo/control group; and also as an adjunctive treatment in comparison to the same control group. They considered individuals with all depression subtypes excepting SAD: major depressive disorder; persistent depressive disorder, and BD depression. All forms of BLT (timing of administration, brightness, and duration of light exposure) were included, even though most studies ($n = 5$) used bright white light at 10,000 lux in early morning for 30 min/day or 2,500 lux for 120 min/day. They found that BLT was associated with a small to moderate effect in reducing symptoms in adults (11). Interestingly, studies demonstrated twice the reduction in depressive symptoms for BLT than placebo. Moreover, meta-analyses of Perera et al. (11) and Golden et al. (2) both found that BLT may be most effective when applied as an antidepressant monotherapy (and not as an adjunct treatment), when administered in the morning and among out-patients, that may have less severe depressive symptoms and comorbidities than in-patients. So, taken as a whole, patients who are non-responsive or ineligible for pharmacotherapy may benefit from monotherapy BLT, but BLT could also be considered as an effective first line treatment. For the elderly, BLT also seems to be efficient (33–35). Recently a systematic review in non-seasonal geriatric depression found that BLT during 6 weeks, with exposure duration varying between 30 and 60 min and light intensity varying from 1,200 to 10,000 Lux, is an effective treatment for reducing the depression symptoms in the elderly (34).

Finally, regarding safety in non-seasonal depression, side effects are rare and generally mild: nausea, diarrhea, headache, and eye irritation (11). This good safety profile may be of particular interest for women with depression in the perinatal period where medications may be inappropriate or ineffective, and also in the elderly.

Usage in Non-seasonal Depression

Precise recommendations regarding the optimal treatment (i.e., optimal exposure duration and intensity) are difficult because of the heterogeneity of study protocols and absence of comparisions between protocols (32). However, it is possible to say that BLT is confirmed to be efficient both as a mono- or adjunct-therapy in treating non-seasonal depression in his acute phase, with benefits that can be perceived during the first week of treatment. The effects of BLT do not appear to persist after discontinuation with a complete offset of effect after 1 month (36), and this relapse can be prevented when combining BLT with common antidepressant drugs (37). According to previous studies, daily early morning exposures to 2,500 Lux for 2 h (38), 5,000 Lux for 1 h (39), or 10,000 Lux for 30 min (40) all appear efficient in reducing antidepressant symptoms. Finally, BLT is well-tolerated by patients, and possible adverse effects might be headache, eyestrain, nausea, and agitation, that are usually transient and mild (see **Table 1**).

Bright Light Therapy in Acute Bipolar Disorder Depression

BLT as an Effective Treatment in Bipolar Disorder Depression

About 1–4% of the worldwide population suffers from bipolar disorder (BD), which is a severe mental disorder associated with both depressive and manic episodes that may be induced by antidepressants (41, 42). Given the limited treatment options in BD depression, since Lewy's study (43) several researches have focused on investigating BLT in this particular population because BD are increasingly recognized as disorders of the biological clock (44, 45), with circadian dysregulation being evident in both acute and remission phases (46, 47). Indeed, research has shown that patients with BD depression responded robustly to BLT (1). While the efficacy of BLT in monotherapy is non-significant in some studies (48, 49), the combination of BLT with other chronotherapeutic techniques such as sleep deprivation and with lithium salts was proven in BD depression patients (6, 50).

First, Leibenluft et al. showed that BLT at midday could be tailored to counteract depressive swings without exacerbating mania, in course of rapid cycling BD (51). Later, Benedetti et al. showed that morning sunlight reduces length of hospitalization in BD depression by comparing a sample of 415 unipolar and 187 bipolar depression inpatients assigned with eastern or western windows (52). They found that inpatients in eastern rooms exposed to direct sunlight in the morning had a shorter hospitalization than patients in western rooms (52). In 2005, the same team showed that combination of total sleep deprivation and BLT in drug-resistant patients with BD depression was useful in triggering an acute response (6). Since 2005, several randomized controlled studies and meta-analyses of randomized controlled studies focused on BLT efficacy in BD and confirmed that BLT is an effective and safe option as an adjunctive therapy in BD depression (53–56). Indeed, Yorguner Kupeli et al. confirmed in a randomized single blind placebo-controlled study the efficacy of BLT as an add-on treatment for BD depression when it is administered in the mornings at 10,000 lux for 30 min for a 2-week period, sitting 40–70 cm's away from the device (56). Zhou et al. also confirmed in a randomized single blind placebo controlled study the efficacy of 1 h, 5,000 lux, every morning -between 6:30 am and 9 am- of BLT as an add-on therapy, by reduction of depressive symptoms and observed onset efficacy at 4 days (54). Interestingly, no participants experienced symptoms of mania and no serious adverse effects were reported. Regarding midday BLT, Sit et al. performed a 6 week randomized double-blind placebo-controlled trial and found results supporting midday BLT as an efficient therapy in BD depression (55). In this RCT study, light therapy was administered as an add-on therapy (anti-manic or antidepressant medication) to patients with a current moderate or severe depression and showed that the BLT group (7,000 Lux at midday) had significantly higher remission rates (56%) vs. the 50-lux dim red light (14.3%). Duration of light therapy was increased progressively every week by 15 min to attain a target dose of 60 min per day at 4 weeks (55). Again, in this randomized controlled trial, no hypomanic/manic shift was observed, contrary to a previous report from the same team that observed (hypo)manic switches in females with rapid cycling BD and morning exposures (55). Benedetti (57) performed a systematic review of the literature studies reporting effect of antidepressant BLT in BD and their conclusions were limited again by the heterogeneity of treatment modalities between studies. Nevertheless, their review managed to include 799 treated patients and shows that the rate of switch into mania after morning BLT was small and close to the 4.2% expected during the placebo treatment of BD, whereas the rate of switch into mania after antidepressant drug treatment is 15–40% (58).

TABLE 1 | Forms of bright light therapy use in different mood disorders.

	Seasonal affective disorder (SAD)	Non-seasonal unipolar disorder	Non-seasonal bipolar disorder
Light intensity	2,500–10,000 Lux Or low-intensity blue-enriched light	2,500–10,000 Lux	<10,000 Lux
Dose (Exposure durations/Intensity of illumination)	First line: 10,000 Lux for 30 min/day Also consider: 5,000 Lux for 1 h/day or 2,500 Lux for 2 h/day		Slower increase For instance: 5,000 Lux with increase of 15 min per week until 60 min at one month (depending on efficacy and tolerance)
Lamp disposition	lamp at eye level distance of 30–80 cm (depending on the device recommendations)		
Frequency	Daily		Daily
Administration	Mono- or adjunct-therapy		Only with a mood stabilizer with antimanic properties
Time of the day	Early morning (for instance: 8 am, chronotype may be considered)		Midday (especially if there is an history of manic switch) Or Early morning
Onset of response	1 week		
Duration of treatment	Until the period of usual spontaneous remission in the spring or summer	2–5 weeks	Until reduction of depressive symptoms or maintained in case of relapse when stopped
Prevention	Possibility to treat by light therapy a few weeks before the usual seasonal depressive relapse period	NA	NA
Adverse effects	Manic switch and mild side effects (headache, eyestrain, nausea, and agitation)	Mild side effects (headache, eyestrain, nausea, diarrhea, and agitation)	Manic switch and mild side effects (headache, eyestrain, nausea, and agitation)
Contraindications	Ophthalmic disorders (cataract, macular degeneration, glaucoma, retinitis pigmentosa), and disorders affecting the retina (retinopathy, diabetes, herpes, etc.)		

NA, data not available.

Usage in Bipolar Depression

BLT is a robust strategy treatment for bipolar depression and might be considered as a first line option for depressive episode in the course of BD (**Table 1**). Interestingly, BLT acts rapidly (within 4 days), has low side effects and low risk of manic switch in combination with mood stabilizing treatment (54). The most efficient light parameters are not yet fully determined, but it seems that patients are sensitive to light intensities below 10,000 lux, depending on the duration of exposure. Some observations suggest that depression could respond to light intensities as low as 300–500 lux (48, 50). Studies support both midday or morning BLT as an efficient therapy in BD depression and duration of light therapy could be increased progressively every week by 15 min to attain a target dose of 60 min per daily at 4 weeks (55). Furthermore, BLT should always be combined with a mood stabilizer, first to prevent manic switch in BD, but also to enhance and sustain the acute antidepressant effects of BLT (6).

BLT for Sleep and Circadian Rhythm Abnormalities in Chronic Mood Disorders

BLT as an Effective Treatment in sleep and Circadian Rhythms Abnormalities

Light may act as a therapeutic mood stabilizer in patients with mood disorders during remission by stabilizing sleep alterations (like insomnia or longer sleep duration), and circadian rhythms (like evening chronotype or sleep phase delayed) (10). Indeed light exerts strong effects on mood through different pathways. First, light may affect mood through phase shifting of circadian rhythms (59–61). This circadian effect of light on mood results from its effect on the optimal alignment vs. misalignment of different circadian rhythms, which may be mediated through the phase shifting effects of light and modifying the duration of nocturnal melatonin secretion (59–61). This effect of light on mood via the circadian system is well-illustrated by SAD. SAD involves an internal misalignment of the circadian system and responds positively to treatments that resynchronize the biological clock, such as BLT. So, in addition to increasing the monoaminergic tone, application of BLT in the morning causes phase advance of endogenous circadian rhythms. These effects of light exposure on mood via modulation of the circadian system are not restricted to patients with SAD, but also in non-seasonal depression (both unipolar and bipolar), with available data that shows that BLT is an effective antidepressant or mood stabilizer (6).

Secondly, light exerts an effect on alertness, a parameter-influencing mood (62, 63). Impaired alertness is a common symptom in many affective disorders such as MDD, BD, or SAD (10). Increasing alertness has also been an effective strategy for improving mood (64–66). Light stimulates alertness through the synchronization of the homeostatic and circadian drives, and through melatonin suppression (10). And light has direct effect on alertness via the melanopsin retinal ganglion cells by impinging on the sleep-active neurons: through simultaneous inhibition of the sleep-inducing VLPO and activation of the

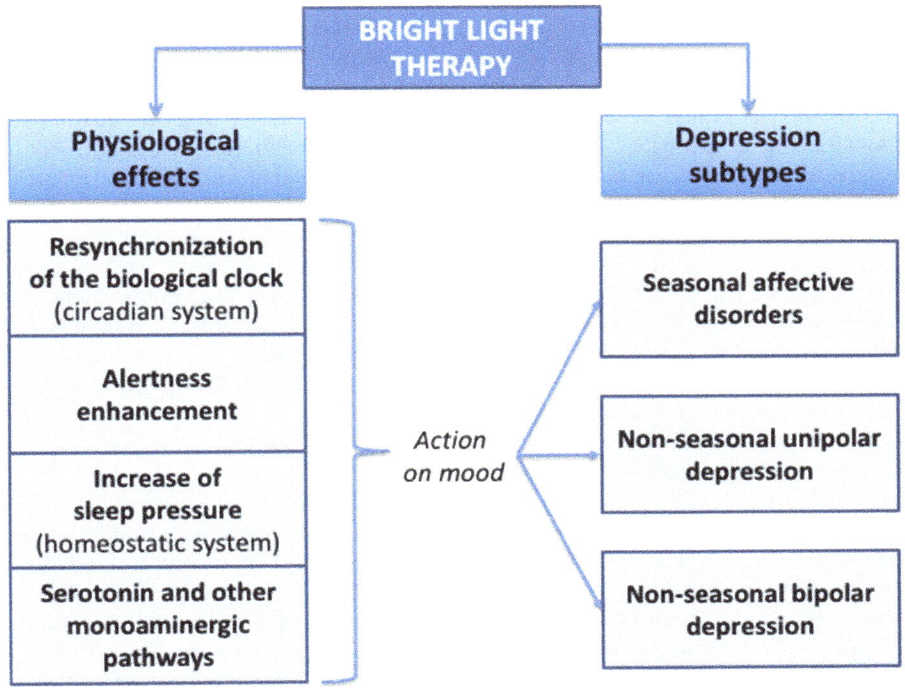

FIGURE 1 | Effects of bright light therapy in mood disorders.

monoaminergic arousal systems that are also involved in control of mood (10).

Thirdly, light may regulate mood disorders by improving sleep homeostasis with direct positive effect on the EEG delta sleep activity via the secretion of melanopsin, which is a photopigment expressed in a subset of retinal ganglion cells that activates the VLPO and improve by this way sleep homeostasis (10, 67, 68). This is again well-illustrated in studies with SAD patients that have a lower delta activity and lower sleep efficiency (69). Indeed, sleep deprivation combined with chronotherapeutics such as BLT have an antidepressant effect by improving sleep pressure (69).

All these data support an impact of BLT by resynchronizing the biological clock (circadian system), and/or enhancing alertness, and/or increasing sleep pressure (homeostatic system), acting consequently on mood both in acute and remission phases (**Figure 1**).

Recommendations for Use in Patients With BD in Remission

Sleep and circadian rhythm abnormalities are frequent in mood disorders, even between acute episodes, contributing to poor functioning, and relapses (70, 71). For instance, in BD, studies of actigraphy and DMLO identify higher prevalence of delayed sleep phase (72) and exhibit greater variability in sleep duration, fragmentation, later, and more variable bedtimes than healthy controls (71). In this context, we suggest treating and applying recommendations for comorbid delayed phase sleep, insomnia, or hypersomnia in individuals suffering from mood disorders, even in remission. Recommending BLT in the context of such circadian and sleep comorbidities in mood disorders may thus be similar to recommendations for previous different subtype of depression detailed previously (**Table 1**).

DISCUSSION

This review draws up an inventory of scientific knowledge about the use of BLT in mood disorders thanks to a growing evidence about BLT evolving as an effective depression treatment not only to be used in SAD but also in non-seasonal depression and in BD. BLT is efficient on depression, acts rapidly, with low rates of manic switch, and can be easily prescribed combined or not with mood-stabilizing antidepressant, or other chronotherapeutic treatments such as sleep deprivation or lithium (6, 73). **Table 1** summarizes different forms of BLT use in the different mood disorders subtypes. This review also highlights several shortcomings in the scientific literature, and paves the way for further studies to clarify the management of BLT across mood disorders by comparing different initiation protocols depending on depression subtypes, to validate its use as a maintenance treatment, and also to identify predictive biomarkers of response and tolerability.

First, there is a great heterogeneity of management of BLT across studies making it difficult to make recommendations for good practices of BLT (2, 11). For instance, whereas recent studies such as Lam et al. (40) that directly compared mono or adjunct therapies found larger effect of BLT/SSRI combination, some meta-analyses suggest on the other hand that monotherapy may be more effective (2, 11), maybe because of limitations previously advocated.

Secondly, where the lamp should be placed relative to the eye varies between available devices and across studies. Nevertheless, for most traditional BLT devices, it should be placed at eye level and a distance of 30–80 cm, in an adequately lighted room (where a newspaper may be read easily). The distance depends of the device and should be closely respected since Lux decreased quickly. Others new BLT devices should be placed as glasses and are easy to placed.

Thirdly, the vast majority of data are from review or meta-analyses in which the distinction is not made between unipolar disorder or BD, but also between seasonal characteristics or not, mostly because of lacking data and small sample sizes (55).

Nevertheless, our review aimed to propose global therapeutic strategies to use BLT in SAD, unipolar and bipolar disorders without seasonal characteristic and so, allows only partially personalizing BLT in mood disorder.

Because of the heterogeneity of study protocols and absence of comparisions between protocols, proper guidelines are difficult to define. In this context of absence of comparisons between protocols, we propose in BD to increase more slowly duration of exposure by 15 min every week to attain a target dose of 60 min per day at 4 weeks in case of insufficient response. In BD, a midday exposure might be safer with regards to manic switch, and should be preferred in cases where individuals have a history of antidepressant manic switch (74). BLT studies do not propose personalized BLT use modalities for bipolar disorder with seasonal pattern. For instance BLT studies assess only the effects of bright light therapy on SAD, which is a transdiagnostic disorder that may affect patients with unipolar and bipolar disorders, and proposed early morning administration with exposure duration of 30 min, using a light intensity of 10,000 lux.

Future studies will likely need to distinguish the use of BLT between bipolar disorder with seasonal pattern and unipolar disorder with seasonal pattern because patients with bipolar disorder with seasonal pattern are able to switch into mania (75). As patients with bipolar disorder without seasonal pattern, they are likely to need a midday utilization of BLT or a more progressive titration, and always in combination with an anti-manic treatment (75).

Finally, evidence suggests that light may play a role in the mood stabilizers therapeutic action by improving sleep quality, and stabilizing circadian rhythms (76). The role of sleep or circadian disturbances as disease course modifiers is well-established, mainly due to their association with treatment-refractory or prolonged mood phases and as predictors of early relapse (70). This review highlights the urgent need for good quality RCTs of BLT in BD during remission for relapses prevention through a potential improvement of sleep quality and stabilization of circadian rhythms.

CONCLUSION

BLT should be considered as a stand-alone treatment option in patient with SAD, but also non-seasonal unipolar or bipolar depression. BLT in treating mood disorders is characterized by rapid and sustained effects both in mono- or adjunct-therapy, combined with antidepressant, or mood stabilizing drugs. However, the management of BLT needs to be clarified across mood disorders and future studies are expected to compare different dose-titration protocols, to validate its use as a maintenance treatment, and also to identify predictive biomarkers of response and tolerance. Finally, BLT may also be useful to improve sleep quality, decreased alertness, abnormalities in circadian rhythms such as sleep phase delay syndrome, that are frequently associated in mood disorders, in order to prevent mood early relapses and recurrences.

AUTHOR CONTRIBUTIONS

JM and PAG performed the literature search and analysis, and both contributed in the manuscript's redaction. JM wrote the first draft of the manuscript. PAG made the figure and the table.

REFERENCES

1. Geoffroy PA, Schroder CM, Bourgin P. Light treatment in depression: an antique treatment with new insights. *Sleep med rev.* (2018) 40:218–9. doi: 10.1016/j.smrv.2018.03.002
2. Golden RN, Gaynes BN, Ekstrom RD, Hamer RM, Jacobsen FM, Suppes T, et al. The efficacy of light therapy in the treatment of mood disorders: a review and meta-analysis of the evidence. *Am j psychiatry.* (2005) 162:656–62. doi: 10.1176/appi.ajp.162.4.656
3. Terman M, Terman JS. Light therapy for seasonal and non-seasonal depression: efficacy, protocol, safety, and side effects. *CNS spectr.* (2005) 10:647–63; quiz 72. doi: 10.1017/S1092852900019611
4. Terman M. Evolving applications of light therapy. *Sleep med rev.* (2007) 11:497–507. doi: 10.1016/j.smrv.2007.06.003
5. Rosenthal NE, Sack DA, Gillin JC, Lewy AJ, Goodwin FK, Davenport Y, et al. Seasonal affective disorder. A description of the syndrome and preliminary findings with light therapy. *Arch general psychiatry.* (1984) 41:72–80. doi: 10.1001/archpsyc.1984.01790120076010
6. Benedetti F, Barbini B, Fulgosi MC, Colombo C, Dallaspezia S, Pontiggia A, et al. Combined total sleep deprivation and light therapy in the treatment of drug-resistant bipolar depression: acute response and long-term remission rates. *J clin psychiatry.* (2005) 66:1535–40. doi: 10.4088/JCP.v66n1207
7. Martiny K, Lunde M, Unden M, Dam H, Bech P. Adjunctive bright light in non-seasonal major depression: results from patient-reported symptom and well-being scales. *Acta psychiatr Scand.* (2005) 111:453–9. doi: 10.1111/j.1600-0447.2005.00532.x
8. Maruani J, Anderson G, Etain B, Lejoyeux M, Bellivier F, Geoffroy PA. The neurobiology of adaptation to seasons: relevance and correlations in bipolar disorders. *Chronobiol int.* (2018) 35:1335–53. doi: 10.1080/07420528.2018.1487975
9. Tyrer AE, Levitan RD, Houle S, Wilson AA, Nobrega JN, Meyer JH. Increased seasonal variation in serotonin transporter binding in seasonal affective disorder. *Neuropsychopharmacology.* (2016) 41:2447–54. doi: 10.1038/npp.2016.54
10. Stephenson KM, Schroder CM, Bertschy G, Bourgin P. Complex interaction of circadian and non-circadian effects of light on mood: shedding new light on an old story. *Sleep med rev.* (2012) 16:445–54. doi: 10.1016/j.smrv.2011.09.002
11. Perera S, Eisen R, Bhatt M, Bhatnagar N, de Souza R, Thabane L, et al. Light therapy for non-seasonal depression: systematic review and meta-analysis. *BJPsych open.* (2016) 2:116–26. doi: 10.1192/bjpo.bp.115.001610

12. Tuunainen A, Kripke DF, Endo T. Light therapy for non-seasonal depression. *Cochr database syst rev.* (2004) 2:CD004050. doi: 10.1002/14651858.CD004050.pub2
13. Magnusson A. An overview of epidemiological studies on seasonal affective disorder. *Acta psychiatr Scand.* (2000) 101:176–84. doi: 10.1034/j.1600-0447.2000.101003176.x
14. Geoffroy PA, Bellivier F, Scott J, Etain B. Seasonality and bipolar disorder: a systematic review, from admission rates to seasonality of symptoms. *J affect disorders.* (2014) 168:210–23. doi: 10.1016/j.jad.2014.07.002
15. Terman M, Terman JS, Quitkin FM, McGrath PJ, Stewart JW, Rafferty B. Light therapy for seasonal affective disorder. A review of efficacy. *Neuropsychopharmacology.* (1989) 2:1–22. doi: 10.1016/0893-133X(89)90002-X
16. Ravindran AV, Balneaves LG, Faulkner G, Ortiz A, McIntosh D, Morehouse RL, et al. Canadian network for mood and anxiety treatments (CANMAT) 2016 clinical guidelines for the management of adults with major depressive disorder: section 5. Complementary and alternative medicine treatments. *Can j psychiatry Revue canad psychiatr.* (2016) 61:576–87. doi: 10.1177/0706743716660290
17. Lam RW, Levitt AJ, Levitan RD, Enns MW, Morehouse R, Michalak EE, et al. The Can-SAD study: a randomized controlled trial of the effectiveness of light therapy and fluoxetine in patients with winter seasonal affective disorder. *Am j psychiatry.* (2006) 163:805–12. doi: 10.1176/ajp.2006.163.5.805
18. Ravaris CL, Elliott B, Hegel M, Rose R, Schiffman J, Singer J. A simple portable ocular light device for phototherapy of seasonal affective disorder. *Biomed instrument technol.* (1994) 28:484–9.
19. Bragard I, Coucke PA. [Impact of the use of Luminette(R) on well-being at work in a radiotherapy department]. *Cancer radiother.* (2013) 17:731–5. doi: 10.1016/j.canrad.2013.05.014
20. Eastman CI, Young MA, Fogg LF, Liu L, Meaden PM. Bright light treatment of winter depression: a placebo-controlled trial. *Arch general psychiatry.* (1998) 55:883–9. doi: 10.1001/archpsyc.55.10.883
21. Terman M, Terman JS, Ross DC. A controlled trial of timed bright light and negative air ionization for treatment of winter depression. *Arch general psychiatry.* (1998) 55:875–82. doi: 10.1001/archpsyc.55.10.875
22. Meesters Y, Dekker V, Schlangen LJ, Bos EH, Ruiter MJ. Low-intensity blue-enriched white light (750 lux) and standard bright light (10,000 lux) are equally effective in treating SAD. A randomized controlled study. *BMC psychiatry.* (2011) 11:17. doi: 10.1186/1471-244X-11-17
23. Terman M, Terman JS. Bright light therapy: side effects and benefits across the symptom spectrum. *J clin psychiatry.* (1999) 60:799–808; quiz 9. doi: 10.4088/JCP.v60n1113
24. Labbate LA, Lafer B, Thibault A, Sachs GS. Side effects induced by bright light treatment for seasonal affective disorder. *J clin psychiatry.* (1994) 55:189–91.
25. Partonen T, Lonnqvist J. Prevention of winter seasonal affective disorder by bright-light treatment. *Psychol med.* (1996) 26:1075–80. doi: 10.1017/S003329170003539X
26. Meesters Y, Beersma DG, Bouhuys AL, van den Hoofdakker RH. Prophylactic treatment of seasonal affective disorder (SAD) by using light visors: bright white or infrared light? *Biol psychiatry.* (1999) 46:239–46. doi: 10.1016/S0006-3223(98)00252-2
27. Nussbaumer B, Kaminski-Hartenthaler A, Forneris CA, Morgan LC, Sonis JH, Gaynes BN, et al. Light therapy for preventing seasonal affective disorder. *Cochr database syst rev.* (2015) 11:CD011269. doi: 10.1002/14651858.CD011269.pub2
28. Murray CJ, Lopez AD. Evidence-based health policy–lessons from the global burden of disease study. *Science.* (1996) 274:740–3. doi: 10.1126/science.274.5288.740
29. Connolly KR, Thase ME. If at first you don't succeed: a review of the evidence for antidepressant augmentation, combination and switching strategies. *Drugs.* (2011) 71:43–64. doi: 10.2165/11587620-000000000-00000
30. Kripke DF. Light treatment for non-seasonal depression: speed, efficacy, and combined treatment. *J affect disorders.* (1998) 49:109–17. doi: 10.1016/S0165-0327(98)00005-6
31. Benedetti F, Colombo C, Pontiggia A, Bernasconi A, Florita M, Smeraldi E. Morning light treatment hastens the antidepressant effect of citalopram: a placebo-controlled trial. *J clin psychiatry.* (2003) 64:648–53. doi: 10.4088/JCP.v64n0605
32. Al-Karawi D, Jubair L. Bright light therapy for non-seasonal depression: meta-analysis of clinical trials. *J affect disorders.* (2016) 198:64–71. doi: 10.1016/j.jad.2016.03.016
33. Lieverse R, Van Someren EJ, Nielen MM, Uitdehaag BM, Smit JH, Hoogendijk WJ. Bright light treatment in elderly patients with non-seasonal major depressive disorder: a randomized placebo-controlled trial. *Arch general psychiatry.* (2011) 68:61–70. doi: 10.1001/archgenpsychiatry.2010.183
34. Zhao X, Ma J, Wu S, Chi I, Bai Z. Light therapy for older patients with non-seasonal depression: a systematic review and meta-analysis. *J affect disorders.* (2018) 232:291–9. doi: 10.1016/j.jad.2018.02.041
35. Sondergaard MP, Jarden JO, Martiny K, Andersen G, Bech P. Dose response to adjunctive light therapy in citalopram-treated patients with post-stroke depression. A randomised, double-blind pilot study. *Psychother psychosomat.* (2006) 75:244–8. doi: 10.1159/000092895
36. Martiny K, Lunde M, Unden M, Dam H, Bech P. The lack of sustained effect of bright light, after discontinuation, in non-seasonal major depression. *Psychol med.* (2006) 36:1247–52. doi: 10.1017/S0033291706008105
37. Martiny K. Adjunctive bright light in non-seasonal major depression. *Acta psychiatr Scand Supplement.* (2004) 110:7–28. doi: 10.1111/j.1600-0447.2004.00460_2.x
38. Kripke DF, Mullaney DJ, Klauber MR, Risch SC, Gillin JC. Controlled trial of bright light for non-seasonal major depressive disorders. *Biol psychiatry.* (1992) 31:119–34. doi: 10.1016/0006-3223(92)90199-A
39. Even C, Schroder CM, Friedman S, Rouillon F. Efficacy of light therapy in non-seasonal depression: a systematic review. *J affect disorders.* (2008) 108:11–23. doi: 10.1016/j.jad.2007.09.008
40. Lam RW, Levitt AJ, Levitan RD, Michalak EE, Cheung AH, Morehouse R, et al. Efficacy of bright light treatment, fluoxetine, and the combination in patients with non-seasonal major depressive disorder: a randomized clinical trial. *JAMA psychiatry.* (2016) 73:56–63. doi: 10.1001/jamapsychiatry.2015.2235
41. Collins PY, Patel V, Joestl SS, March D, Insel TR, Daar AS, et al. Grand challenges in global mental health. *Nature.* (2011) 475:27–30. doi: 10.1038/475027a
42. Merikangas KR, Akiskal HS, Angst J, Greenberg PE, Hirschfeld RM, Petukhova M, et al. Lifetime and 12-month prevalence of bipolar spectrum disorder in the national comorbidity survey replication. *Arch general psychiatry.* (2007) 64:543–52. doi: 10.1001/archpsyc.64.5.543
43. Lewy AJ, Kern HA, Rosenthal NE, Wehr TA. Bright artificial light treatment of a manic-depressive patient with a seasonal mood cycle. *Am j psychiatry.* (1982) 139:1496–8. doi: 10.1176/ajp.139.11.1496
44. Harvey AG. Sleep and circadian rhythms in bipolar disorder: seeking synchrony, harmony, and regulation. *Am j psychiatry.* (2008) 165:820–9. doi: 10.1176/appi.ajp.2008.08010098
45. Gonzalez R. The relationship between bipolar disorder and biological rhythms. *J clin psychiatry.* (2014) 75:e323–31. doi: 10.4088/JCP.13r08507
46. Boudebesse C, Lajnef M, Geoffroy PA, Bellivier F, Nieto I, Gard S, et al. Chronotypes of bipolar patients in remission: validation of the French version of the circadian type inventory in the FACE-BD sample. *Chronobiol int.* (2013) 30:1042–9. doi: 10.3109/07420528.2013.798330
47. Geoffroy PA, Scott J, Boudebesse C, Lajnef M, Henry C, Leboyer M, et al. Reply: sleep in patients with remitted bipolar disorders: analyses stratified on actigraphy devices, age and gender. *Acta psychiatr Scand.* (2015) 131:400. doi: 10.1111/acps.12400
48. Deltito JA, Moline M, Pollak C, Martin LY, Maremmani I. Effects of phototherapy on non-seasonal unipolar and bipolar depressive spectrum disorders. *J affect disorders.* (1991) 23:231–7. doi: 10.1016/0165-0327(91)90105-2
49. Dauphinais DR, Rosenthal JZ, Terman M, DiFebo HM, Tuggle C, Rosenthal NE. Controlled trial of safety and efficacy of bright light therapy vs. negative air ions in patients with bipolar depression. *Psychiatry res.* (2012) 196:57–61. doi: 10.1016/j.psychres.2012.01.015
50. Colombo C, Lucca A, Benedetti F, Barbini B, Campori E, Smeraldi E. Total sleep deprivation combined with lithium and light therapy in the treatment of bipolar depression: replication of main effects and interaction. *Psychiatry res.* (2000) 95:43–53. doi: 10.1016/S0165-1781(00)00164-5
51. Leibenluft E, Turner EH, Feldman-Naim S, Schwartz PJ, Wehr TA, Rosenthal NE. Light therapy in patients with rapid cycling bipolar disorder: preliminary results. *Psychopharmacol bull.* (1995) 31:705–10.

52. Benedetti F, Colombo C, Barbini B, Campori E, Smeraldi E. Morning sunlight reduces length of hospitalization in bipolar depression. *J affect disorders.* (2001) 62:221–3. doi: 10.1016/S0165-0327(00)00149-X
53. Tseng PT Chen YW, Tu KY, Chung W, Wang HY, Wu CK, et al. Light therapy in the treatment of patients with bipolar depression: a meta-analytic study. *Eur neuropsychopharmacol.* (2016) 26:1037–47. doi: 10.1016/j.euroneuro.2016.03.001
54. Zhou TH, Dang WM, Ma YT, Hu CQ, Wang N, Zhang GY, et al. Clinical efficacy, onset time and safety of bright light therapy in acute bipolar depression as an adjunctive therapy: a randomized controlled trial. *J affect disorders.* (2018) 227:90–6. doi: 10.1016/j.jad.2017.09.038
55. Sit DK, McGowan J, Wiltrout C, Diler RS, Dills JJ, Luther J, et al. Adjunctive bright light therapy for bipolar depression: a randomized double-blind placebo-controlled trial. *Am j psychiatry.* (2018) 175:131–9. doi: 10.1176/appi.ajp.2017.16101200
56. Yorguner Kupeli N, Bulut NS, Carkaxhiu Bulut G, Kurt E, Kora K. Efficacy of bright light therapy in bipolar depression. *Psychiatry res.* (2017) 260:432–8. doi: 10.1016/j.psychres.2017.12.020
57. Benedetti F. Rate of switch from bipolar depression into mania after morning light therapy: a historical review. *Psychiatry Res.* (2018) 261:351–56. doi: 10.1016/j.psychres.2018.01.013
58. Goldberg JF. When do antidepressants worsen the course of bipolar disorder? *J psychiatr pract.* (2003) 9:181–94. doi: 10.1097/00131746-200305000-00002
59. Boivin DB, Czeisler CA, Dijk DJ, Duffy JF, Folkard S, Minors DS, et al. Complex interaction of the sleep-wake cycle and circadian phase modulates mood in healthy subjects. *Arch general psychiatry.* (1997) 54:145–52. doi: 10.1001/archpsyc.1997.01830140055010
60. Boivin DB. Influence of sleep-wake and circadian rhythm disturbances in psychiatric disorders. *J psychiatry neurosci.* (2000) 25:446–58.
61. Danilenko KV, Cajochen C, Wirz-Justice A. Is sleep *per se* a zeitgeber in humans? *J biol rhythms.* (2003) 18:170–8. doi: 10.1177/0748730403251732
62. Revell VL Burgess HJ, Gazda CJ, Smith MR, Fogg LF, Eastman CI. Advancing human circadian rhythms with afternoon melatonin and morning intermittent bright light. *J clin endocrinol metab.* (2006) 91:54–9. doi: 10.1210/jc.2005-1009
63. Lockley SW, Evans EE, Scheer FA, Brainard GC, Czeisler CA, Aeschbach D. Short-wavelength sensitivity for the direct effects of light on alertness, vigilance, and the waking electroencephalogram in humans. *Sleep.* (2006) 29:161–8. doi: 10.1093/sleep/29.2.161
64. Penetar D McCann U, Thorne D, Kamimori G, Galinski C, Sing H, et al. Caffeine reversal of sleep deprivation effects on alertness and mood. *Psychopharmacology.* (1993) 112:359–65. doi: 10.1007/BF02244933
65. DeBattista C, Doghramji K, Menza MA, Rosenthal MH Fieve RR, Modafinil in Depression Study G. Adjunct modafinil for the short-term treatment of fatigue and sleepiness in patients with major depressive disorder: a preliminary double-blind, placebo-controlled study. *J clin psychiatry.* (2003) 64:1057–64. doi: 10.4088/JCP.v64n0911
66. Even C, Thuile J, Santos J, Bourgin P. Modafinil as an adjunctive treatment to sleep deprivation in depression. *J psychiatry neurosci.* (2005) 30:432–3.
67. Tsai JW, Hannibal J, Hagiwara G, Colas D, Ruppert E, Ruby NF, et al. Melanopsin as a sleep modulator: circadian gating of the direct effects of light on sleep and altered sleep homeostasis in Opn4(-/-) mice. *PLoS biol.* (2009) 7:e1000125. doi: 10.1371/journal.pbio.1000125
68. Gaus SE, Strecker RE, Tate BA, Parker RA, Saper CB. Ventrolateral preoptic nucleus contains sleep-active, galaninergic neurons in multiple mammalian species. *Neuroscience.* (2002) 115:285–94. doi: 10.1016/S0306-4522(02)00308-1
69. Benedetti F, Barbini B, Colombo C, Smeraldi E. Chronotherapeutics in a psychiatric ward. *Sleep med rev.* (2007) 11:509–22. doi: 10.1016/j.smrv.2007.06.004
70. Bellivier F, Geoffroy PA, Etain B, Scott J. Sleep- and circadian rhythm-associated pathways as therapeutic targets in bipolar disorder. *Expert opin ther targets.* (2015) 19:747–63. doi: 10.1517/14728222.2015.1018822
71. Geoffroy PA, Scott J, Boudebesse C, Lajnef M, Henry C, Leboyer M, et al. Sleep in patients with remitted bipolar disorders: a meta-analysis of actigraphy studies. *Acta psychiatr Scand.* (2015) 131:89–99. doi: 10.1111/acps.12367
72. Robillard R, Naismith SL, Rogers NL, Ip TK, Hermens DF, Scott EM, et al. Delayed sleep phase in young people with unipolar or bipolar affective disorders. *J affect disorders.* (2013) 145:260–3. doi: 10.1016/j.jad.2012.06.006
73. Moreira J, Geoffroy PA. Lithium and bipolar disorder: impacts from molecular to behavioural circadian rhythms. *Chronobiol int.* (2016) 33:351–73. doi: 10.3109/07420528.2016.1151026
74. Sit D, Wisner KL, Hanusa BH, Stull S, Terman M Light therapy for bipolar disorder: a case series in women. *Bipolar disorders.* (2007) 9:918–27. doi: 10.1111/j.1399-5618.2007.00451.x
75. Geoffroy PA, Abbassi EMBE, Maruani J, Etain B, Lejoyeux M, Amad A, et al. Bright light therapy in the morning or at mid-day in the treatment of non-seasonal bipolar depressive episodes (LuBi): study protocol for a dose research phase I/II trial. *Psychiatry Investig.* (2018) 15:1188–202. doi: 10.30773/pi.2018.09.27.1
76. Geoffroy PA. Clock genes and light signaling alterations in bipolar disorder: when the biological clock is off. *Biol Psychiatry.* (2018) 84:775–7. doi: 10.1016/j.biopsych.2018.09.006

Growth Factor Proteins and Treatment-Resistant Depression: A Place on the Path to Precision

Alice Pisoni[1†], Rebecca Strawbridge[1†], John Hodsoll[2], Timothy R. Powell[3], Gerome Breen[3], Stephani Hatch[1], Matthew Hotopf[1,4], Allan H. Young[1,4] and Anthony J. Cleare[1,4]*

[1] Department of Psychological Medicine, Institute of Psychiatry, Psychology and Neuroscience, King's College London, London, United Kingdom, [2] Department of Biostatistics, Institute of Psychiatry, Psychology and Neuroscience, King's College London, London, United Kingdom, [3] Social, Genetic and Developmental Psychiatry Centre, Institute of Psychiatry, Psychology and Neuroscience, King's College London, London, United Kingdom, [4] South London and Maudsley NHS Foundation Trust, London, United Kingdom

***Correspondence:**
Rebecca Strawbridge
becci.strawbridge@kcl.ac.uk

†Joint first authors

Background: Since the neurotrophic hypothesis of depression was formulated, conflicting results have been reported regarding the role of growth factor proteins in depressed patients, including whether there are state or trait alterations found in patients compared to controls and whether they represent predictors of treatment response. Recently it has been hypothesized that heterogeneity of findings within this literature might be partly explained by participants' history of treatment-resistant depression. This study aimed to investigate the role of growth factor proteins in patients with treatment-resistant depression (TRD) undergoing an inpatient intervention.

Methods: Blood samples were collected from 36 patients with TRD and 36 matched controls. Patients were assessed both at admission and discharge from a specialist inpatient program. We examined serum biomarker differences between patients and non-depressed matched controls, longitudinal changes after inpatient treatment and relationship to clinical outcomes. Additionally, the influence of potential covariates on biomarker levels were assessed.

Results: Patients displayed lower serum levels of brain-derived neurotrophic factor (OR = 0.025; 95% CI = 0.001, 0.500) and vascular endothelial growth factor-C (VEGFC; OR = 0.083, 95% CI = 0.008, 0.839) as well as higher angiopoietin-1 receptor (Tie2; OR = 2.651, 95% CI = 1.325, 5.303) compared to controls. Patients were stratified into responders (56%) and non-responders (44%). Lower VEGFD levels at admission predicted subsequent non-response (OR = 4.817, 95% CI = 1.247, 11.674). During treatment, non-responders showed a decrease in VEGF and VEGFC levels, while responders showed no significant changes.

Conclusion: TRD patients demonstrate a deficit of peripheral growth factors and our results suggest that markers of the VEGF family might decline over time in chronically depressed patients in spite of multidisciplinary treatment. The action of angiogenic proteins may play an important role in the pathophysiology of TRD, and pending comprehensive investigation may provide important insights for the future of precision psychiatry.

Keywords: depression, neurogenesis, growth factor, brain derived neurotrophic factor, treatment-resistant depression, biomarker, precision medicine

INTRODUCTION

Major Depressive Disorder (MDD) is now considered the leading cause of disability worldwide (1). Understanding the pathophysiology of this disorder is essential to optimizing treatment, however the underlying neurobiological mechanisms are still not fully understood. The neurotrophic and neurogenic hypothesis of depression (2) postulates that stress-induced alterations in neurotrophic action mediate reduced adult neurogenesis and volume reductions in the hippocampus which ultimately increase risk for mood disorders (3). Antidepressant use is hypothesized to reverse this process and increase the proliferation of progenitor cells by stimulating the production of growth factors, molecules responsible for neurogenesis and maintenance of neural networks (4, 5).

Evidence for a role of growth factors in the pathophysiology of depression has come from clinical studies mainly investigating brain derived neurotrophic factor (BDNF), a neurotrophin involved in processes of neuronal maturation, synapse formation and synaptic plasticity (3), and vascular endothelial growth factor (VEGF or VEGFA), an angiogenic factor also possessing neurotrophic and neuroprotective properties (6, 7).

Research has reported lower BDNF levels in post-mortem brains of depressed patients compared to non-depressed controls (8–10), although these appear to be higher in those patients who had taken antidepressants (11). Low levels of BDNF have also been found in the blood of depressed patients, with increases reported following antidepressant treatment (12–14).

On the contrary, levels of VEGF tend to be elevated in depressed patients (15, 16), although a number of studies have reported no significant differences compared with non-depressed controls (see (17) for a review). The effects of antidepressants on VEGF are also not clear-cut, with some studies reporting no changes (18–21), one reporting a decrease (22) and one reporting an increase correlated with improvement of depressive symptomatology (23).

Recently, resistance to treatment has been suggested as a potential confounding factor in this field of research (17). Treatment-resistant depression (TRD) is common and contributes substantially to the burden of depression (24). More pronounced reductions of proteins central to cellular growth and proliferation might be expected in patients with TRD, which could be a risk factor and/or consequence of an unsuccessfully treated affective illness. Indeed, limited research has found lower BDNF levels in TRD than both non-depressed controls and treatment-responsive patients (25). Measuring a similar cohort to the present study, Carvalho et al. identified non-significantly lower VEGF levels in participants with TRD who did not go on to respond to an inpatient treatment package than responder participants [$p = 0.058$; (26)].

Research to date has not identified sufficiently consistent effects to progress the pathway toward precision medicine, perhaps in part due to studying heterogeneous depressed groups and limited trophic biomarker panels. We aimed to address these drawbacks by examining a severe TRD population (alongside non-depressed, matched controls) and monitoring them during a naturalistic course of inpatient treatment in addition to a long-term follow-up. Alongside the well-researched BDNF and VEGF, we also considered six growth factors that play a role in neurogenesis and maintenance of neural connections but have never been investigated in TRD; due to the scant evidence in our possession surrounding their role in depression, these comparisons were exploratory in nature. We therefore test three main two-tailed hypotheses: First, that patients and controls would differ in levels of growth factors; second, that growth factor levels would change between pre- and post-treatment assessments; and third, that protein levels would differ between subsequent responders and non-responders to inpatient treatment.

MATERIALS AND METHODS

This study was approved by the Camberwell & St. Giles NHS Research Ethics Committee (TRD patients; reference 322/03) and King's College London Research Ethics Committee (non-depressed controls; reference PNM/12/13-152). In accordance with the recommendations of the Declaration of Helsinki, all participants provided written informed consent prior to participation.

Participants

TRD Patients

A cohort of 36 TRD patients were naturalistically recruited and treated within a specialist inpatient unit for treatment-resistant mood disorders (National Affective Disorders Unit, South London and Maudsley NHS Foundation Trust, UK). Assessments took place as close as possible after admission, and before discharge; mean treatment duration 6 months. Patients met inclusion criteria if they had a primary diagnosis of an affective disorder (unipolar or bipolar) and were currently depressed, defined as a score ≥ 8 using the Hamilton Depression Rating Scale [HDRS-17; (27)]. The diagnosis was defined following DSM-IV and ICD-10 criteria, assessed using the Mini International Neuropsychiatric Interview [MINI; (28)] and confirmed by two psychiatrists and a screening of patients' records. Upon admission, all patients were treatment-resistant, defined by a score >7.5 using the Maudsley Staging Method [MSM; (29)], and taking medications. Patients underwent a multidisciplinary intervention, including pharmacological, psychological and occupational treatment, as well as electroconvulsive therapy (ECT) in some cases, however not all participants underwent all types of treatment. All patients completed non-biological measures at both time points, and blood collection at admission; 7 patients were unavailable for venepuncture measurement at the discharge time point.

Control Participants

36 non-depressed controls were selected from the South East London Community Health study (SELCoH) based on closeness of matching to the TRD sample in age, gender and BMI [see (30) for more information regarding the SELCoH study]. Control participants did not meet criteria for current psychiatric disorders measured using the Clinical Interview Schedule-Revised (31) and did not have significant depressive symptoms as indicated by a score <10 on the Patient Health Questionnaire (32).

Measures

Biomarkers

Levels of eight different biomarkers were measured: angiopoietin-1 receptor (Tie2), brain-derived neurotrophic factor (BDNF), vascular endothelial growth factor (VEGF), vascular endothelial growth factor-C (VEGFC), vascular endothelial growth factor-D (VEGFD), placental growth factor (PlGF), basic fibroblast growth factor (bFGF), and soluble fms-like tyrosine kinase-1 (sFlt1; also termed soluble VEGF receptor-1). Blood for serum samples (1 × 5ml tube) was collected in the morning between 9 and 11 a.m. Following complete clotting, the tubes were centrifuged and serum extracted, transferred into cryovials and frozen (between −40° and −80°C). Serum concentrations of biomarkers were assayed in duplicate with ultra-high sensitivity Meso Scale Discovery (MSD) V-plex kits (Meso Scale Diagnostics, Maryland, USA), shown to be a reliable measurement tool (33). Unless otherwise stated, protein levels are reported in pg/ml.

Non-biological Assessments

These were conducted in the TRD group only. Depression severity was measured using a clinician-administered rating scale [HDRS-17; (27)], with treatment response defined as more than 50% reduction in scores between admission and discharge time points. Severity of treatment resistance was assessed at admission using the Maudsley Staging Method [MSM; (29)]. History of childhood adversity was measured using the Childhood Trauma Questionnaire [CTQ; (34)]. Cognitive impairment was assessed at admission using the Mini-Mental State Examination [MMSE; (35)]. Physical health was assessed at admission using the Modified Cumulative Illness Rating Scale [MCIRS; (36)], with the total score calculated excluding the item pertaining to mental health. Demographic data was obtained at admission. Number of medications were recorded at each time point, and changes during treatment were noted at discharge.

Statistical Analyses

Raw biomarker data was standardized using logarithmic transformation (base log10) before undergoing analyses. All data analyses were carried out using bootstrapping, with 1000 generated samples.

Primary Analyses

Logistic regressions and paired *t*-tests were used to test the primary null hypotheses, testing differences between responders and non-responders. Conditional logistic regressions compared the differences in biomarker levels between individually matched TRD patients and controls at each time point, accounting for gender, age and BMI. Other covariates were individuated using correlational analyses (see below; secondary analyses) and added to the relevant regression model if both correlations and unadjusted analyses were significant. Repeated measures ANOVAs were performed to identify changes in biomarker levels after treatment, using time as the within-subject variable.

Due to the number of comparisons, a False Discovery Rate (FDR) control for multiple testing was applied to primary analyses to reduce the probability of type I error. Thus, uncorrected p values < 0.05 are reported as tentatively significant findings and q values < 0.1 as significant (37).

Secondary Analyses

Paired sample *t*-tests were performed to examine longitudinal changes in the responder and non-responder groups individually. Pearson's correlations tested for possible association between different biomarkers, as well as between biomarkers and potential covariates in the TRD group, namely depression severity at admission and discharge, childhood trauma, cognitive impairment, physical health, severity of treatment-resistance, number of medications, and number of medication changes during inpatient treatment (i.e., starting or stopping an antidepressant medication, but not changes in dosage).

RESULTS

Sample Characteristics

There was a preponderance of female participants (n = 42; male = 30). Mean age at admission was 54.54 (SD = 13.85). Mean BMI was 28.19 (SD = 5.16). Descriptive statistics for demographic and biomarker data can be found in **Table 1**. 20 patients (55.6%) were classified as responders, and 16 patients as non-responders (44.4%). The two subgroups did not differ in other clinical or sociodemographic factors. Mean values for all measures, including scores from questionnaires, can be found in supplementary material (**Supplementary Table 1**).

Biomarker Characteristics

As BDNF levels obtained for one participant in the control group did not reach the lowest limit of detection (LLOD, 30 pg/mL; Meso Scale Diagnostics, Maryland, USA), this datum was initially replaced by half of the LLOD (38), but the dataset became highly skewed, thus this datum was excluded from the dataset. No other biomarker data was outside of detectable limits. Several variables had slightly skewed or kurtotic distributions; where

TABLE 1 | Participant characteristics.

		Non-depressed controls (n = 36)		TRD patients (n = 36)		*p*-value
		Log-mean (SD)	**Range**	**Log-mean (SD)**	**Range**	
Age		54.48 (13.78)	28–80	54.55 (14.30)	26–83	0.970
BMI		28.11 (4.64)	20.20–41.60	28.22 (5.75)	18.00–46.00	0.930
Biomarker levels (log-pg/ml)						
Pre-treatment	Tie2	3.57 (0.12)	3.32–3.84	3.66 (0.07)	3.38–3.84	0.006*
	PIGF	1.44 (0.15)	1.16–1.82	1.43 (0.13)	1.04–1.71	0.547
	VEGF	2.50 (0.30)	1.84–3.05	2.53 (0.41)	1.55–3.31	0.652
	VEGFC	2.55 (0.15)	2.30–2.91	2.45 (0.29)	1.72–2.85	0.045*
	VEGFD	2.87 (0.19)	2.29–3.16	2.77 (0.20)	2.21–3.46	0.087
	bFGF	0.70 (0.31)	−0.10–1.23	0.53 (0.63)	−1.22–1.94	0.084
	sFlt1	1.90 (0.13)	1.65–2.30	1.89 (0.12)	1.51–2.17	0.627
	BDNF	4.28 (0.17)	3.68–4.63	4.04 (0.37)	3.02–4.42	0.012*
Biomarker levels (log-pg/ml)						
Post-treatment	Tie2			3.68 (0.08)	3.57–3.88	0.010*
	PIGF			1.48 (0.08)	1.30–1.64	0.295
	VEGF			2.44 (0.57)	1.57–3.37	0.728
	VEGFC			2.28 (0.48)	1.07–2.80	0.007*
	VEGFD			2.79 (0.19)	2.08–3.22	0.196
	bFGF			0.66 (0.53)	−0.39–1.77	0.572
	sFlt1			1.87 (0.13)	1.52–2.10	0.354
	BDNF			4.10 (0.25)	2.98–4.40	0.126

**Different between patients and controls ($p < 0.05$)*
Other factors did not differ between patient and control groups, as indicated by p-values. For TRD patients as a whole group, no biomarker changes occurred during treatment.

this affected statistical test assumptions, the relevant variable was standardized using z scores prior to regression analyses.

Differences Between Patients and Controls

Conditional logistic regressions demonstrated three biomarkers as significantly different between the TRD and control groups at both time points. Tie2 was significantly higher in TRD patients [admission: $X^2_{(1)} = 11.67$, $p = 0.006$, $q = 0.048$; discharge: $X^2_{(1)} = 11.82$, $p = 0.010$, $q = 0.070$]. VEGFC was significantly lower in the TRD group [admission: $X^2_{(1)} = 3.33$, $p = 0.045$, $q = 0.270$; discharge: $X^2_{(1)} = 7.85$, $p = 0.007$, $q = 0.056$]. Lower BDNF was also found in TRD participants [admission: $X^2_{(1)} = 11.92$, $p = 0.012$, $q = 0.084$) but was not significant at discharge [$X^2_{(1)} = 5.56$, $p = 0.126$]. Visual representations of these differences are depicted in **Figure 1**. **Table 2** details the conditional logistic regressions used to compare protein levels between these matched groups of TRD and non-depressed groups. Finally, due to the wide age range we presented scatter plots of BDNF, Tie2 and VEGFC in correlation with age in patients and controls; these were not significantly related (see **Supplementary Figure 1**).

Biomarkers as Predictors of Response

High admission VEGFD predicted response with tentative significance (responder 2.83 ± 0.17 vs. non-responder 2.69 ± 0.21, respectively), as shown in **Figure 2** [$X^2_{(1)} = 5.38$, $p = 0.014$, $q = 0.112$]. A trend for higher BDNF levels in responders at admission was also found, however it did not reach significance ($p = 0.067$, $q = 0.462$).

Changes Following Inpatient Treatment

Analyses revealed no significant overall differences between biomarker levels at admission and discharge (pre- and post-treatment protein levels are outlined in **Table 1**). However, after stratifying based on response, paired samples t-tests showed that non-responders experienced a decrease in VEGF and VEGFC during treatment [VEGF: $t_{(11)} = 2.87$ $p = 0.015$, $q = 0.120$; VEGFC: $t_{(11)} = 2.71$, $p = 0.020$, $q = 0.140$], while responders' levels did not change (VEGF: p =.491; VEGFC: p =.957); see **Figure 3**.

Secondary Analyses

Two independent samples t-tests compared biomarker levels between patients diagnosed with unipolar and bipolar depression, both at inpatient admission and discharge. bFGF levels at admission were higher in unipolar (M =.69, SD =.58) compared to bipolar patients (M = 0.22, SD = 0.65); $t_{(34)} = 2.19$, p =0.038. No significant differences were identified at discharge.

Most biomarkers were inter-correlated, with the exception of BDNF which was not correlated with any other proteins.

Importantly, levels of biomarkers were not associated with depression severity at either time point. Significant correlations were found between biomarkers and other covariates: Tie-2 levels at admission positively correlated with BMI (r = 0.46, p = 0.024), while admission VEGFC levels were negatively

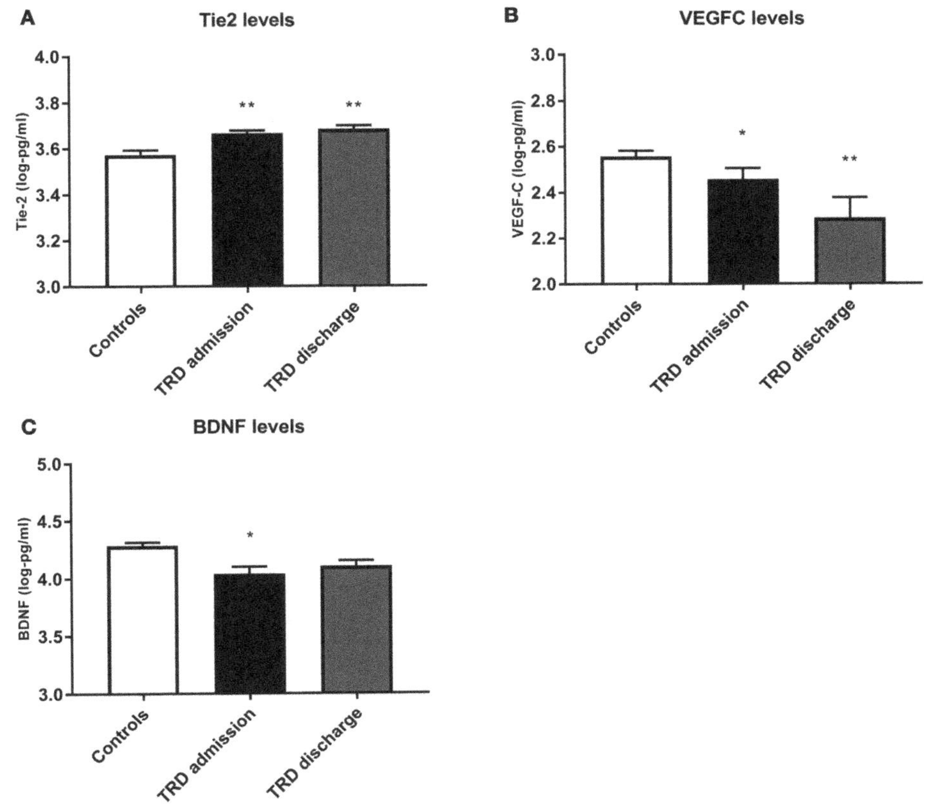

FIGURE 1 | Comparison of protein levels between controls (white bar) and TRD patients on admission (black bar) and discharge (gray bar) from the inpatient unit, for **(A)** Tie2, **(B)** VEGF C and **(C)** BDNF. Error bars show standard error. Note that axes have been cut according to protein levels expressed to clearly depict group differences. *, significantly different from controls at $p < 0.05$. **, significantly different from controls at $p < 0.01$.

correlated with both BMI ($r = -0.45$, $p = 0.027$) and poorer physical health score ($r = -0.47$, $p = 0.022$). PlGF levels at admission positively correlated with both number of medications ($r = 0.50$, $p = 0.013$) and number of changes in medications that occurred subsequently during treatment ($r = 0.44$, $p = 0.029$). Similarly, bFGF levels at admission positively correlated with number of medications taken ($r = 0.50$, $p = 0.013$) and levels at discharge negatively correlated with number of changes in medication that had taken place since the baseline research assessment ($r = -0.55$, $p = 0.014$). Non-biological variables did not differ between responders and non-responders (see **Supplementary Table 1**).

DISCUSSION

The findings from this study may have notable implications for more personalized, predictive approaches to treatment selection for people with depression who have not responded to multiple treatments. Results from the main analyses showed that Tie2 levels were higher in TRD patients than controls, while VEGFC and BDNF were lower in the TRD participants. The BDNF finding replicates two previous clinical studies on TRD (25, 39), which appear to indicate an association between resistance to pharmacological treatment and extremely low levels of BDNF, with implications for the role of neurogenesis and neuroplasticity in therapeutic response. If BDNF expression mediates the action of antidepressants on neural birth and maintenance, patients with low availability of this growth factor may necessitate other forms of therapy in order to elicit a meaningful response. The minimisation of this difference by discharge from this specialist inpatient program support this theory, although we note there were not differences identified between responders and non-responders.

Interestingly, levels of VEGF were not significantly different between patients and controls. Previous work has found levels of VEGF in depressed patients to be either higher than or the same as those found in controls (15–17), and TRD has been proposed as a potential confounder responsible for this heterogeneity. It has been suggested that patients with non-resistant depression display higher VEGF levels, representing a neuroprotective attempt by specific brain structures in response to stress (17). On the other hand, patients with TRD fail to present this automated reaction, preventing response to antidepressants. Our data could support this hypothesis by indicating no difference between VEGF levels in TRD patients and controls, though responders and non-responders also did not differ in VEGF levels.

TABLE 2 | Conditional logistic regression of biomarker levels (TRD vs. control group; $N = 72$).

Biomarker	OR	X^2	95% Confidence intervals		*p*
			Lower	Upper	
PRE-TREATMENT					
Tie2	2.651	11.672	1.325	5.303	0.006*
PlGF	0.344	0.383	0.011	10.386	0.547
VEGF	1.365	0.216	0.366	5.089	0.652
VEGFC	0.159	3.327	0.018	1.362	0.045*
VEGFD	0.118	3.738	0.011	1.220	0.087
bFGF	0.288	2.949	0.124	1.209	0.084
sFlt1	0.377	0.273	0.009	15.098	0.627
BDNF	0.025	11.921	0.001	0.500	0.012*
POST-TREATMENT					
Tie2	3.008	11.823	1.308	6.917	0.010*
PlGF	1.326	1.156	0.781	2.251	0.295
VEGF	0.818	0.123	0.266	2.519	0.728
VEGFC	0.083	7.853	0.008	0.839	0.007*
VEGFD	0.128	2.064	0.007	2.475	0.196
bFGF	0.681	0.413	0.209	2.220	0.572
sFlt1	0.201	0.809	0.006	7.007	0.354
BDNF	0.028	5.557	0.001	1.338	0.126

**Different between patients and controls, at both $p < 0.05$ and $q < 0.1$.*
OR, odds ratio; χ^2, Chi-square.
Other factors did not differ between patient ($n = 36$) and control groups ($n = 36$) following FDR control for multiple comparisons.

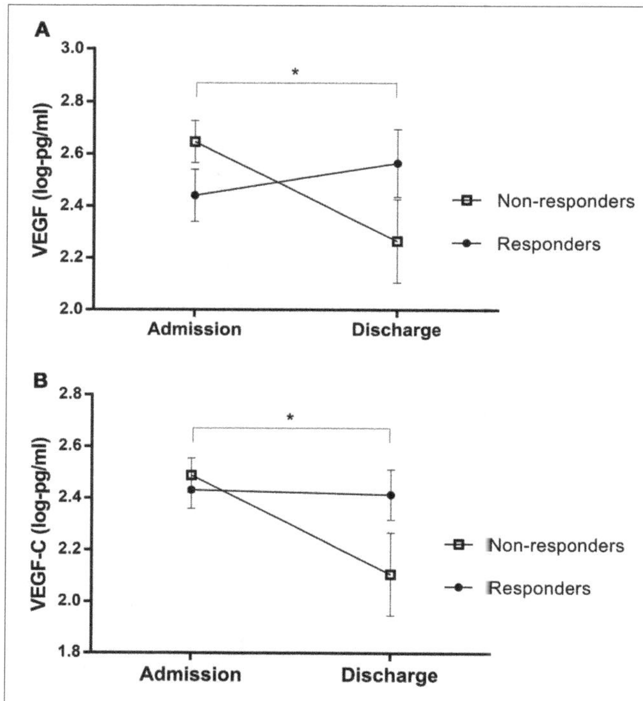

FIGURE 3 | Protein changes in non-responders and responders pre- and post-treatment, for **(A)** VEGF and **(B)** VEGF-C levels. Error bars show standard error. Note that axes have been cut according to protein levels expressed to depict differences clearly. *, The interactions of response status were significant at $p < 0.05$, rather than cross-sectional differences between responder and non-responder patients.

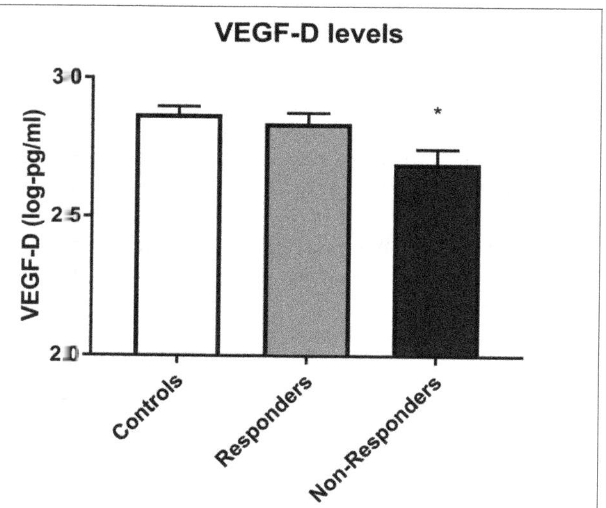

FIGURE 2 | VEGF D levels in controls, responders and non-responders before starting treatment. Error bars show standard error. Note that axes have been cut according to protein levels expressed to depict differences clearly. Lower VEGFD predicted subsequent non-response to treatment ($p = 0.014$).
*, subsequent non-responders significantly different from responders at $p < 0.05$.

VEGFC levels were lower in TRD patients than controls. VEGFC has not yet, to our knowledge, been investigated in depression, however it belongs to the same protein family of VEGF, and the two were highly correlated ($p < 0.001$). This could indicate that low availability of growth factors belonging to the VEGF network may be associated with TRD.

Finally, Tie2 was found to be higher in TRD patients compared to controls. Despite the paucity of data surrounding Tie2's function in depression (and absence of data in TRD), this result may be representative of increased inflammatory signaling (40), as would be expected in these patients (41, 42).

After stratifying participants based on treatment response, analyses indicated a decrease of VEGF and VEGFC over time, only in non-responders. Previous studies have found response not to interact with VEGF changes during pharmacological treatment for non-TRD depressed samples (18, 19, 21). Our result could suggest that while an increase in VEGF is not necessary for the therapeutic effects of antidepressants, the non-responders' decrease may represent a progressive loss of neurotrophic action. It is notable here that the treatment period averaged at 6 months, which is of longer duration than the majority of previous research studies within this literature.

No changes were seen in levels of BDNF following antidepressant treatment, contrasting theories that an increase in the availability of this biomarker is a key mechanism in antidepressant action (43). It is likely that these inconsistencies stem in part from heterogeneity of type of treatment, as well as clinical profile and time length between measurement points, as appears to pervade biological research in depression (44). Specifically, all patients were taking multiple pharmacotherapy throughout the admission and for the majority of patients this included mood stabilizer medications, which in this sample were far more frequently taken (27/36 patients) than monoaminergic medications (20/36 patients), although both have been posited to upregulate BDNF (43).

Non-responders displayed significantly lower levels of VEGFD at admission compared to responders. This is, to our knowledge, the first study to examine VEGFD levels in patients with depression, but in addition to its angiogenic and lymphangiogenic functions, this protein also helps to restore and maintain dendritic complexity in the hippocampus (45). Thus lower levels before antidepressant treatment may have contributed to the reduced clinical benefits for non-responder patients. In similar vein, VEGF has been studied as a potential predictor of antidepressant response, twice in TRD samples. In a recent study by Clark-Raymond et al. (18) involving 38 MDD patients, higher VEGF levels were found in remitters, compared to patients who did not respond to pharmacological therapy. Likewise, Carvalho et al. (26) found a trend for lower levels of VEGF in a small sample of non-responder TRD patients, and Minelli et al. (46) found that lower levels of VEGF predicted lack of response to ECT in a large cohort of 67 TRD patients. In the latter study, VEGF predicted response to ECT but not for another subgroup of MDD patients receiving pharmacological treatment. The authors argue that these results indicate a predictive potential of VEGF specific to TRD Interestingly, higher levels of VEGF have been found to downregulate the activity of multi-drug resistance transporter at the blood-barrier (47), resulting in increased concentrations of exogenous compounds in the brain, including antidepressants (48). Thus, a greater availability of VEGF may result in larger quantity of antidepressant reaching the brain, while low levels of VEGF in TRD patients (discussed above) may contribute to a low cerebral concentration of antidepressants, insufficient to produce a therapeutic response (46). The authors argue that ECT boosts VEGF availability, thus increasing the effectiveness of antidepressants. However, a challenge to this hypothesis comes from the observation that amelioration of symptoms following ECT is not associated with an increase in VEGF (49). Thus, the temporal relationship between these two events with regards to the blood-barrier hypothesis need to be further investigated, as well as the role played by VEGFD.

Limitations and Future Directions

Not all potentially significant results survived the FDR control for multiple comparisons. It may be that the smaller effects of biomarkers predicting response in this study were false positive findings, or that the small sample size and lack of consistently strong inter-correlations between proteins caused these comparisons to be non-significant after FDR control. It is our hope that future studies will help to elucidate this.

The naturalistic approach adopted in this study allowed for an unbiased observation of patients within a realistic clinical environment. The methodological challenges that this presents should be considered when interpreting these findings. Particularly, data on the type of medication prescribed for each patient and which treatments were undertaken during the inpatient program were highly variable and thus challenging to model. The vast majority of TRD participants were undergoing concomitant treatment with antipsychotics and/or mood stabilizers in addition to monoaminergic antidepressants, and such combinations may have unknown and unpredictable effects on growth factor levels. Moreover, data on participation in ECT would have been essential to explore the hypothesis that ECT leads to greater percentage of medication entering the brain following a moderation of the permeability of the blood-barrier by VEGF (46). These issues require further clarification and should be addressed by future studies on TRD. It is also important to consider that growth factor levels are known to fluctuate in response to a number of variables, including food intake (50), exercise and sedentary behavior (51, 52), and even the menstrual cycle (53), representing a common limitation in this type of clinical study. Furthermore, it is important to consider that the TRD and control samples were obtained from two separate studies; as such, differences in sampling conditions may have affected the results. Finally, reduced follow-up biomarker data for patients and the small sample size of our study represent clear limitations. Thus, future research should focus on replicating these findings in larger samples to confirm the importance of the VEGF protein family and Tie2, as factors displaying angiogenic properties have the potential to play a role in the psychopathology of TRD. Furthermore, in order to shed light on potential differences between TRD and non-refractory depression, controlled studies comparing these two clinical groups are desirable, possibly adopting a longitudinal design to monitor changes following discharge. Finally, it has been suggested that our current lack of information on TRD stems mainly from the *post-hoc* design of many studies. To solve this issue, it would be helpful to examine patients at the time of their initial contact with mental health services, and follow them to identify whether biomarker levels represent a predictor of risk of TRD (54).

In conclusion, the present study provides support that compounds such as BDNF and VEGF are important markers in treatment-resistant depression and provides new information on the dynamics of growth factors in TRD. Specifically, longitudinal activity of VEGF-family members might represent candidates for stratifying patients based on likelihood of response. Results have highlighted the importance of angiogenic proteins, which have the potential to represent unique biomarkers of TRD and may be involved in mechanisms of response. Although replication studies in larger samples are needed before definitive conclusions can be drawn, findings from this study characterize novel trophic biomarkers that hold promise as new targets for mood disorder treatment strategies.

AUTHOR CONTRIBUTIONS

AP contributed to study conception and conducted data analysis, interpretation and writing of the manuscript. RS was involved in the study's conception, data collection, analysis, interpretation, and writing of the manuscript. JH contributed to the design and supervision of statistical analysis and interpretation of data. TP, GB, SH, MH, and AY were involved with study conception and/or design. TP undertook laboratory work and generated the protein data. AC was substantially involved with study conception and design and interpretation of data. Additionally, all authors contributed to drafting/revising the article and approved the final version for publication.

ACKNOWLEDGMENTS

The authors are grateful to the participants and staff in the ADU and SELCoH studies who engaged their time and effort into these projects. This research was supported by the Biomedical Research Nucleus data management and informatics facility at South London and Maudsley NHS Foundation Trust, which is funded by the National Institute for Health Research (NIHR) Mental Health Biomedical Research Centre at South London and Maudsley NHS Foundation Trust and King's College London and a joint infrastructure grant from Guy's and St Thomas' Charity and the Maudsley Charity. TP is funded by a Medical Research Council Skills Development Fellowship (MR/N014863/1). The biomarker work was supported by an LRAP grant from Eli Lilly. These funders had no involvement in study design, data collection, analysis or the decision to submit for publication. The views expressed are those of the author(s) and not necessarily those of the NHS, the NIHR or the Department of Health.

REFERENCES

1. World Health Organization. *Depression and Other Common Mental Disorders.* Global Health Estimates (2017). Available online at: http://apps.who.int/iris/bitstream/10665/254610/1/WHO-MSD-MER-2017.2-eng.pdf?ua=1&ua=1
2. Duman RS, Heninger GR, Nestler EJ. A molecular and cellular theory of depression. *Arch General Psychiatry* (1997) 54:597–606. doi: 10.1001/archpsyc.1997.01830190015002
3. Duman RS, Monteggia LM. A neurotrophic model for stress-related mood disorders. *Biol Psychiatry* (2006) 59:1116–27. doi: 10.1016/j.biopsych.2006.02.013
4. Banasr M, Dwyer JM, Duman RS. Cell atrophy and loss in depression: reversal by antidepressant treatment. *Curr Opin Cell Biol.* (2011) 23:730–7. doi: 10.1016/j.ceb.2011.09.002
5. Castren E. Neurotrophic effects of antidepressant drugs. *Curr Opin Pharmacol.* (2004) 4:58–64. doi: 10.1016/j.coph.2003.10.004
6. Nowacka MM, Obuchowicz E. Vascular endothelial growth factor (VEGF) and its role in the central nervous system: a new element in the neurotrophic hypothesis of antidepressant drug action. *Neuropeptides* (2012) 46:1–10. doi: 10.1016/j.npep.2011.05.005
7. Fournier NM, Duman RS. Role of vascular endothelial growth factor in adult hippocampal neurogenesis: implications for the pathophysiology and treatment of depression. *Behav Brain Res.* (2012) 227:440–9. doi: 10.1016/j.bbr.2011.04.022
8. Pandey GN, Ren X, Rizavi HS, Conley RR, Roberts RC, Dwivedi Y. Brain-derived neurotrophic factor and tyrosine kinase B receptor signalling in post-mortem brain of teenage suicide victims. *Int J Neuropsychopharmacol.* (2008) 11:1047–61. doi: 10.1017/S1461145708009000
9. Karege F, Vaudan G, Schwald M, Perroud N, La Harpe R. Neurotrophin levels in postmortem brains of suicide victims and the effects of antemortem diagnosis and psychotropic drugs. *Mol Brain Res.* (2005) 136:29–37. doi: 10.1016/j.molbrainres.2004.12.020
10. Dwivedi Y, Rizavi HS, Conley RR, Roberts RC, Tamminga CA, Pandey GN. Altered gene expression of brain-derived neurotrophic factor and receptor tyrosine kinase B in postmortem brain of suicide subjects. *Arch General Psychiatry* (2003) 60:804–15. doi: 10.1001/archpsyc.60.8.804
11. Chen B, Dowlatshahi D, MacQueen GM, Wang JF, Young LT. Increased hippocampal BDNF immunoreactivity in subjects treated with antidepressant medication. *Biol. Psychiatry* (2001) 50:260–5. doi: 10.1016/S0006-3223(01)01083-6
12. Molendijk ML, Spinhoven P, Polak M, Bus BAA, Penninx BWJH, Elzinga BM. Serum BDNF concentrations as peripheral manifestations of depression: evidence from a systematic review and meta-analyses on 179 associations (N= 9484). *Mol Psychiatry* (2014) 19:791–800. doi: 10.1038/mp.2013.105
13. Sen S, Duman R, Sanacora G. Serum brain-derived neurotrophic factor, depression, and antidepressant medications: meta-analyses and implications. *Biol Psychiatry* (2008) 64:527–32. doi: 10.1016/j.biopsych.2008.05.005
14. Brunoni AR, Lopes M, Fregni F. A systematic review and meta-analysis of clinical studies on major depression and BDNF levels: implications for the role of neuroplasticity in depression. *Int J Neuropsychopharmacol.* (2008) 11:1169–80. doi: 10.1017/S1461145708009309
15. Carvalho AF, Köhler CA, McIntyre RS, Knöchel C, Brunoni AR, Thase ME, et al. Peripheral vascular endothelial growth factor as a novel depression biomarker: A meta-analysis. *Psychoneuroendocrinology* (2015) 62:18–26. doi: 10.1016/j.psyneuen.2015.07.002
16. Tseng PT, Cheng YS, Chen YW, Wu CK, Lin PY. Increased levels of vascular endothelial growth factor in patients with major depressive disorder: a meta-analysis. *Eur Neuropsychopharmacol.* (2015) 25:1622–30. doi: 10.1016/j.euroneuro.2015.06.001
17. Clark-Raymond A, Halaris A. VEGF and depression: a comprehensive assessment of clinical data. *J Psychiatr Res.* (2013) 47:1080–7. doi: 10.1016/j.jpsychires.2013.04.008
18. Clark-Raymond A, Meresh E, Hoppensteadt D, Fareed J, Sinacore J, Garlenski B, et al. Vascular endothelial growth factor: potential predictor of treatment response in major depression. *World J Biol Psychiatry* (2016) 18:575–85. doi: 10.3109/15622975.2015.1117655
19. Halmai Z, Dome P, Dobos J, Gonda X, Szekely A, Sasvari-Szekely M, et al. Peripheral vascular endothelial growth factor level is associated with antidepressant treatment response: results of a preliminary study. *J Affect Disord.* (2013) 144:269–73. doi: 10.1016/j.jad.2012.09.006
20. Dome P, Halmai Z, Dobos J, Lazary J, Gonda X, Kenessey I, et al. Investigation of circulating endothelial progenitor cells and angiogenic and inflammatory cytokines during recovery from an episode of major depression. *J Affect Disord.* (2012) 136:1159–63. doi: 10.1016/j.jad.2011.09.027
21. Ventriglia M, Zanardini R, Pedrini L, Placentino A, Nielsen MG, Gennarelli M, et al. VEGF serum levels in depressed patients during SSRI antidepressant treatment. *Prog Neuro-Psychopharmacol Biol Psychiatry* (2009) 33:146–9. doi: 10.1016/j.pnpbp.2008.11.009
22. Buttenschøn HN, Foldager L, Elfving B, Poulsen PH, Uher R, and Mors O. Neurotrophic factors in depression in response to treatment. *J Affect Disord.* (2015) 183:287–94. doi: 10.1016/j.jad.2015.05.027
23. Ibrahim L, Duncan W, Luckenbaugh DA, Yuan P, Machado-Vieira R, Zarate CA. Rapid antidepressant changes with sleep deprivation in major depressive disorder are associated with changes in vascular endothelial growth factor (VEGF): a pilot study. *Brain Res Bull.* (2011) 86:129–33. doi: 10.1016/j.brainresbull.2011.06.003
24. Fekadu A, Wooderson SC, Markopoulo K, Donaldson C, Papadopoulos A, Cleare AJ. What happens to patients with treatment-resistant depression? A systematic review of medium to long term outcome studies. *J Affect Disord.* (2009) 116:4–11. doi: 10.1016/j.jad.2008.10.014
25. Hong W, Fan J, Yuan C, Zhang C, Hu Y, Peng D, et al. Significantly decreased mRNA levels of BDNF and MEK1 genes in treatment- resistant depression. *Neuroreport* (2014) 25:753–5. doi: 10.1097/WNR.0000000000000165
26. Carvalho LA, Torre JP, Papadopoulos AS, Poon L, Juruena MF, Markopoulou K, et al. Lack of clinical therapeutic benefit of antidepressants is associated overall activation of the inflammatory system. *J Affect Disord.* (2013) 148:136–40. doi: 10.1016/j.jad.2012.10.036

27. Hamilton M. A rating scale for depression. *J Neurol Neurosurg Psychiatry* (1960) 23:56–62. doi: 10.1136/jnnp.23.1.56
28. Sheehan D, Lecrubier Y, Sheehan KH, Sheehan K, Amorim P, Janavs J, et al. Diagnostic psychiatric interview for DSM-IV and ICD- 10. *J Clin Psychiatry* (1998) 59:22–33.
29. Fekadu A, Wooderson S, Donaldson C, Markopoulou K, Masterson B, Poon L, et al. A multidimensional tool to quantify treatment resistance in depression: the maudsley staging method. *J Clin Psychiatry* (2009) 70:177–84. doi: 10.4088/JCP.08m04309
30. Hatch SL, Frissa S, Verdecchia M, Stewart R, Fear NT, Reichenberg A, et al. Identifying socio-demographic and socioeconomic determinants of health inequalities in a diverse London community: the South East London Community Health (SELCoH) study. *BMC Public Health* (2011) 11:861. doi: 10.1186/1471-2458-11-861
31. Lewis G, Pelosi AJ, Araya R, Dunn G. Measuring psychiatric disorder in the community: a standardized assessment for use by lay interviewers. *Psychol Med.* (1992) 22:465–86. doi: 10.1017/S0033291700030415
32. Kroenke K, Spitzer RL. The PHQ-9: A new depression diagnostic and severity measure. *Psychiatr Ann.* (2002) 32:509–15. doi: 10.3928/0048-5713-20020901-06
33. Dabitao D, Margolick JB, Lopez J, Bream JH. Multiplex measurement of proinflammatory cytokines in human serum: comparison of the meso scale discovery electrochemiluminescence assay and the cytometric bead array. *J Immunol Methods* (2011) 372:71–7. doi: 10.1016/j.jim.2011.06.033
34. Bernstein DP, Fink L, Handelsman L, Foote J, Lovejoy M, Wenzel K, et al. Initial reliability and validity of a new retrospective measure of child abuse and neglect. *Am J Psychiatry* (1994) 151:1132. doi: 10.1176/ajp.151.8.1132
35. Folstein MF, Robins LN, Helzer JE. The mini-mental state examination. *Arch General Psychiatry* (1983) 40:812. doi: 10.1001/archpsyc.1983.01790060110016
36. Salvi F, Miller MD, Grilli A, Giorgi R, Towers AL, Morichi V, et al. A manual of guidelines to score the modified cumulative illness rating scale and its validation in acute hospitalized elderly patients. *J Am Geriatrics Soc.* (2008) 56 1926–31. doi: 10.1111/j.1532-5415.2008.01935.x
37. Benjamini Y, Hochberg Y. Controlling the false discovery rate: a practical and powerful approach to multiple testing. *J R Stat Soc.* (1995) 57:289–300.
38. Hornung RW, Reed LD. Estimation of average concentration in the presence of nondetectable values. *Appl Occup Environ Hygiene* (1990) 5:46–51. doi: 10.1080/1047322X.1990.10389587
39. Bilgen AE, Zincir SB, Zincir S, Özdemir B, Mehmet AK, Aydemir E, et al. Effects of electroconvulsive therapy on serum levels of brain-derived neurotrophic factor and nerve growth factor in treatment resistant major depression. *Brain Res Bull.* (2014) 104:82–7. doi: 10.1016/j.brainresbull.2014.04.005
40. Willam C, Koehne P, Jürgensen JS, Gräfe M, Wagner KD, Bachmann S, et al. Tie2 receptor expression is stimulated by hypoxia and proinflammatory cytokines in human endothelial cells. *Circ Res.* (2000) 87:370–7. doi: 10.1161/res.87.5.370
41. Zunszain PA, Hepgul N, Pariante CM. Inflammation and depression. *Behav Neurobiol Depression Treatment* (2012) 14:135–51. doi: 10.1007/7854_2012_211
42. Strawbridge R, Arnone D, Danese A, Papadopoulos A, Vives AH, Cleare AJ. Inflammation and clinical response to treatment in depression: a meta-analysis. *Eur Neuropsychopharmacol.* (2015) 25:1622–30. doi: 10.1016/j.euroneuro.2015.06.007
43. Masi G, Brovedani P. The hippocampus, neurotrophic factors and depression. *CNS Drugs* (2011) 25:913–31. doi: 10.2165/11595900-000000000-00000
44. Strawbridge R, Young AH, Cleare AJ. Biomarkers for depression: recent insights, current challenges and future prospects. *Neuropsychiatr Dis Treatment* (2017) 13:1245. doi: 10.2147/NDT.S114542
45. Mauceri D, Freitag HE, Oliveira AM, Bengtson CP, Bading H. Nuclear calcium- VEGFD signaling controls maintenance of dendrite arborization necessary for memory formation. *Neuron* (2011) 71:117–30. doi: 10.1016/j.neuron.2011.04.022
46. Minelli A, Maffioletti E, Bortolomasi M, Conca A, Zanardini R, Rillosi L, et al. Association between baseline serum vascular endothelial growth factor levels and response to electroconvulsive therapy. *Acta Psychiatr Scand.* (2014) 129:461–6. doi: 10.1111/acps.12187
47. Hawkins BT, Sykes DB, Miller DS. Rapid, reversible modulation of blood–brain barrierP-glycoprotein transport activity by vascular endothelial growth factor. *J Neurosci.* (2010) 30:1417–25. doi: 10.1523/JNEUROSCI.5103-09.2010
48. O'Brien FE, Dinan TG, Griffin BT, Cryan JF. Interactions between antidepressants and P-glycoprotein at the blood–brain barrier: clinical significance of *in vitro* and *in vivo* findings. *Br J Pharmacol.* (2012) 165:289–312. doi: 10.1111/j.1476-5381.2011.01557.x
49. Minelli A, Zanardini R, Abate M, Bortolomasi M, Gennarelli M, Bocchio-Chiavetto L. Vascular endothelial growth factor (VEGF) serum concentration during electroconvulsive therapy (ECT) in treatment resistant depressed patients. *Prog Neuropsychopharmacol Biol Psychiatry* (2011) 35:1322–5. doi: 10.1016/j.pnpbp.2011.04.013
50. Rosas-Vargas H, Martínez-Ezquerro JD, Bienvenu T. Brain-derived neurotrophic factor, food intake regulation, and obesity. *Arch Med Res.* (2011) 42:482–94. doi: 10.1016/j.arcmed.2011.09.005
51. Kraus RM, Stallings HW, Yeager RC, Gavin TP. Circulating plasma VEGF response to exercise in sedentary and endurance-trained men. *J Appl Physiol.* (2004) 96:1445–50. doi: 10.1152/japplphysiol.01031.2003
52. Cotman CW, Berchtold NC. Exercise: A behavioral intervention to enhance brain health and plasticity. *Trends Neurosci.* (2002) 25:295–301. doi: 10.1016/S0166-2236(02)02143-4
53. Begliuomini S, Casarosa E, Pluchino N, Lenzi E, Centofanti M, Freschi L, et al. Influence of endogenous and exogenous gender hormones on plasma brain-derived neurotrophic factor. *Hum Repr.* (2007) 22:995–1002. doi: 10.1093/humrep/del479
54. Smith DF. Quest for biomarkers of treatment-resistant depression: shifting the paradigm toward risk. *Front Psychiatry* (2013) 4:57. doi: 10.3389/fpsyt.2013.00057

10

Putative Astroglial Dysfunction in Schizophrenia: A Meta-Analysis of ^{1}H-MRS Studies of Medial Prefrontal Myo-Inositol

Tushar Kanti Das[1,2,3], *Avyarthana Dey*[1,2], *Priyadharshini Sabesan*[1], *Alborz Javadzadeh*[1], *Jean Théberge*[3,4], *Joaquim Radua*[5] *and Lena Palaniyappan*[1,2,3,4*]

[1] Department of Psychiatry, University of Western Ontario, London, ON, Canada, [2] Robarts Research Institute, London, ON, Canada, [3] Lawson Health Research Institute, London, ON, Canada, [4] Department of Medical Biophysics, University of Western Ontario, London, ON, Canada, [5] FIDMAG Germanes Hospitalàries, CIBERSAM, Sant Boi de Llobregat & Institut d'Investigacions Biomediques August Pi i Sunyer (IDIBAPS), Barcelona, Spain

***Correspondence:**
Lena Palaniyappan
lpalaniy@uwo.ca

Background: Several lines of evidence support a role for astroglial pathology in schizophrenia. Myo-inositol is particularly abundant in astroglia. Many small sized studies have reported on myo-inositol concentration in schizophrenia, but to date these have not been pooled to estimate a collective effect size.

Methods: We reviewed all proton magnetic resonance spectroscopy (1H-MRS) studies reporting myo-inositol values for patients satisfying DSM or ICD based criteria for schizophrenia in comparison to a healthy controls group in the medial prefrontal cortex published until February 2018. A random-effects model was used to calculate the pooled effect size using *metafor* package. A meta-regression analysis of moderator variables was also undertaken.

Results: The literature search identified 19 studies published with a total sample size of 585 controls, 561 patients with schizophrenia. Patients with schizophrenia had significantly reduced medial prefrontal myo-inositol compared to controls (RFX standardized mean difference = 0.19, 95% CI [0.05–0.32], $z = 2.72$, $p = 0.0067$; heterogeneity $p = 0.09$). Studies with more female patients reported more notable schizophrenia-related reduction in myo-inositol ($z = 2.53$, $p = 0.011$).

Discussion: We report a small, but significant reduction in myo-inositol concentration in the medial prefrontal cortex in schizophrenia. The size of the reported effect indicates that the biological pathways affecting the astroglia are likely to operate only in a subset of patients with schizophrenia. MRS myo-inositol could be a useful tool to stratify and investigate such patients.

Keywords: myo-inositol, astroglia, schizophrenia, inflammation, spectroscopy

INTRODUCTION

A role for astroglial pathology has been long suspected in schizophrenia (1–3). Astrocytes are critical for reducing oxidative stress and restoring redox balance in the brain, thus preventing neurotoxicity (4, 5). Astrocytes enable the crucial glutamate-glutamine cycle that helps clear extracellular glutamate from synaptic space as well as reduce the deleterious cellular ammonia content (6, 7). In addition, two crucial indicators of neuronal connectivity—synaptic maintenance and myelination—appear to rely on astrocytic guidance (8–10). Thus, abnormalities in astrocytic function can produce neuronal dysconnectivity as well as glutamatergic abnormalities that are known to occur in schizophrenia (11). Indeed, converging genetic and molecular evidence now supports the case for a primary role of astroglial dysfunction in schizophrenia (10, 12).

In vivo imaging of astrocytic integrity holds promise in clarifying the nature of its dysfunction in schizophrenia. ^{1}H-MRS does not specifically differentiate between brain cell types, nevertheless, given that myo-inositol is particularly abundant in astroglia rather than the neurons and other cells, it can be considered an astroglial marker (13, 14). The MRS measure of myo-inositol predominantly reflects astrocytic intracellular compartment, where it has osmotic functions (15, 16). An increase in MRS myo-inositol resonance relates to markers of astroglial activation (17, 18), associated with gliosis (19, 20), and occurs in response to brain injury (21, 22), thus reflecting an inflammatory response. On the other hand, myo-inositol also has an important role as an intracellular second messenger in calcium mediated glutamatergic signaling (23). Reduced myo-inositol resonance may relate to astroglial dysfunction and consequently, aberrant extracellular glutamate clearance from synaptic space. Thus, low levels of myo-inositol may in turn facilitate excitotoxic damage and local inflammatory processes that are currently subjects of investigation in the pathophysiology of schizophrenia (1).

Many small sized studies have reported on myo-inositol concentration in schizophrenia, but to date these have not been pooled to estimate a collective effect size (24). Examining the state of myo-inositol abnormalities will aid in our understanding of the role of astroglial cells in schizophrenia. We reviewed MRS studies reporting myo-inositol resonance in schizophrenia and conducted a meta-analysis to synthesize the nature of myo-inositol abnormalities in the medial prefrontal cortex of patients with schizophrenia. We focussed on the medial prefrontal cortex as most MRS studies in schizophrenia have placed voxels in this brain region (24).

METHODS

Search Process

We followed the guidelines set out by the consensus statement from PRISMA group (25). Our literature search started with the MEDLINE electronic database to identify journal articles published until 28 February 2018. We used the following Medical Subject Headings and freeform search terms: (schizophrenia OR schizo* OR psychos* OR psychot*) AND ("1H-MRS" OR "1H NMRS" OR "1HMRS" OR "MRS" OR "Magnetic resonance spectroscopy" OR "Spectroscopy" OR "proton magnetic resonance spectroscopy") AND ("myo-inositol" OR "inositol" OR "myo-inositol"). We noted that in many reports, myo-inositol was reported as a secondary measure, and not included in keywords or abstracts. As a result, we used the terms ("glutathione" OR "NAA" OR "n-acetyl aspartate" OR "glutamine" OR "GSH" OR "neurometabolic" OR "Glutamate" OR "Glu" OR "GABA" OR "Lactate" OR "creatinine") instead of the 3 terms denoting myo-inositol in order to identify all eligible studies. We attempted to contact authors whenever the individual studies indicated that myo-inositol resonance of adequate quality was measured in the brain region of interest (see below) but when the data was not published. We also undertook a manual search of reference lists of review articles and eligible full text articles. Third, we repeated the search with Google Scholar to identify journal articles that were not indexed on MEDLINE. Finally, we also searched the citation records of Google Scholar for all identified full text articles in order to locate in press articles that are not yet indexed. Two authors (AD and PS) undertook independent searches using the inclusion and exclusion criteria without any exchange of notes.

Inclusion/Exclusion Criteria

Peer-reviewed articles in English language reporting myo-inositol concentrations in the brain in patients with schizophrenia or schizoaffective disorder in comparison with a healthy control group were included. We did not include studies that only report on patients with bipolar disorder or depression related psychosis. We selected studies where the largest proportion of MRS voxel was placed on the medial prefrontal cortex, anterior to the posterior commissure, as per the cingulate boundaries defined by Vogt et al. (26). This ensured that both caudal and rostral ACC placements were included, but posterior cingulate voxels were excluded. In line with Egerton et al. (27), we will use the term medial frontal cortex (mFC) to describe this region of distributed voxel placement.

We excluded 1H-MRS studies that reported within-subject changes in myo-inositol without the required group comparison contrast and studies that excluded adult samples of age >16. If a single study was reported as 2 samples, the largest sample was included. In case of partial overlap, both studies were included with weighting based only on the non-overlapping sample for the smaller study (28, 29). We also excluded studies where no information was available on voxel placement (30) or when study-specific Cramer-Rao Lower Bound (a measure of MRS signal quality and reliability) was exceeded for myo-inositol signal (31).

We extracted the study-specific mean and standard deviation of 1H-MRS myo-inositol concentration for the control and patient groups. As the meta-analysis was based on effect size from group differences, we included absolute as well as ratio measures of myo-inositol concentrations, as long as both patients and controls in a dataset had identical metrics reported. When a study reported on more than 1 demographically stratified patient group, all contrasts were included in the meta-analysis (29); when groups were stratified according to clinical characteristics (e.g., treatment response) but compared against a single control group, the contrasts were combined to form a single dataset (weighted mean and pooled SD for a single patient group) (32). When voxels were split into 2 hemispheres, average values were computed (mean value from the 2 hemispheres and pooled SD) We contacted authors when these values were not reported or if moderator variables for meta-regression were not available.

Meta-analysis was conducted using the *metafor* package of R CRAN (33). We used a random-effects model to calculate the pooled effect size, with 95% confidence limits. This approach enables more robust inferences when there is a notable heterogeneity among individual studies. We assessed heterogeneity using I^2 statistics for quantification and Cochran's Q for statistical significance test. Potential publication bias was quantified using Egger's test. Sensitivity testing was carried out using a jack-knife approach. During each of the iterations of this leave-one-out jack-knife testing, one study was left out and the meta-analytical estimate for (n-1) studies was recalculated. Meta-regression analyses were undertaken to investigate the effect of (1) age (based on mean age of patients) (2) gender (based on % female patients) (3) medication status (based on % unmedicated patients) (4) scanner strength (in Tesla) and (5) duration of illness (based on mean years of illness).

RESULTS

Search Results

The literature search identified 19 studies (one with 2 eligible contrasts (29)), published between 2002 and 2018, with a total of 561 patients and 585 controls (PRISMA flow diagram presented **Figure 1**) (29, 32, 34–49). The sample sizes ranged from 10 to 75 for controls and 9–72 for patients (**Table 1**). Mean illness duration varied between 0.49 and 27.4 years.

The voxel placement of individual studies is shown in **Figure 2**. MRS parameters for individual studies are shown in **Table 2**.

Meta-Analysis Results

The estimate of heterogeneity had a trend level statistical significance ($I^2 = 14.61\%$; Cochran's $Q = 27.64$, $p = 0.09$) among the 20 datasets eligible for analysis. Random effects analysis revealed reduced myo-inositol content in patients

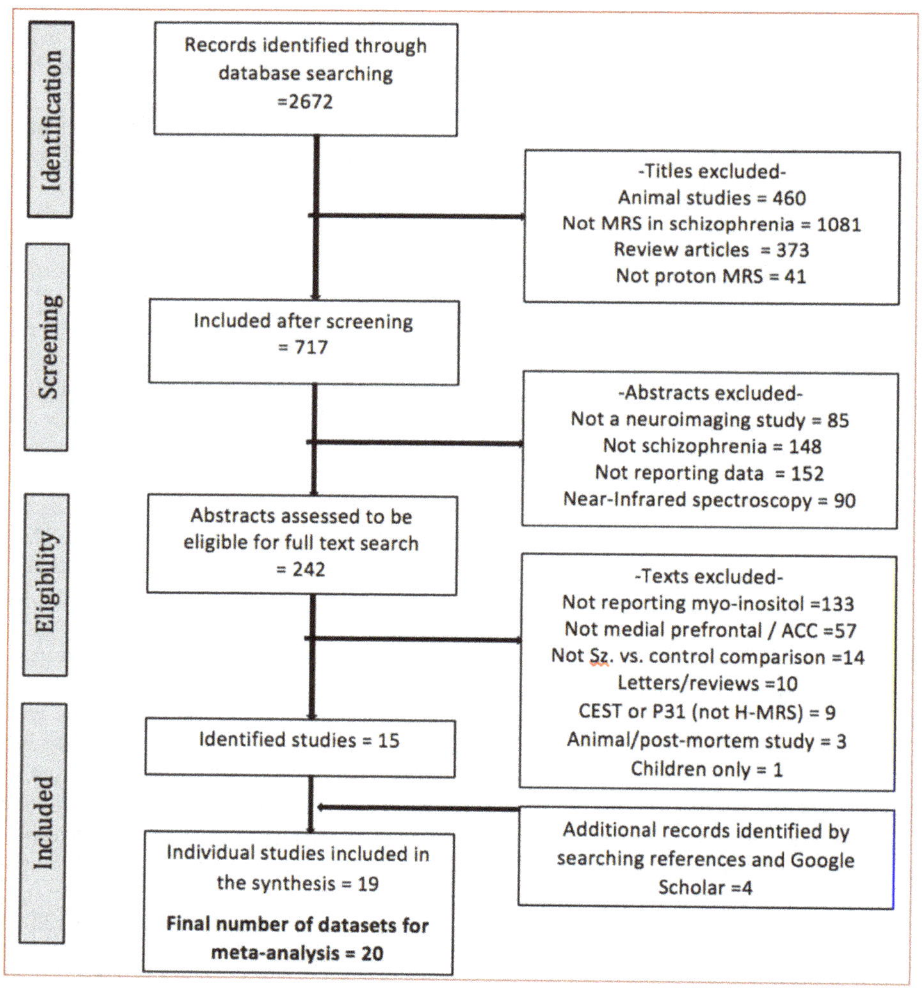

FIGURE 1 | The literature search process.

TABLE 1 | Clinical and demographic features of studies included in the meta-analysis.

Study	Year	Number of patients/controls	Patients mean ml (SD)	Controls Mean ml (SD)	% Female patients	Age patient Mean (SD) in years	Age controls Mean (SD) in years	Unmedicated patients in %	Illness duration Mean (SD) in years
Theberge	2002	20/20	8.82 (3.92)	8.72 (2.71)	35.00	25.40 (7.20)	25.52 (7.29)	100	1.75 (2.00)
Delamillieure	2002	17/14	0.63(0.19)	0.66(0.13)	17.65	31.25(6.09)	30.14(6.39)	29.41	8.42(5.45)
Theberge	2003	21/21	9.73 (3.1)	8.74 (3.38)	4.76	37.10 (10.60)	33.30 (11.73)	0	15.6 (8.92)
Yasukawa	2005	15/20	0.98 (0.28)	1.29 (0.24)	46.67	32 (4.9)	36.1 (6.8)	13.33	1.7 (2.10)
Ongur	2008	17/21	0.92(0.33)	1.09(0.32)	41.18	41.8 (9.8)	34.3(10)	0	NA
Tayoshi	2009	30/25	6.73 (2.2)	8.22 (2.35)	53.33	33.8 (9.5)	34.9 (10.7)	0	10.3 (8.7)
Ongur	2010	21/19	0.25 (0.03)	0.27 (0.04)	33.33	39 (10.8)	36.3 (9.8)	13.33	21.1 (7.3)
Shirayama	2010	19/18	5.7 (0.68)	5.55 (0.72)	36.84	30.5 (5.6)	31.4 (8.4)	5.26	7.3 (5.2)
Lutkenhoff	2010	9/21	7.90(1.73)	8.26(2.65)	44.44	48.8(11.5)	55.7(3.8)	0	27.4(11.1)
Bustillo	2014	72/75	10.97 (5.47)	11.03 (4.96)	15.28	36.43 (14.25)	35.04 (12.17)	3.7	15.9 (5.5)
Demjaha	2014	14/10	6.88 (1.66)	6.39 (1.07)	54.17	44.8 (10.9)	44.2 (8.9)	0	16.2(9.4)
Chiappelli	2015	59/69	6.84 (0.84)	6.94 (0.60)	30.51	37.1 (10.6)	33.3 (11.73)	5.08	NA
Brandt	2016	24/24	6.36 (1.34)	6.69 (0.88)	20.83	37.5 (16.7)	36.6 (14.6)	0.00	NA
Rowland	2016a	45/53	6.8 (0.9)	6.90 (0.60)	35.56	37.7 (12.8)	37.1 (13.1)	8.9	14.7 (12.1)
Rowland	2016b	27/29	5.8 (0.64)	5.80 (0.42)	37.04	34.4 (13.1)	29.7 (9.4)	18.52	13.1 (12.1)
Chiu	2017	19/14	5.13 (2.65)	7.71 (1.63)	42.11	29.11 (6.68)	27.71 (5.88)	0	1.47 (1.23)
Taylor	2017	16/18	8.4 (1.3)	8.00 (0.80)	18.75	22.7 (2.9)	23.9 (4.6)	6.06	2.46 (1.31)
Wijtenburg (young)	2017	48/54	6.6 (0.7)	6.72 (0.50)	29.17	25.2 (4.5)	25.2 (4.8)	8.33	6.1 (5.8)
Wijtenburg (older)	2017	47/39	6.82 (0.9)	7.00 (0.80)	44.68	49.5 (5.4)	51.2 (5.7)	4.26	25.4 (9.3)
Reid	2018	21/21	4.88 (0.47)	5.03 (0.50)	23.81	23.2 (4.4)	23.5 (4.5)	4.76	0.49 (0.86)

ml, myo-inositol (absolute or ratio measure of concentration).

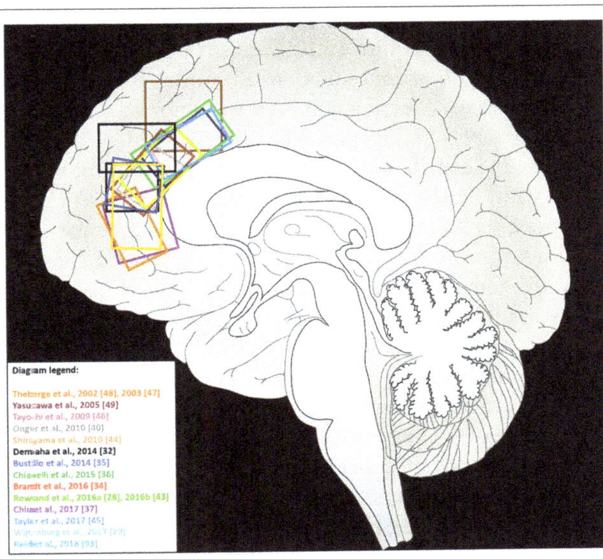

FIGURE 2 | Voxel locations in medial frontal cortex for 1H-MRS studies of myo-inositol included in this meta-analysis. Studies from which a sagittal view of the MRS voxel could not be obtained are not included in this illustration.

with schizophrenia compared to healthy controls (effect estimate = 0.19, 95% CI [0.05–0.32], $z = 2.72$, $p = 0.0067$). These results are displayed in the forest plot **Figure 3**.

Sensitivity/Bias Analysis

All the 16 iterations of the leave-one out analyses were statistically significant, indicating that the meta-analytical estimates were reliable and not influenced by any single study. Egger's test for funnel plot asymmetry (**Figure 4**) was not statistically significant ($t = 0.77$, $p = 0.45$), indicating low probability of publication bias.

Meta-Regression Analysis

There was a statistically significant moderator effect of the percentage of female patients included in the samples in the effect size for myo-inositol ($z = 2.53$, $p = 0.011$). With this moderator, heterogeneity significantly decreased (Cochran's Q = 21.2, $p = 0.27$). Specifically, studies with more female patients were more likely to report reduced myo-inositol concentrations in patients compared to controls (**Figure 5**). We did not find any statistically significant moderator effect of the proportion of unmedicated patients ($z = -0.60$, $p = 0.55$), scanner strength ($z = -1.21$, $p = 0.22$), echo time ($z = 1.59$, $p = 0.11$), repetition time ($z = 0.13$, $p = 0.9$), age of patients ($z = -0.05$, $p = 0.95$), and duration of illness ($z = -0.94$, $p = 0.34$).

DISCUSSION

The main finding from this meta-analysis is the observation of a small, but statistically significant reduction in myo-inositol concentration in the medial frontal cortex in schizophrenia. There is a notable heterogeneity across MRS studies; a substantial

TABLE 2 | MRS parameters of individual studies.

Study	Year	Field strength (T)	MRS fitting model	Voxel size/volume (cm × cm × cm) or cc	MRS sequences	TE/TR (ms)
Theberge	2002	4	fitMAN	1.0 × 1.5 × 1.0	STEAM	20/2,000
Delamillieure	2002	1.5	In-house analysis	3 × 1.5 × 2.5	STEAM	30/1,500
Theberge	2003	4	fitMAN	1.0 × 1.5 × 1.0	STEAM	20/2,000
Yasukawa	2005	1.5	In-house analysis	1.8 cc	PRESS	30/1,500
Ongur	2008	4	LCModel	2.0 × 2.0 × 2.0	PRESS	48/2,000
Tayoshi	2009	3	LCModel	1.7 × 1.7 × 1.5	STEAM	18/5,000
Ongur	2010	4	LCModel	2.3 × 2.2 × 2.3	MEGA-PRESS	30/5,000
Shirayama	2010	3	LCModel	2.8 × 3.0 × 2.2	PRESS	68/2,000
Lutkenhoff	2010	3	LCModel	2.0 × 2.0 × 2.0	PRESS	30/3,000
Bustillo	2014	3	LCModel	2.0 × 2.0 × 3.0	PRESS	40/1,500
Demjaha	2014	3	LCModel	2.0 × 2.0 × 2.0	PRESS	30/3,000
Chiappelli	2015	3	LCModel	4.0 × 3.0 × 2.0	PR-STEAM	6.5/2,000
Brandt	2016	7	LCModel	3.0 × 2.0 × 1.2	STEAM	28/3,000
Rowland	2016a	3	LCModel, GannetFit	4.0 × 3.0 × 2.0	PR-STEAM	14/3,000
Rowland	2016b	7	LCModel	3.0 × 2.0 × 2.0	STEAM	6.5/2,000
Chiu	2017	3	GannetFit	3.0 × 3.0 × 3.0	MEGA-PRESS	68/2,000
Taylor	2017	7	fitMAN	2.0 × 2.0 × 2.0	STEAM	10/3,000
Wijtenburg (young)	2017	3	In house analysis	3.0 × 4.0 × 2.0	PR-STEAM	6.5/2,000
Wijtenburg (older)	2017	3	In house analysis	3.0 × 4.0 × 2.0	PR-STEAM	6.5/2,000
Reid	2018	7	LCModel	2.7 × 2.0 × 1.0	STEAM	5/10,000

LCModel, Linear Combination Model; STEAM, STimulated Echo Acquisition Mode; PRESS, Point REsolved Spectroscopic Sequence; MEGA-PRESS, MEscher-GArwood Point RESolved Spectroscopy; PR-STEAM, Phase Rotation STimulated Echo Acquisition Mode; TE/TR, Echo Time/Repetition Time.

proportion of this heterogeneity is explained by the sex distribution in individual studies. In studies with higher number of female patients, the myo-inositol reduction is much more pronounced. We found no evidence of publication bias, and the meta-analytic estimates were sensitive to removal of any of the individual studies. These results indicate that myo-inositol reduction in medial frontal cortex occurs in some patients with schizophrenia, especially in a subset that is more likely to include female patients.

To our knowledge, this is the first meta-analysis of MRS myo-inositol studies in schizophrenia. Post-mortem studies in schizophrenia indicate a reduction in frontal myo-inositol (50) as well as reduced glial cell count (51), of 32–35% in layer 5 (52, 53) and 20% in layer 6 of the prefrontal cortex (54), though contradicting results indicating normal (55, 56) or increased glial cell counts also exist (57, 58). In this context, reduced myo-inositol resonance reported in our meta-analysis, when taken together with reduced glutamate levels reported in established cases of schizophrenia (59), may reflect deficits in astrocyte activation and recruitment [as proposed in (21)], rather than an actual reduction in the cell count.

Our meta-regression analysis indicates that studies with female subjects are more likely to report lower myo-inositol resonance among patients. An association between sex and myo-inositol has not been reported so far in schizophrenia (36, 46). Interestingly, Chiappeli et al. reported that depressive symptoms, rather than sex, are associated with lower myo-inositol in schizophrenia (36). Both reductions in myo-inositol (60) and glial loss (61) in the medial prefrontal cortex are reported in depressive disorder. Given that one-third of patients with schizophrenia require antidepressant treatments (62), it is possible that myoinositol reduction is prominent in a subgroup of patients prone to depression. We were not able to test this notion, as except for Chiappeli et al. other MRS studies have not reported on the distribution of affective symptom severity among patients with schizophrenia. Nevertheless, it is worth noting that depression is much more common among women, than men with schizophrenia (63). Sex-specific epigenetic differences have been noted in the enzymes that regulate myo-inositol turnover in rat tissues (64). Importantly, astrocytes exhibit sexual dimorphism during development (65) and in their response to inflammation in later life (66, 67). Further investigations in larger samples of female human subjects, and in patients with and without affective symptoms are warranted.

Meta-analyses of medial prefrontal MRS studies suggest that glutamate (68), N-acetyl aspartate levels (69) are reduced in schizophrenia indicating possible dendritic reduction (70), while no consistent changes are noted in GABA concentration (27) or pH levels (71). Glutamate levels are higher during early stages of schizophrenia, but appear reduced in older cohorts with more established illness (68). We did not observe any age- or illness duration related effects on myo-inositol reduction, suggesting that astroglial dysfunction could be an invariant feature of schizophrenia, possibly contributing to the observed course of glutamatergic abnormalities. Preclinical studies suggest that at excitotoxic levels of glutamatergic signaling, inositol

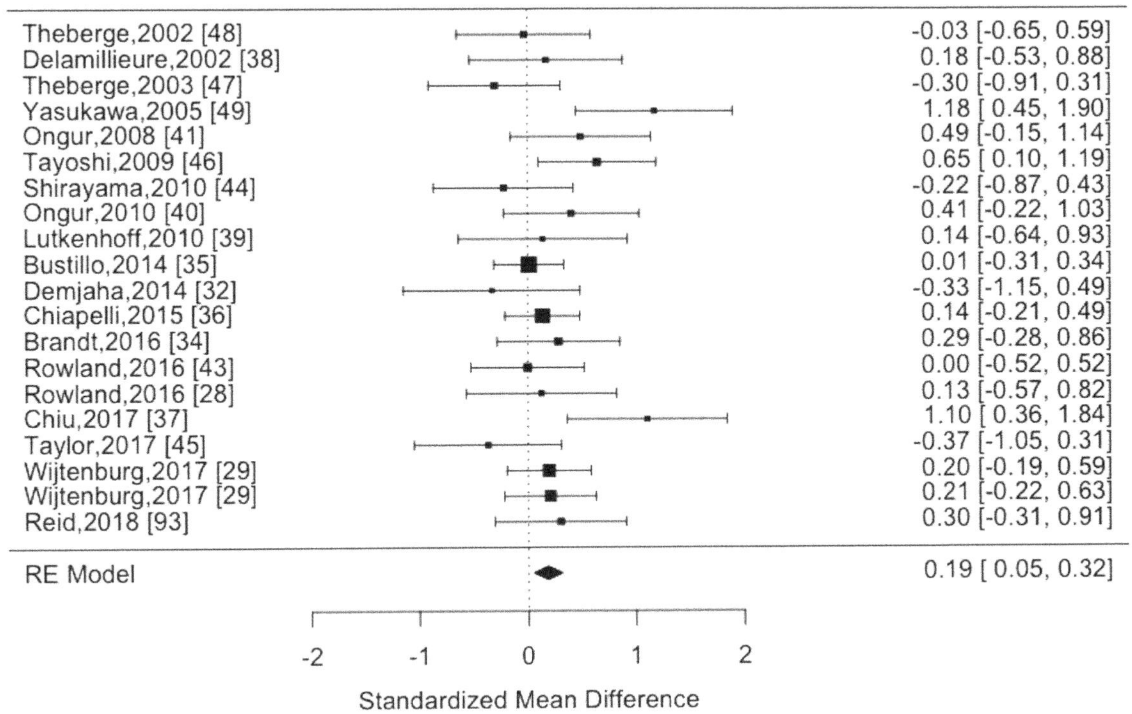

FIGURE 3 | Forest plot of MRS myo-inositol studies comparing schizophrenia vs. healthy controls.

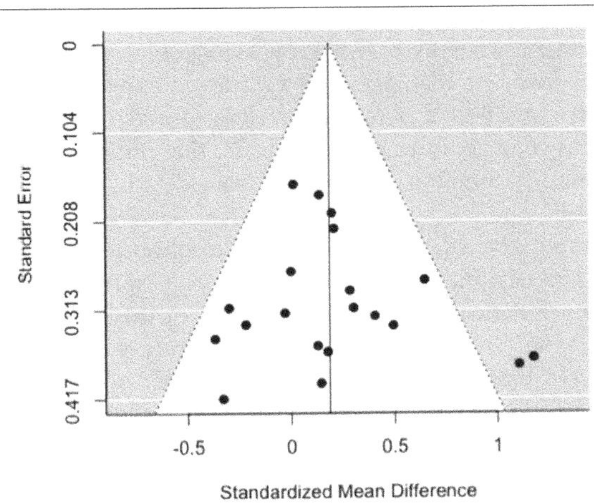

FIGURE 4 | Funnel plot of MRS myo-inositol studies comparing schizophrenia vs. healthy controls.

turnover could be notably reduced. In this context, the putative dysfunction of synaptic transmission in schizophrenia could share a common origin, simultaneously affecting the neuron-astroglia network. Similar to NAA, myo-inositol also reflects cellular membrane integrity. Thus a combined NAA and myo-inositol changes could reflect the status of dendritic spine development or loss, as shown in preclinical studies (72). While the existing MRS literature cannot be taken as conclusive due to several technical limitations (as highlighted in the meta-analyses cited above), the observations to date make a compelling case to consider astrocytic dysfunction in further detail in schizophrenia.

There are several caveats that need to be considered when interpreting the results reported here. We limited our analysis to medial prefrontal cortex, as the number of studies examining other brain regions is limited and voxel placements are more diverse. As a result, the observed myo-inositol reduction may not be generalizable to other brain regions. In fact, an increase in MRS myo-inositol signal has been reported in regions such as basal ganglia (73) and parietal lobe (74) in patients with schizophrenia, while a reduction occurs in medial temporal white matter (75). Secondly, mood stabilizers acutely deplete inositol levels (76). None of the included studies reported on the use of mood stabilizer drugs in the patient samples. The effect of antipsychotics on myo-inositol concentration is hitherto unknown. Antipsychotics can reduce astrocyte count, and thus contribute to reduced myo-inositol concentration (77), though regional differences can be expected from existing data (78). We did not find any systematic association between either unmedicated patient numbers or duration of illness (which often relates also to cumulative antipsychotic exposure in clinical settings) to the reported effect sizes. Furthermore, both schizophrenia and antipsychotics can affect metabolite relaxation rates (mostly T1, but likely also T2) (79–81). Therefore, the choice of acquisition technique, at a given field strength, could affect the ability to detect a difference between patients and controls. Nevertheless, we did not observe any linear relationship

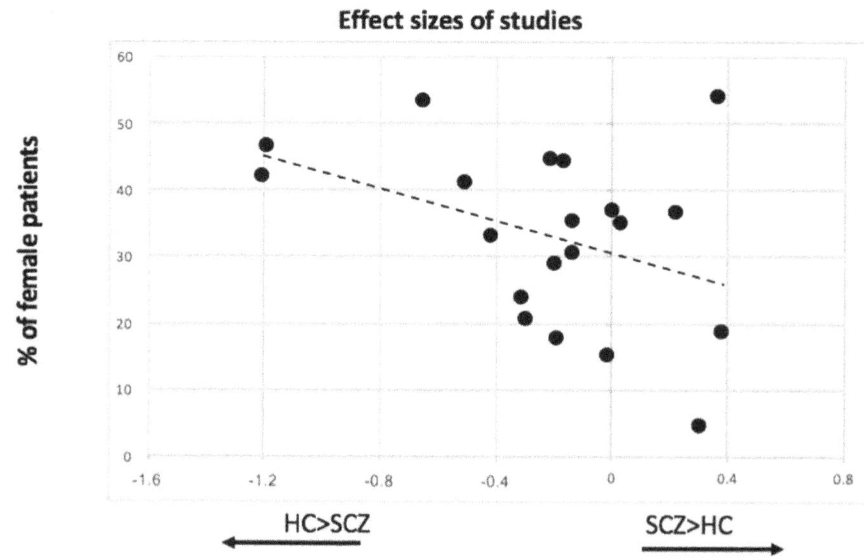

FIGURE 5 | Association between proportion of female patients included in individual MRS studies and the effect size of myo-inositol resonance.

between echo time, scanner strength, repetition time and effect sizes reported in individual studies. We noted several studies where MRS sequences were suitable to extract myo-inositol concentrations alongside other metabolites, but myo-inositol levels were not measured or reported. Though our estimate of publication bias was low, it is likely that MRS myo-inositol concentration is largely underreported in the literature. Finally, we did not include analysis that primarily contrasted bipolar disorder or depression with psychosis with healthy controls or patients with schizophrenia. Thus, the observed changes in myo-inositol cannot be taken to be specific for schizophrenia.

Prenatal exposure to maternal immune activation (MIA) reduces cingulate cortex myo-inositol in mice, which in turn relates to physiological markers of schizophrenia phenotype such as deficits in pre-pulse inhibition and reduced glutamic acid decarboxylase (GAD_{67}) levels (82). These changes were reversed when the offspring were exposed to a *n-3 polyunsaturated fatty acid* (PUFA) enriched post-weaning diet (82). Consistent with this observation, healthy human subjects who have reduced omega-3 fatty acid profile (measured from erythrocytes), show reduced medial prefrontal myo-inositol and exhibit slower reaction times in a continuous performance task (83). We speculate that these observations, considered alongside the reported reduction in myo-inositol levels in schizophrenia, may indicate a specific developmental perturbation. It is worth noting that dietary replacements may not have the same intended effect across disorders; for example, in major depressive disorder where myo-inositol level is reduced, inositol supplementation appears to be beneficial (84, 85), though similar effects have not been observed in schizophrenia (86, 87). Studies that investigate the effect of dietary interventions on brain myo-inositol levels in specific diagnostic subgroups are warranted to further understand the translational potential of such approaches.

It is important to note that both increased (21, 22) and reduced (88–91) brain myo-inositol levels have been noted in various inflammatory states. Thus, the reduced myo-inositol level noted in schizophrenia does not contradict the role of neuroinflammation in this illness. In fact, this observation adds an important clarification that the inflammatory changes observed to date may be secondary to a permissive astrocytic environment, whereby reduced myo-inositol levels in astrocytes facilitate osmotic damage, as well as glutamatergic excess. Without longitudinal data that tracks pre-psychotic and post-psychotic changes in same individuals, this notion of primary astrocytic dysfunction should be considered to be merely speculative.

In summary, in patients with schizophrenia, a small but statistically significant reduction in medial prefrontal myo-inositol resonance is observable. The size of the reported effect indicates that the biological pathways affecting the myo-inositol system are likely to operate only in a subset of patients with schizophrenia. In this regard, MRS myo-inositol could be a useful tool to parse heterogeneity as well as to explore treatment stratification in schizophrenia. Furthermore, combining MRS myo-inositol measurement with *in-vivo* probes of astroglial function (e.g., PET ligands selective for the astrocytic imidazoline binding sites (92)) could take this investigation further in the near future.

AUTHOR CONTRIBUTIONS

LP conceived, designed, supervised the analysis, and wrote the draft manuscript. TD undertook the statistical analysis, prepared figures and tables, and contributed to writing the manuscript. JR undertook the statistical analysis and contributed to writing the manuscript. AD and AJ undertook literature search, prepared figures/tables, and contributed to writing the manuscript. PS undertook literature search, verified extracted data, and contributed to writing the manuscript. JT contributed to the conception of the review and contributed to writing the manuscript.

FUNDING

This work was funded by the Canadian Institute of Health Research (Foundation Grant 375104 to LP), Bucke Family Fund (LP and PS), and the Academic Medical Organization of South Western Ontario (LP). This work was also supported by Miguel Servet contract from the Carlos III Health Institute (Spain) to JR (CP14/00041).

ACKNOWLEDGMENTS

We acknowledge the authors who provided data on request: Dr. Juan Bustillo.

REFERENCES

1. Bernstein H-G, Steiner J, Bogerts B. Glial cells in schizophrenia: pathophysiological significance and possible consequences for therapy. *Exp Rev Neurother.* (2009) 9:1059–71. doi: 10.1586/ern.09.59
2. Harrison PJ. Neuropathology of schizophrenia. *Psychiatry* (2005) 4:18–21. doi: 10.1383/psyt.2005.4.10.18
3. Schnieder TP, Dwork AJ. Searching for neuropathology: gliosis in Schizophrenia. *Biol Psychiatr.* (2011) 69:134–9. doi: 10.1016/j.biopsych.2010.08.027
4. Bélanger M, Allaman I, Magistretti PJ. Brain energy metabolism: focus on astrocyte-neuron metabolic cooperation. *Cell Metab.* (2011) 14:724–38. doi: 10.1016/j.cmet.2011.08.016
5. Dringen R, Pfeiffer B, Hamprecht B. Synthesis of the antioxidant glutathione in neurons: supply by astrocytes of cysgly as precursor for neuronal glutathione. *J Neurosci.* (1999) 19:562–9. doi: 10.1523/JNEUROSCI.19-02-00562.1999
6. Rose CF, Verkhratsky A, Parpura V. Astrocyte glutamine synthetase: pivotal in health and disease. *Biochem Soc Trans.* (2013) 41:1518–24. doi: 10.1042/BST20130237
7. Schousboe A, Scafidi S, Bak LK, Waagepetersen HS, McKenna MC. Glutamate metabolism in the brain focusing on astrocytes. *Adv Neurobiol.* (2014) 11:13–30. doi: 10.1007/978-3-319-08894-5_2
8. Bélanger M, Magistretti PJ. The role of astroglia in neuroprotection. *Dialog Clin Neurosci.* (2009) 11:281–95.
9. Volterra A, Meldolesi J. Astrocytes, from brain glue to communication elements: the revolution continues. *Nat Rev Neurosci.* (2005) 6:626–40. doi: 10.1038/nrn1722
10. Windrem MS, Osipovitch M, Liu Z, Bates J, Chandler-Militello D, Zou L, et al. Human iPSC glial mouse chimeras reveal glial contributions to schizophrenia. *Cell Stem Cell* (2017) 21:195–208.e6. doi: 10.1016/j.stem.2017.06.012
11. Xia M, Abazyan S, Jouroukhin Y, Pletnikov M. Behavioral sequelae of astrocyte dysfunction: focus on animal models of schizophrenia. *Schizophrenia Res.* (2016) 176:72–82. doi: 10.1016/j.schres.2014.10.044
12. Duncan LE, Holmans PA, Lee PH, O'Dushlaine CT, Kirby AW, Smoller JW, et al. Pathway analyses implicate glial cells in schizophrenia. *PLoS ONE* (2014) 9:e89441. doi: 10.1371/journal.pone.0089441
13. Granville NT, Byers DM, Cook HW, Spence MW, Palmer FBSC. Differences in the metabolism of inositol and phosphoinositides by cultured cells of neuronal and glial origin. *Biochim Biophys. Acta* (1989) 1004:169–79. doi: 10.1016/0005-2760(89)90265-8
14. Hattingen E, Raab P, Franz K, Zanella FE, Lanfermann H, Pilatus U. Myo-inositol: a marker of reactive astrogliosis in glial tumors? *NMR Biomed.* (2008) 21:233–41. doi: 10.1002/nbm.1186
15. Brand A, Richter-Landsberg C, Leibfritz D. Multinuclear NMR studies on the energy metabolism of glial and neuronal cells. *Dev Neurosci.* (1993) 15:289–98. doi: 10.1159/000111347
16. Griffin JL, Bollard M, Nicholson JK, Bhakoo K. Spectral profiles of cultured neuronal and glial cells derived from HRMAS (1)H NMR spectroscopy. *NMR Biomed.* (2002) 15:375–84. doi: 10.1002/nbm.792
17. Filibian M, Frasca A, Maggioni D, Micotti E, Vezzani A, Ravizza T. *In vivo* imaging of glia activation using ^{1}H-magnetic resonance spectroscopy to detect putative biomarkers of tissue epileptogenicity. *Epilepsia* (2012) 53:1907–16. doi: 10.1111/j.1528-1167.2012.03685.x
18. Rothermundt M, Ohrmann P, Abel S, Siegmund A, Pedersen A, Ponath G, et al. Glial cell activation in a subgroup of patients with schizophrenia indicated by increased S100B serum concentrations and elevated myo-inositol. *Prog Neuro-Psychopharmacol Biol Psychiatr.* (2007) 31:361–4. doi: 10.1016/j.pnpbp.2006.09.013
19. Geiszler PC, Ugun-Klusek A, Lawler K, Pardon M-C, Yuchun D, Bai L, et al. Dynamic metabolic patterns tracking neurodegeneration and gliosis following 26S proteasome dysfunction in mouse forebrain neurons. *Sci Rep.* (2018) 8:4833. doi: 10.1038/s41598-018-23155-2
20. Pardon M-C, Yanez Lopez M, Yuchun D, Marjanska M, Prior M, Brignell C, et al. Magnetic resonance spectroscopy discriminates the response to microglial stimulation of wild type and Alzheimer's disease models. *Sci Rep.* (2016) 6:19880. doi: 10.1038/srep19880
21. Harris JL, Choi I-Y, Brooks WM. Probing astrocyte metabolism *in vivo*: proton magnetic resonance spectroscopy in the injured and aging brain. *Front Aging Neurosci.* (2015) 7:202. doi: 10.3389/fnagi.2015.00202
22. Kierans AS, Kirov II, Gonen O, Haemer G, Nisenbaum E, Babb JS, et al. Myoinositol and glutamate complex neurometabolite abnormality after mild traumatic brain injury. *Neurology* (2014) 82:521–8. doi: 10.1212/WNL.0000000000000105
23. Kim H, McGrath BM, Silverstone PH. A review of the possible relevance of inositol and the phosphatidylinositol second messenger system (PI-cycle) to psychiatric disorders–focus on magnetic resonance spectroscopy (MRS) studies. *Hum Psychopharmacol.* (2005) 20:309–26. doi: 10.1002/hup.693
24. Schwerk A, Alves FDS, Pouwels PJW, van Amelsvoort T. Metabolic alterations associated with schizophrenia: a critical evaluation of proton magnetic resonance spectroscopy studies. *J Neurochem.* (2014) 128:1–87. doi: 10.1111/jnc.12398
25. Moher D, Liberati A, Tetzlaff J, Altman DG, The PRISMA Group preferred reporting items for systematic reviews and meta-analyses: the PRISMA statement. *PLoS Med.* (2009) 6:e1000097. doi: 10.1371/journal.pmed.1000097
26. Vogt BA, Nimchinsky EA, Vogt LJ, Hof P. Human cingulate cortex: surface features, flat maps, and cytoarchitecture. *J Compar Neurol.* (2004) 359:490–506. doi: 10.1002/cne.903590310
27. Egerton A, Modinos G, Ferrera D, McGuire P. Neuroimaging studies of GABA in schizophrenia: a systematic review with meta-analysis. *Transl Psychiatr.* (2017) 7:e1147. doi: 10.1038/tp.2017.124
28. Rowland LM, Summerfelt A, Wijtenburg SA, Du X, Chiappelli JJ, Krishna N, et al. Frontal glutamate and γ-aminobutyric acid levels and their associations with mismatch negativity and digit sequencing task performance in schizophrenia. *JAMA Psychiatr.* (2016) 73:166–74. doi: 10.1001/jamapsychiatry.2015.2680
29. Wijtenburg SA, Wright SN, Korenic SA, Gaston FE, Ndubuizu N, Chiappelli J, et al. Altered glutamate and regional cerebral blood flow levels in schizophrenia: A1H-MRS and pCASL study. *Neuropsychopharmacology* (2017) 42:562–71. doi: 10.1038/npp.2016.172
30. Delamillieure P, Fernandez J, Constans J-M, Brazo P, Benali K, Abadie P, et al. Proton magnetic resonance spectroscopy of the medial prefrontal cortex in patients with deficit schizophrenia: preliminary report. *Am J Psychaitry* (2000) 157:641–3. doi: 10.1176/appi.ajp.157.4.641
31. Théberge J, Williamson KE, Aoyama N, Drost DJ, Manchanda R, Malla AK, et al. Longitudinal grey-matter and glutamatergic losses in first-episode schizophrenia. *Br J Psychiatry* (2007) 191:325–34. doi: 10.1192/bjp.bp.106.033670

32. Demjaha A, Egerton A, Murray RM, Kapur S, Howes OD, Stone JM, et al. Antipsychotic treatment resistance in schizophrenia associated with elevated glutamate levels but normal dopamine function. *Biol Psychiatry* (2014) 75:e11–13. doi: 10.1016/j.biopsych.2013.06.011
33. Viechtbauer W. Conducting meta-analyses in R with the metafor package. *J Stat Softw.* (2010) 36:1–48. doi: 10.18637/jss.v036.i03
34. Brandt AS, Unschuld PG, Pradhan S, Lim IAL, Churchill G, Harris AD, et al. Age-related changes in anterior cingulate cortex glutamate in schizophrenia: a (1)H MRS Study at 7Tesla. *Schizophr Res.* (2016) 172:101–5. doi: 10.1016/j.schres.2016.02.017
35. Bustillo JR, Chen H, Jones T, Lemke N, Abbott C, Qualls C, et al. Increased glutamine in patients undergoing long-term treatment for schizophrenia: a proton magnetic resonance spectroscopy study at 3 T. *JAMA Psychiatry* (2014) 71:265–72. doi: 10.1001/jamapsychiatry.2013.3939
36. Chiappelli J, Rowland LM, Wijtenburg SA, Muellerklein F, Tagamets M, McMahon RP, et al. Evaluation of myo-inositol as a potential biomarker for depression in schizophrenia. *Neuropsychopharmacology* (2015) 40:2157–64. doi: 10.1038/npp.2015.57
37. Chiu PW, Lui SSY, Hung KSY, Chan RCK, Chan Q, Sham PC, et al. *In vivo* gamma-aminobutyric acid and glutamate levels in people with first-episode schizophrenia: a proton magnetic resonance spectroscopy study. *Schizophr Res.* (2017) 193:295–303. doi: 10.1016/j.schres.2017.07.021
38. Delamillieure P, Constans J-M, Fernandez J, Brazo P, Benali K, Courthéoux P, et al. Proton magnetic resonance spectroscopy (1H MRS) in schizophrenia: investigation of the right and left hippocampus, thalamus, and prefrontal cortex. *Schizophr Bull.* (2002) 28:329–39. doi: 10.1093/oxfordjournals.schbul.a006942
39. Lutkenhoff ES, van Erp TG, Thomas MA, Therman S, Manninen M, Huttunen MO, et al. Proton MRS in twin pairs discordant for schizophrenia. *Mol Psychiatry* (2010) 15:308–18. doi: 10.1038/mp.2008.87
40. Ongür D, Prescot AP, McCarthy J, Cohen BM, Renshaw PF. Elevated gamma-aminobutyric acid levels in chronic schizophrenia. *Biol Psychiatry* (2010) 68:667–70. doi: 10.1016/j.biopsych.2010.05.016
41. Ongür D, Jensen JE, Prescot AP, Stork C, Lundy M, Cohen BM, et al. Abnormal glutamatergic neurotransmission and neuronal-glial interactions in acute mania. *Biol Psychiatry* (2008) 64:718–26. doi: 10.1016/j.biopsych.2008.05.014
42. Reid MA, Stoeckel LE, White DM, Avsar KB, Bolding MS, Akella NS, et al. Assessments of function and biochemistry of the anterior cingulate cortex in schizophrenia. *Biol Psychiatry* (2010) 68:625–33. doi: 10.1016/j.biopsych.2010.04.013
43. Rowland LM, Pradhan S, Korenic S, Wijtenburg SA, Hong LE, Edden RA, et al. Elevated brain lactate in schizophrenia: a 7 T magnetic resonance spectroscopy study. *Transl Psychiatry* (2016) 6:e967. doi: 10.1038/tp.2016.239
44. Shirayama Y, Obata T, Matsuzawa D, Nonaka H, Kanazawa Y, Yoshitome E, et al. Specific metabolites in the medial prefrontal cortex are associated with the neurocognitive deficits in schizophrenia: a preliminary study. *Neuroimage* (2010) 49:2783–90. doi: 10.1016/j.neuroimage.2009.10.031
45. Taylor R, Osuch EA, Schaefer B, Rajakumar N, Neufeld RWJ, Théberge J, et al. Neurometabolic abnormalities in schizophrenia and depression observed with magnetic resonance spectroscopy at 7 T. *BJ Psych Open* (2017) 3:6–11. doi: 10.1192/bjpo.bp.116.003756
46. Tayoshi S, Sumitani S, Taniguchi K, Shibuya-Tayoshi S, Numata S, Iga J, et al. Metabolite changes and gender differences in schizophrenia using 3-Tesla proton magnetic resonance spectroscopy (1H-MRS). *Schizophr Res.* (2009) 108:69–77. doi: 10.1016/j.schres.2008.11.014
47. Theberge J, Al-Semaan Y, Williamson PC, Menon RS, Neufeld RWJ, Rajakumar N, et al. Glutamate and glutamine in the anterior cingulate and thalamus of medicated patients with chronic schizophrenia and healthy comparison subjects measured with 4.0-T proton MRS. *Am J Psychiatry* (2003) 160:2231–3. doi: 10.1176/appi.ajp.160.12.2231
48. Théberge J, Bartha R, Drost DJ, Menon RS, Malla A, Takhar J, et al. Glutamate and glutamine measured with 4.0 T proton MRS in never-treated patients with schizophrenia and healthy volunteers. *Am J Psychiatry* (2002) 159:1944–6. doi: 10.1176/appi.ajp.159.11.1944
49. Yasukawa R, Miyaoka T, Mizuno S, Inagaki T, Horiguchi J, Oda K, et al. Proton magnetic resonance spectroscopy of the anterior cingulate gyrus, insular cortex and thalamus in schizophrenia associated with idiopathic unconjugated hyperbilirubinemia (Gilbert's syndrome). *J Psychiatry Neurosci.* (2005) 30:416–22.
50. Shimon H, Sobolev Y, Davidson M, Haroutunian V, Belmaker RH, Agam G. Inositol levels are decreased in postmortem brain of schizophrenic patients. *Biol Psychiatry* (1998) 44:428–32. doi: 10.1016/S0006-3223(98)00071-7
51. Benes FM, Davidson J, Bird ED. Quantitative cytoarchitectural studies of the cerebral cortex of schizophrenics. *Arch Gen Psychiatry* (1986) 43:31–5. doi: 10.1001/archpsyc.1986.01800010033004
52. Cotter D, Mackay D, Chana G, Beasley C, Landau S, Everall IP. Reduced neuronal size and glial cell density in area 9 of the dorsolateral prefrontal cortex in subjects with major depressive disorder. *Cereb Cortex* (2002) 12:386–94. doi: 10.1093/cercor/12.4.386
53. Rajkowska G, Miguel-Hidalgo JJ, Makkos Z, Meltzer H, Overholser J, Stockmeier C. Layer-specific reductions in GFAP-reactive astroglia in the dorsolateral prefrontal cortex in schizophrenia. *Schizophr Res.* (2002) 57:127–38. doi: 10.1016/S0920-9964(02)00339-0
54. Cotter D, Mackay D, Landau S, Kerwin R, Everall I. Reduced glial cell density and neuronal size in the anterior cingulate cortex in major depressive disorder. *Arch Gen Psychiatry* (2001) 58:545–53. doi: 10.1001/archpsyc.58.6.545
55. Öngür D, Drevets WC, Price JL. Glial reduction in the subgenual prefrontal cortex in mood disorders. *Proc Natl Acad Sci USA.* (1998) 95:13290–5.
56. Selemon LD Rajkowska G, Goldman-Rakic PS. Abnormally high neuronal density in the schizophrenic cortex: a morphometric analysis of prefrontal area 9 and occipital area 17. *Arch Gen Psychiatry* (1995) 52:805–18. doi: 10.1001/archpsyc.1995.03950220015005
57. Harrison PJ. Postmortem studies in schizophrenia. *Dialog Clin Neurosci.* (2000) 2:349–57.
58. Schneider M, Koch M. Behavioral and morphological alterations following neonatal excitotoxic lesions of the medial prefrontal cortex in rats. *Exp Neurol.* (2005) 195:185–98. doi: 10.1016/j.expneurol.2005.04.014
59. Merritt K, Egerton A, Kempton MJ, Taylor MJ, McGuire PK. Nature of glutamate alterations in schizophrenia: a meta-analysis of proton magnetic resonance spectroscopy studies. *JAMA Psychiatry* (2016) 73:665–74. doi: 10.1001/jamapsychiatry.2016.0442
60. Coupland NJ, Ogilvie CJ, Hegadoren KM, Seres P, Hanstock CC, Allen PS. Decreased prefrontal myo-inositol in major depressive disorder. *Biol Psychiatry* (2005) 57:1526–34. doi: 10.1016/j.biopsych.2005.02.027
61. Smiałowska M, Szewczyk B, Wozniak M, Wawrzak-Wleciał A, Domin H. Glial degeneration as a model of depression. *Pharmacol Rep.* (2013) 65:1572–9. doi: 10.1016/S1734-1140(13)71518-4
62. Gregory A, Mallikarjun P, Upthegrove R. Treatment of depression in schizophrenia: systematic review and meta-analysis. *Br J Psychiatry* (2017) 211:198–204. doi: 10.1192/bjp.bp.116.190520
63. McGlashan TH, Bardenstein KK. Gender differences in affective, schizoaffective, and schizophrenic disorders. *Schizophr Bull.* (1990) 16:319–29.
64. Seelan RS, Pisano MM, Greene RM, Casanova MF, Parthasarathy RN. Differential methylation of the gene encoding myo-inositol 3-phosphate synthase (Isyna1) in rat tissues. *Epigenomics* (2011) 3:111–24. doi: 10.2217/epi.10.73
65. McCarthy MM. Sex differences in neuroimmunity as an inherent risk factor. *Neuropsychopharmacology* (2018). doi: 10.1038/s41386-018-0138-1. [Epub ahead of print].
66. Santos-Galindo M, Acaz-Fonseca E, Bellini MJ, Garcia-Segura LM. Sex differences in the inflammatory response of primary astrocytes to lipopolysaccharide. *Biol Sex Differ.* (2011) 2:7. doi: 10.1186/2042-6410-2-7
67. Acaz-Fonseca E, Avila-Rodriguez M, Garcia-Segura LM, Barreto GE. Regulation of astroglia by gonadal steroid hormones under physiological and pathological conditions. *Prog Neurobiol.* (2016) 144:5–26. doi: 10.1016/j.pneurobio.2016.06.002
68. Marsman A, van den Heuvel MP, Klomp DWJ, Kahn RS, Luijten PR, Hulshoff Pol HE. Glutamate in schizophrenia: a focused review and meta-analysis of 1H-MRS Studies. *Schizophr Bull.* (2011) 39:120–9. doi: 10.1093/schbul/sbr069
69. Kraguljac NV, Reid M, White D, Jones R, den Hollander J, Lowman D, et al. Neurometabolites in schizophrenia and bipolar disorder – a systematic review and meta-analysis. *Psychiatry Res.* (2012) 203:111–25. doi: 10.1016/j.pscychresns.2012.02.003

70. Glausier JR, Lewis DA. Dendritic spine pathology in schizophrenia. *Neuroscience* (2013) 251:90–107. doi: 10.1016/j.neuroscience.2012.04.044
71. Dogan AE, Yuksel C, Du F, Chouinard V-A, Öngür D. Brain lactate and pH in schizophrenia and bipolar disorder: a systematic review of findings from magnetic resonance studies. *Neuropsychopharmacology* (2018) 43:1681–90. doi: 10.1038/s41386-018-0041-9
72. Shi D, Xu S, Waddell J, Scafidi S, Roys S, Gullapalli RP, et al. Longitudinal *in vivo* developmental changes of metabolites in the hippocampus of Fmr1 knockout mice. *J Neurochem.* (2012) 123:971–81. doi: 10.1111/jnc.12048
73. Plitman E, Fuente-Sandoval C de la, Reyes-Madrigal F, Chavez S, Gómez-Cruz G, León-Ortiz P, et al. Elevated myo-inositol, choline, and glutamate levels in the associative striatum of antipsychotic-naive patients with first-episode psychosis: a proton magnetic resonance spectroscopy study with implications for glial dysfunction. *Schizophr Bull.* (2015) 42:415–24. doi: 10.1093/schbul/sbv118
74. Auer DP, Wilke M, Grabner A, Heidenreich JO, Bronisch T, Wetter TC. Reduced NAA in the thalamus and altered membrane and glial metabolism in schizophrenic patients detected by 1H-MRS and tissue segmentation. *Schizophr Res.* (2001) 52:87–99. doi: 10.1016/S0920-9964(01)00155-4
75. Chang L, Friedman J, Ernst T, Zhong K, Tsopelas ND, Davis K. Brain metabolite abnormalities in the white matter of elderly schizophrenic subjects: implication for glial dysfunction. *Biol Psychiatry* (2007) 62:1396–404. doi: 10.1016/j.biopsych.2007.05.025
76. Harwood AJ. Lithium and bipolar mood disorder: the inositol-depletion hypothesis revisited. *Mol Psychiatry* (2005) 10:117–26. doi: 10.1038/sj.mp.4001618
77. Konopaske GT, Dorph-Petersen K-A, Sweet RA, Pierri JN, Zhang W, Sampson AR, et al. Effect of chronic antipsychotic exposure on astrocyte and oligodendrocyte numbers in macaque monkeys. *Biol Psychiatry* (2008) 63:759–65. doi: 10.1016/j.biopsych.2007.08.018
78. Szulc A, Galinska B, Tarasow E, Dzienis W, Kubas B, Konarzewska B, et al. The effect of risperidone on metabolite measures in the frontal lobe, temporal lobe, and thalamus in schizophrenic patients. a proton magnetic resonance spectroscopy (1H MRS). *Pharmacopsychiatry* (2005) 38:214–9. doi: 10.1055/s-2005-873156
79. Bracken BK, Rouse ED, Renshaw PF, Olson DP. T2 relaxation effects on apparent N-acetylaspartate concentration in proton magnetic resonance studies of schizophrenia. *Psychiatry Res.* (2013) 213:142–53. doi: 10.1016/j.pscychresns.2013.03.005
80. Öngür D, Prescot AP, Jensen JE, Rouse ED, Cohen BM, Renshaw PF, et al. T2 relaxation time abnormalities in bipolar disorder and schizophrenia. *Magn Reson Med.* (2010) 63:1–8. doi: 10.1002/mrm.22148
81. Williamson P, Pelz D, Merskey H, Morrison S, Karlik S, Drost D, et al. Frontal, temporal, and striatal proton relaxation times in schizophrenic patients and normal comparison subjects. *Am J Psychiatry* (1992) 149:549–51. doi: 10.1176/ajp.149.4.549
82. Li Q, Leung YO, Zhou I, Ho LC, Kong W, Basil P, et al. Dietary supplementation with n-3 fatty acids from weaning limits brain biochemistry and behavioural changes elicited by prenatal exposure to maternal inflammation in the mouse model. *Transl Psychiatry* (2015) 5:e641. doi: 10.1038/tp.2015.126
83. McNamara RK, Jandacek R, Tso P, Weber W, Chu W-J, Strakowski SM, et al. Low docosahexaenoic acid status is associated with reduced indices in cortical integrity in the anterior cingulate of healthy male children: a 1H MRS Study. *Nutr Neurosci.* (2013) 16:183–90. doi: 10.1179/1476830512Y.0000000045
84. Mukai T, Kishi T, Matsuda Y, Iwata N. A meta-analysis of inositol for depression and anxiety disorders. *Hum Psychopharmacol.* (2014) 29:55–63. doi: 10.1002/hup.2369
85. Levine J, Barak Y, Gonzalves M, Szor H, Elizur A, Kofman O, et al. Double-blind, controlled trial of inositol treatment of depression. *Am J Psychiatry* (1995) 152:792–4. doi: 10.1176/ajp.152.5.792
86. Levine J, Umansky R, Ezrielev G, Belmaker RH. Lack of effect of inositol treatment in chronic schizophrenia. *Biol Psychiatry* (1993) 33:673–5. doi: 10.1016/0006-3223(93)90112-Q
87. Firth J, Stubbs B, Sarris J, Rosenbaum S, Teasdale S, Berk M, et al. The effects of vitamin and mineral supplementation on symptoms of schizophrenia: a systematic review and meta-analysis. *Psychol Med.* (2017) 47:1515–27. doi: 10.1017/S0033291717000022
88. Elberling TV, Danielsen ER, Rasmussen AK, Feldt-Rasmussen U, Waldemar G, Thomsen C. Reduced myo-inositol and total choline measured with cerebral MRS in acute thyrotoxic Graves' disease. *Neurology* (2003) 60:142–5. doi: 10.1212/01.WNL.0000038911.07643.BF
89. Haris M, Cai K, Singh A, Hariharan H, Reddy R. *In vivo* mapping of brain myo-inositol. *Neuroimage* (2011) 54:2079–85. doi: 10.1016/j.neuroimage.2010.10.017
90. Howes OD, McCutcheon R. Inflammation and the neural diathesis-stress hypothesis of schizophrenia: a reconceptualization. *Transl Psychiatry* (2017) 7:e1024. doi: 10.1038/tp.2016.278
91. Shawcross DL, Balata S, Olde Damink SWM, Hayes PC, Wardlaw J, Marshall I, et al. Low myo-inositol and high glutamine levels in brain are associated with neuropsychological deterioration after induced hyperammonemia. *Am J Physiol Gastrointest Liver Physiol.* (2004) 287:G503–9. doi: 10.1152/ajpgi.00104.2004
92. Parker CA, Nabulsi N, Holden D, Lin S, Cass T, Labaree D, et al. Evaluation of 11C-BU99008, a PET ligand for the imidazoline2 binding sites in rhesus brain. *J Nucl Med.* (2014) 55:838–44. doi: 10.2967/jnumed.113.131854
93. Reid MA, Salibi N, White DM, Gawne TJ, Denney TS, Lahti AC. 7T Proton magnetic resonance spectroscopy of the anterior cingulate cortex in first-episode schizophrenia. *Schizophr Bull.* (2018). doi: 10.1093/schbul/sbx190. [Epub ahead of print].

11

Myoclonic Jerks and Schizophreniform Syndrome

**Dominique Endres[1,2], Dirk-M. Altenmüller[3], Bernd Feige[1,2], Simon J. Maier[1,2], Kathrin Nickel[1,2], Sabine Hellwig[1,2], Jördis Rausch[1,2], Christiane Ziegler[2], Katharina Domschke[2], John P. Doerr[2], Karl Egger[4] and Ludger Tebartz van Elst[1,2]*

[1] Section for Experimental Neuropsychiatry, Department of Psychiatry and Psychotherapy, Medical Center — University of Freiburg, Faculty of Medicine, University of Freiburg, Freiburg, Germany, [2] Department of Psychiatry and Psychotherapy, Medical Center — University of Freiburg, Faculty of Medicine, University of Freiburg, Freiburg, Germany, [3] Department of Neurosurgery, Medical Center — University of Freiburg, Faculty of Medicine, University of Freiburg, Freiburg, Germany, [4] Department of Neuroradiology, Medical Center — University of Freiburg, Faculty of Medicine, University of Freiburg, Freiburg, Germany

***Correspondence:**
Ludger Tebartz van Elst
tebartzvanelst@uniklinik-freiburg.de

Background: Schizophreniform syndromes can be divided into primary idiopathic forms as well as different secondary organic subgroups (e.g., paraepileptic, epileptic, immunological, or degenerative). Secondary epileptic explanatory approaches have often been discussed in the past, due to the high rates of electroencephalography (EEG) alterations in patients with schizophrenia. In particular, temporal lobe epilepsy is known to be associated with schizophreniform symptoms in well-described constellations. In the literature, juvenile myoclonic epilepsy has been linked to emotionally unstable personality traits, depression, anxiety, and executive dysfunction; however, the association with schizophrenia is largely unclear.

Case presentation: We present the case of a 28-year-old male student suffering from mild myoclonic jerks, mainly of the upper limbs, as well as a predominant paranoid-hallucinatory syndrome with attention deficits, problems with working memory, depressive-flat mood, reduced energy, fast stimulus satiation, delusional and audible thoughts, tactile hallucinations, thought inspirations, and severe sleep disturbances. Cerebral magnetic resonance imaging and cerebrospinal fluid analyses revealed no relevant abnormalities. The routine EEG and the first EEG after sleep deprivation (under treatment with oxazepam) also returned normal findings. Video telemetry over one night, which included a partial sleep-deprivation EEG, displayed short generalized spike-wave complexes and polyspikes, associated with myoclonic jerks, after waking in the morning. Video-EEG monitoring over 5 days showed over 100 myoclonic jerks of the upper limbs, frequently with generalized spike-wave complexes with left or right accentuation. Therefore, we diagnosed juvenile myoclonic epilepsy.

Discussion: This case report illustrates the importance of extended EEG diagnostics in patients with schizophreniform syndromes and myoclonic jerks. The schizophreniform symptoms in the framework of epileptiform EEG activity can be interpreted as a (para)epileptic mechanism due to local area network inhibition (LANI). Following the LANI hypothesis, paranoid hallucinatory symptoms are not due to primary excitatory activity (as myoclonic jerks are) but rather to the secondary process of hyperinhibition triggered by epileptic activity. Identifying subgroups of schizophreniform patients with comorbid epilepsy is important because of the potential benefits of optimized pharmacological treatment.

Keywords: juvenile myoclonic epilepsy, myoclonic jerks, Janz syndrome, schizophrenia, paraepileptic, LANI-hypothesis

BACKGROUND

Schizophreniform syndromes are characterized by delusions, hallucinations, thought disorders, cognitive impairment, and social withdrawal (1). Besides the primary, idiopathic, and polygenetic forms, different secondary pathophysiological mechanisms (e.g., immunological, degenerative, monogenetic, metabolic, epileptic, or paraepileptic) can be assumed (2, 3). Epileptic or paraepileptic explanatory approaches have traditionally been used due to the high rates of electroencephalography (EEG) alterations in patients with schizophreniform syndromes (4–8). In line with this assumption, we have reported the case of a young patient with a schizophreniform syndrome and generalized spike-wave complexes, but without seizures. This patient achieved full psychotic remission under treatment with valproate (9, 10). More recently, we have also reported a case of a female patient with schizophreniform syndrome and generalized 3 Hz polyspike wave complexes, but without seizures. This patient reached complete remission under treatment with levetiracetam (11). While a pathogenetic link between temporal lobe epilepsy and schizophreniform symptoms has been extensively discussed in the literature (12)—an observation that had led to the temporal lobe hypothesis for schizophrenia (13, 14)—a pathophysiological connection between primary generalized forms of epilepsy and schizophrenia is rarely proposed (7).

The association between juvenile myoclonic epilepsy (also called Janz syndrome) and schizophreniform syndromes is largely unclear. Janz syndrome is a frequent, age-related, and inheritable disorder with prevalence estimated to be 5–10% of all epilepsies and approximately 18% of idiopathic generalized epilepsies (15). It is characterized by seizures with bilateral, arrhythmic myoclonic jerks, mainly of the arms, without disturbance of consciousness (16). Psychiatric symptoms include emotionally unstable personality traits with rapid mood changes, depression, anxiety, substance abuse, and executive dysfunction (16, 17). Often, generalized tonic-clonic seizures can be observed; their absence is less frequent. In addition, about a third of patients with Janz syndrome have typical absence seizures. Myoclonic jerks typically occur after awakening and are pronounced after sleep deprivation. In the interictal and ictal EEG, generalized spike-wave complexes and polyspikes waves are commonly found (16).

CASE PRESENTATION

We present the case of a 28-year-old male student who had suffered from fluctuating paranoid-hallucinatory symptoms over the last seven years (since the age of 21 years) and who had been psychiatrically hospitalized five times due to this condition. On first admission to our department at the age of 25, the patient reported increasing problems, with difficulties in studying and social withdrawal, over the past several weeks. He reported attention and concentration deficits, as well as problems with "working memory." Formal thought processes were slowed, the mood was depressive-flat, and energy was decreased. The patient displayed suspicious behavior and sensory overload phenomena. Moreover, he reported ideas of reference and delusional thoughts thinking somebody might poison him. Other psychotic features included dysmorphic delusions, acouasms, thought reading, broadcasting and insertions plus tactile hallucinations. The patient also reported severe sleep disturbances with sleep-onset insomnia and a sleep phase delay, as well as suicidal thoughts. Approximately three years (at the age of 24 years) after the beginning of paranoid-hallucinatory symptoms, the patient developed myoclonic jerks. During the first occurrence of myoclonic jerks, the patient was treated with fluoxetine and zopiclone. Before onset of first myoclonic jerks the patient was already treated with different neuroleptics (aripiprazole, olanzapine, promethazine, quetiapine), as well as the antidepressant duloxetine and the benzodiazepine oxazepam. All these neuroleptics and duloxetine were not tolerated and only prescribed for short time. The myoclonic jerks mostly affected the right arm, but sometimes also the left arm and occasionally the legs. He described "electric shock feelings" in his body while having the myoclonic jerks. At the age of 26, the patient had one isolated bilateral tonic-clonic seizure (during the tapering of oxazepam). Treatment with different neuroleptics led to an increase of the myoclonic jerks. Sleep deprivation also led to an increase in myoclonic jerks. In addition, they were specifically triggered by writing.

Developmental, Somatic, and Family History

The patient's developmental history was negative for *in utero* or birth complications, febrile convulsions, and inflammatory brain diseases. At the age of 11, he experienced a mild cerebral contusion. In primary school, he was affected by symptoms of attention deficit hyperactivity disorder. No autistic features or tic symptoms were reported. At the age of 14, he had problems at school and abused cannabis and alcohol. After graduating from high school, he started studying economics. His medical history revealed only bronchial hyper-reactivity. The family history was negative for myoclonic jerks or epilepsy; however, the mother was described as having an emotionally unstable personality.

Investigations

Most of the investigations were performed during the patient's first stay in our department when he was 25. Blood analyses showed a vitamin D deficiency; renal, liver, and thyroid functions were normal. Thyroid autoantibodies (*against thyroglobulin, thyroid peroxidase, and thyroid-stimulating hormone*), antibodies against intracellular onconeural antigens (*Yo, Hu, CV2/CRMP5, Ri, Ma1/2, SOX1*), and intracellular synaptic antigens (*GAD, amphiphysin*) showed no abnormalities. Cerebrospinal fluid (CSF) analyses were essentially normal with a regular white cell count (1 μL; reference <5 μL), no blood-brain barrier dysfunction (protein concentration: 341; reference <450 mg/L; albumin quotient of 4; age-dependent reference $<6.5 \times 10^{-3}$), and no oligoclonal bands. CSF antibodies against neuronal cell surface antigens (*NMDAR, AMPA-R, GABA-B-R, VGKC-complex [LGI1, Caspr2]*) were negative. The initial contrast-enhanced cerebral magnetic resonance imaging (cMRI) as well as the 2-year follow-up epilepsy-specific cMRI including high-resolution 2D- and isotropic 3D-MRI-sequences showed an isolated and uncomplicated developmental venous anomaly (DVA) in the right temporal lobe (**Figure 1**). There was no associated epileptogenic lesion, such as cavernoma or cortical dysplasia. Taken together, we did not find any evidence of an immunological encephalopathy or other relevant inflammatory diseases. The routine EEG was normal. The first EEG after sleep deprivation also showed no slow or epileptic activity; however, the patient had been treated with oxazepam at that time. Therefore, we performed a 24h video telemetry (under treatment with amisulpride 600 mg and escitalopram 10 mg) including a partial sleep EEG, in combination with measurement of melatonin levels. During this measurement, the patient was awake until 3:00 a.m. Subsequently, he slept for 5 h. During the whole period, the patient reported three mild myoclonic jerks of the right arm. These myoclonic jerks were not associated with epileptic activity in the EEG. However, in the following period, after awakening in the morning, the patient reported six myoclonic jerks of the right arm. All of these presented with simultaneous epileptic activity in the EEG characterized by brief (<3 s) trains of generalized polyspikes and spike-wave complexes with left fronto-central maximum. For syndrome diagnosis, additional long-term video-EEG monitoring (under treatment with clozapine 75 mg, escitalopram 20 mg, oxcarbazepine gradually reduced, and brivaracetam stopped) was carried out when the patient was 27. The monitoring was performed over 5 days and, during this period, the patient showed over 100 myoclonic jerks of the upper limbs (right, left, and bilaterally synchronous), frequently associated with generalized spike-wave complexes (**Figure 2**) and occasionally with left or right accentuation. All clinical events were praxis-induced (by writing with the right or left hand). Additional absences or bilateral tonic-clonic seizures were not documented. The interictal EEG showed frequent intermittent generalized theta slowing, but no clear-cut epileptiform activity. Intermittent photic stimulation did not evoke photoparoxysmal responses.

Differential Diagnosis

In light of the ictal generalized epileptiform activity, the seizure semiology characterized by praxis-induced myoclonic jerks of both arms with worsening after sleep deprivation, and the history of one additional bilateral tonic-clonic seizure, we diagnosed juvenile myoclonic epilepsy (Janz syndrome). The generalized EEG activity, the absence of any potentially epileptogenic lesion in the cMRI, and the semiology with myoclonic jerks of both arms suggested that the epilepsy was not focal. Psychotropic drugs might have triggered or strengthened the symptoms due to genetic vulnerability; however, it is unlikely that the persistent myoclonic jerks are only a side effect of psychotropic drugs because myoclonic jerks also occurred over longer periods with solely antiepileptic treatment with carbamazepine. Myoclonic jerks could also be due to paraneoplastic or non-paraneoplastic inflammatory processes such as immunological encephalopathies or opsoclonus-myoclonus syndrome. In our case, the normal cMRI and CSF findings speak against this idea. Normal copper and ceruloplasmin levels and the normal cMRI findings are not compatible with Morbus Wilson. We also found no neurological signs of progressive myoclonus epilepsies such as Unverricht-Lundborg disease or Lafora disease. Clinically, there were no signs (e.g., labyrinthine deafness, optic atrophy, or myopathy), pointing to a mitochondrial myoclonic epilepsy (e.g., with ragged red fibers or MERRF syndrome). However, a new mitochondrial disease cannot be completely ruled out. The extensive investigation was performed because of the atypical neuropsychiatric presentation with paranoid hallucinatory symptoms and myoclonic jerks. The psychiatric symptoms formally fulfilled the criteria of paranoid-hallucinatory schizophrenia following the International Statistical Classification of Diseases and Related Health Problems (10th revision; ICD-10). Due to the temporal association regarding the development of myoclonic jerks and schizophreniform symptoms, as well as the partial improvement of the psychiatric symptoms with antiepileptic treatment, we suspected a common (para-)epileptic pathomechanism. Alternatively, the presence of Janz syndrome can be a simple comorbidity in primary schizophrenia.

Therapy and Outcome

Initially, the patient was treated unsuccessfully with different antidepressants (bupropion, duloxetine, fluoxetine, mirtazapine, and venlafaxine) and neuroleptics (amisulpride, aripiprazole, olanzapine, promethazine, quetiapine, and risperidone). During treatment with amisulpride, quetiapine, and risperidone, an increased rate of myoclonic jerks was reported. The treatment of early dyskinesia with biperiden led to a dramatic increase in the myoclonic jerks. Oxazepam quickly reduced the rate of myoclonic jerks and was taken by the patient over a longer period. Promethazine also led to an increased rate of myoclonic jerks.

Since his first stay in our department, when the patient was 25, we have prescribed various anticonvulsants. However,

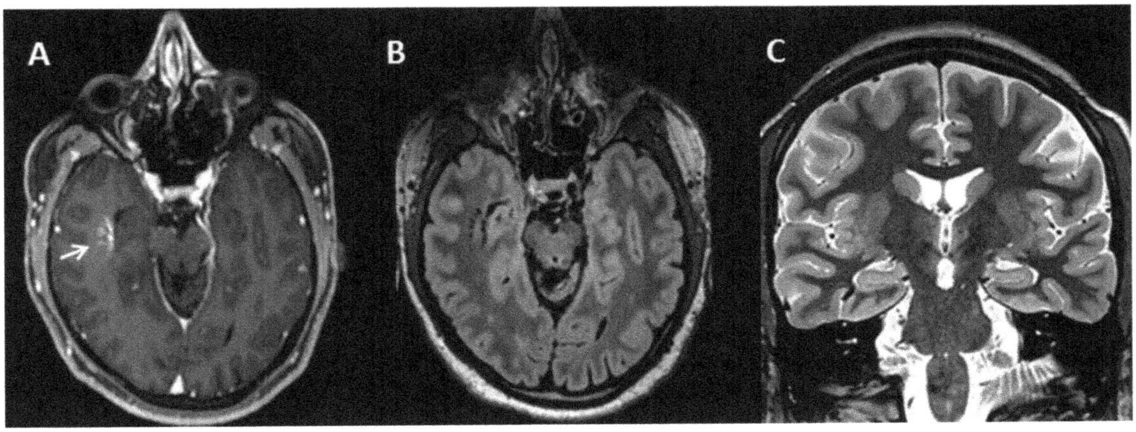

FIGURE 1 | Cerebral magnetic resonance imaging (cMRI) showing an isolated uncomplicated developmental venous anomaly in the right temporal lobe (white arrow) on the contrast enhanced initial axial MPRAGE **(A)** and on the 2 year follow-up epilepsy specific high-resolution T2-weighted axial reformatted 3D-FLAIR **(B)** and coronal T2-weighted STIR **(C)** images. cMRI scans were acquired on a Siemens 3T scanner TRIO **(A)** and PRISMA **(B,C)**.

many antiepileptic drugs were not tolerated (valproate due to an increase of pancreatic enzymes, topiramate due to subjectively experienced cognitive deficits, levetiracetam due to daily tiredness, and perampanel due to dizziness and daily tiredness). Of these, topiramate led to a rapid reduction of myoclonic jerks, even at low doses of 25 mg; however, psychiatric symptoms persisted. Under the sole treatment with carbamazepine (up to 900 mg), the myoclonic jerks and paranoid hallucinatory symptoms temporarily improved; however, they did not disappear completely and ongoing. Zonisamide (up to 100 mg) was tolerated but had no relevant positive effects. Oxazepam (different doses) and clobazam (up to 20 mg) led to the reduction of myoclonic jerks. Oxcarbazepine (up to 2,400 mg) was well tolerated, though its effect was unclear. In combination with brivaracetam (200–250 mg), the myoclonic jerks were reduced in frequency and severity.

Over one year, the patient was treated with clozapine (75 mg), brivaracetam (200–250 mg), and oxcarbazepine (2,400 mg). Clozapine led to a reduction in delusions, hallucinations, and thought inspirations, though these psychotic symptoms did not disappear completely. Higher doses were not tolerated due to an increased frequency of myoclonic jerks. A hypochondriac personality type, together with delusions and dysmorphophobic tendencies, persisted as well as mood fluctuations and concentration deficits. Furthermore, the patient still had about 10 writing-induced myoclonic jerks per day.

DISCUSSION

We presented the case of a patient with paranoid-hallucinatory syndrome in the context of juvenile myoclonic epilepsy.

Previous Findings

In a retrospective study analyzing 100 patients with Janz syndrome, nearly 50% suffered from Axis I psychiatric disorders. Anxiety (23%) and mood disorders (19%) were most frequent, while 7% suffered from somatoform disorders and three cases (3%) were reported to have schizophrenia. The temporal association between the occurrence of myoclonic jerks and schizophrenia was not reported. Seventeen cases fulfilled the "Structured Clinical Interview for DSM Disorders" (SCID) II criteria for cluster B personalities (histrionic, borderline, and passive-aggressive) (17). In an older study of 170 patients, only 26.5% suffered from a comorbid psychiatric disorder. Psychotic disorders were found in 2.9%; however, only one case (0.6%) fulfilled criteria for paranoid-hallucinatory schizophrenia. Depressive disorders (1.8%) and anxiety disorders (3.5%) were less frequent in this study. Personality disorders were found in 14.1% of cases, mainly with BPD (18). In the study from Somayajula et al., analyzing 165 patients with juvenile myoclonic epilepsy in India, 47% were diagnosed with psychiatric disorders, which were mostly anxiety disorders (30.4%) and depression (15.7%). Only one patient (0.6%) suffered from schizophrenia (19). In summary, schizophrenia seems to be infrequent in Janz syndrome. The individual cases of patients with Janz syndrome and schizophrenia, reported in the larger studies mentioned above, are not presented in detail. No case reports are available analyzing this important association. Therefore, in our opinion, case studies like the present one are necessary.

Diagnostic Process

After the initial normal routine and sleep-deprivation EEG, one could have speculated that the myoclonic jerks were merely psychogenic especially because the patient described them as "electric shocks" in his body. However, patients with Janz syndrome often describe the seizures as comparable with "electric shocks." Therefore, this syndrome often has a meaningful delay in the diagnosis because myoclonic jerks are not recognized. Usually patients seek for a medical consultation only after the first generalized-tonic clonic seizure. Therefore, directly asking the patients about myoclonic seizures is a key procedure for diagnosis. Normal interictal EEGs are possible in patients with

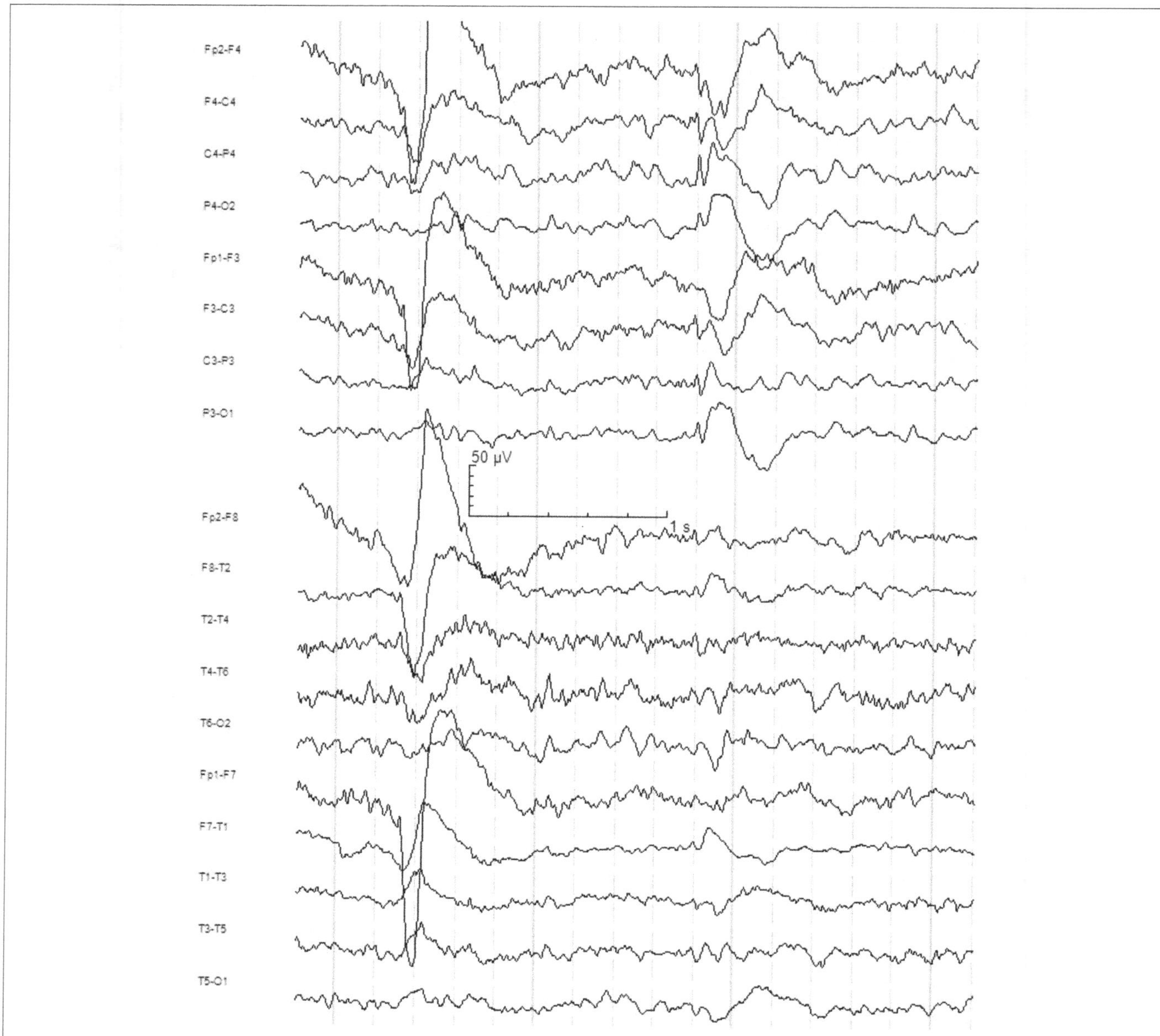

FIGURE 2 | Ictal EEG recording during long-term video-EEG monitoring: Generalized spike-wave complex with fronto-central maximum associated with a habitual myoclonic jerk of the right hand during writing. Longitudinal bipolar montage, 50 Hz notch filter, low-pass filter 30 Hz, high-pass filter 1 Hz.

Janz syndrome. Therefore, a detailed anamnesis and extended EEG analyses including video-telemetry may help in correct diagnostic identification, as we did in our patient.

Pathophysiological Interpretation

Schizophreniform syndromes and epilepsy may share common genetic susceptibility (20, 21). The LANI hypothesis could explain a potential causal relationship between epileptiform EEG activity, myoclonic jerks, and schizophreniform syndromes. The genetically determined and pathologically enhanced excitatory network activity seen in the surface EEG in the form of generalized epileptiform potentials presenting clinically with (praxis-induced) myoclonic seizures and a bilateral tonic-clonic seizure might lead to consecutive inhibitory processes in a homoeostatic, electrophysiological attempt to stabilize cerebral networks. In our patient, we found recurrent excitatory activity (primarily epileptiform activity, but also interictal intermittent generalized theta slowing) that could have exceeded a critical threshold, leading to successive hyperinhibition of cerebral networks. Following this theory, schizophreniform symptoms would not be due to primary excitatory activity as represented by myoclonic jerks, but to the secondary homoeostatic process of hyperinhibition. Frontal hyperinhibition might have led to attention and concentration deficits, and temporal hyperinhibition might have led to hallucinations or memory deficits (7, 10). The LANI hypothesis allows an explanation of short-term schizophreniform symptoms in the present patient. It needs to be further investigated using animal studies, as well as imaging and electrophysiological measurements. Longer-lasting personality traits and cognitive deficits in patients with Janz syndrome might alternatively be interpreted as a form of an epileptic encephalopathy (22, 23).

Treatment Strategies

Identifying schizophreniform subgroups of patients with such (para-)epileptic pathomechanisms may allow new treatment options with antiepileptics for these individuals. For patients with Janz syndrome, treatment alternatives include valproate, lamotrigine, levetiracetam, topiramate, or zonisamide (24). All these substances were tried in our patient except for lamotrigine, which can sometimes worsen myoclonic jerks (24) and which needs a long period for dosage increase. Carbamazepine and oxcarbazepine are also known to aggravate myoclonic jerks (24); however, this was not the case in our patient who showed temporary improvement especially under treatment with carbamazepine. Interestingly, the antiepileptics valproate and lamotrigine are already approved for augmentative therapy in schizophrenia (25–27). It can be assumed that patients with (para)epileptic pathomechanisms and comorbidity may benefit more from such anticonvulsive augmentation strategies than other subgroups (e.g., polygenetic subtypes). Moreover, it is important to recognize that different neuroleptics and biperiden can reduce the seizure threshold (7) and, therefore, may push this pathophysiology and worsen myoclonic jerks in patients with a relevant predisposition (especially because the first myoclonic jerks occurred at first after treatment with psychotropic drugs in our case report patient).

This reaction was the reason for the intolerance of neuroleptic monotherapy in the history of our patient. Moreover, following the general assumptions of the LANI model, the improvement that followed a low dose of clozapine treatment can be explained by its proconvulsive properties, which might have overcome hyperinhibitory network states, although it is likely to improve the causative excitatory activity.

CONCLUSION

This case report shows the importance of the clinical history in patients with myoclonic jerks, which should be taken from the patients and at least one person who witnessed the seizures. Moreover, it shows that EEG diagnostic is very useful in psychiatric patients. In unclear cases with clinical suspicion of mild Janz syndrome with predominant psychiatric manifestations, a sleep-deprivation EEG and long-term video-EEG monitoring may help with the diagnosis of Janz syndrome in the case of normal routine EEG. Identifying subgroups of schizophreniform patients with (para)epileptic pathomechanisms is important because these patients might improve under antiepileptic treatment and might deteriorate under isolated neuroleptic medication.

AUTHOR CONTRIBUTIONS

DE, D-MA and LTvE treated the patient. DE wrote the Paper. All authors were crucial involved in the theoretical discussion and the preparation of the manuscript. All authors read and approved the final version of the manuscript.

FUNDING

The article processing charge was funded by the German Research Foundation (DFG) and the University of Freiburg in the funding program Open Access Publishing.

REFERENCES

1. Owen M, Sawa A, Mortensen P. Schizophrenia. *Lancet* (2016) **388**:86–97. doi: 10.1016/S0140-6736(15)01121-6
2. Lishman A. *Lishman's - Organic Psychiatry - A Textbook of Neuropsychiatry, 4th Edn*. Chichester: Wiley-Blackwell (2009).
3. Tebartz van Elst L. *Vom Anfang und Ende der Schizophrenie: Eine neuropsychiatrische Perspektive auf das Schizophrenie-Konzept*. Stuttgart: Kohlhammer (2017).
4. Trimble M. The relationship between epilepsy and schizophrenia: a biochemical hypothesis. *Biol Psychiatry* (1977) **12**:299–304.
5. Hughes JR. A review of the usefulness of the standard EEG in psychiatry. *Clin Electroencephalogr* (1996) **27**:35–9. doi: 10.1177/155005949602700106
6. Shelley BP, Trimble MR, Boutros NN. Electroencephalographic cerebral dysrhythmic abnormalities in the trinity of nonepileptic general population, neuropsychiatric, and neurobehavioral disorders. *J Neuropsychiatry Clin Neurosci* (2008) **20**:7–22. doi: 10.1176/jnp.2008.20.1.7
7. Tebartz van Elst L, Perlov E. *Epilepsie und Psyche: Psychische Störungen bei Epilepsie - epileptische Phänomene in der Psychiatrie*, 1st ed. Stuttgart: Kohlhammer (2013).
8. Endres D, Perlov E, Feige B, Fleck M, Bartels S, Altenmüller D, et al. Electroencephalographic findings in schizophreniform and affective disorders. *Int J Psychiatry Clin Pract.* (2016) **20**:157–64. doi: 10.1080/13651501.2016.1181184
9. van Elst LT, Schulze-Bonhage A, Altenmüller D, Ebert D. Generalised spike-and-slow-wave complexes without seizures in schizophrenia. *Br J Psychiatry* (2011) **199**:253–4. doi: 10.1192/bjp.199.3.253a
10. Tebartz van Elst L, Krishnamoorthy ES, Schulze-Bonhage A, Altenmüller DM, Richter H, Ebert D, et al. (2011). Local area network inhibition: a model of a potentially important paraepileptic pathomechanism in neuropsychiatric disorders. *Epilepsy Behav.* **22**:231–9. doi: 10.1016/j.yebeh.2011.06.016
11. Endres D, Perlov E, Feige B, Altenmüller D, Venhoff N, Tebartz van Elst L. Schizophrenia associated with epileptiform discharges without seizures successfully treated with levetiracetam. *Front Psychiatry* (2017) **8**:12. doi: 10.3389/fpsyt.2017.00012
12. Trimble MR. Interictal psychoses of epilepsy. *Adv Neurol.* (1991) **55**:143–52.
13. Slater E, Berad AW, Glithero E. The schizophrenialike psychoses of epilepsy. *Br J Psychiatry.* (1963) **109**:95–150. doi: 10.1192/bjp.109.458.95
14. Gibbs FA. Ictal and non-ictal psychiatric disorders in temporal lobe epilepsy. *J Nerv Ment Dis.* (1951) **113**:522–8.
15. Camfield CS, Striano P, Camfield PR. Epidemiology of juvenile

myoclonic epilepsy. *Epilepsy Behav.* (2013) **28**(Suppl. 1):S15–7. doi: 10.1016/j.yebeh.2012.06.024

16. Wolf P, Yacubian E, Avanzini G, Sander T, Schmitz B, Wandschneider B, et al. Juvenile myoclonic epilepsy: a system disorder of the brain. *Epilepsy Res.* (2015) **114**:2–12. doi: 10.1016/j.eplepsyres.2015.04.008
17. de Araújo Filho G, Pascalicchio T, Sousa Pda S, Lin K, Ferreira Guilhoto L, Yacubian E. Psychiatric disorders in juvenile myoclonic epilepsy: a controlled study of 100 patients. *Epilepsy Behav.* (2007) **10**:437–41. doi: 10.1016/j.yebeh.2007.01.016
18. Gélisse P, Genton P, Samuelian J, Thomas P, Bureau M. Psychiatric disorders in juvenile myoclonic epilepsy. *Epilepsia* (2007) **48**:1032–3. doi: 10.1111/j.1528-1167.2007.01009_4.x
19. Somayajula S, Vooturi S, Jayalakshmi S. Psychiatric disorders among 165 patients with juvenile myoclonic epilepsy in India and association with clinical and sociodemographic variables. *Epilepsy Behav.* (2015) **8**:37–42. doi: 10.1016/j.yebeh.2015.09.024
20. Vonberg FW, Bigdeli TB. Genetic Correlation Between Schizophrenia and Epilepsy. *JAMA Neurol.* (2016) **73**:125–6. doi: 10.1001/jamaneurol.2015.3480
21. Fujisao EK, Cristaldo NR, da Silva Braga AM, Cunha PR, Yamashita S, Betting LE. Hippocampal Damage and Atrophy Secondary to Status Epilepticus in a Patient with Schizophrenia. *Front Neurol.* (2017) **8**:24. doi: 10.3389/fneur.2017.00024
22. Holmes G, Lenck-Santini PP. Role of interictal epileptiform abnormalities in cognitive impairment. *Epilepsy Behav.* (2006) **8**:504–15. doi: 10.1016/j.yebeh.2005.11.014
23. Ghacibeh G, Fields C. Interictal epileptiform activity and autism. *Epilepsy Behav.* (2015) **47**:158–62 doi: 10.1016/j.yebeh.2015.02.025
24. Crespel A, Gelisse P, Reed R, Ferlazzo E, Jerney J, Schmitz B, et al. Management of juvenile myoclonic epilepsy. *Epilepsy Behav.* (2013) **28**:S81–6. doi: 10.1016/j.yebeh.2013.01.001
25. Basan A, Kissling W, Leucht S. Valproate as an adjunct to antipsychotics for schizophrenia: a systematic review of randomized trials. *Schizophr Res.* (2004) **70**:33–7. doi: 10.1016/j.schres.2004.01.016
26. Tiihonen J, Wahlbeck K, Kiviniemi V. The efficacy of lamotrigine in clozapine-resistant schizophrenia: a systematic review and meta-analysis. *Schizophr Res.* (2009) **109**:10–14. doi: 10.1016/j.schres.2009.01.002
27. Dold M, Leucht S. Pharmacotherapy of treatment-resistant schizophrenia: a clinical perspective. *Evid Based Ment Health.* (2014) **17**:33–7. doi: 10.1136/eb-2014-101813

12

Can an Integrated Science Approach to Precision Medicine Research Improve Lithium Treatment in Bipolar Disorders?

Jan Scott[1,2,3*], *Bruno Etain*[2,3,4,5,6,7] *and Frank Bellivier*[3,4,5,6,7]

[1] Institute of Neuroscience, Newcastle University, Newcastle upon Tyne, United Kingdom, [2] Centre for Affective Disorders, Institute of Psychiatry, Psychology and Neuroscience, King's College London, London, United Kingdom, [3] Faculté de Médecine, Université Paris Diderot, Paris, France, [4] AP-HP, Groupe Hospitalier Saint-Louis-Lariboisière-Fernand Widal, Paris, France, [5] INSERM, Unité UMR-S 1144, Variabilité de Réponse aux Psychotropes, Université Paris Descartes-Paris Diderot, Paris, France, [6] AP-HP, Groupe Henri Mondor-Albert Chenevier, Pôle de Psychiatrie, Créteil, France, [7] INSERM, Unité 955, IMRB, Equipe de Psychiatrie Translationnelle, Créteil, France

***Correspondence:**
Jan Scott
jan.scott@newcastle.ac.uk

Clinical practice guidelines identify lithium as a first line treatment for mood stabilization and reduction of suicidality in bipolar disorders (BD); however, most individuals show sub-optimal response. Identifying biomarkers for lithium response could enable personalization of treatment and refine criteria for stratification of BD cases into treatment-relevant subgroups. Existing systematic reviews identify potential biomarkers of lithium response, but none directly address the conceptual issues that need to be addressed to enhance translation of research into precision prescribing of lithium. For example, although clinical syndrome subtyping of BD has not led to customized individual treatments, we emphasize the importance of assessing clinical response phenotypes in biomarker research. Also, we highlight the need to give greater consideration to the quality of prospective longitudinal monitoring of illness activity and the differentiation of non-response from partial or non-adherence with medication. It is unlikely that there is a single biomarker for lithium response or tolerability, so this review argues that more research should be directed toward the exploration of biosignatures. Importantly, we emphasize that an integrative science approach may improve the likelihood of discovering the optimal combination of clinical factors and multimodal biomarkers (e.g., blood omics, neuroimaging, and actigraphy derived-markers). This strategy could uncover a valid lithium response phenotype and facilitate development of a composite prediction algorithm. Lastly, this narrative review discusses how these strategies could improve eligibility criteria for lithium treatment in BD, and highlights barriers to translation to clinical practice including the often-overlooked issue of the cost-effectiveness of introducing biomarker tests in psychiatry.

Keywords: bipolar disorders, lithium, mood stabilizers, prediction, response, phenotype, biomarkers, personalized

INTRODUCTION

Although Hippocrates (fourth century BC) is often described as the "Father of Modern Medicine," the reality is that the science of disease prevention and treatment is a relatively recent phenomenon. Until the twentieth century, careful observation and clinical judgement underpinned most medical practice. In the twenty first century, clinical practice guidelines (CPGs) began to appear with increasing frequency. These CPGs were based on the principles of evidence-based medicine (EBM) and emphasized that treatment recommendations for physical and mental disorders should be founded on systematic assessment of the strength of evidence available (which was graded hierarchically e.g., meta-analyses were ranked above individual studies, etc) (1, 2). Whilst CPGs were an improvement on subjective opinions, treatments were invariably recommended based on the "average response" amongst individuals recruited to randomized controlled trials (RCTs) and it became increasingly clear that this "one size fits all" approach did not meet the needs of some of the most disabled patients (1, 2). Recently, attention has shifted toward the potential utility of personalized or precision medicine in clinical practice (3, 4). There are subtle differences in the meaning of these terms (see **Table 1**), but both personalized and precision medicine share the same goal, namely to tailor diagnostic and treatment decisions to each patient by utilizing information about individual phenotypes and genotypes (3, 4).

Precision medicine has yielded important breakthroughs in several branches of medicine, such as the development of drugs that target cells containing large amounts of HER2 (human epidermal growth factor receptor 2) in breast cancer (5). However, there are many clinical, methodological, and regulatory challenges to the translation of data about individualized profiles and diagnostics into personalized interventions (4, 5). Recognition of these challenges and concerns about delays in the introduction of more effective, tailored interventions for patients led the European Union (EU) to propose a new funding stream for the development of personalized approaches to complex diseases with high prevalence and high economic impact (6, 7). Most major mental disorders match this description, and there is an acknowledged need to provide reliable assistance to clinicians to help them to customize treatment decisions in psychiatry (7, 8). For example, psychiatrists, patients, their families and significant others would welcome a more nuanced approach to the use of mood stabilizers in individuals with bipolar disorders (BD), especially greater precision in prescribing of long-term treatment with lithium in bipolar-I-disorder (BD-I).

There are several systematic reviews of potential biomarkers of response to lithium and emerging ideas on research strategies that may aid identification of biomarkers or treatment selection. However, we did not identify any reviews that specifically focused on the broader conceptual and strategic issues (e.g., how to integrate high quality biomarker research with more reliable and valid clinical observations; whether to search for single biomarkers or multi-modal sets of markers). In essence, this paper does not review new findings, but rather reconsiders the state of the art and what can be learnt and applied to future research in the field of biomarker research. Given this apparent gap in the literature, we undertook a narrative review to consider these broader, but potentially critical issues and how they may inform efforts to translate research findings in precision prescribing.

TABLE 1 | Definitions of key concepts.

Concept	Definitions and Observations
Evidence-Based Medicine (EBM)	EBM is an approach to medical practice intended to optimize decision-making by integrating the best research evidence with clinical expertise and patient values (1, 2). Sackett et al. (1) state that evidence is viewed epistemologically e.g., only strong evidence (from meta-analyses, systematic reviews, and randomized controled trials) can yield strong recommendations. However, Perna et al. (7) note that EBM emphasizes the use of scientific evidence regarding the most effective intervention for the "average" patient with a specific diagnosis, leading to criticism of the utility of EBM in day-to-day practice (2).
Personalized Medicine	Personalized Medicine proposes to establish clinical decisions based upon a patient's individual profile, tailoring the treatment to their characteristics and needs (4, 7). It is argued that the term "personalized" should be replaced by "precision" as the former term may also be used e.g., in psychotherapy to describe the formulation of an individual's problems or as a generic term referring to clinical management (i.e., it does not specify the links to pathophysiological mechanisms).
Precision Medicine	The Precision Medicine Initiative defined precision medicine as "an emerging approach for disease treatment and prevention that considers individual variability in genes, environment, and lifestyle for each person" (4).
Stratified Medicine	Stratified medicine focuses on the identification of biomarkers or psychological tests to stratify patients in smaller treatment relevant subgroups. Wium-Andersen et al. (3) note that, unlike precision medicine, stratification does not require complete understanding of the etiology of the underlying illness and that it may coexist alongside conventional diagnostic systems, where patients are first diagnosed and later stratified into putative treatment subgroups.

This review begins by briefly highlighting the arguments for, but difficulties in, applying precision medicine first to the diagnosis of BD subtypes and second to the prescribing of mood stabilizers. Next, we consider core components and underlying principles that could inform viable research into precision psychiatry, using the example of the prescription of lithium in BD-I. Several publications have highlighted details of and evidence for putative biomarkers [e.g., (9–12)], so rather than replicate those reviews, we primarily focus on broader, strategic issues regarding the application of precision medicine research to psychiatry. We describe these in terms of "bottom-up" approaches (namely, the under-rated role of systematic assessment of baseline characteristics, clinical phenotypes and longitudinal monitoring of illness activity and treatment response, etc.) and the importance of combining these with "top-down" approaches (highlighting some of the guiding principles for examining biomarkers). We conclude by identifying some of the key considerations in implementing "precision" that may be relevant to BD research, to psychiatry and potentially to general medicine as well.

MATERIALS AND METHODS

Literature searches were undertaken to identify publications (reviews, discussion papers, individual studies, policy documents, conference proceedings, etc.) addressing the topics of BD (diagnosis, prediction of treatment response, and outcome), mood stabilizers (prescribing, efficacy, and prediction of response to lithium), and precision, personalized, or stratified medicine (as defined in **Table 1**). Relevant information was extracted, and key concepts were synthesized under the headings reported in this narrative review. However, we explicitly focused on broader conceptual and methodological issues and aimed to avoid reporting information or evidence that had been reviewed in other publications. Additionally, the authors incorporated some of the insights gained from the development of a multicentre grant application entitled R-LiNK (Response to Lithium Network); that has received EU funding (http://www.r-link.eu.com). Lastly, the extant literature was examined to identify some key lessons that have been learnt or may need to be learned to enable precision in psychiatry and in the treatment of BD.

RESULTS

We begin by commenting on the diagnosis of BD and the more narrowly defined subtype of BD-I, then consider definitions of and prescribing of mood stabilizers, before focusing on precision medicine approaches to the prediction of response to lithium in BD-I.

Bipolar Disorders

The term BD refers to a group of disorders that are primarily characterized by changes in mood, activity and energy (13). The two main subtypes are BD-I (characterized by at least one episode of mania) and BD-II (characterized by at least one episode of major depression and of hypomania), but other variants, referred to as the BD spectrum, are recognized. The morbidity associated with BD can partly be explained by the early peak age of onset (of 15–25 years), the prevalence (1–4% of the global population depending on range of BD spectrum included) and the high rates of physical and mental comorbidities; also, BD is a leading cause of suicide (14, 15). Overall, BD is ranked 6th in the global burden of diseases in working age adults (14) and 4th amongst youth aged less than 25 years (15).

As well as the clinical and social impairments experienced by individuals with BD and the stress and distress experienced by their families and significant others, a recent study from the USA estimated the total economic cost of BD-I was greater than $200 billion (16). The largest contributors to excess costs were caregiving, direct health care and unemployment; findings that highlight the importance of early diagnosis and the need to optimize therapeutic strategies.

Early diagnosis of BD is hampered by the lack of objective laboratory tests in psychiatry. As such, accurate diagnosis of any mental disorder is dependent on careful observation of presenting signs and symptoms, skillful history-taking, and clinical expertise. Unfortunately, even when international criteria are employed, the reliability of diagnoses varies significantly (17). Diagnostic precision is diminished because the symptoms and signs of one mental disorder may overlap considerably with several other diagnostic categories (18). In BD, this problem is compounded by the fact that symptoms vary greatly between the different syndromes included within the BD spectrum. Although there are shared clinical features across the BD spectrum, current research indicates that these disorders probably represent heterogeneous syndromes resulting from multiple etiological processes, rather than comprising a specific disease category (19, 20).

Given the lack of diagnostic reliability and limited biological validity of the broad category of BD and its spectrum, further important research continues as in the long-term precision approaches in psychiatry will aim to commence with precision diagnostics. However, the majority of current studies of the application of precision medicine in BD should be limited to a more narrowly defined subgroup. The obvious subtype to target is BD-I as this is one of the three most reliable diagnoses in psychiatry (17) and objective measurements are available of current mental state, such as activation and sleep-wake cycle (21). However, it must be emphasized that this relatively more clinically homogeneous BD-I diagnostic subtype lacks a disease signature and current animal models demonstrate low predictive power (5); so personalized diagnostics are not viable and will remain an aspiration for the foreseeable future for BD. As such, we suggest that efforts might best be directed toward the identification of "treatment-relevant" subgroups (also referred to as stratified medicine; see **Table 1**) for prescribing recommended medications for BD-I, such as mood stabilizers.

Mood Stabilizers

It is generally accepted that the term mood stabilizer refers to a category of medication that shows at least two of the three following properties: anti-manic, antidepressant and prophylactic, without increasing the risk of episodes of the opposite polarity (22). International CPGs repeatedly identify lithium as a "gold standard" mood stabilizer treatment, with robust evidence for its efficacy in preventing BD relapses and rehospitalizations and reducing suicidality (23–25). Lithium is also prescribed as an acute treatment for mania and as an adjunct to traditional antidepressants in acute major depressive episodes. Another potential advantage is that a 1-month supply of lithium only costs about one dollar compared with $15 per month for olanzapine and $60 per month for valproic acid (26).

Despite being regarded as a first line, cost-effective treatment, there is a significant gap between the research efficacy and clinical effectiveness of lithium. Only about 30% of lithium-treated patients show an excellent long-term response and the short-term benefits of acute lithium treatment do not reliably predict the outcome of prophylaxis. Overall, it can take 18–24 months to determine that there has been a significant reduction in the frequency or severity of BD episodes or a clinically meaningful decrease in illness activity. The extended time frame for ascertaining a true positive "good response," the prevalence of sub-optimal outcomes and the narrow therapeutic window for lithium, plus its perception as less safe than newer compounds, have all probably contributed to the reported decline in lithium use (26–28).

Robust biological predictors of continuation and maintenance treatment response (or of tolerability) remain elusive (26). Further, the clinical predictors identified by psychiatrists (e.g., family history of lithium response, BD subtype, etc.) are not consistently supported by the empirical literature (26, 29–31) and cannot be employed as reliable eligibility criteria for lithium prescribing. Critics of EBM and CPGs argue that they do not assist in the identification of moderators and mediators of lithium response or of non-response because they focus on highly selected samples of patients recruited to RCTs. Overall, findings from these current approaches lack external validity or generalizability to real world clinical settings (32).

Presently, many clinicians and patients are dependent on a "trial and error" approach to prescribing lithium and determining its effectiveness. This strategy is problematic as the prolonged trial combined with concerns about side-effects may increase the risk of lithium non-adherence, which compounds the likelihood of treatment failure (33, 34). Understandably, there is an increased impetus toward research that enables targeting of lithium treatment toward subgroups of patients who are most likely to benefit. Given the complexity of BD-I and the limited understanding of the mechanisms of action of lithium (28), the search for these "responder/non-responder" subgroups or phenotypes needs to combine the systematic exploration of socio-demographics, clinical characteristics, and course of illness, with genetics, omics, neuro-imaging, and other biomarker tests, etc. This might allow clinicians and patients to predict the likelihood of response (or of non-response or intolerance) to lithium prior to the initiation of mood stabilizer treatment or within the first few months of its commencement.

An Integrated Science Approach to Response Prediction

As precision psychiatry research is in its infancy, we describe some of the options for studying precision or stratified medicine approaches to the prediction of response to lithium in BD-I. We suggest that it is more realistic for research programs to integrate clinical assessment and monitoring (so-called "bottom up") approaches with applied biological research and analytic approaches (so-called "top down") (35, 36). Each strategy is insufficient for identifying putative predictors of response alone, but their joint application may lead to progress. We briefly highlight some key considerations, beginning with clinical strategies.

Bottom-Up Approaches

Three relevant clinical considerations are (i) sample selection; (ii) assessment of past history and current diagnosis, and prospective longitudinal monitoring of symptoms and illness dimensions (including patient related outcomes); (iii) assessment of lithium response and strategies for minimizing confounding of treatment non-response with non-adherence.

Sampling

A recognized problem of studies of predictors and biomarkers for treatment response is that they are largely based on secondary analyses of data from samples included in efficacy RCTs (37). This, plus other limitations in the recruitment process (such as convenience sampling and small sample sizes) has produced a number of biases in reported findings (38). Whilst data from efficacy studies will show a better signal-to-noise ratio, there is an argument that predictors of treatment response in psychiatry might best be identified from prospective cohort studies of large clinically representative samples that are purposefully designed. This approach is being used in R-LiNK which is a project that is being undertaken in 15 clinical centers across eight EU countries that aims to study individuals with BD-I who clinicians have identified as candidates for a trial of lithium (according to the recommendations in the CPG employed at those centers). Whilst the pragmatic design has some drawbacks, the prospective assessment of treatment response in about 300 patients over 2 years will offer important insights into the real-world effectiveness of lithium, which increases the translational potential of any findings regarding early predictors of response.

Clinical assessments

Although clinical syndrome subtypes are insufficient for personalizing psychiatric treatment (3), they are still relevant for developing a detailed clinical picture of each persons' experience of the disorder being studied. This includes structured clinical interviews that allow longitudinal assessment of lifetime and current diagnoses as well as allowing researchers to reconstruct the illness trajectory, prior history, etc. In BD-I, this includes determination of precursors and patterns of illness episodes (e.g., antecedents and symptom profiles of familial and non-familial BD), polarity of BD onset, predominant polarity, history of psychotic symptoms, frequency, and severity of episodes, inter-episode symptoms, and functioning, etc.

The choice of diagnostic instrument is not usually contentious (e.g., existing structured clinical interviews offer a detailed assessment of BD as well as other psychiatric comorbidities), and these interview schedules can be combined with tools that screen for medical comorbidities, etc. However, a weakness of previous studies of psychotropic response biomarkers is that they have paid insufficient attention to the rating scales used to assess symptoms and how these change during treatment. Any change in illness activity post-initiation of lithium needs to be captured by measures that enable observers to determine the evolution of symptoms and syndromes and ensure a detailed picture of BD-I before and after the introduction of lithium can be constructed. This is important as precision psychiatry research should aim to be compatible with other approaches to identifying treatment response phenotypes, such as the R-DOC framework (39) which highlights the importance of examining trans-diagnostic illness dimensions that are grounded in neuroscience e.g., cognitive, arousal, and regulatory systems, etc.

Regarding BD-I studies, the rating scales selected for monitoring disease progression during exposure to lithium treatment need to clearly reflect the core dimensions of the current diagnostic criteria (mood, activity, energy) and give adequate weighting to the symptoms that are especially likely to change during lithium treatment, as these may represent clinical markers of response. It should be borne in mind that most mania and depression rating scales were developed about 30–40 years ago and demonstrate considerable heterogeneity in the range of symptoms assessed and in the underlying assumptions about the nature of BD episodes (21, 38). For example, the Young Mania Rating Scale (YMRS) was introduced at a time when elation or irritability were the criterion A symptoms for BD (not mood and activation as described currently) (13) and, unsurprisingly, YMRS ratings correlate poorly with objective measures of activation (21, 40–42). Likewise, the 6-item version of the Hamilton Rating Scale for Depression (HRSD-6) and the 15-item version of Inventory of Depressive Symptoms give equal weighting to each core dimension of depression and have better psychometric, IRT (item response theory) and clinimetric profiles than other scales used to assess depression in BD (40, 43, 44). These may seem like lower order issues, but they take on greater significance when considered in the context of the fact that change in activation or sleep-wake cycle may occur early in lithium responders or may be early warning signs of relapse when lithium is withdrawn (42). Thus, selection of rating scales to monitor illness activity longitudinally is a critical but often overlooked element of biomarker research.

Whilst repeated observer assessments of course of illness and treatment response are important, consideration should be given to how these measures can be supplemented by subjective ratings and patient related outcomes (PRO). Techniques such as PRO can ensure that additional measures of functioning or outcomes that are important to individual patients (such as "personal recovery") are also included (45). Whilst this may extend the range of response categories that are considered for analysis, it improves the likelihood that a study will be valued by patients as well as clinicians and researchers. Symptoms or items that are identified for subjective rating can be included in ecological momentary assessments (EMA) when feasible, to allow more detailed analysis of response patterns and variability in treatment outcomes (21, 46). In BD-I, these measures may be combined with objective real-time monitoring of sleep-wake cycle and activity patterns using actigraphy (21).

Lastly, clinical assessments may extend beyond symptom ratings to include other measurements such as neuropsychological profiles. The latter has been linked to biological measures of response [e.g., structural and functional magnetic resonance imaging (MRI)] and may show direct or indirect (via medication non-adherence) associations with treatment response (47).

Treatment response and adherence

A critical element of any study of treatment response is to carefully operationalize definitions of this concept. As lithium is a prophylactic treatment, then reduction in BD relapses during a demarcated follow-up period is typically the most important parameter. However, some studies categorize lithium response based only on retrospective assessment, and even prospective studies may fail to employ (or describe) any consensus definitions of lithium response.

As a first step, researchers need to decide if response is synonymous with e.g., absence of any illness episodes meeting syndromal criteria over a given timeframe; achieving symptom remission for a specified period; time to remission (or to relapse) after commencing lithium; time to "treatment failure" (e.g., stopping lithium; introduction of another mood stabilizer; etc.). Further, each of these conceptualizations of response may need to be considered in the context of vulnerability to adverse effects or side effects. Thus, researchers need to provide a detailed description of the criteria employed to define response so that others can consider the reliability and validity of the definitions (against which the biomarkers are bench-marked), the applicability to their own clinical or research setting and to ensure that findings from other studies can be compared and contrasted accordingly.

Another overlooked element of the definition of treatment non-response is that it is not always sufficiently differentiated from non-adherence. Whilst these concepts overlap, it is worth noting that if a patient is non-adherent with lithium but appears to have a good outcome during prospective monitoring, then any identified predictors may be markers of illness trajectory (i.e., the predictor variables may be identifying individuals with a good prognosis independent of the treatment being assessed). Further, existing evidence, e.g., from genetics studies, suggests that the way in which these two variables (response and adherence) are considered may influence reported findings and which markers may be regarded as significant (48, 49). Interestingly, the TRIPP (treatment response and resistance in the psychosis) working group advocate obtaining measures of medication adherence and employing minimum adherence criteria before classifying patients as non-responders (50). In R-LiNK, measures of plasma levels of lithium and observer and self-reported assessments of medication adherence will be employed. These will be used alongside regular measurement of health beliefs that have previously been shown to identify individuals at high risk of becoming partially or non-adherent in the near future (51). In this way, it is possible to minimize confounding of non-response and non-adherence (50) and to consider the introduction of simple evidence-based clinical strategies to optimize medication adherence (52).

Top Down Approaches

There has been a rapid expansion in research into precision psychiatry, especially regarding biomarkers (measurable characteristics that reflect biologic function or dysfunction, response to a therapeutic measure, or indication of the natural progression of disease) (12). A scoping exercise of biological predictors of lithium response indicates that researchers usually explore one or more of three types of biomarkers (53):

- functional markers, which can be measured e.g., by neurocognitive tests or neuro-imaging of neural networks;
- structural markers that assess the topography of brain architecture;
- metabolic/molecular markers, such as omics and including microRNAs that reflect glial and neuronal dysfunction.

To date, many lithium biomarker studies are domain specific (e.g., focused only on neuroimaging or omics, etc.). Although this research contributes to the overall understanding of the state of the art, there are potential problems in interpretability of multiple individual studies (38). We concur with Trivedi et al. (54), who suggest that it is unlikely that there is a single biomarker for psychotropic response or non-response that is based only on a single dimension or modality (e.g., genetics, omics, neuroimaging, neuropsychology, or clinical presentation). As such, the rest of this section focuses on three important considerations for research on precision prescribing: multidimensional phenotyping; analytic strategies for response prediction; and cost-effectiveness.

Multidimensional phenotyping

It is suggested that the robust heritability of BD may extend to familial patterns of lithium response and several international consortia are investigating the genetics and pharmacogenomics of BD and its treatment [e.g., (26, 55)]. The R-LiNK study uses several "omic" approaches (transcriptomics, microRNA, methylomics, metabolomics, proteomics, etc.), employing a strategy that is sometimes referred to as "convergent functional omics" (56), to try to detect a molecular signature associated with biological pathways or networks underlying treatment response (57–59). However, even convergent functional omics ought not be undertaken in isolation, as a contemporary approach to integrative biology should ideally extend to a range of systems. This is especially true for a medication such as lithium, which appears to be implicated in a wide range of processes at all levels (58–60). For example, it is hypothesized that lithium inhibition of GSK-3 may result in neuroprotection and attenuation of cognitive deficits (57) as well as modification of circadian clock machinery (28), etc. Findings on neuroplasticity build a bridge to neuro-imaging research which in turn examine neuro-anatomical and biochemical abnormalities associated with a diagnosis of BD and the effects of lithium on brain structure, biochemistry, and connectivity in BD-I [e.g., (61–63)]. Likewise, hypotheses regarding circadian rhythms may be linked to actigraphic examination of sleep-wake cycles [e.g., (64, 65)]. Merging findings within and across these dimensions may lead to the identification of combinations of biomarkers or biosignatures, with greater predictive value than isolated markers (54).

Several research groups have suggested that it is worthwhile to extend the search for phenotypes beyond the established architypes (66). In R-LiNK, this includes strategies such as exploring the heterogeneity in brain lithium distribution and whether this differs in responders and non-responders (67). However, it may extend further to new paradigms such as smartphone apps and wearable technologies, which can be employed to assess digital phenotypes (a term that describes health data collected from individual monitoring, social media use, and measurement of interactions with technology e.g. the combination of self-rated PRO, EMA, and actigraphy) (68, 69). In BD, this has the potential for real-time recording of mood, activation and sleep-wake cycle, and the early detection of any changes in symptoms or health status parameters that are associated with lithium treatment (42, 46).

Whilst multidimensional precision modeling for response to lithium in BD-I is in its infancy, it is noteworthy that this strategy is employed increasingly in psychiatry research. For example, some research on suicidality has examined clinical and biological markers and combined these into an algorithm for predicting suicide attempts (70). With this in mind, **Figure 1** offers a diagrammatic representation of the steps involved in using this approach for precision prescribing of lithium. The figure tries to include core elements of the top-down and bottom-up approaches as shows approximately the point at which each of these elements might be considered.

Analytic strategies for response prediction

A biosignature can be based on a combination of biomarkers and clinical characteristics (71) and their joint contributions to

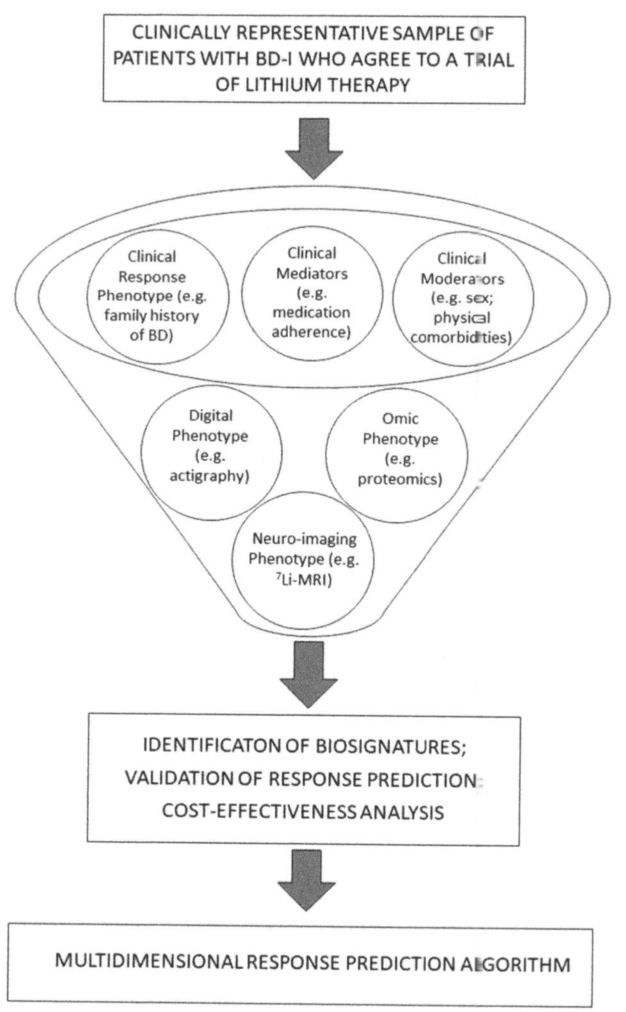

FIGURE 1 | A diagrammatic representation of integrated, bottom-up and top-down approaches and their potential role in the development of precision prescribing pf lithium in BD-I.

the prediction of different dimensions of treatment response. As shown in **Figure 1**, these may be further examined from the perspective of moderators and mediators (72); e.g., moderators of treatment effects may include baseline clinical characteristics (e.g., gender, family history of BD, etc.). Likewise, early markers of lithium response may be derived from tests undertaken in the weeks or early months after treatment is initiated (e.g., brain lithium distribution after 12 weeks of lithium). Potential mediators of lithium effects may include changes in omics or neuroimaging markers that occur over a short timeframe (e.g., changes in variables measured immediately prior to and 12 weeks after commencing lithium) but could also include early changes in sleep-wake cycles as shown by actigraphy recordings or EMA symptom ratings (21, 42, 46).

Statistical analyses in precision psychiatry research are complicated by the fact that many studies rely on "high dimensional data," i.e., many measured variables (repeated measures of multiple putative biomarkers) collected in a relatively restricted clinical sample (of a few hundred participants or sometimes less). Whilst it is feasible to construct a treatment decision algorithm from such data, considerable statistical expertise is required to address the challenges arising regarding data management, harmonization of data on biomarkers derived from different systems and handling missing data within and across domains, as well as avoiding "over-fitting" of statistical models, such as machine learning (73). The latter is increasingly being applied to psychiatry in general and BD in particular to aid diagnostic and treatment selection (74, 75).

Many researchers argue that discovery science strategies may be justifiable approaches to analyzing data in precision psychiatry as these are both hypothesis generating as well as hypothesis-testing [e.g., (56, 76, 77)]. For instance, a comprehensive stepwise statistical approach to outcome prediction (starting with discovery, prioritization and validation, followed by further examination of selected predictors) may lead to the discovery of novel biomarkers as well as replicating findings from previous research and ultimately lead to the development of a prediction tool (70). A similar strategy may be useful for R-LiNK or comparable studies, which attempt to quantify the predictive value of putative biomarkers and to determine which combinations of markers have additive or interactive effects for identifying an individuals' likelihood of treatment response.

In practice, we suggest that contemporary studies may need to combine discovery science approaches for the identification of putative early predictors of lithium response (defined as a categorical outcome) with more targeted analyses focused on the exploration of markers of different measures of response (e.g., time to achieve a response category; continuous measures of response such as number of days ill per annum for 2 years before and after lithium initiation). This strategy allows researchers to consider the level of precision of biomarkers by using predetermined approaches to analyzing any biosignatures associated with different definitions of response. For example, machine learning is now widely employed for pattern recognition, and multivariate logistic regression or mixed models might be used for analyses of categorical measures of response. Other concepts of response, such as the analysis of PRO might focus on temporal changes in quality of life or employ "mirror-image" approaches to change in symptoms or health status over time. More subtle notions of response, such as intra-individual, day-to-day symptom variability (as measured by the digital phenotype) will require different statistical models and, e.g., actigraphy data may be best explored using non-linear dynamics.

Cost-effectiveness

Another, so far ignored issue in precision prescribing in psychiatry, is the need to determine whether the cost of biomarker-driven treatments will be economically as well as clinically justifiable. For example, even if a multidimensional predictor tool or algorithm is developed for predicting response to lithium and shows external validity in replication studies, very expensive testing of large populations may complicate value assessments and, in some instances, may indicate that the use of the tool is unlikely to be cost-effective (78).

To better inform clinical decision-making, precision psychiatry research will need to determine which biomarkers or biosignatures can be transferred most efficaciously from bench to bedside. This translation should be assessed from several perspectives, including the positive and negative predictive values of different sets of biomarkers, additivity, or redundancy in employing multimodal biosignatures, access to and interpretability of tests, as well as patient acceptability or burden associated with testing, etc. This process represents a critical step and needs greater acknowledgment in research planning and reporting of findings in future publications. These translational steps can be considered alongside cost-effectiveness by constructing simulation models that estimate the expected lifetime costs of treatment for BD-I (of which lithium is one element) compared to the predicted outcomes in terms of Quality Adjusted Life Years.

DISCUSSION

Clinical syndrome subtyping has failed to inform personalization of treatments in psychiatry (10, 19, 79). This is partly because even more narrowly defined clinical presentations, such as those included in the BD-I category still represent heterogeneous endpoints of different underlying causal pathways. The latter may include clinical, demographic and environmental factors, and genetic, epigenetic and other biological processes (19, 20); but this diversity also offers a plausible reason to promote personalized approaches rather than avoid exploring them (8, 19).

The search for biomarkers of psychotropic treatment response is in its infancy (80), but there are encouraging emerging findings form individual studies and useful up-to-date syntheses of the data in several existing systematic reviews (8–12, 38). This narrative review seeks to argue that now is an ideal time to consider the development of a robust template for such studies so that the approach can be applied to research on existing treatments and then to much needed new drug developments in the future (81). Although the prediction of lithium response remains ambiguous (26), it is hoped that the identification of a combination of clinical and biological markers may inform the development of a composite prediction algorithm that could guide treatment decisions in BD-I (37, 72). The additional advantage of considering lithium is that we have some information on plasma levels associated with therapeutic response as well as toxicity, which is not the case for most other putative mood stabilizers (82). However, even starting this process involves making further progress on a consensus of how to best monitor illness activity (to assess changes between pre-to-post-lithium initiation periods) and best define response. This step is needed to enhance not only the quality of research (validation of putative predictors) but also to assist in the translation of findings from biomarker research into the clinical application of biosignatures in day-to-day practice.

Precision prescribing of lithium holds the promise of reducing the duration of a treatment trail from about 18–24 months to 3 months or less (as response might be predicted prior to commencing lithium or within the typical timeframe for titration of the dose of lithium). However, widespread dissemination into clinical practice of one or more biomarkers or biosignatures will require synergy between academia and industry and government (83). The incremental cost effectiveness of these strategies is likely to change significantly over time, as the cost of biomarker assays may reduce, but the cost of introducing new medications increases. Thus, markers that increase the prediction of treatment response are likely to become more valuable over time. Furthermore, as noted by Fernandes et al. (18), merging research findings into EBM-driven or "personalized" CPG will require the addition of new sections within the guidelines that specify how any newly developed technologies should be employed and further evaluated in clinical settings.

This review was undertaken in order to more fully appreciate the broader concepts and emerging strategies being employed in biomarker research. This was deemed important because nearly all existing reviews on this topic in BD focused on study findings rather than considering whether the research strategy or methodology was a source of confounding or variance between studies. Overall, this narrative review suggests that the opportunities for research and development of precision prescribing of lithium in BD-I must be balanced by a realistic appraisal of the complexity of analyzing high dimensional data, the robustness of any putative biosignatures identified and the potential barriers that will then arise when moving forward to clinical implementation. Currently, high quality biological research will be undermined, and translational options will be reduced without additional consideration of integrative approaches, including the clinical evaluation, analytic strategy and how biosignature findings can be introduced efficiently into real world settings.

ETHICS STATEMENT

The R-Link study is being carried out in accordance with the Declaration of Helsinki; ethical approval for each of the centres is granted by the relevant ethics committee in that country.

AUTHOR CONTRIBUTIONS

All authors contributed substantially to the preparation of the manuscript. JS and FB undertook the literature review. JS wrote the first draft of the manuscript, BE revised the draft manuscript. FB (the chief investigator for R-LiNK) added relevant insights gained from the development of the R-LiNK project. All authors contributed to writing the submitted draft and approved the final version of the manuscript.

FUNDING

The R-LiNK study of biomarkers of lithium response in bipolar disorders is supported by the EU H2020 initiative (H2020-EU.3.1.1.—Understanding health, wellbeing, and disease): https://cordis.europa.eu/project/rcn/212676_en.html; with Grant No 754907. Further details regarding the study are available at http://www.r-link.eu.com.

REFERENCES

1. Sackett D, Rosenberg W, Gray J, Haynes R, Richardson W. Evidence based medicine: what it is and what it isn't. *BMJ* (1996) 312:71–2.
2. Greenhalgh T, Howick J, Maskrey N, for the Evidence Based Medicine Renaissance Group. Evidence based medicine: a movement in crisis? BMJ (2014) 348:g3725. doi: 10.1136/bmj.g3725
3. Wium-Andersen IK, Vinberg M, Kessing LV, McIntyre RS. Personalized medicine in psychiatry. *Nord J Psychiatry* (2017) 71:12–9. doi: 10.1080/08039488.2016.1216163
4. Collins F, Varmus H. A new initiative on precision medicine. *N Engl J Med.* (2015) 372:793–5. doi: 10.1056/NEJMp1500523
5. Peer D. Precision medicine–delivering the goods? *Cancer Lett.* (2014) 352:2–3. doi: 10.1016/j.canlet.2014.04.011
6. European Commission. *European Perspectives in Personalised Medicine. Conference Report, 12-13 May 2011.* Luxembourg: Publications Office of the European Union (2011). p. 36. Available online at: https://ec.europa.eu/research/health/pdf/personalised-medicine-conference-report_en.pdf
7. Perna G, Grassi M, Caldirola D, Nemeroff CB. The revolution of personalized psychiatry: will technology make it happen sooner? *Psychol Med.* (2018) 48:705–13. doi: 10.1017/S0033291717002859
8. Schumann G, Binder EB, Holte A, de Kloet ER, Oedegaard KJ, Robbins TW, et al. Stratified medicine for mental disorders. *Eur Neuropsychopharmacol.* (2014) 24:5–50. doi: 10.1016/j.euroneuro.2013.09.010
9. Bellivier F, Geoffroy PA, Scott J, Schurhoff F, Leboyer M, Etain B. Biomarkers of bipolar disorder: specific or shared with schizophrenia? *Front Biosci.* (2013) E5:845–63. doi: 10.2741/E665
10. Hasler G, Wolf A. Toward stratified treatments for bipolar disorders. *Eur Neuropsychopharmacol.* (2015) 25:283–94. doi: 10.1016/j.euroneuro.2014.12.006
11. Alda M, Manchia M. Personalized management of bipolar disorder. *Neurosci Lett.* (2018) 669:3–9. doi: 10.1016/j.neulet.2017.12.005
12. Frey BN, Andreazza AC, Houenou J, Jamain S, Goldstein BI, Frye MA, et al. Biomarkers in bipolar disorder: a positional paper from the International Society for Bipolar Disorders Biomarkers Task Force. *Aust N Z J Psychiatry* (2013) 47:321–32. doi: 10.1177/0004867413478217

13. American Psychiatric Association. *Diagnostic and Statistical Manual of Mental Disorders*. 5th Ed. Arlington, VA: American Psychiatric Association (2013). 432p.
14. Whiteford HA, Degenhardt L, Rehm J, Baxter AJ, Ferrari AJ, Erskine HE, et al. Global burden of disease attributable to mental and substance use disorders: findings from the Global Burden of Disease Study 2010. *Lancet* (2013) 382:1575–86. doi: 10.1016/S0140-6736(13)61611-6
15. Gore FM, Bloem PJ, Patton GC, Ferguson J, Joseph V, Coffey C, et al. Global burden of disease in young people aged 10-24 years: a systematic analysis. *Lancet* (2011) 377:2093–102. doi: 10.1016/S0140-6736(11)60512-6
16. Cloutier M, Greene M, Guerin A, Touya M, Wu E. The economic burden of bipolar I disorder in the United States in 2015. *J. Affect. Disord.* (2018) 226:45–51. doi: 10.1016/j.jad.2017.09.011
17. First MB. The importance of developmental field trials in the revision of psychiatric classifications. *Lancet Psychiatry* (2016) 3:579–84. doi: 10.1016/S2215-0366(16)00048-1
18. Fernandes BS, Williams LM, Steiner J, Leboyer M, Carvalho AF, Berk M. The new field of "precision psychiatry". *BMC Med.* (2017) 15:80. doi: 10.1186/s12916-017-0849-x
19. Fraguas D, Diaz-Caneja CM, State MW, O'Donovan MC, Gur RE, Arango C. Mental disorders of known aetiology and precision medicine in psychiatry: a promising but neglected alliance. *Psychol Med.* (2017) 47:193–7. doi: 10.1017/S0033291716001355
20. Paulus MP, Stein MB, Craske MG, Bookheimer S, Taylor CT, Simmons AN, et al. Latent variable analysis of positive and negative valence processing focused on symptom and behavioral units of analysis in mood and anxiety disorders. *J Affect Disord.* (2017) 216:17–29. doi: 10.1016/j.jad.2016.12.046
21. Scott J, Murray G, Henry C, Morken G, Scott E, Angst J, et al. Activation in bipolar disorders: a systematic review. *JAMA Psychiatry* (2017) 74:189–96. doi: 10.1001/jamapsychiatry.2016.3459
22. Bauer MS, Mitchner I. What is a "mood stabilizer"? an evidence-based response. *Am J Psychiatry* (2004) 161:3–18. doi: 10.1176/appi.ajp.161.1.3
23. Severns E, Taylor MJ, Sauer C, Pfennig A, Ritter P, Bauer M, Geddes JR. Lithium for prevention of mood episodes in bipolar disorders: systematic review and meta-analysis. *Int J Bipolar Disord.* (2014) 20:15. doi: 10.1186/s40345-014-0015-8
24. Kessing L, Bauer M, Nolen W, Severus E, Goodwin G, Geddes J. Effectiveness of maintenance therapy of lithium vs other mood stabilizers in monotherapy and in combinations: a systematic review of evidence from observational studies. *Bipolar Disord.* (2018). doi: 10.1111/bdi.12623. [Epub ahead of print].
25. Roberts E, Cipriani A, Geddes J, Nierenberg AA, Young AH. The evidence for lithium in suicide prevention. *Br J Psychiatry* (2017) 211:396. doi: 10.1192/bjp.211.6.396
26. Oedegaard KJ, Alda M, Anand A, Andreassen OA, Balaraman Y, Berrettini WH, et al. The Pharmacogenomics of Bipolar Disorder study (PGBD): identification of genes for lithium response in a prospective sample. *BMC Psychiatry* (2016) 16:129. doi: 10.1186/s12888-016-0732-x
27. Zivanovic O. Lithium: a classic drug-frequently discussed, but, sadly, seldom prescribed!. *Aust N Z J Psychiatry* (2017) 51:886–96. doi: 10.1177/0004867417695889
28. Pisanu C, Heilbronner U, Squassina A. The role of pharmacogenomics in bipolar disorder: moving towards precision medicine. *Mol Diagn Ther.* (2018) 22:409–20. doi: 10.1007/s40291-018-0335-y
29. Scott J, Geoffroy PA, Sportiche S, Brichant-Petit-Jean C, Gard S, Kahn JP, et al. Cross-validation of clinical characteristics and treatment patterns associated with phenotypes for lithium response defined by the Alda scale. *J Affect Disord.* (2017) 208:62–7. doi: 10.1016/j.jad.2016.08.069
30. Kleindienst N, Engel R, Greil W. Which clinical factors predict response to prophylactic lithium? A systematic review for bipolar disorders. *Bipolar Disord.* (2005) 7:404–17. doi: 10.1111/j.1399-5618.2005.00244.x
31. Montlahuc C, Curis E, Grillault Laroche D, Bagoe G, Etain B, Bellivier F, et al. Response to lithium in patients with bipolar disorder: what are psychiatrists' experiences and practices compared to literature review? *Pharmacopsychiatry* (2018). doi: 10.1055/s-0044-100521. [Epub ahead of print].
32. Scott, J. Cognitive-behavioural therapy for severe mental disorders: back to the future? *Br J Psychiatry* (2008) 192:401–3. doi: 10.1192/bjp.bp.108.053876
33. Hayes J, Marston L, Walters K, Geddes J, King M, Osborn D. Lithium vs. valproate vs. olanzapine vs. quetiapine as maintenance monotherapy for bipolar disorder: a population-based UK cohort study using electronic health records. *World Psychiatry* (2016) 15:53–8. doi: 10.1002/wps.20298
34. Scott J, Pope M. Self-reported adherence to treatment with mood stabilizers, plasma levels, and psychiatric hospitalization. *Am J Psychiatry* (2002) 159:1927–9. doi: 10.1176/appi.ajp.159.11.1927
35. Wu Z, Pang W, Coghill GM. An integrative top-down and bottom-up qualitative model construction framework for exploration of biochemical systems. *Soft comput.* (2015) 19:1595–610. doi: 10.1007/s00500-014-1467-6
36. Lee JH, Choi JH, Youn JS, Cha YJ, Song W, Park AJ. Comparison between bottom-up and top-down approaches in the estimation of measurement uncertainty. *Clin Chem Lab Med.* (2015) 53:1025–32. doi: 10.1515/cclm-2014-0801
37. Petkova E, Ogden RT, Tarpey T, Ciarleglio A, Jiang B, Su Z, et al. Statistical analysis plan for Stage 1 EMBARC (Establishing Moderators and Biosignatures of Antidepressant Response for Clinical Care) Study. *Contemp Clin Trials Commun.* (2017) 6:22–30. doi: 10.1016/j.conctc.2017.02.007
38. Carvalho AF, Kohler CA, Fernandes BS, Quevedo J, Miskowiak KW, Brunoni AR, et al. Bias in emerging biomarkers for bipolar disorder. *Psychol Med.* (2016) 46:2287–97. doi: 10.1017/S0033291716000957
39. Cuthbert BN, Insel TR. Toward the future of psychiatric diagnosis: the seven pillars of RDoC. *BMC Med.* (2013) 11:126. doi: 10.1186/1741-7015-11-126
40. Scott J, Murray G. Are rating scales for bipolar disorders fit for purpose? *Br. J. Psychiatry.* (in press).
41. Presciandaro JJ, Tolliver BK. An item response theory evaluation of the young mania rating scale and the Montgomery-Asberg depression rating scale in the systematic treatment enhancement program for bipolar disorder (STEP-BD). *J Affect Disord.* (2016) 205:73–80. doi: 10.1016/j.jad.2016.06.062
42. Klein E, Lavie P, Meiraz R, Sadeh A, Lenox R.H. Increased motor activity and recurrent manic episodes: predictors of rapid relapse in remitted bipolar disorder patients after lithium discontinuation. *Biol Psychiatry* (1992) 31:279–84. doi: 10.1016/0006-3223(92)90051-Z
43. Bagby RM, Ryder AG, Schuller DR, Marshall MB. The Hamilton depression rating scale: has the gold standard become a lead weight? *Am J Psychiatry* (2004) 161:2163–77. doi: 10.1176/appi.ajp.161.12.2163
44. Timmerby N, Andersen JH, Sondergaard S, Ostergaard SD, Bech P. A systematic review of the clinimetric properties of the 6-Item version of the Hamilton depression rating scale (HAM-D6). *Psychother Psychosom.* (2017) 86:141–49. doi: 10.1159/000457131
45. Jonas D, Mansfield A, Curtis P, Gilmore J, Watson L, Brode S, et al. Identifying priorities for patient-centered outcomes research for serious mental illness. *Psychiatr Serv.* (2012) 63:1125–130. doi: 10.1176/appi.ps.201100369
46. Moskowitz DS, Young SN. Ecological momentary assessment: what it is and why it is a method of the future in clinical psychopharmacology. *J Psychiatry Neurosci.* (2006) 31:13–20.
47. Wu MJ, Mwangi B, Bauer IE, Passos IC, Sanches M, Zunta-Soares GB, et al. Identification and individualized prediction of clinical phenotypes in bipolar disorders using neurocognitive data, neuroimaging scans and machine learning. *Neuroimage* (2017) 145(Pt. B):254–64. doi: 10.1016/j.neuroimage.2016.02.016
48. Hou L, Heilbronner U, Degenhardt F, Adli M, Akiyama K, Akula N, et al. Genetic variants associated with response to lithium treatment in bipolar disorder: a genome-wide association study. *Lancet* (2016) 387:1085–93. doi: 10.1016/S0140-6736(16)00143-4
49. Chen C, Lee C, Chen H, Wu L, Chang J, Liu C, et al. GADL1 variant and medication adherence in predicting response to lithium maintenance treatment in bipolar I disorder. *BJPsych Open* (2016) 2:301–6. doi: 10.1192/bjpo.bp.116.002881
50. Howes OD, McCutcheon R, Agid O, de Bartolomeis A, van Beveren NJ, Birnbaum ML, et al. Treatment-Resistant Schizophrenia:Treatment Response and Resistance in Psychosis (TRRIP) working group consensus guidelines on diagnosis and terminology. *Am J Psychiatry* (2017) 174:216–29. doi: 10.1176/appi.ajp.2016.16050503
51. Clatworthy J, Bowskill R, Parham R, Rank T, Scott J, Horne R. Understanding medication non-adherence in bipolar disorders using a Necessity-Concerns Framework. *J Affect Disord.* (2009) 116:51–5. doi: 10.1016/j.jad.2008.11.004

52. Scott J, Tacchi MJ. A pilot study of concordance therapy for individuals with bipolar disorders who are non-adherent with lithium prophylaxis. *Bipolar Disord.* (2002) 4:386–92. doi: 10.1034/j.1399-5618.2002.02242.x
53. Dambinova SA, Sowell RL, Maroon JC. Gradual return to play: potential role of neurotoxicity biomarkers in assessment of concussions severity. *J Mol Biomark Diagn* (2013) S3:003. doi: 10.4172/2155-9929.S3-003
54. Trivedi MH, McGrath PJ, Fava M, Parsey RV, Kurian BT, Phillips ML, et al. Establishing moderators and biosignatures of antidepressant response in clinical care (EMBARC): rationale and design. *J Psychiatr Res.* (2016) 78:11–23. doi: 10.1016/j.jpsychires.2016.03.001
55. Schulze TG, Alda M, Adli M, Akula N, Ardau R, Bui ET, et al. The International Consortium on Lithium Genetics (ConLiGen): an initiative by the NIMH and IGSLI to study the genetic basis of response to lithium. *Neuropsychobiology* (2010) 62:72–8. doi: 10.1159/000314708
56. Le-Niculescu H, Kurian SM, Yehyawi N, Dike C, Patel SD, Edenberg HJ, et al. Identifying blood biomarkers for mood disorders using convergent functional genomics. *Mol Psychiatry.* (2009) 14:156–74. doi: 10.1038/mp.2008.11
57. Amare AT, Schubert K, Baune BT. Pharmacogenomics in the treatment of mood disorders: strategies and opportunities for personalized psychiatry. *EPMA J.* (2017) 8:211–17. doi: 10.1007/s13167-017-0112-8
58. Amare AT, Schubert KO, Hou L, Clark SR, Papiol S, Heilbronner U, et al. Association of polygenic score for schizophrenia and HLA antigen and inflammation genes with response to lithium in bipolar affective disorder: a Genome-Wide Association Study. *JAMA Psychiatry* (2018) 75:65–74. doi: 10.1001/jamapsychiatry.2017.3433
59. Moreira J, Courtin C, Geoffroy PA, Curis E, Bellivier F, Marie-Claire C. Lithium response in bipolar disorder: no difference in GADL1 gene expression between cell lines from excellent-responders and non-responders. *Psychiatry Res.* (2017) 251:217–20. doi: 10.1016/j.psychres.2017.02.022.
60. Roux M, Dosseto A. From direct to indirect lithium targets: a comprehensive review of omics data. *Metallomics* (2017) 9:1326–51. doi: 10.1039/c7mt00203c
61. Sassi RB, Brambilla P, Hatch JP, Nicoletti MA, Mallinger AG, Frank E, et al. Reduced left anterior cingulate volumes in untreated bipolar patients. *Biol Psychiatry* (2004) 56:467–75. doi: 10.1016/j.biopsych.2004.07.005
62. Silverstone PH, Bell EC, Willson MC, Dave S, Wilman AH. Lithium alters brain activation in bipolar disorder in a task- and state-dependent manner: an fMRI study. *Ann Gen Psychiatry* (2005) 4:14. doi: 10.1186/1744-859X-4-14
63. Hallahan B, Newell J, Soares JC, Brambilla P, Strakowski SM, Fleck DE, et al. Structural magnetic resonance imaging in bipolar disorder: an international collaborative mega-analysis of individual adult patient data. *Biol Psychiatry* (2011) 69:326–35. doi: 10.1016/j.biopsych.2010.08.029
64. Brochard H, Godin O, Geoffroy PA, Yeim S, Boudebesse C, Benizri C, et al. Metabolic syndrome and actigraphy measures of sleep and circadian rhythms in bipolar disorders during remission. *Acta Psychiatr Scand.* (2018). doi: 10.1111/acps.12910. [Epub ahead of print].
65. Scott J, Naismith S, Grierson A, Carpenter J, Hermens D, Scott E, et al. Sleep-wake cycle phenotypes in young people with familial and non-familial mood disorders. *Bipolar Disord.* (2016) 18:642–9. doi: 10.1111/bdi.12450
66. Dawkins, R. *The Extended Phenotype: the Gene as the Unit of Selection.* Oxford: Oxford University Press (1982). 273p.
67. Smith FE, Thelwall PE, Necus J, Flowers CJ, Blamire AM, Cousins DA. 3D (7)Li magnetic resonance imaging of brain lithium distribution in bipolar disorder. *Mol Psychiatry* (2018). doi: 10.1038/s41380-018-0016-6. [Epub ahead of print].
68. Jain S, Powers B, Hawkins J, Brownstein J. The digital phenotype. *Nat Biotechnol.* (2015) 33:462–3. doi: 10.1038/nbt.3223
69. Faurholt-Jepsen M, Vinberg M, Frost M, Debel S, Margrethe Christensen E, Bardram JE, et al. Behavioral activities collected through smartphones and the association with illness activity in bipolar disorder. *Int J Methods Psychiatr Res.* (2016) 25:309–23. doi: 10.1002/mpr.1502
70. Niculescu A, Le-Niculescu H, Levey D, Phalen P, Dainton H, Roseberry K, et al. Precision medicine for suicidality: from universality to subtypes and personalization. *Mol Psychiatry* (2017) 22:1250–73. doi: 10.1038/mp.2017.128
71. Demjaha A. On the brink of precision medicine for psychosis: treating the patient, not the disease. *Schizophr Res.* (2018) 193:487–88. doi: 10.1016/j.schres.2017.08.011
72. Kraemer HC, Frank E, Kupfer DJ. How to assess the clinical impact of treatments on patients, rather than the statistical impact of treatments on measures. *Int J Methods Psychiatr Res.* (2011) 20:63–72. doi: 10.1002/mpr.340
73. Wellek S, Schumann G. Statistical confirmation of results of association studies in genetic epidemiology. *Am J Med Genet B Neuropsychiatr Genet.* (2004) 128B:126–30. doi: 10.1002/ajmg.b.30012
74. Iniesta R, Stahl D, McGuffin P. Machine learning, statistical learning and the future of biological research in psychiatry. *Psychol Med.* (2016) 46:2455–65. doi: 10.1017/S0033291716001367.
75. Librenza-Garcia D, Kotzian BJ, Yang J, Mwangi B, Cao B, Pereira Lima LN, et al. The impact of machine learning techniques in the study of bipolar disorder: a systematic review. *Neurosci Biobehav Rev.* (2017) 80:538–54. doi: 10.1016/j.neubiorev.2017.07.004
76. Trivedi MH. Modeling predictors, moderators and mediators of treatment outcome and resistance in depression. *Biol Psychiatry* (2013) 74:2–4. doi: 10.1016/j.biopsych.2013.05.009
77. Mennes M. Commentary: leveraging discovery science to advance child and adolescent psychiatric research–a commentary on Zhao and Castellanos 2016. *J Child Psychol Psychiatry* (2016) 57:440–2. doi: 10.1111/jcpp.12538
78. Fugel HJ, Nuijten M, Faulkner E. The application of economics concepts to stratified medicine–use of health economics data to support market access for stratified medicine interventions. *J Med Econ.* (2014) 17:305–11. doi: 10.3111/13696998.2014.902842
79. Joyce DW, Kehagia AA, Tracy DK, Proctor J, Shergill SS. Realising stratified psychiatry using multidimensional signatures and trajectories. *J Transl Med.* (2017) 15:15. doi: 10.1186/s12967-016-1116-1
80. Krishnan V, Nestler EJ. The molecular neurobiology of depression. *Nature* (2008) 455:894–902. doi: 10.1038/nature07455
81. European Medicines Agency. *Concept Paper on the Need for Revision of the Note for Guidance on Clinical Investigation of Medicinal Products for the Treatment and Prevention of Bipolar Disorder.* Committee for Medicinal products for Human Use. (2015) EMA/CHMP/318360/2015.
82. Musenga A, Saracino MA, Sani G, Raggi MA. Antipsychotic and antiepileptic drugs in bipolar disorder: the importance of therapeutic drug monitoring. *Curr Med Chem.* (2009) 16:1463–81. doi: 10.2174/092986709787909604
83. Ashley EA. The precision medicine initiative: a new national effort. *JAMA* (2015) 313:2119–20. doi: 10.1001/jama.2015.3595

13

Precision Medicine for Frontotemporal Dementia

Mu-N Liu[1,2,3]*, Chi-Ieong Lau*[4,5,6] *and Ching-Po Lin*[1,7,8*]

[1] Institute of Brain Science, National Yang-Ming University, Taipei, Taiwan, [2] Department of Psychiatry, Taipei Veterans General Hospital, Taipei, Taiwan, [3] Department of Neurology, Memory and Aging Centre, University of California, San Francisco, San Francisco, CA, United States, [4] Department of Neurology, Shin Kong Wu Ho-Su Memorial Hospital, Taipei, Taiwan, [5] Applied Cognitive Neuroscience Group, Institute of Cognitive Neuroscience, University College London, London, United Kingdom, [6] College of Medicine, Fu-Jen Catholic University, Taipei, Taiwan, [7] Institute of Neuroscience, National Yang-Ming University, Taipei, Taiwan, [8] Aging and Health Research Center, National Yang Ming University, Taipei, Taiwan

***Correspondence:**
Ching-Po Lin
chingpolin@gmail.com

Frontotemporal dementia (FTD) is a common young-onset dementia presenting with heterogeneous and distinct syndromes. It is characterized by progressive deficits in behavior, language, and executive function. The disease may exhibit similar characteristics to many psychiatric disorders owing to its prominent behavioral features. The concept of precision medicine has recently emerged, and it involves neurodegenerative disease treatment that is personalized to match an individual's specific pattern of neuroimaging, neuropathology, and genetic variability. In this paper, the pathophysiology underlying FTD, which is characterized by the selective degeneration of the frontal and temporal cortices, is reviewed. We also discuss recent advancements in FTD research from the perspectives of clinical, imaging, molecular characterizations, and treatment. This review focuses on the approach of precision medicine to manage the clinical and biological complexities of FTD.

Keywords: frontotemporal dementia, frontotemporal lobar degeneration, genetics, precision medicine, neuroimaging, primary progressive aphasia

INTRODUCTION

Frontotemporal dementia (FTD) is an insidious neurodegenerative clinical syndrome that is characterized by progressive disturbances in behavior as well as deficits in executive function and language. FTD is a common early-onset dementia (occurring in patients aged <65 years), has a prevalence rate of 3–26%, and is one of the most common forms of dementia across all age groups (1). Arnold Pick, a Czech psychiatrist, first identified the clinical syndrome of FTD in 1892 (2). He described a patient with aphasia, focal frontal and temporal lobar atrophy, and presenile dementia. Alois Alzheimer, a German psychiatrist and neuropathologist, later characterized Pick bodies as being associated with FTD and named the disorder Pick's disease in 1911 (3). Although, the term Pick's disease initially referred to both the clinical syndrome and the pathological diagnosis, modern nomenclature designates Pick's disease as only the pathological diagnosis, whereas a clinical diagnosis for prominent behavioral changes is known as behavioral-variant FTD (bvFTD). Mesulam described primary progressive aphasia (PPA), the language subtype of FTD, in 1982 (4). Revised diagnostic criteria were issued in 2011 (5, 6).

Precision medicine, also called "personalized medicine" or "individualized medicine," is a rapidly advancing field in medical, clinical, and research settings. It aims to optimize the effectiveness of disease prevention and treatment and simultaneously minimize side effects in individuals who are less likely to respond to a particular therapy, by considering an individual's specific makeup with regard to genetics, biomarkers, phenotype, and psychosocial characteristics. In this review, we discuss the precision medicine of FTD, from clinical phenotypes, epidemiology, genetics, neuroimaging to neuropathological biomarkers. We further review recent advancements in therapeutic strategies and potential personalized treatment for FTD (7–13). This review improves the understanding of accurate diagnosis and personalized effective disease treatment strategies.

COGNITIVE AND BEHAVIORAL MARKERS

FTD is an umbrella term for three recognizable clinical syndromes, namely bvFTD, semantic-variant PPA (svPPA), and non-fluent-variant PPA (nfvPPA) (**Table 1**). FTD also frequently overlaps clinically with three neurodegenerative diseases that exhibit motor deficits, namely corticobasal degeneration (CBD), progressive supranuclear palsy (PSP), and amyotrophic lateral sclerosis (1–4).

Behavioral-Variant Frontotemporal Dementia

The symptoms of bvFTD include progressive personality and behavioral changes, apathy, and disinhibition in interpersonal interactions. Patients may experience early changes in disinhibition, stereotypic behavior, alterations in food preferences and eating behavior, alterations in empathy, apathy, and dysexecutive symptoms (5, 15). Some of these early symptoms, such as decreased empathy, may have diagnostic value for bvFTD, but they have not been ascertained in clinical practice. Apathy may manifest as reduced interest in work, hobbies, social interaction, and hygiene; however, apathy can be misdiagnosed as depression.

Symptoms similar to those detected in psychiatric disorders are frequently observed in patients with bvFTD. Thus, discriminating the behavioral features of bvFTD from those of primary psychiatric disorders such as depression, schizophrenia, bipolar disorder, and borderline personality disorder may be challenging (16, 17). Although psychotic symptoms such as hallucinations and delusions are rare in bvFTD, cases of these symptoms have been reported (17), particularly in patients carrying the chromosome 9 open reading frame 72 *(C9orf72)* repeat expansion (18).

Primary Progressive Aphasia

Patients with PPA exhibit a progressive decline in linguistic skills during the early phase of the disease. Language dysfunction is the main symptom during the first 2 years of PPA. Deficits in object naming, syntax, or word comprehension may become apparent during conversation or may be identified using speech and language assessment. The subtypes of PPA are differentiated by specific types of speech or language deficits. The three PPA subtypes are the semantic, non-fluent, and logopenic variants (19). Each subtype has a distinct pattern of language deficits. Naming difficulty is common to all three subtypes; therefore, it is not a distinguishing feature. The non-fluent (or agrammatic) variant and the semantic variant are classified as FTD, whereas the logopenic variant, most often associated with temporoparietal atrophy, is typically due to underlying Alzheimer's pathology; hence, it is not discussed in this review.

Semantic-Variant Primary Progressive Aphasia

In svPPA, a syndrome characterized by semantic aphasia and associative agnosia, anterior temporal lobe degeneration disrupts semantic memory (**Table 1**) (6). Anomia and single-word comprehension deficits, starting with low-frequency items, are essential for diagnosis (20). In contrast to patients with nfvPPA, those with svPPA maintain fluent speech and correct grammar during the early stages of this disease. Early symptoms of semantic PPA include anomia, word-finding difficulties, and repetitive speech, whereas early behavioral syndrome presents with irritability and emotional distance or coldness.

Non-fluent/Agrammatic-Variant Primary Progressive Aphasia

Articulation deficits resulting in slow, labored, and halting speech production as well as incorrect grammar or syntax (agrammatism) characterize nfvPPA. The core criteria of nfvPPA are agrammatism and effortful speech, and at least one of the criteria should be present (**Table 1**) (6). Patients tend to exhibit motor speech disorders characterized by a slow speech rate, abnormal prosody, and distorted sound substitutions, additions, repetitions, and prolongations, which are occasionally accompanied by groping, trial-and-error articulatory movements (21), or agrammatic errors. Repetition is less impaired than is spontaneous speech, and semantic knowledge for words typically remains well-preserved throughout the disease process.

Motor Symptoms

The three FTD-spectrum motor syndromes are FTD with motor neuron disease (FTD-MND) and two variants with parkinsonism, namely corticobasal syndrome (CBS) and progressive supranuclear palsy syndrome (PSP-S). Up to 15% of patients with FTD have concomitant MND, and nearly 30% of patients present with mild features of MND (9, 22). MND may include upper motor neuron signs (hyperreflexia, extensor plantar response, and spasticity), lower motor neuron signs (weakness, muscle atrophy, and fasciculations), dysarthria, dysphagia, and pseudobulbar affect (22). Up to 20% of patients with FTD present with parkinsonism, which is most often observed in patients with bvFTD, followed by those with nfvPPA (23). Patients with FTD may exhibit features of CBS or PSP-S. CBS is a heterogeneous syndrome featuring behavioral, cognitive, and motor changes. The clinical criteria for probable CBS include asymmetric presentation with any two symptoms among (A) limb rigidity or akinesia, (B) limb dystonia, and (C) limb myoclonus, as well as any two symptoms among (D) orobuccal or limb apraxia, (E) cortical sensory deficit, and (F) alien limb phenomena (more than simple levitation) (24). Finally, PSP-S is characterized by atypical parkinsonism with axial and symmetrical rigidity, supranuclear gaze palsy (most prominent in the vertical plane), decreased saccadic velocity, early postural instability with falls, and prominent frontal lobe dysfunction (25, 26).

TABLE 1 | Clinical features of bvFTD, svPPA, and nfvPPA (5, 6).

Syndrome	Possible diagnosis with clinical evidence	Probable diagnosis with imaging evidence	Definite diagnosis with pathological or genetic support	Exclusionary criteria
bvFTD	At least three of the following: • Behavioral disinhibition (socially inappropriate behavior; Loss of manners or decorum; impulsive, rash or careless actions) within the first 3 years. • Apathy or inertia within the first 3 years • Lack of empathy or sympathy (loss of response to other people's needs and feelings; loss of social interest, interrelatedness or personal warmth) within the first 3 years • Perseverations, stereotypies or compulsions (simple repetitive movements; complex, compulsive or ritualistic behaviors; stereotypy of speech) within the first 3 years • Dietary habit changes or hyperorality (altered food preferences; binge eating, increased consumption of alcohol or cigarettes; oral exploration or consumption of inedible objects) • Executive-predominant deficits on neuropsychological profile with relative sparing of episodic memory and visuospatial skills	All of the following: • Meets possible diagnostic criteria • Significant functional deficit (according to Clinical Dementia Rating Scale, Functional Activities Questionnaire scores, or caregiver report) • Imaging consistent with bvFTD (predominant frontal and/or anterotemporal atrophy, hypoperfusion and/or hypometabolism)	All of the following: • Meets possible or probable diagnostic criteria • Histopathological proof of FTLD pathology and/or existence of a known pathogenic mutation	Deficits or disturbances are not better explained by other disorders (neurodegenerative, non-degenerative nervous system, psychiatric, or medical diseases)
svPPA	Both of the following core features: • Impaired confrontation naming • Impaired single-word comprehension • At least three of the following four features: • Impaired object knowledge (particularly for low familiar or frequent items) • Surface dyslexia or dysgraphia • Spared repetition • Spared grammar and motor speech (speech production)	All of the following: • Meets possible diagnostic criteria • Imaging consistent with svPPA (predominant anterior temporal lobe atrophy, hypoperfusion and/or hypometabolism)	All of the following: • Meets possible or probable diagnostic criteria • Histopathological proof of FTLD pathology and/or existence of a known pathogenic mutation	• Deficits are not better explained by other disorders (non-degenerative nervous system, psychiatric, or medical diseases) • Prominent initial symptoms are not episodic memory, visuospatial impairments, or behavioral disturbance
nfvPPA	At least one of the following two core features: • Agrammatism • Effortful, halting speech with inconsistent sound errors and distortions (apraxia of speech) • At least two of the following three features: • Impaired comprehension of syntactically complex sentences • Spared single-word comprehension • Spared object knowledge	All of the following: • Meets possible diagnostic criteria • Imaging consistent with nfvPPA • (predominant left posterior frontoinsular atrophy, hypoperfusion and/or hypometabolism)	All of the following: • Meets possible or probable diagnostic criteria • Histopathological proof of FTLD pathology and/or existence of a known pathogenic mutation	• Deficits are not better explained by other disorders (non-degenerative nervous system, psychiatric, or medical diseases) • Prominent initial symptoms are not episodic memory, visuospatial impairments, or behavioral disturbance

BvFTD, behavioral-variant frontotemporal dementia; svPPA, semantic-variant primary progressive aphasia; and nfvPPA, non-fluent variant primary progressive aphasia.

Taken together, the vast heterogeneity and overlap of clinical phenotypes in FTD often poses diagnostic challenges for clinicians, in particular the presenting psychiatric symptoms that may easily be mistaken for psychiatric disorders. The accurate diagnosis of each subtype of FTD, therefore, requires a precision medicine approach.

IMAGING BIOMARKERS

Neuroimaging has the potential to aid the differential diagnosis of FTD. For example, FTD is characterized by predominant frontal or temporal atrophy, particularly in the frontoinsular region, as revealed by structural brain imaging (**Figure 1**; **Table 2**) (8). Using voxel-based morphometry, Rosen et al. demonstrated that core neuropsychiatric symptoms of bvFTD, including apathy, disinhibition, and aberrant motor behavior, are localized to the right frontal structures. Moreover, atrophy in the right-hemispheric anterior cingulate cortex and adjacent ventromedial superior frontal gyrus, posterior ventromedial prefrontal cortex, lateral middle frontal gyrus, caudate head, orbitofrontal cortex, and anterior insula was correlated with symptom severity (27). Very mild bvFTD targets paralimbic networks, including the anterior cingulate, insular, medial frontal, and orbitofrontal cortices (28). Specifically, atrophy of the right ventromedial

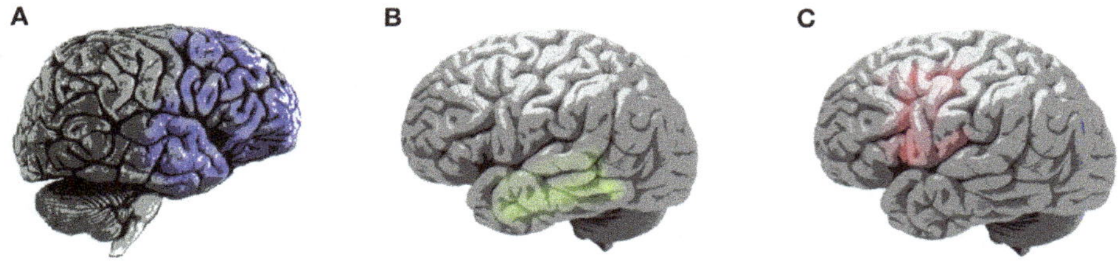

FIGURE 1 | Patterns of brain atrophy in clinical subtypes of frontotemporal dementia (7–9). **(A)** Areas of brain atrophy in behavioral-variant frontotemporal dementia (blue), right hemisphere lateral view; **(B)** Areas of brain atrophy in semantic-variant primary progressive aphasia(green), left hemisphere lateral view; **(C)** Areas of brain atrophy in non-fluent variant primary progressive aphasia, left hemisphere lateral view.

TABLE 2 | Imaging and pathological characteristics of frontotemporal dementia (7–9).

Three types FTD		**Genetic and pathological characteristics**	**Imaging characteristics**
Behavior variant	bvFTD	*C9orf72, MAPT,* and *GRN* mutations; tau and TDP-43 proteinopathy	Prefrontal and anterior temporal cortex loss, particularly in the right hemisphere; reduced white matter fractional anisotropy in uncinate fasciculus striatum, thalamus, anterior cingulate, and insula atrophy; reduced fractional anisotropy in superior and inferior longitudinal fasciculi, inferior fronto-occipital fasciculus, genu of corpus callosum and cingulum
Language variant	svPPA	Rare genetic mutations; tau and TDP-43 (majority) proteinopathy	Brain atrophy in inferior temporal and fusiform gyri, temporal pole, parahippocampal cortex, entorhinal cortex, particularly in the left hemisphere; reduced fractional anisotropy in left superior longitudinal fasciculus and corpus callosum; brain atrophy also affecting anterior cingulate, orbitofrontal, inferior frontal, and insular cortices; reduced fractional anisotropy in left cingulum, left orbitofrontal, inferior frontal, anterior temporal, inferior parietal white matter regions
	nfvPPA	*GRN* mutations; tau (majority), and TDP-43 proteinopathy	Brain atrophy in the inferior frontal, prefrontal and temporal cortices, caudate and putamen, particularly in the left hemisphere; reduced fractional anisotropy in left uncinate fasciculus, corpus callosum, cingulum, and inferior longitudinal fasciculus tract

BvFTD, behavioral-variant frontotemporal dementia; svPPA, semantic-variant primary progressive aphasia; nfvPPA, non-fluent variant primary progressive aphasia; C9orf72, chromosome 9 open reading frame 72; MAPT, microtubule-associated protein tau; GRN, progranulin mutations; and TDP-43, transactive response (TAR) DNA-binding protein of 43 kDa.

superior frontal gyrus was associated with apathy; atrophy of the right ventromedial prefrontal cortex was associated with disinhibition (27); and atrophy of the dorsolateral prefrontal was associated with executive deficit (7). A widespread alteration in white matter connectivity between the frontal and temporal lobes was noted using diffusion tensor imaging. The uncinate fasciculus, anterior parts of the superior and inferior longitudinal fasciculi, genu of the corpus callosum, cingulum, and inferior fronto-occipital fasciculus were affected (**Table 2**) (10, 29).

By contrast, language symptoms are usually localized to the left hemisphere and are associated with a deficit of the language circuit. Degeneration of the left anterior temporal lobe is associated with linguistic semantic loss, whereas that of the right anterior temporal lobe is associated with prominent behavioral and personality changes, including lack of empathy and increased rigidity (30). Patients with PPA present with focal and asymmetric changes in specific networks fundamental to language processing.

Patients with svPPA present with semantic memory deficit that is localized to the anterior temporal lobes. Abnormalities in white matter connectivity are predominantly distributed over the left fronto-temporal areas, including the uncinate fasciculus, inferior longitudinal fasciculus, corpus callosum, and cingulum (**Figure 1**; **Table 2**) (10, 31, 32). The occipital lobe, cerebellum, and brainstem are spared (10, 31). The left temporal lobe variant is approximately three times more common than the right temporal lobe variant (33). Eventually, degeneration spreads to the other side; accordingly, patients with svPPA develop right temporal pole atrophy (and vice versa). The following observations are relatively likely to be associated with major right temporal atrophy and difficulty with person identification (34). Patients with the right temporal variant may have difficulty recognizing famous faces because of semantic loss. As the disease spreads from the temporal lobes into the orbitofrontal cortex, the patients start exhibiting behavioral changes, such as irritability, emotional withdrawal, insomnia, strict or selective eating (often focusing on one particular type of food), and occasionally depression (30). Despite the loss of semantic knowledge in the left temporal lobe variant, functions such as visual attention on the right side are sometimes enhanced. Patients with the left temporal lobe variant are more likely to develop visual compulsions such as repetitions in activities, collecting brightly colored objects, jewelry beading, gardening, or painting (30, 35). By contrast, individuals with the right temporal lobe variant develop verbal

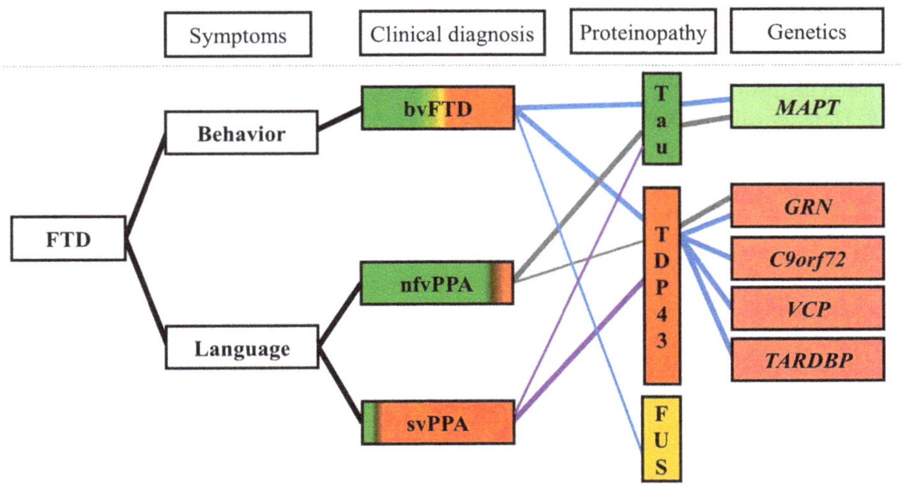

FIGURE 2 | Clinical, pathological, and genetic associations in FTD (7–9, 37). Clinical symptoms are shown at left, colored regions of clinical diagnosis represent relative percentages of patients found to have each underlying neuropathological diagnosis. Blue line, genetic and pathological aspects of bvFTD; gray line, genetic, and pathological aspects of nfvPPA; purple line, genetic, and pathological aspects of svPPA. bvFTD, behavioral-variant frontotemporal dementia; svPPA, semantic-variant primary progressive aphasia; nfvPPA, non-fluent variant primary progressive aphasia; FUS, fused in sarcoma; TDP-43, transactive response (TAR) DNA-binding protein of 43 kDa; *C9orf72,* chromosome 9 open reading frame 72; *GRN,* progranulin mutations; *MAPT,* microtubule-associated protein tau; and *VCP*, valosin-containing protein.

compulsions on words and symbols (such as compulsively writing letters, playing solitaire, writing telephone numbers, and making puns). In summary, left temporal atrophy has been associated with loss of verbal semantic knowledge, whereas behavioral symptoms dominate the right temporal variant.

In nfvPPA, the deficits target the frontoinsular cortex. Atrophy is most frequently noted in the left inferior frontal and insular cortices, which disrupts language fluency and grammar (7, 35). White matter abnormalities are predominantly distributed over the left frontal-temporal-parietal regions, including the left superior longitudinal fasciculus, corpus callosum, cingulum, inferior and orbital frontal, anterior temporal, and inferior parietal areas (**Figure 1**; **Table 2**) (10, 36). Except for structural MRI, functional MRI, fluorodeoxyglucose (FDG)- PET, and single-photon-emission computed tomography all show disturbances in perfusion and metabolism over these areas (8, 10). In summary, due to cerebral hemispheric differences, patients with right-predominant patterns of atrophy tend to present with behavioral disturbance, such as bvFTD and right-sided svPPA, whereas patients with left-predominant atrophy may lead to language-related impairment, such as left-sided svPPA and nfvPPA.

NEUROPATHOLOGICAL BIOMARKERS: TAU, TDP-43, AND FUSED IN SARCOMA

FTD is caused by FTLD, a pathological process of cortical and subcortical degeneration over the frontal and temporal areas. Abnormal intracellular aggregates of tau and transactive response (TAR) DNA-binding protein of 43 kDa (TDP-43) are the leading causes of FTD (accounting for ~90% of cases). Fused in sarcoma (FUS), characterized by abnormal intracellular FUS inclusions, is associated with most of the remaining cases (**Figure 2**) (7).

Frontotemporal Lobar Degeneration -Tau Pathology

FTLD-tau accounts for one-third to one-half of all cases of FTLD, characterized by neuronal and glial tau aggregation (8, 38). Tau is critical for cellular morphology and function by binding to and stabilizing microtubules. In neurodegenerative disorders, tau becomes excessively hyperphosphorylated, dissociates from microtubules, and aberrantly aggregates within neurons and glia. Tau is encoded by microtubule-associated protein tau (*MAPT*). *MAPT* mutations mainly result in FTLD-tau pathology (**Figure 2**). Alternative splicing of *MAPT* mRNA leads to the production of three or four microtubule-binding domain repeats (3R or 4R). FTLD-tau is further subdivided into 3R, 4R, and 3R/4R tauopathies. Pick's disease, a 3R tauopathy, accounts for up to 30% of FTLD-tau cases (8, 38). A striking atrophy over the frontal, cingulate, and temporal gyri was noted (8). CBD, a 4R tauopathy, has been observed in approximately 35% of patients with FTLD-tau and involves the dorsal prefrontal cortex, supplemental motor area, perirolandic cortex, and subcortical nuclei (8, 38). PSP, also a 4R tauopathy, accounts for approximately 30% of patients with FTLD-tau (38). PSP is associated with frontal atrophy and with subcortical atrophy of the globus pallidus, subthalamic nucleus, and brainstem nuclei (8).

Approximately half of all bvFTD patients and the majority of nfvPPA patients have FTLD-tau pathology (**Figure 2**) (11). Furthermore, in most bvFTD or nfvPPA cases, the presence of extrapyramidal symptoms suggestive of CBS/PSP likely reflect an underlying tauopathy (12). Behavioral changes seen in bvFTD, or non-fluent motor speech difficulties in nfvPPA, may be presented in patients with CBS/PSP clinical syndrome before or after development of movement disorder. PSP neuropathology is strongly associated with patients with PSP clinical syndrome, particularly presence of the supranuclear vertical gaze palsy and early postural instability (11). Thus, PSP patients have become popular for the emergence of tau-targeting therapies in precision medicine. On the other hand, CBS is a highly variable clinical syndrome. In contrast, only 23% of the clinical CBS patients possessed Alzheimer's disease (AD) neuropathology, 13% with PSP neuropathology and 35% with CBD neuropathology in a large series of autopsy (39).

Frontotemporal Lobar Degeneration-TDP Pathology

FTLD-TDP accounts for approximately half of all patients with FTLD (38). TDP-43, a nuclear protein, is crucial for exon skipping and transcription regulation (40). In FTLD-TDP, TDP-43 becomes aberrantly localized from the nucleus to the cytoplasm, where it forms cytoplasmic inclusions (41). The cytoplasmic inclusions cause neurodegeneration though the potential toxicity of pathological TDP-43 aggregates and loss of normal TDP-43 function (i.e., nuclear clearance, RNA regulation) (11, 42). Four subtypes of FTLD-TDP (types A, B, C, and D) are recognized on the basis of the shape and distribution of TDP-43-positive lesions within the associative cortex (8). Type A accounts for approximately half of nfvPPA patients, one-quarter of suspected CBD patients, and one-quarter of bvFTD patients. Type C accounts for the majority of svPPA patients (**Figure 2**) (8).

Frontotemporal Lobar Degeneration -FUS Pathology

FUS is an RNA-binding protein involved in splicing and nuclear export of mRNA. FTLD-FUS has the following three subtypes: atypical FTLD with ubiquitin-positive inclusions, neuronal intermediate filament inclusion disease, and basophilic inclusion body disease (11, 43). A majority of patients with FTLD-FUS pathology are diagnosed as having bvFTD, characterized by sporadic early-onset FTD with behavioral disturbance, disinhibition, and psychotic symptoms (**Figure 2**) (44).

Collectively, the diversity of pathology FTLD gives rise to a vast complexity of clinical phenotypes, with often overlapping neuropsychiatric features. Understanding the underlying neuropathological biomarkers, through personalized medicine, may in the future, offer more targeted and precise therapeutic options (**Figure 2**).

GENETICS BIOMARKERS

Up to 40% of FTLD patients have a family history of dementia, thus suggesting a familial transmission; however, a clear autosomal-dominant history accounts for only 10% of all patients (45). To date, mutations in *MAPT*, chromosome 9 open reading frame 72 *(C9orf72)*, and progranulin (*GRN*) have accounted for more than half of patients in FTLD families with a strong autosomal-dominant history (8). Mutations in *MAPT* and *GRN* account for 5–20% of patients with familial FTLD; *C9orf72* mutations account for approximately 13–50% of familial FTLD patients and is a common genetic cause of FTD (8, 46, 47).

MAPT

MAPT mutations cause impaired microtubule assembly, impaired axonal transport, and increased pathological tau aggregation (48). As mentioned above, pathological tau formation in the cortical and subcortical brain areas results in neurodegeneration and is neuroanatomically correlated with the development of clinical symptoms (13). Patients with *MAPT* mutations are relatively young at onset (<50 years) and have a relatively short duration of illness (compared with those with other mutations), characterized by psychiatric and behavioral features (i.e., disinhibition, stereotyped repetitive behavior, and obsessions), parkinsonism, and oculomotor dysfunction (13, 49, 50). Neuroimaging studies revealed brain atrophy in the anterior temporal, orbitofrontal, caudate, insula, and anterior cingulate cortices (51), and different *MAPT* mutations may target different brain areas. For example, the medial temporal lobe indicates mutations in the splicing of exon 10, whereas mutations affecting the coding region target the lateral temporal lobe (52).

C9orf72

The expansion of a noncoding GGGGCC hexanucleotide repeat in *C9orf72* is the most common cause of inherited FTD worldwide, and it accounts for a relatively small proportion of sporadic cases (47, 53). Normally, the number of GGGGCC hexanucleotide repeats is <20; however, the presence of 65 or more repeats is considered pathogenic. Typically, the number of pathogenic repeats is in the hundreds (54). These expansion mutations are highly associated with TDP-43 pathology (13). FTD patients with the *C9orf72* expansion mutation commonly present with bvFTD, MND, or a combination of the two, characterized by behavioral features (i.e., apathy, loss of empathy, and disinhibition), complex stereotyped behaviors, executive dysfunction, and Parkinson-like symptoms (i.e., gait disturbance, tremor, and rigidity) (13). Approximate 38% of patients present with psychotic symptoms, characterized by delusions, hallucinations, somatic symptoms, agitation, and anxiety (13, 55). Imaging-genetic studies in FTD patients with *C9orf72* expansions have revealed a distributed symmetric pattern of brain atrophy in the frontal lobe (medial, dorsolateral, and orbitofrontal FTD patients with the *C9orf72* expansion may have a more rapid cognitive decline related to cortical atrophy compared with other forms of FTLD-TDP (56, 57), and most *C9orf72* expansion carriers with Parkinson-like symptoms respond poorly to levodopa usage (13). Therefore, *C9orf72* genotyping could potentially be useful for precision medicine approach, not only to classify patients with FTLD but also offer prognostic values.

GRN

Progranulin is a secreted protein involved in cell-cycle regulation, wound repair, axonal growth, and inflammation modulation (58). *GRN* mutations are associated with haploinsufficiency and the reduction of progranulin production and secretion (59). They are clinically associated with bvFTD, nfvPPA, and CBS, thus conferring relatively low penetrance until 70 years (60, 61). Psychiatric symptoms, including delusions, hallucinations, ritualistic behaviors, apathy, and social withdrawal, are common. Language function is involved early in FTD patients with *GRN* mutations compared with patients with *C9orf72* or *MAPT* mutations (13). Imaging study results showed asymmetric atrophy in the inferior frontal, temporal, and inferior parietal lobes whereas *C9orf72 or MAPT* mutations are associated with symmetrical brain atrophy (62).

Other Genetic Biomarkers

Mutations in TAR DNA-binding protein (*TARDBP*), valosin-containing protein (*VCP*), *TIA1*, *TBK1*, and *CCNF* genes (associated with TDP-43 pathology); and *FUS* and *CHMP2B* (associated with tau-negative, TDP-negative, ubiquitin-positive inclusions) account for a minority of familial FTD (8). Mutations of *TARDBP* are commonly associated with ALS and FTD-ALS, and may be associated with PSP-like symptoms and chorea. Patients with "ALS-plus" symptom (clinical features extending beyond pyramidal and neuromuscular systems) have an increased likelihood of carrying a pathogenic *TARDBP*, *C9orf72*, or *VCP* mutation in contrast with sporadic cases (63).

Accordingly, genetic assessment for the above known genetic variants may improve diagnosis of FTD amid an overly complicated clinical picture. In addition, it may offer biological information to predict personal disease risk, understand underlying pathophysiology, identify presymptomatic individuals at risk for FTD and even provide future options for personalized therapeutics.

APPLICATIONS OF FTD BIOMARKERS FOR PRECISION MEDICINE

Although abnormal tau and TDP protein deposits may not be the only cause of FTD pathogenesis, they can define FTD as a unique neurodegenerative disease in the differential diagnosis of dementia. In addition, the initial differentiation of FTD from atypical AD using FTD precision medicine is crucial because FTD symptoms may become more severe following the application of approved AD therapies (64). A research framework focusing on biomarker diagnosis of FTD is urgently required because of the complex clinicopathological relationships of the disease. With the advent of biomarkers diagnostic techniques such as neuroimaging, biofluid dynamics, and genetics, FTD pathology can be identified; this can greatly improve diagnostic precision regarding the underlying pathophysiology of clinical syndromes. The National Institute on Aging and Alzheimer's Association recently introduced a new research framework for AD diagnosis based on biomarkers (65). A future diagnostic framework for FTD could adopt a similar approach for precision medicine. The best neuroimaging approach to separate AD from FTD is by FDG-PET, as evident by the diffuse posterior temporoparietal hypometabolism in AD vs. the focal frontotemporal hypometabolism in FTD (8, 10). Although a high proportion of FTLD patients have low levels of comorbid AD neuropathology and amyloid-beta ($A\beta_{1-42}$) imaging is non-specific, amyloid PET scanning may still be useful for such differentiation (11). However, total tau (t-tau) and $A\beta_{1-42}$ are extensively studied cerebrospinal fluid (CSF) biomarkers that may be used to accurately distinguish autopsy-confirmed FTD from AD (66); FTD patients have lower t-tau–$A\beta_{1-42}$ ratios (37). The CSF t-tau–$A\beta_{1-42}$ ratio may lead to substantial improvement in clinical diagnosis for differentiating FTD from atypical AD (67). Levels of CSF biomarkers of axonal injury and neuronal loss such as neurofilament light chains are reportedly elevated in clinical FTD cohorts compared with cohorts of other neurodegenerative diseases (68, 69) and have been associated with FTD disease severity (69).

A key task is to distinguish FTD from transmissible spongiform encephalopathies [i.e., Creutzfeldt-Jakob disease (CJD)], especially when early symptoms are subtle. CJD is a typical human prion disease caused by the aggregation and propagation of scrapie prion protein (PrP^{SC})—a misfolded form of normal prion protein (PrP^{C}). CJD has many forms, including familial, variant, iatrogenic, and sporadic. Sporadic is the most common form (appropriately 85%) (70). Symptoms include myoclonus, rapidly progressive dementia, pyramidal/extrapyramidal signs, visual/cerebellar symptoms, and akinetic mutism. Clinical diagnosis of sporadic CJD (sCJD) is supported by the identification of 14-3-3 protein in CSF, periodic sharp electroencephalographic spikes, or MRI T2 FLAIR or diffusion-weighted imaging hyperintensities in the basal ganglia and cerebral or cerebellar cortex (71, 72). Compared with FTD, in sCJD, the CSF t-tau level is higher and the p-tau-t-tau ratio is lower (73). The aforementioned clinical, imaging, and biofluid markers are helpful in discriminating patients with FTD from those with CJD when clinical images are early and subtle.

Based on protein-targeting therapies such as those targeting tau (74), differentiation of FTLD-tau from FTLD-TDP after the exclusion of other neurodegenerative diseases (i.e., atypical AD and CJD) is the third step. Compared with FTLD-TDP and ALS, FTLD-tau has a higher p-tau level and higher p-tau-t-tau ratio (11). FTLD-TDP does not have significant p-tau pathology, and thus less p-tau may be released into the CSF compared with FTLD-tau (68, 75). The quantitative immunoprecipitation approach has been developed to detect specific forms of tau [extended (55 kDa) and truncated (33 kDa)] (76) to differentiate FTLD-tau from its subtypes. Through the exploratory proteomics-based approach, many novel CSF biomarkers have been identified for discriminating FTLD-tau from the main FTLD pathological subtypes as well as from non-demented controls and other forms of dementia with maximal accuracy (77). Studies to demonstrate the use of non-invasive methods such as the application of tau-specific radio ligands to identify FTLD-tau cases are ongoing (78, 79). Imaging and CSF biomarkers may assist in the development of successful therapies by facilitating the appropriate selection of cases for clinical trials targeting specific proteinopathies.

The longitudinal progression of biomarkers at early disease stages may be understood through the investigation of presymptomatic individuals within families that possess pathogenic mutations such as an earlier age of FTLD-tau onset with *MAPT* mutations (64). Brain network dysfunction has been observed in presymptomatic FTD with *GRN* (80) and *C9orf72* (81) mutations. *C9orf72* disease exhibits additional protein inclusion, additional clinical symptoms, and worse prognosis compared with its sporadic forms (11).

In line with the popular use of the *APOE* genotype in AD clinical trials, hereditary FTLD may be a popular choice for clinical trial development of therapies specific to this mutation. An autopsy-confirmed sporadic FTLD genetic study revealed several single-nucleotide polymorphisms (SNPs) that were overexpressed in patients with FTLD-tau and those with FTLD-TDP (82). The risk allele in the FTLD-tau-related SNP was associated with a shorter disease duration and white matter loss in the midbrain and long association fibers in sporadic bvFTD (83). This indicates the usefulness of SNP genotyping as a diagnostic and prognostic tool. A syndrome constitutes a clinical outcome of one or multiple diseases as opposed to an etiology. Similar to AD, a biological definition of FTD as opposed to a syndromal one is a superior means of enhancing the understanding of the underlying mechanisms of the clinical expression of FTD (65). Future precision-medicine approaches for FTD treatment must include biologically defined targets alongside the establishment of biomarker profiles and categories.

TREATMENTS

Nonpharmacological interventions are considered for the management of dementia before the use of pharmacological treatments that may exacerbate medical comorbidities affecting elderly patients. Healthy lifestyle changes, social connections, physical activity, and environmental intervention may mitigate the effects of dementia (42, 43). The main purpose of nonpharmacological interventions is to prevent disruptive behaviors, provide symptom remission, and reduce caregiver distress. For example, environmental approaches (i.e., reduction of noise, limitation of stimuli, and simplification of daily activities and social parameters) intend to reduce irritability, aggression, and anxiety caused by daily external stimuli.

Currently, no disease-modifying drugs approved by the U.S. Food and Drug Administration are available for the treatment of FTD. Most treatments are focused on the management of behavioral symptoms. The use of selective serotonin reuptake inhibitors can reduce the severity of agitation, aggressiveness, impulsivity, aberrant eating behaviors, and compulsions (8). Herrmann et al. reported that behavioral and psychiatric symptoms (including irritability, disinhibition, and depression) were alleviated after citalopram treatment at a target dose of 40 mg once daily; furthermore, they observed a decrease in the overall Neuropsychiatric Inventory and Frontal Behavioral Inventory scores (84). The findings suggest that antidepressants may be beneficial in the treatment of neuropsychiatric and behavioral disturbances in FTD.

Behavioral disturbance (agitation or impulsivity) may also be controlled using atypical antipsychotics such as risperidone, olanzapine, and quetiapine. However, these medications could have side effects and increase the risk of mortality in patients with FTD (13, 85). In FTD patients with *C9orf72* expansion, antipsychotic drugs cause noticeable adverse effects, and the adverse effects could not be reversed in some patients even after drug withdrawal (86, 87). In summary, low doses of atypical antipsychotic drugs may be useful for managing behavioral disturbance (8), but such drugs should be used with caution in patients with FTD because of the risk of mortality associated with cardiac events and falls secondary to the side effects (88).

Cholinesterase inhibitors, such as donepezil, do not alleviate but can even exacerbate behavioral disturbance in patients with FTD (89). This is likely because cholinergic deficit may not contribute to the pathophysiology of FTD (90). Memantine, an *N*-methyl-d-aspartate (NMDA) antagonist, has been reported to have no benefits in alleviating or delaying the progression of FTD symptoms, but it is generally well-tolerated by patients (91, 92). In summary, cholinesterase inhibitors and NMDA antagonist have no clinical efficacy in the treatment of FTD, and they potentially have detrimental effects on cognitive performance and behavioral symptoms (91, 93). Therefore, preferred management options should be based on risk assessment, and nonpharmacological interventions and caregiver support are preferred for first-line interventions (93).

TAU-TARGETING THERAPEUTICS

Due to knowledge advancements in molecular biology, pathophysiology, and neuropathology, precision medicine could be applied in FTD treatment by targeting the underlying pathogenesis (85). Based on the knowledge of the pathological tau protein spreading through prion-like propagation, the prevention of transneuronal spreading of pathological abnormalities is potentially an effective therapeutic strategy (94, 95). Administering tau aggregation inhibitors (i.e., methylthioninium chloride), microtubule-stabilizing drugs, tau-targeted immunotherapy, and tau vaccines may be useful therapeutic approaches in patients with tau pathology (96, 97).

Multiple approaches are available for tau-targeting therapeutics. First, tau aggregation and the various tau species formed (monomers, oligomers, prefilaments, granules, fibrils, and insoluble aggregates) during aggregation are of interest for potential therapeutic intervention. Hence, tau aggregation inhibitors have been proven effective in various *in vitro* studies (98). A proprietary formulation of non-neuroleptic phenothiazine methylene blue (methylthioninium chloride), which is used to treat malaria (99), has risen in the ranks in clinical development in recent years. This compound readily crosses the blood-brain barrier and prevents tau aggregation *in vitro* as well as in cell and animal models (100, 101). Safety and efficacy in a randomized, double-blind, placebo-controlled, multinational, and parallel-group clinical trial was demonstrated in 220 patients with bvFTD after 12 months of oral treatment; the results are yet to be published (74). Clarifying the efficacy of tau aggregation inhibitors *in vivo* is critical for preventing cognitive decline.

Second, microtubule stabilizers may be used as FTLD-tau therapeutic agents. Detachment of tau from microtubules leads to the loss of normal microtubule-stabilizing function, resulting in axonal transport defects and synaptic dysfunction. Davunetide—an eight-amino-acid peptide that arises from an activity-dependent neuroprotective protein-exerted substantial effects on behavior and cognition in tau-transgenic mice (102). In addition, intranasal or intravenous administration of davunetide established the safety and tolerability profile of davunetide in patients with mild cognitive impairment (103). However, whether microtubule destabilization is directly related to tau toxicity in tauopathies remains unclear. No therapeutic effect of davunetide for PSP treatment was detected in a double-blind, placebo-controlled, randomized phase II/III clinical trial (104).

Third, various anti-tau immunotherapy strategies have been successfully tested, suggesting that such strategies could be feasible options for clearing toxic protein species in tauopathies (105). Targeting abnormally phosphorylated tau epitopes (or pathologically relevant conformational epitopes) may be favorable for inducing antibody responses that promote tau clearance, as suggested by evidence found in animal models (106) The humanized anti-tau monoclonal antibody named ABBV-8E12 is also available for PSP treatment. A satisfactory safety and tolerability profile for ABBV-8E12 was demonstrated in a placebo-controlled, double-blind, phase I single-ascending-dose trial of 30 patients with PSP (107). Finally, modulating tau phosphorylation and targeting other posttranslational tau modifications (i.e., tau acetylation inhibitors) are also potential therapeutic strategies for FTLD-tau and other tauopathies (74). However, the current consensus is that tau-centric targeted treatment has no marked effect on long-term clinical outcomes (108, 109); further research is required to elucidate the potential roles of such therapies in treating FTD.

Other targets for therapy include disrupting the downstream effects of *C9orf72* and *GRN* mutations. An approach that entails developing antisense oligonucleotides to reduce the concentrations of potentially toxic *C9orf72* mRNAs has been applied to FTD patients (110, 111). This approach has also been implicated in the reduction of the total amount of pathological tau species (112). Because *GRN* mutation is related to progranulin haploinsufficiency and reduced progranulin concentrations, studies are attempting to adopt molecular approaches to prevent the reduction of progranulin concentrations and instead increase progranulin concentrations; such approaches include applying the histone deacetylase inhibitor suberoylanilide hydroxamic acid, which enhances progranulin transcription and alkalizing compounds that stimulate progranulin production (113, 114). Collectively, advances in the understanding of genetic mutations causing FTD have created new potential therapeutic targets for the development of effective disease-modifying drugs (85). These findings may enable physicians to develop precision medicine for the treatment of FTD patients with *C9orf72, MAPT, or GRN* mutations at a single-patient levels (10, 115).

Future Direction- Treatment Through Personalized Medicine

The implication of precision medicine is to enable physicians to identify highly selective and effective treatments with relatively few side effects for patients with specific illness. Currently, precision medicine is applied to FTD diagnosis and treatment. Based on advances in neuroimaging and genomic research that has explored underlying genetic risk variants and cerebral structural and functional change in order to determine specific molecular pathways and pathophysiological processes, precision medicine is currently applied in clinical trials; such trials focus on subgroups of individuals and the development of therapeutic targets with known genetic risk for FTD (116). For example, in patients with clinical diagnosis of bvFTD, tau-targeting therapeutics (e.g., tau aggregation inhibitors) may be administered in those with suspected FTLD-tau pathology. On the other hand, in bvFTD patients with suspected FTLD-TDP pathology, progranulin -related therapies may be a viable treatment for those with *GRN* mutation. Likewise, for those with *C9orf72* repeat expansions, candidate antisense therapeutics could be used to reduce C9ORF72 expression. However, this is only the beginning of the precision medicine approach targeting the clinical process and treatment response of FTD. Collaboration among parents, family caregivers, and professionals (e.g., clinicians, scientists, and medical technologists) is crucial for identifying the pathological processes underlying FTD and for developing new interventions for successful application of precision medicine.

AUTHOR CONTRIBUTIONS

All authors listed have made a substantial, direct and intellectual contribution to the work, and approved it for publication.

FUNDING

This research was supported by V108B-009, MOST 107-2634-F-010-001, MOST 107-2420-H-010 -001, MOST 104-2218-E-010-007-MY3, and NHRI-EX106-10611EI.

ACKNOWLEDGMENTS

The authors acknowledge the support received from the MRI Core Laboratory of National Yang-Ming University, Taiwan. M-NL enormously grateful to the UCSF Memory and Aging Center to offer training for the clinical assessment of frontotemporal dementia.

REFERENCES

1. Vieira RT, Caixeta L, Machado S, Silva AC, Nardi AE, Arias-Carrion O, et al. Epidemiology of early-onset dementia: a review of the literature. *Clin Pract Epidemiol Ment Health* (2013) 9:88–95. doi: 10.2174/1745017901309010088
2. Pick A. Über die Beziehungen der senilen Hirnatrophie zur Aphasie. *Prager Med Wochenschr.* (1892) 17:165–67.
3. Alzheimer A. Über eigenartige Krankheitsfälle der späteren Alters. *Z Gesamte Neurol Psychiatr.* (1911) 4:356–85.
4. Mesulam MM. Primary progressive aphasia. *Ann Neurol.* (2001) 49:425–32. doi: 10.1002/ana.91
5. Rascovsky K, Hodges JR, Knopman D, Mendez MF, Kramer JH, Neuhaus J, et al. Sensitivity of revised diagnostic criteria for the behavioural variant of frontotemporal dementia. *Brain* (2011) 134(Pt 9):2456–77. doi: 10.1093/brain/awr179
6. Gorno-Tempini ML, Hillis AE, Weintraub S, Kertesz A, Mendez M, Cappa SF, et al. Classification of primary progressive aphasia and its variants. *Neurology* (2011) 76:1006–14. doi: 10.1212/WNL.0b013e31821103e6
7. Elahi FM, Miller BL. A clinicopathological approach to the diagnosis of dementia. *Nat Rev Neurol.* (2017) 13:457–76. doi: 10.1038/nrneurol.2017.96
8. Bang J, Spina S, Miller BL. Frontotemporal dementia. *Lancet* (2015) 386:1672–82. doi: 10.1016/S0140-6736(15)00461-4
9. Olney NT, Spina S, Miller BL. Frontotemporal dementia. *Neurol Clin.* (2017) 35:339–74. doi: 10.1016/j.ncl.2017.01.008
10. Gordon E, Rohrer JD, Fox NC. Advances in neuroimaging in frontotemporal dementia. *J Neurochem.* (2016) 138(Suppl. 1):193–210. doi: 10.1111/jnc.13656
11. Irwin DJ, Cairns NJ, Grossman M, McMillan CT, Lee EB, Van Deerlin VM, et al. Frontotemporal lobar degeneration: defining phenotypic diversity through personalized medicine. *Acta Neuropathol.* (2015) 129:469–91. doi: 10.1007/s00401-014-1380-1
12. Forman MS, Farmer J, Johnson JK, Clark CM, Arnold SE, Coslett HB, et al. Frontotemporal dementia: clinicopathological correlations. *Ann Neurol.* (2006) 59:952–62. doi: 10.1002/ana.20873
13. Young JJ, Lavakumar M, Tampi D, Balachandran S, Tampi RR. Frontotemporal dementia: latest evidence and clinical implications. *Ther Adv Psychopharmacol.* (2018) 8:33–48. doi: 10.1177/2045125317739818
14. Rogalski E, Cobia D, Martersteck A, Rademaker A, Wieneke C, Weintraub S, et al. Asymmetry of cortical decline in subtypes of primary progressive aphasia. *Neurology* (2014) 83:1184–91. doi: 10.1212/WNL.0000000000000824
15. Garcin E, Lillo P, Hornberger M, Piguet O, Dawson K, Nestor PJ, et al. Determinants of survival in behavioral variant frontotemporal dementia. *Neurology* (2009) 73:1656–61. doi: 10.1212/WNL.0b013e3181c1dee7
16. Rankin KP, Santos-Modesitt W, Kramer JH, Pavlic D, Beckman V, Miller BL. Spontaneous social behaviors discriminate behavioral dementias from psychiatric disorders and other dementias. *J Clin Psychiatry* (2008) 69:60–73. doi: 10.4088/JCP.v69n0109
17. Velakoulis D, Walterfang M, Mocellin R, Pantelis C, McLean C. Frontotemporal dementia presenting as schizophrenia-like psychosis in young people: clinicopathological series and review of cases. *Br J Psychiatry* (2009) 194:298–305. doi: 10.1192/bjp.bp.108.057034
18. Sha SJ, Takada LT, Rankin KP, Yokoyama JS, Rutherford NJ, Fong JC, et al. Frontotemporal dementia due to C9ORF72 mutations: clinical and imaging features. *Neurology* (2012) 79:1002–11. doi: 10.1212/WNL.0b013e318268452e
19. Gorno-Tempini ML, Brambati SM, Ginex V, Ogar J, Dronkers NF, Marcone A, et al. The logopenic/phonological variant of primary progressive aphasia. *Neurology* (2008) 71:1227–34. doi: 10.1212/01.wnl.0000320506.79811.da
20. Kramer JH, Jurik J, Sha SJ, Rankin KP, Rosen HJ, Johnson JK, et al. Distinctive neuropsychological patterns in frontotemporal dementia, semantic dementia, and Alzheimer disease. *Cogn Behav Neurol.* (2003) 16:211–8. doi: 10.1097/00146965-200312000-00002
21. Josephs KA, Duffy JR, Strand EA, Whitwell JL, Layton KF, Parisi JE, et al. Clinicopathological and imaging correlates of progressive aphasia and apraxia of speech. *Brain* (2006) 129(Pt 6):1385–98. doi: 10.1093/brain/awl078
22. Burrell JR, Kiernan MC, Vucic S, Hodges JR. Motor neuron dysfunction in frontotemporal dementia. *Brain* (2011) 134(Pt 9):2582–94. doi: 10.1093/brain/awr195
23. Le Ber I, Guedj E, Gabelle A, Verpillat P, Volteau M, Thomas-Anterion C, et al. Demographic, neurological and behavioural characteristics and brain perfusion SPECT in frontal variant of frontotemporal dementia. *Brain* (2006) 129(Pt 11):3051–65. doi: 10.1093/brain/awl288
24. Armstrong MJ, Litvan I, Lang AE, Bak TH, Bhatia KP, Borroni B, et al. Criteria for the diagnosis of corticobasal degeneration. *Neurology* (2013) 80:496–503. doi: 10.1212/WNL.0b013e31827f0fd1
25. Hoglinger GU, Respondek G, Stamelou M, Kurz C, Josephs KA, Lang AE, et al. Clinical diagnosis of progressive supranuclear palsy: the movement disorder society criteria. *Mov Disord.* (2017) 32:853–64. doi: 10.1002/mds.26987
26. Litvan I, Agid Y, Calne D, Campbell G, Dubois B, Duvoisin RC, et al. Clinical research criteria for the diagnosis of progressive supranuclear palsy (Steele-Richardson-Olszewski syndrome): report of the NINDS-SPSP international workshop. *Neurology* (1996) 47:1–9. doi: 10.1212/WNL.47.1.1
27. Rosen HJ, Allison SC, Schauer GF, Gorno-Tempini ML, Weiner MW, Miller BL. Neuroanatomical correlates of behavioural disorders in dementia. *Brain* (2005) 128(Pt 11):2612–25. doi: 10.1093/brain/awh628
28. Seeley WW, Crawford R, Rascovsky K, Kramer JH, Weiner M, Miller BL, et al. Frontal paralimbic network atrophy in very mild behavioral variant frontotemporal dementia. *Arch Neurol.* (2008) 65:249–55. doi: 10.1001/archneurol.2007.38
29. Diehl-Schmid J, Onur OA, Kuhn J, Gruppe T, Drzezga A. Imaging frontotemporal lobar degeneration. *Curr Neurol Neurosci Rep.* (2014) 14:489. doi: 10.1007/s11910-014-0489-x
30. Seeley WW, Bauer AM, Miller BL, Gorno-Tempini ML, Kramer JH, Weiner M, et al. The natural history of temporal variant frontotemporal dementia. *Neurology* (2005) 64:1384–90. doi: 10.1212/01.WNL.0000158425.46019.5C
31. Lam BY, Halliday GM, Irish M, Hodges JR, Piguet O. Longitudinal white matter changes in frontotemporal dementia subtypes. *Hum Brain Mapp.* (2014) 35:3547–57. doi: 10.1002/hbm.22420
32. Tu S, Leyton CE, Hodges JR, Piguet O, Hornberger M. Divergent longitudinal propagation of white matter degradation in logopenic and semantic variants of primary progressive aphasia. *J Alzheimers Dis.* (2016) 49:853–61. doi: 10.3233/JAD-150626
33. Thompson SA, Patterson K, Hodges JR. Left/right asymmetry of atrophy in semantic dementia: behavioral-cognitive implications. *Neurology* (2003) 61:1196–203. doi: 10.1212/01.WNL.0000091868.28557.B8
34. Chan D, Anderson V, Pijnenburg Y, Whitwell J, Barnes J, Scahill R, et al. The clinical profile of right temporal lobe atrophy. *Brain* (2009) 132(Pt 5):1287–98. doi: 10.1093/brain/awp037
35. Gorno-Tempini ML, Dronkers NF, Rankin KP, Ogar JM, Phengrasamy L, Rosen HJ, et al. Cognition and anatomy in three variants of primary progressive aphasia. *Ann Neurol.* (2004) 55:335–46. doi 10.1002/ana.10825
36. Galantucci S, Tartaglia MC, Wilson SM, Henry ML, Filippi M, Agosta F, et al. White matter damage in primary progressive aphasias: a diffusion tensor tractography study. *Brain* (2011) 134(Pt 10):3011–29. doi: 10.1093/brain/awr099
37. Struyfs H, Niemantsverdriet E, Goossens J, Fransen E, Martin JJ, De Deyn PP, et al. Cerebrospinal fluid P-Tau181P: biomarker for improved differential dementia diagnosis. *Front Neurol.* (2015) 6:138. doi: 10.3389/fneur.2015.00138
38. Josephs KA, Hodges JR, Snowden JS, Mackenzie IR, Neumann M, Mann DM, et al. Neuropathological background of phenotypical variability in frontotemporal dementia. *Acta Neuropathol.* (2011) 122:137–53. doi: 10.1007/s00401-011-0839-6
39. Lee SE, Rabinovici GD, Mayo MC, Wilson SM, Seeley WW, DeArmond SJ, et al. Clinicopathological correlations in corticobasal degeneration. *Ann Neurol.* (2011) 70:327–40. doi: 10.1002/ana.22424
40. Bhardwaj A, Myers MP, Buratti E, Baralle FE. Characterizing TDP-43 interaction with its RNA targets. *Nucleic Acids Res.* (2013) 41:5062–74. doi: 10.1093/nar/gkt189
41. Neumann M, Sampathu DM, Kwong LK, Truax AC, Micsenyi MC, Chou TT, et al. Ubiquitinated TDP-43 in frontotemporal lobar

degeneration and amyotrophic lateral sclerosis. *Science* (2006) 314:130–3. doi: 10.1126/science.1134108
42. Lee EB, Lee VM, Trojanowski JQ. Gains or losses: molecular mechanisms of TDP43-mediated neurodegeneration. *Nat Rev Neurosci.* (2011) 13:38–50. doi: 10.1038/nrn3121
43. Mackenzie IR, Munoz DG, Kusaka H, Yokota O, Ishihara K, Roeber S, et al. Distinct pathological subtypes of FTLD-FUS. *Acta Neuropathol.* (2011) 121:207–18. doi: 10.1007/s00401-010-0764-0
44. Riedl L, Mackenzie IR, Forstl H, Kurz A, Diehl-Schmid J. Frontotemporal lobar degeneration: current perspectives. *Neuropsychiatr Dis Treat.* (2014) 10:297–310. doi: 10.2147/NDT.S38706
45. Rohrer JD, Guerreiro R, Vandrovcova J, Uphill J, Reiman D, Beck J, et al. The heritability and genetics of frontotemporal lobar degeneration. *Neurology* (2009) 73:1451–6. doi: 10.1212/WNL.0b013e3181bf997a
46. Rademakers R, Neumann M, Mackenzie IR. Advances in understanding the molecular basis of frontotemporal dementia. *Nat Rev Neurol.* (2012) 8:423–34. doi: 10.1038/nrneurol.2012.117
47. DeJesus-Hernandez M, Mackenzie IR, Boeve BF, Boxer AL, Baker M, Rutherford NJ, et al. Expanded GGGGCC hexanucleotide repeat in noncoding region of C9ORF72 causes chromosome 9p-linked FTD and ALS. *Neuron* (2011) 72:245–56. doi: 10.1016/j.neuron.2011.09.011
48. Hutton M, Lendon CL, Rizzu P, Baker M, Froelich S, Houlden H, et al. Association of missense and 5'-splice-site mutations in tau with the inherited dementia FTDP-17. *Nature* (1998) 393:702–5. doi: 10.1038/31508
49. Ng AS. Genetics of frontotemporal dementia in Asia: advancing knowledge through collaboration. *Neurology* (2015) 85:2060–2. doi: 10.1212/WNL.0000000000002045
50. Boeve BF, Hutton M. Refining frontotemporal dementia with parkinsonism linked to chromosome 17: introducing FTDP-17 (MAPT) and FTDP-17 (PGRN). *Arch Neurol.* (2008) 65:460–4. doi: 10.1001/archneur.65.4.460
51. Ghetti B, Oblak AL, Boeve BF, Johnson KA, Dickerson BC, Goedert M. Invited review: frontotemporal dementia caused by microtubule-associated protein tau gene (MAPT) mutations: a chameleon for neuropathology and neuroimaging. *Neuropathol Appl Neurobiol.* (2015) 41:24–46. doi: 10.1111/nan.12213
52. Whitwell JL, Jack CR Jr, Boeve BF, Senjem ML, Baker M, Ivnik RJ, et al. Atrophy patterns in IVS10+16, IVS10+3, N279K, S305N, P301L, and V337M MAPT mutations. *Neurology* (2009) 73:1058–65. doi: 10.1212/WNL.0b013e3181b9c8b9
53. Renton AE, Majounie E, Waite A, Simon-Sanchez J, Rollinson S, Gibbs JR, et al. A hexanucleotide repeat expansion in C9ORF72 is the cause of chromosome 9p21-linked ALS-FTD. *Neuron* (2011) 72:257–68. doi: 10.1016/j.neuron.2011.09.010
54. Loy CT, Schofield PR, Turner AM, Kwok JB. Genetics of dementia. *Lancet* (2014) 383:828–40. doi: 10.1016/S0140-6736(13)60630-3
55. Snowden JS, Rollinson S, Thompson JC, Harris JM, Stopford CL, Richardson AM, et al. Distinct clinical and pathological characteristics of frontotemporal dementia associated with C9ORF72 mutations. *Brain* (2012) 135(Pt 3):693–708. doi: 10.1093/brain/awr355
56. Floeter MK, Gendron TF. Biomarkers for amyotrophic lateral sclerosis and frontotemporal dementia associated with hexanucleotide expansion mutations in C9orf72. *Front Neurol.* (2018) 9:1063. doi: 10.3389/fneur.2018.01063
57. Irwin DJ, McMillan CT, Brettschneider J, Libon DJ, Powers J, Rascovsky K, et al. Cognitive decline and reduced survival in C9orf72 expansion frontotemporal degeneration and amyotrophic lateral sclerosis. *J Neurol Neurosurg Psychiatry* (2013) 84:163–9. doi: 10.1136/jnnp-2012-303507
58. Toh H, Chitramuthu BP, Bennett HP, Bateman A. Structure, function, and mechanism of progranulin; the brain and beyond. *J Mol Neurosci.* (2011) 45:538–48. doi: 10.1007/s12031-011-9569-4
59. Shankaran SS, Capell A, Hruscha AT, Fellerer K, Neumann M, Schmid B, et al. Missense mutations in the progranulin gene linked to frontotemporal lobar degeneration with ubiquitin-immunoreactive inclusions reduce progranulin production and secretion. *J Biol Chem.* (2008) 283:1744–53. doi: 10.1074/jbc.M705115200
60. Gass J, Cannon A, Mackenzie IR, Boeve B, Baker M, Adamson J, et al. Mutations in progranulin are a major cause of ubiquitin-positive frontotemporal lobar degeneration. *Hum Mol Genet.* (2006) 15:2988–3001. doi: 10.1093/hmg/ddl241
61. Mackenzie IR, Neumann M. Molecular neuropathology of frontotemporal dementia: insights into disease mechanisms from postmortem studies. *J Neurochem.* (2016) 138 (Suppl 1):54–70. doi: 10.1111/jnc.13588
62. Rohrer JD, Ridgway GR, Modat M, Ourselin S, Mead S, Fox NC, et al. Distinct profiles of brain atrophy in frontotemporal lobar degeneration caused by progranulin and tau mutations. *Neuroimage* (2010) 53:1070–6. doi: 10.1016/j.neuroimage.2009.12.088
63. McCluskey L, Vandriel S, Elman L, Van Deerlin VM, Powers J, Boller A, et al. ALS-Plus syndrome: non-pyramidal features in a large ALS cohort. *J Neurol Sci.* (2014) 345:118–24. doi: 10.1016/j.jns.2014.07.022
64. Boxer AL, Gold M, Huey E, Hu WT, Rosen H, Kramer J, et al. The advantages of frontotemporal degeneration drug development (part 2 of frontotemporal degeneration: the next therapeutic frontier). *Alzheimers Dement.* (2013) 9:189–98. doi: 10.1016/j.jalz.2012.03.003
65. Jack CR Jr, Bennett DA, Blennow K, Carrillo MC, Dunn B, Haeberlein SB, et al. NIA-AA research framework: toward a biological definition of Alzheimer's disease. *Alzheimers Dement.* (2018) 14:535–62. doi: 10.1016/j.jalz.2018.02.018
66. Irwin DJ, Trojanowski JQ, Grossman M. Cerebrospinal fluid biomarkers for differentiation of frontotemporal lobar degeneration from Alzheimer's disease. *Front Aging Neurosci.* (2013) 5:6. doi: 10.3389/fnagi.2013.00006
67. Irwin DJ, McMillan CT, Toledo JB, Arnold SE, Shaw LM, Wang LS, et al. Comparison of cerebrospinal fluid levels of tau and Abeta 1-42 in Alzheimer disease and frontotemporal degeneration using 2 analytical platforms. *Arch Neurol.* (2012) 69:1018–25. doi: 10.1001/archneurol.2012.26
68. Kortvelyessy P, Heinze HJ, Prudlo J, Bittner D. CSF biomarkers of neurodegeneration in progressive non-fluent aphasia and other forms of frontotemporal dementia: clues for pathomechanisms? *Front Neurol.* (2018) 9:504. doi: 10.3389/fneur.2018.00504
69. Scherling CS, Hall T, Berisha F, Klepac K, Karydas A, Coppola G, et al. Cerebrospinal fluid neurofilament concentration reflects disease severity in frontotemporal degeneration. *Ann Neurol.* (2014) 75:116–26. doi: 10.1002/ana.24052
70. Danev SI, St Stoyanov D. Early noninvasive diagnosis of neurodegenerative diseases. *Folia Med.* (2010) 52:5–13. doi: 10.2478/v10153-010-0041-y
71. Zerr I, Kallenberg K, Summers DM, Romero C, Taratuto A, Heinemann U, et al. Updated clinical diagnostic criteria for sporadic Creutzfeldt-Jakob disease. *Brain* (2009) 132(Pt 10):2659–68. doi: 10.1093/brain/awp191
72. Vitali P, Maccagnano E, Caverzasi E, Henry RG, Haman A, Torres-Chae C, et al. Diffusion-weighted MRI hyperintensity patterns differentiate CJD from other rapid dementias. *Neurology* (2011) 76:1711–9. doi: 10.1212/WNL.0b013e31821a4439
73. Riemenschneider M, Wagenpfeil S, Vanderstichele H, Otto M, Wiltfang J, Kretzschmar H, et al. Phospho-tau/total tau ratio in cerebrospinal fluid discriminates Creutzfeldt-Jakob disease from other dementias. *Mol Psychiatry* (2003) 8:343–7. doi: 10.1038/sj.mp.4001220
74. Medina M. An Overview on the clinical development of tau-based therapeutics. *Int J Mol Sci.* (2018) 19:E1160. doi: 10.3390/ijms19041160
75. Hu WT, Watts K, Grossman M, Glass J, Lah JJ, Hales C, et al. Reduced CSF p-Tau181 to Tau ratio is a biomarker for FTLD-TDP. *Neurology* (2013) 81:1945–52. doi: 10.1212/01.wnl.0000436625.63650.27
76. Borroni B, Gardoni F, Parnetti L, Magno L, Malinverno M, Saggese E, et al. Pattern of Tau forms in CSF is altered in progressive supranuclear palsy. *Neurobiol Aging* (2009) 30:34–40. doi: 10.1016/j.neurobiolaging.2007.05.009
77. Teunissen CE, Elias N, Koel-Simmelink MJ, Durieux-Lu S, Malekzadeh A, Pham TV, et al. Novel diagnostic cerebrospinal fluid biomarkers for pathologic subtypes of frontotemporal dementia identified by proteomics. *Alzheimers Dement.* (2016) 2:86–94. doi: 10.1016/j.dadm.2015.12.004
78. Brendel M, Yousefi BH, Blume T, Herz M, Focke C, Deussing M, et al. Comparison of F-T807 and F-THK5117 PET in a mouse model of tau pathology. *Front Aging Neurosci.* (2018) 10:174. doi: 10.3389/fnagi.2018.00174
79. Goedert M, Yamaguchi Y, Mishra SK, Higuchi M, Sahara N. Tau Filaments and the development of positron emission tomography Tracers. *Front Neurol.* (2018) 9:70. doi: 10.3389/fneur.2018.00070

80. Dopper EG, Rombouts SA, Jiskoot LC, den Heijer T, de Graaf JR, de Koning I, et al. Structural and functional brain connectivity in presymptomatic familial frontotemporal dementia. *Neurology* (2014) 83:e19–26. doi: 10.1212/WNL.0000000000000583
81. Lee SE, Khazenzon AM, Trujillo AJ, Guo CC, Yokoyama JS, Sha SJ, et al. Altered network connectivity in frontotemporal dementia with C9orf72 hexanucleotide repeat expansion. *Brain* (2014) 137(Pt 11):3047–60. doi: 10.1093/brain/awu248
82. McMillan CT, Toledo JB, Avants BB, Cook PA, Wood EM, Suh E, et al. Genetic and neuroanatomic associations in sporadic frontotemporal lobar degeneration. *Neurobiol Aging* (2014) 35:1473–82. doi: 10.1016/j.neurobiolaging.2013.11.029
83. Irwin DJ, McMillan CT, Suh E, Powers J, Rascovsky K, Wood EM, et al. Myelin oligodendrocyte basic protein and prognosis in behavioral-variant frontotemporal dementia. *Neurology* (2014) 83:502–9. doi: 10.1212/WNL.0000000000000668
84. Herrmann N, Black SE, Chow T, Cappell J, Tang-Wai DF, Lanctot KL. Serotonergic function and treatment of behavioral and psychological symptoms of frontotemporal dementia. *Am J Geriatr Psychiatry* (2012) 20:789–97. doi: 10.1097/JGP.0b013e31823033f3
85. Tsai RM, Boxer AL. Therapy and clinical trials in frontotemporal dementia: past, present, and future. *J Neurochem.* (2016) 138 (Suppl. 1):211–21. doi: 10.1111/jnc.13640
86. Landqvist Waldo M, Gustafson L, Nilsson K, Traynor BJ, Renton AE, Englund E, et al. Frontotemporal dementia with a C9ORF72 expansion in a Swedish family: clinical and neuropathological characteristics. *Am J Neurodegener Dis.* (2013) 2:276–86.
87. Ducharme S, Bajestan S, Dickerson BC, Voon V. Psychiatric presentations of C9orf72 mutation: what are the diagnostic implications for clinicians? *J Neuropsychiatry Clin Neurosci.* (2017) 29:195–205. doi: 10.1176/appi.neuropsych.16090168
88. Steinberg M, Lyketsos CG. Atypical antipsychotic use in patients with dementia: managing safety concerns. *Am J Psychiatry* (2012) 169:900–6. doi: 10.1176/appi.ajp.2012.12030342
89. Mendez MF, Shapira JS, McMurtray A, Licht E. Preliminary findings: behavioral worsening on donepezil in patients with frontotemporal dementia. *Am J Geriatr Psychiatry* (2007) 15:84–7. doi: 10.1097/01.JGP.0000231744.69631.33
90. Chow TW. Treatment approaches to symptoms associated with frontotemporal degeneration. *Curr Psychiatry Rep.* (2005) 7:376–80. doi: 10.1007/s11920-005-0040-5
91. Vercelletto M, Boutoleau-Bretonniere C, Volteau C, Puel M, Auriacombe S, Sarazin M, et al. Memantine in behavioral variant frontotemporal dementia: negative results. *J Alzheimers Dis.* (2011) 23:749–59. doi: 10.3233/JAD-2010-101632
92. Boxer AL, Knopman DS, Kaufer DI, Grossman M, Onyike C, Graf-Radford N, et al. Memantine in patients with frontotemporal lobar degeneration: a multicentre, randomised, double-blind, placebo-controlled trial. *Lancet Neurol.* (2013) 12:149–56. doi: 10.1016/S1474-4422(12)70320-4
93. Mocellin R, Scholes A, Walterfang M, Looi JC, Velakoulis D. Clinical update on frontotemporal dementia: diagnosis and treatment. *Australas Psychiatry* (2015) 23:131–7. doi: 10.1177/1039856215582276
94. Sanders DW, Kaufman SK, DeVos SL, Sharma AM, Mirbaha H, Li A, et al. Distinct tau prion strains propagate in cells and mice and define different tauopathies. *Neuron* (2014) 82:1271–88. doi: 10.1016/j.neuron.2014.04.047
95. Yanamandra K, Kfoury N, Jiang H, Mahan TE, Ma S, Maloney SE, et al. Anti-tau antibodies that block tau aggregate seeding *in vitro* markedly decrease pathology and improve cognition *in vivo*. *Neuron* (2013) 80:402–14. doi: 10.1016/j.neuron.2013.07.046
96. Wischik CM, Harrington CR, Storey JM. Tau-aggregation inhibitor therapy for Alzheimer's disease. *Biochem Pharmacol.* (2014) 88:529–39. doi: 10.1016/j.bcp.2013.12.008
97. Coughlin D, Irwin DJ. Emerging diagnostic and therapeutic strategies for tauopathies. *Curr Neurol Neurosci Rep.* (2017) 17:72. doi: 10.1007/s11910-017-0779-1
98. Mancini RS, Wang Y, Weaver DF. Phenylindanes in brewed coffee inhibit amyloid-beta and tau aggregation. *Front Neurosci.* (2018) 12:735. doi: 10.3389/fnins.2018.00735
99. Buchholz K, Schirmer RH, Eubel JK, Akoachere MB, Dandekar T, Becker K, et al. Interactions of methylene blue with human disulfide reductases and their orthologues from Plasmodium falciparum. *Antimicrob Agents Chemother.* (2008) 52:183–91. doi: 10.1128/AAC.00773-07
100. Heard DS, Tuttle CSL, Lautenschlager NT, Maier AB. Repurposing proteostasis-modifying drugs to prevent or treat age-related dementia: a systematic review. *Front Physiol.* (2018) 9:1520. doi: 10.3389/fphys.2018.01520
101. Wischik CM, Edwards PC, Lai RY, Roth M, Harrington CR. Selective inhibition of Alzheimer disease-like tau aggregation by phenothiazines. *Proc Natl Acad Sci USA.* (1996) 93:11213–8. doi: 10.1073/pnas.93.20.11213
102. Matsuoka Y, Jouroukhin Y, Gray AJ, Ma L, Hirata-Fukae C, Li HF, et al. A neuronal microtubule-interacting agent, NAPVSIPQ, reduces tau pathology and enhances cognitive function in a mouse model of Alzheimer's disease. *J Pharmacol Exp Ther.* (2008) 325:146–53. doi: 10.1124/jpet.107.130526
103. Morimoto BH, Schmechel D, Hirman J, Blackwell A, Keith J, Gold M. A double-blind, placebo-controlled, ascending-dose, randomized study to evaluate the safety, tolerability and effects on cognition of AL-108 after 12 weeks of intranasal administration in subjects with mild cognitive impairment. *Dement Geriatr Cogn Disord.* (2013) 35:325–36. doi: 10.1159/000348347
104. Boxer AL, Lang AE, Grossman M, Knopman DS, Miller BL, Schneider LS, et al. Davunetide in patients with progressive supranuclear palsy: a randomised, double-blind, placebo-controlled phase 2/3 trial. *Lancet Neurol.* (2014) 13:676–85. doi: 10.1016/S1474-4422(14)70088-2
105. Pedersen JT, Sigurdsson EM. Tau immunotherapy for Alzheimer's disease. *Trends Mol Med.* (2015) 21:394–402. doi: 10.1016/j.molmed.2015.03.003
106. Medina M, Avila J. New insights into the role of glycogen synthase kinase-3 in Alzheimer's disease. *Expert Opin Ther Targets* (2014) 18:69–77. doi: 10.1517/14728222.2013.843670
107. West T, Hu Y, Verghese PB, Bateman RJ, Braunstein JB, Fogelman I, et al. Preclinical and clinical development of ABBV-8E12, a humanized anti-tau antibody, for treatment of Alzheimer's disease and other tauopathies. *J Prev Alzheimers Dis.* (2017) 4:236–41. doi: 10.14283/jpad.2017.36
108. Panza F, Solfrizzi V, Seripa D, Imbimbo BP, Lozupone M, Santamato A, et al. Tau-centric targets and drugs in clinical development for the treatment of Alzheimer's disease. *Biomed Res Int.* (2016) 2016:3245935. doi: 10.1155/2016/3245935
109. O'Brien JT, Holmes C, Jones M, Jones R, Livingston G, McKeith I, et al. Clinical practice with anti-dementia drugs: a revised (third) consensus statement from the British Association for Psychopharmacology. *J Psychopharmacol.* (2017) 31:147–68. doi: 10.1177/0269881116680924
110. Lagier-Tourenne C, Baughn M, Rigo F, Sun S, Liu P, Li HR, et al. Targeted degradation of sense and antisense C9orf72 RNA foci as therapy for ALS and frontotemporal degeneration. *Proc Natl Acad Sci USA.* (2013) 110:E4530–9. doi: 10.1073/pnas.1318835110
111. Kramer NJ, Carlomagno Y, Zhang YJ, Almeida S, Cook CN, Gendron TF, et al. Spt4 selectively regulates the expression of C9orf72 sense and antisense mutant transcripts. *Science* (2016) 353:708–12. doi: 10.1126/science.aaf7791
112. DeVos SL, Goncharoff DK, Chen G, Kebodeaux CS, Yamada K, Stewart FR, et al. Antisense reduction of tau in adult mice protects against seizures. *J Neurosci.* (2013) 33:12887–97. doi: 10.1523/JNEUROSCI.2107-13.2013
113. Cenik B, Sephton CF, Dewey CM, Xian X, Wei S, Yu K, et al. Suberoylanilide hydroxamic acid (vorinostat) up-regulates progranulin transcription: rational therapeutic approach to frontotemporal dementia. *J Biol Chem.* (2011) 286:16101–8. doi: 10.1074/jbc.M110.193433
114. Capell A, Liebscher S, Fellerer K, Brouwers N, Willem M, Lammich S, et al. Rescue of progranulin deficiency associated with frontotemporal lobar

degeneration by alkalizing reagents and inhibition of vacuolar ATPase. *J Neurosci.* (2011) 31:1885–94. doi: 10.1523/JNEUROSCI.5757-10.2011

115. Whitwell JL, Weigand SD, Boeve BF, Senjem ML, Gunter JL, DeJesus-Hernandez M, et al. Neuroimaging signatures of frontotemporal dementia genetics: C9ORF72, tau, progranulin and sporadics. *Brain* (2012) 135(Pt 3):794–806. doi: 10.1093/brain/aws001

116. Alberici A, Archetti S, Pilotto A, Premi E, Cosseddu M, Bianchetti A, et al. Results from a pilot study on amiodarone administration in monogenic frontotemporal dementia with granulin mutation. *Neurol Sci.* (2014) 35:1215–9. doi: 10.1007/s10072-014-1683-y

14

Metabolic and Microbiota Measures as Peripheral Biomarkers in Major Depressive Disorder

*Rachael Horne[1] and Jane A. Foster[1,2]**

[1] Department of Psychiatry & Behavioural Neurosciences, McMaster University, Hamilton, ON, Canada, [2] Department of Psychiatry, St. Michael's Hospital, Toronto, ON, Canada

***Correspondence:**
Jane A. Foster
jfoster@mcmaster.ca*

Advances in understanding the role of the microbiome in physical and mental health are at the forefront of medical research and hold potential to have a direct impact on precision medicine approaches. In the past 7 years, we have studied the role of microbiota-brain communication on behavior in mouse models using germ-free mice, mice exposed to antibiotics, and healthy specific pathogen free mice. Through our work and that of others, we have seen an amazing increase in our knowledge of how bacteria signal to the brain and the implications this has for psychiatry. Gut microbiota composition and function are influenced both by genetics, age, sex, diet, life experiences, and many other factors of psychiatric and bodily disorders and thus may act as potential biomarkers of the gut-brain axis that could be used in psychiatry and co-morbid conditions. There is a particular need in major depressive disorder and other mental illness to identify biomarkers that can stratify patients into more homogeneous groups to provide better treatment and for development of new therapeutic approaches. Peripheral outcome measures of host-microbe bidirectional communication have significant translational value as biomarkers. Enabling stratification of clinical populations, based on individual biological differences, to predict treatment response to pharmacological and non-pharmacological interventions. Here we consider the links between co-morbid metabolic syndrome and depression, focusing on biomarkers including leptin and ghrelin in combination with assessing gut microbiota composition, as a potential tool to help identify individual differences in depressed population.

Keywords: gut-brain axis, microbiome, leptin, ghrelin, major depression (MDD)

Major depressive disorder (MDD) is a debilitating disorder that affects nearly 15% of the general population and accounts for the greatest disability burden of any disease (1). One of the major challenges in treating MDD is the lack of understanding of the underlying etiology of the disorder. The clinical heterogeneity observed in MDD makes it difficult to select the best treatment approach for an individual (2). Additionally, upwards of 60% of MDD patients will experience at least some form of treatment resistance over the course of the disease (3), with only one third of MDD suffers achieving remission even with optimal pharmacological and patient treatment (4). The onset and progression of depression is thought to result from a complex combination of genetic, environmental and neurochemical factors that differ considerably across patient populations such that the search for robust biomarkers to both characterize depression subtypes and predict treatment response is at the forefront of clinical psychiatry (5, 6).

Recent work over the last two decades has revealed the bidirectional communication between the central nervous system, enteric nervous system and the gastrointestinal tract, often referred to as the gut brain axis (7–12). Emerging evidence now supports the role of the gut microbiota in influencing behavior with specific links to MDD. The diverse population of the gut microbiota has been shown to be heterogeneous between individuals (13, 14), with dominate factors, such as diet (15), environment and host genetics (16–18) shaping the overall composition and function. Heterogeneity of depression has limited the success of efforts aimed at identifying clinical markers of treatment response and clinical subtypes. Treatment and diagnosis of MDD is also complicated by increasingly common comorbidities, resulting in another layer of heterogeneity in the MDD population. Therefore, the identification of robust biomarkers to both identify individual differences within the MDD population, as well as stratify patients into more homogenous subgroups is of critical importance. This approach is utilized by the Canadian Biomarker Integration Network in Depression (www.canbind.ca) that aims to shorten the time that it takes to match patients with the best treatment. By combining multiple molecular markers that can be measured in blood with clinical, imaging, or EEG researchers can identify and link biomarkers to clinical presentation and help predict treatment response (5).

Metabolic syndrome (MetS) is a well-documented in MDD patients, with the risk of MetS in depressed patient at 1.5 times higher than in the non-depressed population (19). Moreover, the prevalence of MetS is 58% higher in psychiatric patients than in the general population (20), with prominent anorexigenic and orexigenic hormones leptin and ghrelin identified to be associated with psychiatric disorders including schizophrenia, bipolar disorder and major depression (21–23). A role for the microbiome in metabolic syndrome has received attention, with studies demonstrating a role for gut microbiota in features of MetS, such as obesity, diabetes, dyslipidemia and hypertension (24, 25). Here we consider the literature related to leptin and ghrelin in MDD and how these molecular markers in combination with gut microbiota have potential to identify individual differences in patients and provide measures of the gut brain axis in MDD.

MICROBIOTA-BRAIN INTERACTIONS ARE IMPORTANT IN DEPRESSION

Research focused on the gut brain axis has gained momentum in recent years and garnered attention from both the scientific community, the public, and the media, with particular interest in understanding how microbes may influence mood. Accumulating evidence from preclinical work in rodents supports a connection between stress, microbiota, and stress-related behaviors (26–36), however, only a handful of studies have examined gut bacteria in individuals with major depressive disorder (7–9, 37–39). Using 16S rRNA gene sequencing, the composition of fecal microbiota in depressed patients was shown to be different from control samples (**Table 1**). The specific taxa differences observed in these studies varied, in part related to differences in sample size and analytical methods, but also related to the heterogeneity in the clinical populations recruited including age, BMI, smoking status, medication, clinical features, and severity of disease (8, 9, 37, 38). Inter-individual differences in microbiota composition in healthy individuals is ~90% (13, 14). Understanding how individual differences in microbiota influences individual differences in health and disease including MDD and other psychiatric disorders is needed.

The compositional data gained from utilizing 16S rRNA gene sequencing in the MDD population represents an accessible biomarker, that provides both compositional data and, with recent advances in bioinformatics, can contribute functional information (40). The potential therapeutic benefits of treatments that target the microbiome, including probiotic and prebiotic administration, have begun to gain creditability for the treatment of psychiatric disorders (41) and the term psychobiotics is commonly used to classify products, such as probiotics and prebiotics, that when given in adequate amounts produce positive psychological effects (42, 43). Several studies show a benefit of probiotic consumption in healthy individuals including improved mood (44), a beneficial effect on anxiety and depressive measures as well as reduced stress hormone levels (45). Less work has been conducted in MDD clinical populations (46), and work to date has not utilized gut-brain biomarkers to identify subgroups within MDD. Metabolism and metabolic markers are of interest in the microbiome field. Here we selected two well-known metabolic markers that have been well-studied in MDD populations and consider their potential as biomarkers in MDD.

LEPTIN AS A POTENTIAL BIOMARKER OF GUT-BRAIN INTERACTIONS IN MDD

Leptin is an adipocyte derived hormone, with a known role in regulating fat mass storage and energy homeostasis. Leptin circulates as a 16 kDa protein, where it crosses the blood brain barrier (BBB) and interacts with multiple regions of the brain including the hypothalamus and hippocampus (47, 48). Over the last decade there has been increasing evidence of leptin's role in regulating mood (23). Work in animal models has revealed a complex role of circulating leptin along with leptin's receptor (lepR) expression levels throughout the brain. Deletion of the lepR in the hippocampus of rats results in depressive behavior (49), as well as inhibits the behavioral effect of serotonin reuptake inhibitor fluoxetine (50). Animal models of chronic stress have been found to reduce circulating leptin, as well as reliably produce depressive behavior. Systematic injection of leptin has been found to have a dose dependent reduction in depressive behaviors in chronically stress mice (51, 52). A study aimed at exploring the relationship between obesity and depression found that, a combination of diet induced obesity and chronic unpredictable mild stress (CUMS) resulted in increased leptin levels but a decrease in LepR expression, along with depressive behaviors (53). The disparity in leptin serum level and receptor expression may be more representative of what occurs in an obese human and may be contributing to the comorbidity of obesity and MDD.

TABLE 1 | Bacterial taxa differences at the family and genus level observed in individuals with major depressive disorder.

References	Family	Genus
Differences in relative abundance		
Naseribafrouei et al. (38)	Lacnopiraceae (down)	*Alistipes* (up)
		Oscillibacter (up)
Jiang et al. (37)	Acidaminoccocaceae (up)	*Alistipes* (up)
Mothur metastats	Enterobacteriaceae (up)	*Blautia* (up)
	Fusobacteriaceae (up)	*Clostridibum XIX* (up)
	Porphyromonadaceae (up)	*Lachnospiacea* (up)
	Rikenellaceae (up)	*Megamonas* (up)
	Bacteroidaceae (down)	*Parabacteroides* (up)
	Erysipelotrichaceae (down)	*Parasutterella* (up)
	Lacnopiraceae (down)	*Phascolarctobacterium* (up)
	Prevotellaceae (down)	*Oscillibacter* (up)
	Ruminococcaceae (down)	*Roseburia* (up)
	Veillonellaceae (down)	*Bacteroides* (down)
		Dialister (down)
		Faecalibacterium (down)
		Prevotella (down)
		Ruminococcus (down)
Jiang et al. (37)	*Polphyromonadaceae* (up)	*Alistipes* (up)
LefSe LDA	*Eneterobacteriaceae* (up)	*Parabacteroides* (up)
Alpha leve = 0.05	*Rikenellaceae* (up)	*Butyricimonas* (up)
Effect size threshold = 2	*Erysipelotrichaceae* (up)	*Flavonifractor* (up)
	Peptostreptococcaceae (down)	*Haemophilus* (down)
	Pasterueliaceae (down)	*Dialister* (down)
	Ruminococcaceae (down)	*Faecalibacterium* (down)
		Escherichia shigella (down)
		Ruminococcus (down)
Kelly et al. (8)	Prevoellaceae (down)	*Prevotella* (down)
Mann-Whitney U test	Thermoanaerobacteriaceae (up)	*Dialister* (down)
FDR adjusted 10%		*Eggerthella* (up)
		Holdemania (up)
		Gelria (up)
		Turicibacter (up)
		Paraprevotella (up)
		Anaerofilum (up)
Lin et al. (9)		*Prevotella*
Wilcoxon's sign rank test		*Steptococcus*
		Clostridibum XIX
Zheng et al. (39)	Actinomycineae (up)	*Parvimonas* (up)
Random forest classifier	Coriobacterineae (up)	*Anerostipes* (up)
	Lactobacillaceae (up)	*Blautia* (up)
	Streptococcaceae (up)	*Dorea* (up)
	Clostridales incertae sedis XI (up)	*Lachnospiraceae incertae sedis* (up)
	Eubacteriaceae (up)	*Clostridium IV* (up)
	Lachnospiraceae (up)	*Alistipes* (down)
	Ruminococcaceae (up)	*Coprococcus* (down)
	Erysipelotrichaceae in certae sedis (up)	*Clostridium XlVa* (down)
	Bacteroidaceae (down)	*Phascolarctobacterium* (down)
	Rikenellaceae (down)	*Megamonas* (down)
	Lachnospiraceae (down)	*Lachnospiraceae incertae sedis* (down)
	Acidaminococcaceae (down)	*Roseburia* (down)
	Vellonellaceae (down)	*Faecalibacterium* (down)
	Sutterellaceae (down)	

Human studies examining leptin levels in MDD have been mixed, some finding elevated leptin in MDD (54, 55) while others finding decreased levels (56, 57). This may be due to the varying role of leptin in lean verse obese conditions but also represents how we expect a biomarker of individual differences to present in a clinical population. Under lean conditions leptin acts as an anti-obesity hormone, signaling through activation of leptin receptors at the hypothalamus to reduce feeding behavior (58). Obesity is characterized by an increase in circulating leptin and a decrease in leptin receptor expression, leading to leptin resistance and disrupted leptin signaling (59). Concurrently, alterations to appetite, as well as weight changes are known clinical features of MDD (2). Interestingly, two meta-analyses have found a significant association of elevated leptin with depression only when controlling for BMI (60, 61). There is also evidence to support the association between atypical features of depression, such as increase appetite and hyposomnia with elevated leptin levels (62, 63). A recent study aimed at identifying subgroups of depression, found that grouping unmedicated patients by increases or decreases in appetite revealed dramatic differences in metabolic signaling, immune signaling and functional brain activity differences (64). Leptin levels were significantly increased in MDD patients with increased appetite, compared to healthy controls or when compared to MDD individuals with decreased appetite, an observation that was not related to BMI (64). The increased appetite subgroup also had alteration to proinflammatory markers and decreases in orexigenic gut hormone ghrelin, suggesting that biological difference may contribute to differences in disease symptomology. Based on the work to date, leptin may be a useful biomarker in a particular subset of MDD patients and may aid in identifying individual differences.

Leptin levels are related to gut microbiota. The secretion of leptin by adipocytes is regulated by microbial-derived metabolites, specifically short-chain fatty acids (SCFA) that signal through GRP41/42 receptors (65). Studies have shown that the gut microbiota can influence leptin levels independent of food intake (66), and that prebiotic treatment can improve leptin sensitivity (67). Antibiotic use, which has been found as a risk factor for the development of depression has also been shown to reduce leptin levels in rodents (68). In line with the predicted relationship between bacterial populations and leptin levels, several studies have found that certain bacterial taxa correlate with circulating leptin levels. A study by Queipo-Ortuño et al. found that bacteria genera *Lactobacillus* and *Bifidobacterium* positively correlate with serum leptin levels, whereas *Clostridium, Bacteroides*, and *Prevotella* were negatively correlated. In a different study, obese and overweight pregnant women were found to have leptin levels that positively correlated with the abundance of the families Lachnospiraceae and Ruminococcaceae, highlighting the association between leptin levels and energy homeostasis (69). The impact of probiotic treatment on leptin levels within the context of depression has recently been evaluated (62). In mice, administration of *Pseudocatenulatum* reduced depressive behavior and improved leptin serum levels and receptor expression in the hippocampus and intestine of mice (59). Considering circulating leptin as a link to both MDD, metabolic disorders and the gut microbiota may advance its use as a biomarker to identify individual differences in MDD patients.

GHRELIN AS A POTENTIAL BIOMARKER OF GUT-BRAIN INTERACTIONS IN MDD

Ghrelin is a gut peptide hormone that is produced by cholinergic cells in the gastrointestinal tract found predominately in the stomach (70). Acylated ghrelin circulates throughout the body and crosses the BBB, where it interacts with acylated ghrelin receptors (GHSR1), expressed by the hypothalamus (71). GHSR1 is also expressed in the dentate gyrus of the hippocampus, CA2 and CA3 regions, substratum nigria and ventral tegmental area (72). Due to the wide spread expression of GHSR1, ghrelin has been shown to play a role, in energy homeostasis, eating behavior, sleeping behavior (73), cognition, reward mechanisms (74), and mood (75), all of which can be altered in MDD. As with leptin, a body of work now supports the role of ghrelin in regulating mood, with close links to depression (73, 76). Ghrelin has a role in response to acute stress in both animals and humans, with acute stress resulting in elevated ghrelin levels and activation of the hypothalamus-pituitary axis (HPA) (77, 78). Preclinical work has shown that ghrelin inhibited the release of serotonin (79), as well as increased serotonin turnover (80), providing evidence of it potential role in serotonin imbalance observed in MDD. Animal studies have found behavioral effects following cerebral injection of ghrelin including decreased anxiety and depressive behaviors (81). It is suggested that ghrelin acts as a survival mechanism when animals are exposed to acute stress, to induce feeding behavior. In support of this suggestion, a study in 2012 showed the elevated ghrelin after acute stress attenuated anxiety-like behaviors, whereas prolonged stress led to chronic increased ghrelin levels, dysregulation of HPA axis and serotonin signaling as well as increased depressive behaviors (78).

Attempts to associate ghrelin levels in humans with MDD has also shown mixed results, with older studies indicating a decrease in ghrelin levels (82) while newer studies are finding an elevation of ghrelin associated with MDD (83–85). Ghrelin has been predicted to alter a number of genes involved in depression with a ghrelin polymorphism found to be associated with the development of depression (86). Three previous studies have shown that ghrelin may act as a measure of treatment response, finding elevated ghrelin levels in MDD non-responders, and a decrease of serum ghrelin levels associated with response to treatment (85, 87, 88). Serum ghrelin has been recently shown to act as a persistent biomarker for chronic stress exposure in both rodents and humans (89) with exposure to chronic stressors resulting in elevated acyl-ghrelin levels for at least 130 days in rats and 4.5 years in adolescent humans. Indicating that those with elevated ghrelin and MDD, may have a chronic stressor as an underlying mechanism of disease progression. Exposure to both chronic and acute stress results in elevated circulating cortisol levels. The same study identified subgroups of MDD based on appetite and found elevated ghrelin and cortisol levels in MDD patients with decreased appetite (64). This finding indicates that in the depressed population elevated ghrelin may have roles outside of increasing eating behavior and may interact to influence the HPA axis resulting in elevated stress response. Furthermore, work by Algul et al. found both acylated and deacylated serum ghrelin level were elevated in MDD patients and increases in ghrelin concentration significantly correlated with disease severity (84).

Ghrelin is primarily produced in the gut, with previous work establishing the role of the vagus nerve in mediating the communication of the peptide to the brain (90). Due to the proximity of the gut microbiota to ghrelin's central location, work has begun to explore the relationship between the gut microbiota and ghrelin expression. Notably, germ-free mice have lower levels of circulating ghrelin, with levels increasing beyond conventional mice after a period of fasting (91). Additionally, serum ghrelin levels significantly negatively correlate to genera *Bifidobacterium, Lactobacillus*, and *B. coccoides-Eubacterium rectale* and positively correlate with *Bacteroides* and *Prevotella* in rodents (92). Treatment with prebiotics has been found to alter ghrelin levels, with lean and obese mice exhibiting a positive response in ghrelin following prebiotic treatment (93). Metabolism of prebiotics by gut bacteria leads to increased SCFAs and, ghrelin production has been found to be regulated by SCFA signaling (94, 95). Activation of the fatty acid receptor 3 by butyrate reduced serum ghrelin levels (94) however; a recent study identified the role of bacteria-derived acetate in activating the parasympathetic nervous system and increasing ghrelin secretion (95). Further, gastric infusion of acetate dramatically increases ghrelin concentrations in plasma, but the effects were lost in vagotomised mice (95), indicating potential bidirectional communication from the gut to the brain in the control of ghrelin secretion from cholinergic cells. Due to ghrelin's increasingly recognize role in mediate mood and potential biomarker status for MDD, along with its connection to the gut microbiota, it makes an optimal biomarker to identify treatment response to prebiotic and probiotic treatment in the MDD population.

IMPLICATION AND FUTURE DIRECTIONS

While much excitement has been recently focused on the role of the gut microbiota in psychiatric disorders, there is a need to gain a better understand clinical heterogeneity in depressed individuals. Research on gut the brain axis has been rapidly progressing, by examining the relationship between the gut microbiota and metabolic states in healthy and depressed individuals a better understanding of how microbes influence mood will be determine. As MDD commonly occurs with co-morbidities, it is important to evaluate how related factors contribute to disease development or progression. As the relationship between metabolic syndrome and depression is bilateral and suggested that the development of one often leads to the other (96) exploring metabolic endocrine signaling in the context of depression and gut microbiota will enable researchers and clinicians to gain a broader understanding of the underlying biological factors that may be contributing to MDD.

As neuroscientists, psychologists, and psychiatrists are starting to appreciate the importance of gut microbiota to mental health, there is a great opportunity to identify biomarkers associated with the gut-brain axis and thereby provide a better understanding of the aspects that may be modifiable with proper intervention in individuals with mental illness. By measuring: leptin and ghrelin levels, both within context of sex and BMI, and in conjunction with gut microbiota composition and MDD symptomology, researchers will be able to stratify the clinical population in more homogenous subgroups. The ability to identify a subgroup of the clinical MDD population based on metabolic status and gut microbiota composition would aid clinical trials to predict treatment response and for development of therapies that target the microbiome.

AUTHOR CONTRIBUTIONS

JF and RH developed the framework for the mini-review. RH wrote the manuscript, JF edited the manuscript. Both authors approved its submission.

FUNDING

This research was conducted as part of the Canadian Biomarker Integration Network in Depression (CAN-BIND), an Integrated Discovery Program supported by the Ontario Brain Institute, which is an independent non-profit corporation, funded partially by the Ontario Government. The opinions, results and conclusions are those of the authors and no endorsement by the Ontario Brain Institute is intended or should be inferred. Graduate stipend funding was provided by the Canadian Institutes of Health Research (CIHR).

REFERENCES

1. Kessler RC, Bromet EJ. The epidemiology of depression across cultures. *Annu Rev Public Health* (2013) 34:119–38. doi: 10.1146/annurev-publhealth-031912-114409
2. American Psychiatric Association. *Diagnostic and Statistical Manual of Mental Disorders*. 5th ed. Washington, DC (2013).
3. Fava M. Diagnosis and definition of treatment-resistant depression. *Biol Psychiatry* (2003) 53:649–59. doi: 10.1016/S0006-3223(03)00231-2
4. Gaynes BN, Warden D, Trivedi MH, Wisniewski SR, Fava M, Rush AJ. What did STAR*D teach us? results from a large-scale, practical, clinical trial for patients with depression. *Psychiatr Serv.* (2009) 60:1439–45. doi: 10.1176/ps.2009.60.11.1439
5. Lam RW, Milev R, Rotzinger S, Andreazza AC, Blier P, Brenner C, et al. Discovering biomarkers for antidepressant response: protocol from the Canadian biomarker integration network in depression (CAN-BIND) and clinical characteristics of the first patient cohort. *BMC Psychiatry* (2016) 16:105. doi: 10.1186/s12888-016-0785-x
6. Oquendo MA, McGrath P, Weissman MM. Biomarker studies and the future of personalized treatment for depression. *Depress Anxiety* (2014) 31:902–5. doi: 10.1002/da.22300
7. Aizawa E, Tsuji H, Asahara T, Takahashi T, Teraishi T, Yoshida S, et al. Possible association of Bifidobacterium and Lactobacillus in the gut microbiota of patients with major depressive disorder. *J Affect Disord.* (2016) 202:254–7. doi: 10.1016/j.jad.2016.05.038
8. Kelly JR, Borre Y, C OB, Patterson E, El Aidy S, Deane J, et al. Transferring the blues: Depression-associated gut microbiota induces neurobehavioural changes in the rat. *J Psychiatr Res.* (2016) 82:109–18. doi: 10.1016/j.jpsychires.2016.07.019
9. Lin P, Ding B, Feng C, Yin S, Zhang T, Qi X, et al. Prevotella and Klebsiella proportions in fecal microbial communities are potential characteristic parameters for patients with major depressive disorder. *J Affect Disord.* (2017) 207:300–4. doi: 10.1016/j.jad.2016.09.051
10. Lurie I, Yang YX, Haynes K, Mamtani R, Boursi B. Antibiotic exposure and the risk for depression, anxiety, or psychosis: a nested case-control study. *J Clin Psychiatry* (2015) 76:1522–8. doi: 10.4088/JCP.15m09961
11. Steenbergen L, Sellaro R, van Hemert S, Bosch JA, Colzato LS. A randomized controlled trial to test the effect of multispecies probiotics on cognitive reactivity to sad mood. *Brain Behav Immun.* (2015) 48:258–64. doi: 10.1016/j.bbi.2015.04.003
12. Tillisch K, Mayer EA, Gupta A, Gill Z, Brazeilles R, Le Neve B, et al. Brain structure and response to emotional stimuli as related to gut microbial profiles in healthy women. *Psychosom Med.* (2017) 79:905–13. doi: 10.1097/PSY.0000000000000493
13. Dorrestein PC, Mazmanian SK, Knight R. Finding the missing links among metabolites, microbes, and the host. *Immunity* (2014) 40:824–32. doi: 10.1016/j.immuni.2014.05.015
14. Ursell LK, Clemente JC, Rideout JR, Gevers D, Caporaso JG, Knight R. The interpersonal and intrapersonal diversity of human-associated microbiota in key body sites. *J Allergy Clin Immunol.* (2012) 129:1204–8. doi: 10.1016/j.jaci.2012.03.010
15. Cotillard A, Kennedy SP, Kong LC, Prifti E, Pons N, Le Chatelier E, et al. Dietary intervention impact on gut microbial gene richness. *Nature* (2013) 500:585–8. doi: 10.1038/nature12480
16. Benson AK, Kelly SA, Legge R, Ma F, Low SJ, Kim J, et al. Individuality in gut microbiota composition is a complex polygenic trait shaped by multiple environmental and host genetic factors. *Proc Natl Acad Sci USA.* (2010) 107:18933–8. doi: 10.1073/pnas.1007028107
17. Goodrich JK, Davenport ER, Beaumont M, Jackson MA, Knight R, Ober C, et al. Genetic determinants of the gut microbiome in UK twins. *Cell Host Microbe* (2016) 19:731–43. doi: 10.1016/j.chom.2016.04.017

18. Goodrich JK, Waters JL, Poole AC, Sutter JL, Koren O, Blekhman R, et al. Human genetics shape the gut microbiome. *Cell* (2014) 159:789–99. doi: 10.1016/j.cell.2014.09.053
19. Ghanei Gheshlagh R, Parizad N, Sayehmiri K. The relationship between depression and metabolic syndrome: systematic review and meta-analysis study. *Iran Red Crescent Med J.* (2016) 18:e26523. doi: 10.5812/ircmj.26523
20. Vancampfort D, Stubbs B, Mitchell AJ, De Hert M, Wampers M, Ward PB, et al. Risk of metabolic syndrome and its components in people with schizophrenia and related psychotic disorders, bipolar disorder and major depressive disorder: a systematic review and meta-analysis. *World Psychiatry* (2015) 14:339–47. doi: 10.1002/wps.20252
21. Tuncel OK, Sarisoy G, Bilgici B, Pazvantoglu O, Cetin E, Tuncel EK. Adipocytokines and ghrelin level of bipolar patients from manic episode to euthymic episode. *Nord J Psychiatry* (2018) 72:150–6. doi: 10.1080/08039488.2017.1402953
22. Takayanagi Y, Cascella NG, Santora D, Gregory PE, Sawa A, Eaton WW. Relationships between serum leptin level and severity of positive symptoms in schizophrenia. *Neurosci Res.* (2013) 77:97–101. doi: 10.1016/j.neures.2013.07.003
23. Zarouna S, Wozniak G, Papachristou AI. Mood disorders: a potential link between ghrelin and leptin on human body? *World J Exp Med.* (2015) 5:103–9. doi: 10.5493/wjem.v5.i2.103
24. Matey-Hernandez ML, Williams FMK, Potter T, Valdes AM, Spector TD, Menni C. Genetic and microbiome influence on lipid metabolism and dyslipidemia. *Physiol Genomics* (2018) 50:117–26. doi: 10.1152/physiolgenomics.00053.2017
25. Li J, Zhao F, Wang Y, Chen J, Tao J, Tian G, et al. Gut microbiota dysbiosis contributes to the development of hypertension. *Microbiome* (2017) 5:14. doi: 10.1186/s40168-016-0222-x
26. Heijtz RD, Wang S, Anuar F, Qian Y, Bjorkholm B, Samuelsson A, et al. Normal gut microbiota modulates brain development and behavior. *Proc Natl Acad Sci USA.* (2011) 108:3047–52. doi: 10.1073/pnas.1010529108
27. Neufeld KM, Kang N, Bienenstock J, Foster JA. Reduced anxiety-like behavior and central neurochemical change in germ-free mice. *Neurogastroenterol Motil.* (2011) 23:255–64, e119. doi: 10.1111/j.1365-2982.2010.01620.x
28. Cryan JF, Dinan TG. Mind-altering microorganisms: the impact of the gut microbiota on brain and behaviour. *Nat Rev Neurosci.* (2012) 13:701–12. doi: 10.1038/nrn3346
29. Clarke G, Grenham S, Scully P, Fitzgerald P, Moloney RD, Shanahan F, et al. The microbiome-gut-brain axis during early life regulates the hippocampal serotonergic system in a sex-dependent manner. *Mol Psychiatry* (2013) 18:666–73. doi: 10.1038/mp.2012.77
30. Foster JA, McVey Neufeld KA. Gut-brain axis: how the microbiome influences anxiety and depression. *Trends Neurosci.* (2013) 36:305–12. doi: 10.1016/j.tins.2013.01.005
31. Borre YE, Moloney RD, Clarke G, Dinan TG, Cryan JF. The impact of microbiota on brain and behavior: mechanisms & therapeutic potential. *Adv Exp Med Biol.* (2014) 817:373–403. doi: 10.1007/978-1-4939-0897-4_17
32. Stilling RM, Ryan FJ, Hoban AE, Shanahan F, Clarke G, Claesson MJ, et al. Microbes & neurodevelopment–absence of microbiota during early life increases activity-related transcriptional pathways in the amygdala. *Brain Behav Immun.* (2015) 50:209–20. doi: 10.1016/j.bbi.2015.07.009
33. Foster JA. Gut microbiome and behavior: focus on neuroimmune interactions. *Int Rev Neurobiol.* (2016) 131:49–65. doi: 10.1016/bs.irn.2016.07.005
34. Foster JA, Lyte M, Meyer E, Cryan JF. Gut microbiota and brain function: an evolving field in neuroscience. *Int J Neuropsychopharmacol.* (2016) 19:pyv114. doi: 10.1093/ijnp/pyv114
35. Bailey MT, Dowd SE, Galley JD, Hufnagle AR, Allen RG, Lyte M. Exposure to a social stressor alters the structure of the intestinal microbiota: implications for stressor-induced immunomodulation. *Brain Behav Immun.* (2011) 25:397–407. doi: 10.1016/j.bbi.2010.10.023
36. Bharwani A, Mian MF, Foster JA, Surette MG, Bienenstock J, Forsythe P. Structural & functional consequences of chronic psychosocial stress on the microbiome & host. *Psychoneuroendocrinology* (2016) 63:217–27. doi: 10.1016/j.psyneuen.2015.10.001
37. Jiang H, Ling Z, Zhang Y, Mao H, Ma Z, Yin Y, et al. Altered fecal microbiota composition in patients with major depressive disorder. *Brain Behav Immun.* (2015) 48:186–94. doi: 10.1016/j.bbi.2015.03.016
38. Naseribafrouei A, Hestad K, Avershina E, Sekelja M, Linlokken A, Wilson R, et al. Correlation between the human fecal microbiota and depression. *Neurogastroenterol Motil.* (2014) 26:1155–62. doi: 10.1111/nmo.12378
39. Zheng P, Zeng B, Zhou C, Liu M, Fang Z, Xu X, et al. Gut microbiome remodeling induces depressive-like behaviors through a pathway mediated by the host's metabolism. *Mol Psychiatry* (2016) 21:786–96. doi: 10.1038/mp.2016.44
40. Langille MG, Zaneveld J, Caporaso JG, McDonald D, Knights D, Reyes JA, et al. Predictive functional profiling of microbial communities using 16S rRNA marker gene sequences. *Nat Biotechnol.* (2013) 31:814–21. doi: 10.1038/nbt.2676
41. Wallace CJK, Milev R. The effects of probiotics on depressive symptoms in humans: a systematic review. *Ann Gen Psychiatry* (2017) 16:14. doi: 10.1186/s12991-017-0138-2
42. Dinan TG, Stanton C, Cryan JF. Psychobiotics: a novel class of psychotropic. *Biol Psychiatry* (2013) 74:720–6. doi: 10.1016/j.biopsych.2013.05.001
43. Sarkar A, Lehto SM, Harty S, Dinan TG, Cryan JF, Burnet PWJ. Psychobiotics and the manipulation of bacteria-gut-brain signals. *Trends Neurosci.* (2016) 39:763–81. doi: 10.1016/j.tins.2016.09.002
44. Benton D, Williams C, Brown A. Impact of consuming a milk drink containing a probiotic on mood and cognition. *Eur J Clin Nutr.* (2007) 61:355–61. doi: 10.1038/sj.ejcn.1602546
45. Messaoudi M, Violle N, Bisson JF, Desor D, Javelot H, Rougeot C. Beneficial psychological effects of a probiotic formulation (Lactobacillus helveticus R0052 and Bifidobacterium longum R0175) in healthy human volunteers. *Gut Microbes* (2011) 2:256–61. doi: 10.4161/gmic.2.4.16108
46. Huang R, Wang K, Hu J. Effect of probiotics on depression: a systematic review and meta-analysis of randomized controlled trials. *Nutrients* (2016) 8: E483. doi: 10.3390/nu8080483
47. Elmquist JK, Bjorbaek C, Ahima RS, Flier JS, Saper CB. Distributions of leptin receptor mRNA isoforms in the rat brain. *J Comp Neurol.* (1998) 395:535–47. doi: 10.1002/(SICI)1096-9861(19980615)395:4<535::AID-CNE9>3.0.CO;2-2
48. Scott MM, Lachey JL, Sternson SM, Lee CE, Elias CF, Friedman JM, et al. Leptin targets in the mouse brain. *J Comp Neurol.* (2009) 514:518–32. doi: 10.1002/cne.22025
49. Guo M, Huang TY, Garza JC, Chua SC, Lu XY. Selective deletion of leptin receptors in adult hippocampus induces depression-related behaviours. *Int J Neuropsychopharmacol.* (2013) 16:857–67. doi: 10.1017/S1461145712000703
50. Guo M, Lu XY. Leptin receptor deficiency confers resistance to behavioral effects of fluoxetine and desipramine via separable substrates. *Transl Psychiatry* (2014) 4:e486. doi: 10.1038/tp.2014.126
51. Lu XY, Kim CS, Frazer A, Zhang W. Leptin: a potential novel antidepressant. Proc Natl Acad Sci U S A. (2006) 103:1593-8. doi: 10.1073/pnas.0508901103
52. Haque Z, Akbar N, Yasmin F, Haleem MA, Haleem DJ. Inhibition of immobilization stress-induced anorexia, behavioral deficits, and plasma corticosterone secretion by injected leptin in rats. *Stress* (2013) 16:353–62. doi: 10.3109/10253890.2012.736047
53. Yang JL, Liu X, Jiang H, Pan F, Ho CS, Ho RC. The effects of high-fat-diet combined with chronic unpredictable mild stress on depression-like behavior and leptin/leprb in male rats. *Sci Rep.* (2016) 6:35239. doi: 10.1038/srep35239
54. Morris AA, Ahmed Y, Stoyanova N, Hooper WC, De Staerke C, Gibbons G, et al. The association between depression and leptin is mediated by adiposity. *Psychosom Med.* (2012) 74:483–8. doi: 10.1097/PSY.0b013e31824f5de0
55. Gecici O, Kuloglu M, Atmaca M, Tezcan AE, Tunckol H, Emul HM, et al. High serum leptin levels in depressive disorders with atypical features. *Psychiatry Clin Neurosci.* (2005) 59:736–8. doi: 10.1111/j.1440-1819.2005.01445.x
56. Kraus T, Haack M, Schuld A, Hinze-Selch D, Pollmacher T. Low leptin levels but normal body mass indices in patients with depression or schizophrenia. *Neuroendocrinology* (2001) 73:243–7. doi: 10.1159/000054641
57. Jow GM, Yang TT, Chen CL. Leptin and cholesterol levels are low in major depressive disorder, but high in schizophrenia. *J Affect Disord* (2006) 90:21–7. doi: 10.1016/j.jad.2005.09.015
58. Wang Q, Bing C, Al-Barazanji K, Mossakowaska DE, Wang, X, McBay DL, et al. Interactions between leptin and hypothalamic neuropeptide Y neurons

in the control of food intake and energy homeostasis in the rat. *Diabetes* (1997) 46:335–41. doi: 10.2337/diab.46.3.335

59. Agusti A, Moya-Perez A, Campillo I, Montserrat-de la Paz S, Cerrudo V, Perez-Villalba A, et al. Bifidobacterium pseudocatenulatum CECT 7765 ameliorates neuroendocrine alterations associated with an exaggerated stress response and anhedonia in obese mice. *Mol Neurobiol.* (2018) 55:5337–52. doi: 10.1007/s12035-017-0768-z
60. Carvalho AF, Rocha DQ, McIntyre RS, Mesquita LM, Kohler CA, Hyphantis TN, et al. Adipokines as emerging depression biomarkers: a systematic review and meta-analysis. *J Psychiatr Res.* (2014) 59:28–37. doi: 10.1016/j.jpsychires.2014.08.002
61. Cao B, Chen Y, Brietzke E, Cha D, Shaukat A, Pan Z, et al. Leptin and adiponectin levels in major depressive disorder: a systematic review and meta-analysis. *J Affect Disord.* (2018) 238:101–10. doi: 10.1016/j.jad.2018.05.008
62. Milaneschi Y, Lamers F, Bot M, Drent ML, Penninx BW. Leptin dysregulation is specifically associated with major depression with atypical features: evidence for a mechanism connecting obesity and depression. *Biol Psychiatry* (2017) 81:807–14. doi: 10.1016/j.biopsych.2015.10.023
63. Lasserre AM, Strippoli MF, Glaus J, Gholam-Rezaee M, Vandeleur CL, Castelao E, et al. Prospective associations of depression subtypes with cardio-metabolic risk factors in the general population. *Mol Psychiatry* (2017) 22:1026–34. doi: 10.1038/mp.2016.178
64. Simmons WK, Burrows K, Avery JA, Kerr KL, Taylor A, Bodurka J, et al. Appetite changes reveal depression subgroups with distinct endocrine, metabolic, and immune states. *Mol Psychiatry* (2018) doi: 10.1038/s41380-018-0093-6. [Epub ahead of print].
65. Zaibi MS, Stocker CJ, O'Dowd J, Davies A, Bellahcene M, Cawthorne MA, et al. Roles of GPR41 and GPR43 in leptin secretory responses of murine adipocytes to short chain fatty acids. *FEBS Lett.* (2010) 584:2381–6. doi: 10.1016/j.febslet.2010.04.027
66. Rajala MW, Patterson CM, Opp JS, Foltin SK, Young VB, Myers MG, Jr. Leptin acts independently of food intake to modulate gut microbial composition in male mice. *Endocrinology* (2014) 155:748–57. doi: 10.1210/en.2013-1085
67. Everard A, Lazarevic V, Derrien M, Girard M, Muccioli GG, Neyrinck AM, et al. Responses of gut microbiota and glucose and lipid metabolism to prebiotics in genetic obese and diet-induced leptin-resistant mice. *Diabetes* (2011) 60:2775–86. doi: 10.2337/db11-0227
68. Lam V, Su J, Koprowski S, Hsu A, Tweddell JS, Rafiee P, et al. Intestinal microbiota determine severity of myocardial infarction in rats. *FASEB J.* (2012) 26:1727–35. doi: 10.1096/fj.11-197921
69. Gomez-Arango LF, Barrett HL, McIntyre HD, Callaway LK, Morrison M, Dekker Nitert M, et al. Connections between the gut microbiome and metabolic hormones in early pregnancy in overweight and obese women. *Diabetes* (2016) 65:2214–23. doi: 10.2337/db16-0278
70. Kojima M, Hosoda H, Date Y, Nakazato M, Matsuo H, Kangawa K. Ghrelin is a growth-hormone-releasing acylated peptide from stomach. *Nature* (1999) 402:656–60. doi: 10.1038/45230
71. Zigman JM, Jones JE, Lee CE, Saper CB, Elmquist JK. Expression of ghrelin receptor mRNA in the rat and the mouse brain. *J Comp Neurol.* (2006) 494:528–48. doi: 10.1002/cne.20823
72. Guan XM, Yu H, Palyha OC, McKee KK, Feighner SD, Sirinathsinghji DJ, et al. Distribution of mRNA encoding the growth hormone secretagogue receptor in brain and peripheral tissues. *Brain Res Mol Brain Res.* (1997) 48:23–9. doi: 10.1016/S0169-328X(97)00071-5
73. Kluge M, Schussler P, Dresler M, Schmidt D, Yassouridis A, Uhr M, et al. Effects of ghrelin on psychopathology, sleep and secretion of cortisol and growth hormone in patients with major depression. *J Psychiatr Res.* (2011) 45:421–6. doi: 10.1016/j.jpsychires.2010.09.002
74. Jerlhag E, Egecioglu E, Landgren S, Salome N, Heilig M, Moechars D, et al. Requirement of central ghrelin signaling for alcohol reward. *Proc Natl Acad Sci USA.* (2009) 106:11318–23. doi: 10.1073/pnas.0812809106
75. Spencer SJ, Emmerzaal TL, Kozicz T, Andrews ZB. Ghrelin's role in the hypothalamic-pituitary-adrenal axis stress response: implications for mood disorders. *Biol Psychiatry* (2015) 78:19–27. doi: 10.1016/j.biopsych.2014.10.021
76. Poretti MB, Rask-Andersen M, Kumar P, Rubiales de Barioglio S, Fiol de Cuneo M, Schioth HB, et al. Ghrelin effects expression of several genes associated with depression-like behavior. *Prog Neuropsychopharmacol Biol Psychiatry.* (2015) 56:227–34. doi: 10.1016/j.pnpbp.2014.09.012
77. Wren AM, Small CJ, Fribbens CV, Neary NM, Ward HL, Seal LJ, et al. The hypothalamic mechanisms of the hypophysiotropic action of ghrelin. *Neuroendocrinology* (2002) 76:316–24. doi: 10.1159/000066629
78. Spencer SJ, Xu L, Clarke MA, Lemus M, Reichenbach A, Geenen B, et al. Ghrelin regulates the hypothalamic-pituitary-adrenal axis and restricts anxiety after acute stress. *Biol Psychiatry* (2012) 72:457–65. doi: 10.1016/j.biopsych.2012.03.010
79. Ghersi MS, Casas SM, Escudero C, Carlini VP, Buteler F, Cabrera RJ, et al. Ghrelin inhibited serotonin release from hippocampal slices. *Peptides* (2011) 32:2367–71. doi: 10.1016/j.peptides.2011.07.015
80. Hansson C, Alvarez-Crespo M, Taube M, Skibicka KP, Schmidt L, Karlsson-Lindahl L, et al. Influence of ghrelin on the central serotonergic signaling system in mice. *Neuropharmacology* (2014) 79:498–505. doi: 10.1016/j.neuropharm.2013.12.012
81. Lutter M, Sakata I, Osborne-Lawrence S, Rovinsky SA, Anderson JG, Jung S, et al. The orexigenic hormone ghrelin defends against depressive symptoms of chronic stress. *Nat Neurosci.* (2008) 11:752–3. doi: 10.1038/nn.2139
82. Barim AO, Aydin S, Colak R, Dag E, Deniz O, Sahin I. Ghrelin, paraoxonase and arylesterase levels in depressive patients before and after citalopram treatment. *Clin Biochem.* (2009) 42:1076–81. doi: 10.1016/j.clinbiochem.2009.02.020
83. Tuncel OK, Akbas S, Bilgici B. Increased ghrelin levels and unchanged adipocytokine levels in major depressive disorder. *J Child Adolesc Psychopharmacol.* (2016) 26:733–9. doi: 10.1089/cap.2015.0149
84. Algul S, Ozcelik O. Evaluating the levels of nesfatin-1 and ghrelin hormones in patients with moderate and severe major depressive disorders. *Psychiatry Investig.* (2018) 15:214–8. doi: 10.30773/pi.2017.05.24
85. Ozsoy S, Besirli A, Abdulrezzak U, Basturk M. Serum ghrelin and leptin levels in patients with depression and the effects of treatment. *Psychiatry Investig.* (2014) 11:167–72. doi: 10.4306/pi.2014.11.2.167
86. Nakashima K, Akiyoshi J, Hatano K, Hanada H, Tanaka Y, Tsuru J, et al. Ghrelin gene polymorphism is associated with depression, but not panic disorder. *Psychiatr Genet.* (2008) 18:257. doi: 10.1097/YPG.0b013e328306c979
87. Ishitobi Y, Kohno K, Kanehisa M, Inoue A, Imanaga J, Maruyama Y, et al. Serum ghrelin levels and the effects of antidepressants in major depressive disorder and panic disorder. *Neuropsychobiology* (2012) 66:185–92. doi: 10.1159/000339948
88. Ricken R, Bopp S, Schlattmann P, Himmerich H, Bschor T, Richter C, et al. Ghrelin serum concentrations are associated with treatment response during lithium augmentation of antidepressants. *Int J Neuropsychopharmacol.* (2017) 20:692–7. doi: 10.1093/ijnp/pyw082
89. Yousufzai M, Harmatz ES, Shah M, Malik MO, Goosens KA. Ghrelin is a persistent biomarker for chronic stress exposure in adolescent rats and humans. *Transl Psychiatry* (2018) 8:74. doi: 10.1038/s41398-018-0135-5
90. Date Y, Murakami N, Toshinai K, Matsukura S, Niijima A, Matsuo H, et al. The role of the gastric afferent vagal nerve in ghrelin-induced feeding and growth hormone secretion in rats. *Gastroenterology* (2002) 123:1120–8. doi: 10.1053/gast.2002.35954
91. Khosravi Y, Seow SW, Amoyo AA, Chiow KH, Tan TL, Wong WY, et al. Helicobacter pylori infection can affect energy modulating hormones and body weight in germ free mice. *Sci Rep.* (2015) 5:8731. doi: 10.1038/srep08731
92. Queipo-Ortuno MI, Seoane LM, Murri M, Pardo M, Gomez-Zumaquero JM, Cardona F, et al. Gut microbiota composition in male rat models under different nutritional status and physical activity and its association with serum leptin and ghrelin levels. *PLoS ONE* (2013) 8:e65465. doi: 10.1371/journal.pone.0065465
93. Parnell JA, Reimer RA. Prebiotic fibres dose-dependently increase satiety hormones and alter Bacteroidetes and Firmicutes in lean and obese JCR:LA-cp rats. *Br J Nutr.* (2012) 107:601–13. doi: 10.1017/S0007114511003163
94. Lin HV, Frassetto A, Kowalik EJ Jr, Nawrocki AR, Lu MM, Kosinski JR, et al. Butyrate and propionate protect against diet-induced obesity and regulate gut

hormones via free fatty acid receptor 3-independent mechanisms. *PLoS ONE* (2012) 7:e35240. doi: 10.1371/journal.pone.0035240
95. Perry RJ, Peng L, Barry NA, Cline GW, Zhang D, Cardone RL, et al. Acetate mediates a microbiome-brain-beta-cell axis to promote metabolic syndrome. *Nature* (2016) 534:213–7. doi: 10.1038/nature18309
96. Akbaraly TN, Ancelin ML, Jaussent I, Ritchie C, Barberger-Gateau P, Dufouil C, et al. Metabolic syndrome and onset of depressive symptoms in the elderly: findings from the three-city study. *Diabetes Care* (2011) 34:904–9. doi: 10.2337/dc10-1644

15

Epigenetics in Personality Disorders: Today's Insights

Dorothee Maria Gescher[1†], Kai G. Kahl[2†], Thomas Hillemacher[3], Helge Frieling[2], Jens Kuhn[4] and Thomas Frodl[1,5]*

[1] Department of Psychiatry and Psychotherapy, Otto-von-Guericke University of Magdeburg, Magdeburg, Germany, [2] Department of Psychiatry, Social Psychiatry and Psychotherapy, Hanover Medical School, Hanover, Germany, [3] Department of Psychiatry, Paracelsus Medical University, Nuremberg, Germany, [4] Department of Psychiatry and Psychotherapy, University of Cologne, Cologne, Germany, [5] German Centre for Neurodegenerative Diseases, Magdeburg, Germany

Correspondence:
Dorothee Maria Gescher
dorothee.gescher@med.ovgu.de

†These authors share first authorship

Objective: Epigenetic mechanisms have been described in several mental disorders, such as mood disorders, anxiety disorders and schizophrenia. However, less is known about the influence of epigenetic mechanisms with regard to personality disorders (PD). Therefore, we conducted a literature review on existing original data with regards to epigenetic peculiarities in connection with personality disorders.

Methods: Systematic literature review using PRISMA guidelines. Search was performed via NCBI PubMed by keywords and their combinations. Used search terms included "epigenetic," "methylation," "acetylation" plus designations of specified personality traits and disorders according to DSM-IV.

Results: Search yielded in total 345 publications, 257 thereof with psychiatric topic, 72 on personality disorder or traits, 43 of which were in humans and epigenetic, 23 thereof were original studies. Lastly, 23 original publications fulfilled the intended search criteria and were included. Those are 13 studies on gene methylation pattern with aggressive, antisocial and impulsive traits, 9 with borderline personality disorder (BPD), and 2 with antisocial personality disorder (ASPD). The results of these studies showed significant associations of PD with methylation aberrances in system-wide genes and suggest evidence for epigenetic processes in the development of personality traits and personality disorders. Environmental factors, of which childhood trauma showed a high impact, interfered with many neurofunctional genes. Methylation alterations in ASPD and BPD repeatedly affected *HTR2A*, *HTR3A*, *NR3C1,* and *MAOA* genes.

Summary: Epigenetic studies in PD seem to be a useful approach to elucidate the interaction of co-working risk factors in the pathogenesis of personality traits and disorders. However, the complexity of pathogenesis leads to divergent results and impedes an explicit interpretation. Differing methylation patterns within the selected PD could indicate subgroups which would benefit from patient-oriented therapeutic adjustments. They might play a major role in the future design and observation of early therapeutic intervention and thus could help to prevent severe dysfunctional conduct or full-blown personality disorder in risk subjects.

Keywords: epigenetic aberrations, personality disorder, personality trait, early childhood adversity, aggression, antisocial, molecular pathobiology, personalized therapy

INTRODUCTION

The epigenetic view on genes presumably associated with psychiatric disorders is gaining increasing academic interest and enables auxiliary insights in the pathogenesis of a particular disease. Severe psychiatric axis-I disorders like major depressive disorder (MDD) are currently widely investigated at the epigenetic level, and results account for a substantial pathogenetic impact of gene epigenetic modifications.

Epigenetic mechanisms in general function to homeostatically control gene accessibility and transcriptional functionality. Thus, gene function can be organized in both a highly programmed and life-enduring, but also in an environmentally-responsive way (1). The transcriptome as the immediate representation of genomic activity is regulated by (i) control of gene access for the transcriptional machinery through chromatin condensation and histone modification such as (de-)acetylation, (de-)phosphorylation, sumoylation, (ii) non-coding and microRNA that influences chromatin formation, as well as RNA translation and degradation, and (iii) covalent DNA changes by methylation of the cytosine nucleotide, which hampers transcriptase accessibility to the methylated region, and which can activate enzymes that interact in silencing the specific gene [reviewed in (2)].

Whereas epigenetic patterns stably determine mitosis-persistent cell differentiation as a precondition for embryonal development without changing DNA sequence, the epigenome also represents a dynamic adaption to environmental conditions. There is growing evidence in the last two decades that early life experience can affect long standing somatic and mental health trajectories in animals and humans by influencing the epigenetic pattern and thus affects structure and accessibility of the genome. Studies in rodents demonstrated the decisive impact of maternal care and early social adversity on the offspring's development and adult phenotypes. Early life adversity (ELA) in rats led to increased hippocampal glucocorticoid receptor (GR) expression, disturbed hypothalamus-pituitary-adrenal (HPA) axis functionality, and changed DNA methylation of the GR gene (*NR3C1*) in the hippocampus (3), of the brain-derived neurotropic factor gene (*BDNF*) promoter in the prefrontal cortex (4) and of the Arginine Vasopressin gene (*AVP*) (5). In humans, ELA was associated with decreased GR mRNA expression and *NR3C1* hypermethylation in post-mortem human brains (6). Hitherto findings indicate that epigenetic patterns found in context with ELA in animals and humans are not restricted to suggestive disease-associated functional genes but are spread genome-wide (7, 8), and are not stringently tissue-specific (9), since peripheral blood cells (PBC), especially T-cell lymphocytes, were shown to reflect epigenetic patterns similar to neuronal cells in culture and in brain tissue (9–11).

The translation of environmental signals into epigenetic information can be triggered by neuronal activity that initiates intracellular pathways such as cAMP signaling mediated histone acetylation or that influences and interacts with other epigenetic processes (12–14). Additionally, activity of the *AVP* promoter is regulated by the methyl-CpG-binding protein 2 (MeCp2), which is phosphorylated and activated by depolarization of hypothalamic neurons and in turn moderates demethylation of the *BDNF* promoter (5, 15, 16). In sum, although many details of molecular mechanisms remain unknown, the present insights substantiate and refine the idea how environmental signals might be translated into intracellular information and molecular memory.

Currently, a considerable number of studies explore epigenetic changes in association with behavior or affect difficulties like aggression or fear in human and animal subjects, particularly in connection with disturbances of the serotonergic system that meanwhile is well-known to be crucial in early brain development. The objective of this work was to review the current original publications on epigenetic modifications associated with personality disorders (PD) in humans.

METHODS

Literature search was performed as a systematic review according the Preferred Recording Items for Systematic Reviews and Meta-Analyses (PRISMA-P) guidelines (17). We based our search on the PubMed Central database of the U.S. National Institutes of Health's National Library of Medicine (NIH/NLM) using terms oriented on the Medical Subject Headings (MeSH) of the NCBI Library.

For the search keywords were inserted in a double or triple combination to yield comprehensive hits. The following keywords were utilized: "personality," "personality disorder," "personality trait," each of them combined with "epigenetic," "methylation," "acetylation," "phosphorylation," "ubiquitation," "sumoylation," "microRNA," "chromatin" and "chromatin remodeling," respectively, as well as with one of the keywords "aggression," "anankastic," "antisocial," "anxious," "avoidant," "borderline," "dependent," "eccentric," "emotionally unstable," "histrionic," "passive-aggressive," "impulsive," "narcissism," "narcissistic," "paranoid," "schizoid," and "schizotypal," respectively. The search included publications until May 15th 2018.

In total, the search yielded 345 different articles. We secondly perused the gained articles by reviewing their titles, abstracts and full texts in order to identify the proper articles matching to our literal research question. Therefore, studies were sequentially selected if they met the criteria (1) psychiatric topic [$n = 257$], (2) personality disorder or specified personality trait [$n = 72$ of (1)], (3) human study subjects [$n = 61$ of (2)], (4) epigenetic analyses [$n = 43$ of (3)], and (5) original study [$n = 23$ of (4)]. Following these selection criteria, it remained 23 articles according to the intended objective of this review (**Figure 1**).

Concomitantly, we used the PubMed search function of f1000prime (Faculty of 1000 Limited, London, UK). Herewith we found one further expedient study that met all of the described inclusion criteria (18). Finally, 24 original studies were included in this review.

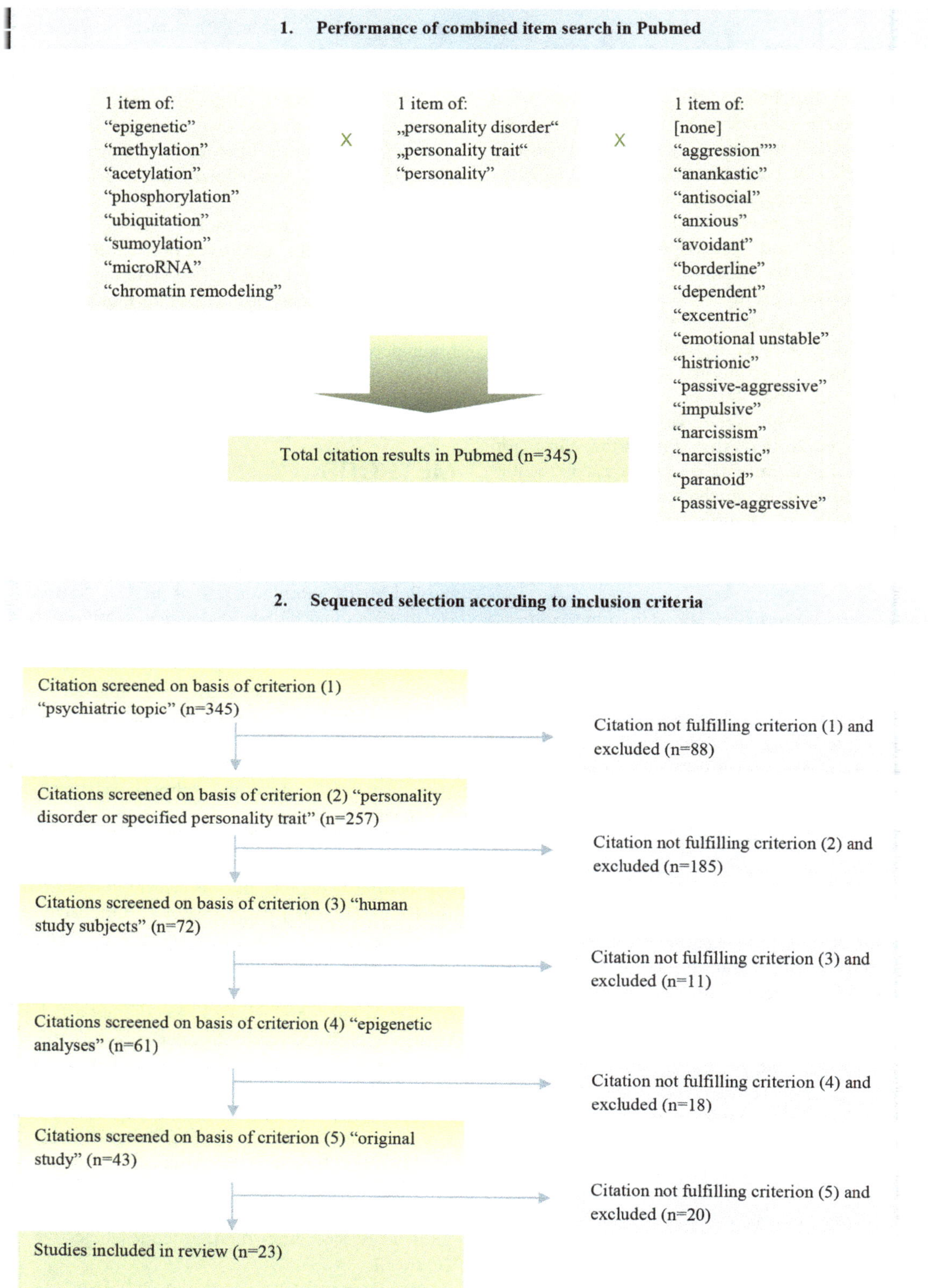

FIGURE 1 | Flow diagram of study search and sequenced selection.

RESULTS

Among the included studies, 13 explored the epigenetic influence on PT (two on impulsiveness, six on antisocial traits, seven on aggression) and 11 studied epigenetic differences in personality disorders (two in antisocial personality disorder (ASPD), 9 in borderline personality disorder (BPD)).

Size, constitution of study groups, and the number of investigated genes varied between the studies and ranged from single gene assays to genome-wide methylation analyses (GWA) with implications for the statistical power.

Personality Disorders

Antisocial Personality Disorder

With regards on antisocial PD, only methylation of the monoamine oxidase A gene (*MAOA*) has been examined. The two studies differed decisively with respect to study design and methylation results.

Philibert et al. considered the known variable nucleotide repeat (VTNR) region of *MAOA* and introduced a new VTNR region upstream of the transcriptional start site (TSS) of the gene (*MAOA* VTNR P2). They found a genotype-dependent methylation level and gene activity, but only in females (19). Within a total of well characterized 571 subjects (312 female) of the Iowa Adoption Study (IAS) they measured ASPD lifetime symptom counts in a linear mode according to DSM-IV criteria. Methylation patterns were analyzed at two promoter-associated CpG islands of *MAOA* in DNA extracted from EBV transformed lymphoblast cell lines from peripheral blood. Sequence analyses of the VTNR P2 revealed five genotypes with each seven to 11 eleven repeats (7R, 8R, 9R, 10R, 11R), of which the 9R genotype showed the lowest methylation in homozygous females, and the greatest gene activity in the functional analysis via luciferase essay. Presence of the low activity allele 10R was associated with higher vulnerability to the harming effects of childhood sexual and physical abuse and it accounted significantly for variances in symptom severity of ASPD in women. In male subjects no significant effect of the P2 genotype on *MAOA* methylation status was found.

In contrast, in a population of incarcerated men ($n = 86$) fulfilling the DSM-IV criteria for ASPD, Checknita et al. found a significant overall hypermethylation of the *MAOA* promoter region in the ASPD group compared with healthy controls ($n = 93$) with significant differences in methylation levels at 34 of 71 distinct *MAOA* promoter CpG sites. In their analysis, they did not consider symptom severity or childhood adversity. Methylation of *MAOA* promoter was associated with decreased gene activity (luciferase-assay) and positively correlated with 5-hydroxytryptophane levels in blood, thus suggesting functional relevance (20).

Borderline Personality Disorder

With respect to epigenetic modifications in BPD, different genes were suggested to be involved during individual development as well as in phenotypic characteristics of the disorder (**Table 1**). Apart from genome wide analyses (GWA), the main focus of theory-driven epigenetic studies was in gene regions coding for BDNF, glucocorticoid receptor (*NR3C1*), dopamine and serotonin receptors, MAOA, and catechol-O-methyltransferase (*COMT*). Most of the studies that focused on targeted genes considered a history of an early child trauma as a confounding factor in their analyses. The diversity in control group definition in the individual studies reflects the struggle for a suitable study design that allows for isolating disorder-specific characteristics. Methylation aberrations were mostly evaluated with diagnostic, but also with predictive concerns (21).

Perroud et al. studied methylation status of the *BDNF* gene in peripheral blood leucocytes and its modulation by a focused therapeutic intervention with intensive dialectical behavior therapy (I-DBT) comprising 4 weeks in outpatients with BPD ($n = 115$). Contrasted with healthy subjects, CpG-rich regions in exon 1 and exon 4 were significantly more highly methylated in BPD subjects before the therapeutic intervention. The number of different types of childhood trauma (CT) according the Childhood Trauma Questionnaire (CTQ) correlated positively with the mean methylation percentage of both CpG-regions. After intensive DBT, methylation status of the considered CpG sites was significantly increased in BPD patients. This effect could be traced back to the non-responders, whereas the responders showed a methylation decrease. However, the comparison of *BDNF* methylation status with peripheral serum protein levels of BDNF revealed no significant association (21).

Regarding studies on *NR3C1* methylation and PD, two studies focused on exon 1F promoter, which is functionally crucial. In a cohort of BPD outpatients ($n = 281$) Martin-Blanco et al. (22) found a significant positive correlation between overall *NR3C1* exon 1F methylation level of peripheral blood leucocytes and clinical severity. Exon 1F methylation was further significantly associated with childhood physical abuse. Individual CpG sites were associated with particular subscores of CTQ.

Perroud et al. (23) considered that a current severe mental illness might have epigenetic implications *per se* and could confound analyses that aim to isolating methylation characteristics specific for BPD. Therefore, in a comparison of subjects with BPD ($n = 101$) to those with MDD ($n = 99$) their results showed higher overall *NR3C1* exon 1F methylation levels in BPD than in MDD subjects in peripheral blood leucocytes. Further, methylation was associated with CT scaled by the CTQ, and correlated with childhood sexual, physical and emotional abuse, and physical and emotional neglect, respectively, and the number of these types of CT. *NR3C1* exon 1F hypermethylation in subjects with BPD was still significant when corrected for childhood maltreatment.

Regarding monoamine receptor genes, within a large-scaled study on subjects with bulimia spectrum disorders (BSD) with and without comorbid BPD Groleau et al. (24) found significant but marginally increased methylation of the dopamine D2 receptor gene (*DRD2*) exon 1 promoter region in whole peripheral blood cell (PBC) DNA of subjects with BSD and BPD compared with that of subjects with BSD only.

Methylation of the serotonin receptor 3A gene (*5HTR3A*) was found by Perroud et al. (25) to be correlated to clinical severity of BPD and other psychiatric disorders. The authors

TABLE 1 | Studies on epigenetics in personality disorders.

Author	Year	PD	Gene	Co-factors	Results	Sample	Tissue/DNA	Limitations
Philibert et al. (19)	2011	ASPD	*MAOA*	VNTR-genotype, CA	Identification of five genotypes of *MAOA* VNTR P2 (7R, 8R, 9R, 10R, 11R), 9R allele with the lowest methylation and associated with the highest activity (luciferase assay), 10R allele the lowest. Methylation status of *MAOA* promoter was genotype-dependent. VNTR genotype interacted with CA in predicting ASPD features. The presence of the low activity allele 10R at P2 was associated with significantly greater vulnerability to the impact of CA regarding ASPD symptoms. All results were found in women only.	*Subjects:* adult participants of the Iowa Adoptee Study (IAS), (n = 571, 312 female). *Diagnostics:* DSM-IV, CMI (SA, PA), ASPD lifetime symptom count (0–7). *Methods:* DNA bisulfite treatment, PCR amplification and methylation quantification. Selected methylation analysis of *MAOA* at two promoter-associated CpG islands (18 and 70 CpG sites, respectively). Sequencing VTNR genotype.	EBV-transformed lymphoblast cell lines	
Checknita et al. (20)	2015	ASPD	*MAOA*		Methylation level of *MAOA* promoter region was significantly higher in ASPD subjects. Methylation in 34 of 71 CpG sites was significantly associated with ASPD, 31 of which were hypermethylated. *MAOA* promoter methylation was *in vitro* associated with decreased gene activity (luciferase-assay) and was positively associated with 5-HT plasma levels *in vivo.*	*Subjects:* incarcerated men (n = 86) with ASPD, HC (n = 93). *Diagnostics:* DSM-IV, SCID-I/-II. *Methods:* Genomic DNA bisulfite treatment. Selected methylation analysis of *MAOA* promoter (71 CpG sites, region chrX:4351407-43515991) performed by quantitative mass spectroscopy. *In vitro* functional analysis (luciferase assay). HPLC-analysis of 5-HT serum levels in blood in a subsample (n = 80).	PBC	No consideration of ELA.
Perroud et al. (21)	2013	BPD	*BDNF*	CT	*BDNF* methylation was significantly higher in both exon 1 and exon 4 CpG regions in BPD than in control subjects. The number of CT was significantly positive correlated with methylation levels. In BPD, *BDNF* methylation was significantly increased after I-DBT in both CpG-regions. This increase was decisively caused by the I-DBT nonresponders. I-DBT responders showed a decrease of methylation. No significant association of *BDNF* methylation with protein plasma levels.	*Subjects:* outpatients with BPD (n = 115, 108 female), HC (n = 52, 24 female). All patients received psychotropic medication. *Diagnostics:* DSM-IV, SCID-II, BDI-II, BHS, BIS-10, CTQ. *Methods:* intervention with I-DBT for 4 weeks. Methylation analysis of two CpG regions within *BDNF* exon 1 (9 CpG; chr11:27743473–27744564) and exon 4 (17 CpG; chr11:27723060–27723294). DNA bisulfite treatment, PCR amplification, methylation analysis by high-resolution melt assay. Quantizing BDNF plasma protein levels (ELISA).	Peipheral blood leukocytes	BPD subjects were on psychotropic medication. In HC, no association analysis of CT with methylation status.
Martín-Blanco et al. (22)	2014	BPD	*NR3C1*	CT	Overall methylation of *NR3C1* was significantly positively correlated with CT (in particular PA) and with clinical severity of BPD (in particular DIB-R total score and previous hospitalizations). No significant association between *NR3C1* methylation level and general severity of CT. Methylation of individual CpG sites showed single significance for association with PA and EN (CpG1-3) and with FA (CpG6).	*Subjects:* female outpatients with BPD (n = 281) without current episode of any axis I disorder. *Diagnostics:* DSM-IV, SCID-II, DIP-R, CTQ-SF. *Methods:* DNA bisulfite treatment, PCR amplification and pyrosequencing for selected methylation analysis of *NR3C1* exon 1F (8 CpG sites).	Peipheral blood leukocytes	Only female subjects. No control.

(Continued)

TABLE 1 | Continued

Author	Year	PD	Gene	Co-factors	Results	Sample	Tissue/DNA	Limitations
Perroud et al. (23)	2011	BPD	*NR3C1*	CT	Subjects with BPD, even without CT, showed higher *NR3C1* methylation levels than MDD subjects with the same reported CT. In BPD, childhood SA, PN, and number of types of CT were significantly associated with increased *NR3C1* methylation. No significant association was found between methylation status and childhood PA, EA and EN. In the whole sample, SA, PA, PN, EA, and EN were significantly associated with *NR3C1* methylation. Number of types of CT was significant positively correlated with overall methylation level.	*Subjects:* patients with BPD ($n = 101$, 95 female), MDD ($n = 99$, with low rate of abuses and neglect) and MDD with comorbid PTSD ($n = 15$). All subjects received psychotropic medication. *Diagnostics:* DSM-IV, SCID-II, DGIS, CTQ, BDI-II, clinical interview for detailed characteristics of suffered abuse. *Methods:* DNA bisulfite treatment, PCR amplification and pyrosequencing for selected methylation analysis of *NR3C1* exon 1F (8 CpG sites). Sample validation by confirmation analyses.	Peipheral blood leukocytes	All participants received psychotropic medication. No HC.
Groleau et al. (24)	2014	BPD	*DRD2*	CA	*Impact of BPD:* Significant group effect of methylation levels with BPD status. Mean methylation levels of *DRD2* in BSD/BPD subjects were significantly increased compared to NE, and marginally significant increased compared to BSD/non-BPD. No significant differences between total BSD and NE. Slightly significant (by trend) higher methylation of BSD/SA than NE (but not of BSD/PA).	*Subjects:* female outpatients with BSD ($n = 52$, 8 of which with BPD) and NE ($n = 19$). BSD subjects: $n = 33$ (63.5%) BN-purging subtype, $n = 2$ (3.8%) BN-non purging subtype, $n = 17$ (32.7%) ED n.o.s. *Diagnostics:* DSM-IV, EDE, CTI, SCID-II. *Methods:* DNA bisulfite treatment, PCR amplification and pyrosequencing for selected methylation analysis of *DRD2* exon 1 promoter (10 CpG sites; chr11:113346237-113346328).	PBC	Only female subjects. No HC.
Perroud et al. (25)	2016	BPD	*HTR3A*	SNP genotype, CT	*Severity of disease:* in BPD, BN and ADHD, CT was associated with higher severity of the disease across and within each disorder. BPD subjects showed highest CTQ scores. Particular methylation differences between disorders: in BPD subjects, methylation of specific CpG-sites was significantly increased. In ADHD subjects, two different CpG-sites were significantly hypermethylated (and significantly less methylated in BPD). *Impact of HTR3A genotype on methylation status:* CC carriers showed significantly higher methylation at a specific CpG-site than T allele carriers, independent of CT history. *Impact of CT on methylation status in BPD:* CTQ total and PA were significantly associated with *HTR3A* methylation at different individual CpG-sites. *Impact of methylation on BPD severity:* methylation at cpG2_III was significantly associated with nearly all criteria of BPD severity, CpG5_III with age of BPD onset and number of mood episodes, methylation at CpG1_III was significantly associated with psychotic symptoms.	*Subjects:* outpatients with BPD ($n = 116$, 106 female), BN ($n = 122$, 65 female), ADHD ($n = 111$, 33 female). All subjects were on stable psychopharmacological treatment. *Diagnostics:* DSM-IV, CTQ, SCID-II (BPD), WURS (ADHD), ASRS. *Methods:* DNA bisulfite treatment, PCR amplification and pyrosequencing for selected methylation analysis of *HTR3A* (8 CpG sites). Gene sequencing of rs1062613 variants.	PBC	All participants received psychotropic medication. No HC.

(Continued)

TABLE 1 | Continued

Author	Year	PD	Gene	Co-factors	Results	Sample	Tissue/DNA	Limitations
Dammann et al. (26)	2011	BPD	*COMT, HTR2A, MAOA, MAOB, NR3C1*		Average and individual CpG-site methylation levels of each *HTR2A*, *NR3C1*, *MAOA*, and *COMT* were significantly increased in BPD subjects, *MAOB* by trend. Significantly higher methylation was found in most of the analyzed single CpG sites: *HTR2A* (4 CpG sites), *NR3C1* (2 of 8 CpG sites), *MAOA* (1 of 5 CpG sites), *MAOB* (1 of 6 CpG sites) and *COMT* (2 of 4 CpG sites).	*Subjects:* outpatients with BPD ($n = 26$, 24 female) and HC ($n = 11$, all female). *Diagnostics:* DSM-IV. *Methods:* DNA bisulfite treatment, PCR amplification for selective methylation analysis: bisulfite pyrosequencing of *HTR2A*, *NR3C1*, *MAOA*, *MAOB* and *COMT* promoter regions (27CpG sites), performed in triplicates and averaged.	PBC	Nearly all subjects female. No consideration of ELA.
Teschler et al. (27)	2013	BPD	genome-wide		Methylation differences between BPD and HC subjects comprised a total of 256 significantly hypermethylated CpG sites in BPD, but significance of any of each didn't persist post Bonferroni correction. By selected quantitative analysis, hypermethylation in BPD was significant at particular CpG sites respecting *APBA2*, *APBA3*, *KCNQ1*, *MCF2*, *NINJ2*, *GATA4* compared with HC subjects (*GATA4* was significantly increased only in the bead chip assay).	*Subjects:* outpatients with BPD ($n = 24$, all female) and HC ($n = 11$). *Diagnostics:* DSM-IV, SCID-II. *Methods:* DNA bisulfite treatment, GWA by BeadChip technology, quantitative pyrosequencing.	PBC	Only female subjects. No consideration of ELA.
Teschler et al. (28)	2016	BPD	*PRIMA1 rDNA*		Methylation of the *rDNA* and *PRIMA1* promoter were significantly associated with BPD. In *PRIMA1* all of 6 CpG sites were each significantly hypermethylated in BPD subjects. All of 9 CpG sites within the *rDNA* promoter were each significantly less methylated in BPD subjects.	*Subjects:* outpatients with BPD ($n = 24$, all female) and HC ($n = 11$). *Diagnostics:* DSM-IV, SCID-II. *Methods:* DNA bisulfite treatment, pyrosequencing for selective methylation analysis of *rDNA* 5′ETS (5 CpG sites) and promoter (9 CpG sites), and of *PRIMA1* promoter CpG island (6 CpG sites).	PBC	Only female subjects. No consideration of ELA. All BPD subjects received psychotropic medication.

(Continued)

TABLE 1 | Continued

Author	Year	PD	Gene	Co-factors	Results	Sample	Tissue/DNA	Limitations
Prados et al. (29)	2015	BPD	genome-wide	CT	*Methylation differences between MDD and BPD subjects:* most significant results respected CpG sites associated with *EFNB1*, *SPSB2* and *CST9L* (multivariate analysis), and with *miR124-3*, *WDR60* and *FAM163A* all with *decreased* methylation in BPD subjects (univariate analysis). A high number of aberrantly methylated CpG sits were localized on chromosome X with *higher* methylation and on chromosome 6 with *lower* methylation in BPD. *Impact of CT:* CpG sites significantly associated with CTQ total score were located p.e. in *OCA2*, *MFAP2*, *CST9L*, *EP400*, *KCNQ2*, *A2ML*, *NT5DC2* and *RPH3L* (multivariate analysis) and within IL17RA exon 1, chromosome 6p22.1, and miR137 (highest significance) (univariate analysis). Methylation of *miR124-3* was associated with both severity of CA (higher methylation) and with BPD (lower methylation).	*Subjects:* outpatients with BPD ($n = 96$, 88 female) or with MDD ($n = 93$, 59 female). MDD subjects were selected for low rate of child abuse and neglect by CTQ. *Diagnostics:* DIGS, SKID-II, CTQ. CTQ, history of maltreatment was validated by a defined clinical talk, BIS-10, STAXI, TCI. *Methods:* DNA ($n = 29$ BPD, $n = 18$ MDD); GWA (485 577 CpGs). Specific methylation analysis of cg04927004 (chr20: 61′809′348) (near miR124-3): bisulfite-pyrosequencing performed in duplicates.	Peripheral blood leukocytes	No HC.

5′ETS, 5′ external transcribed spacer; 5-HT, 5-hydroxytryptophane; ADHD, attention deficit hyperactivity disorder; A2ML, alpha-2 macroglobulin-like protein; APBA2(3), Amyloid Beta Precursor Protein Binding Family A Member 2(3) gene; ASPD, Antisocial personality disorder; ASRS, Adult ADHD Self-Report Scale; BDI, Beck Depression Inventory; BDNF, brain-derived neurotrophic factor; BHS, Beck Hopelessness Scale; BIS-10, Barrat Impulsivity Scale; BN, bulimia nervosa; BPD, borderline personality disorder; BSD, bulimia spectrum disorder; CA, childhood abuse; CMI, Childhood Maltreatment Index; COBRA, combined bisulfite restriction analysis; s-COMT, soluble catechol-O-methyltransferase gene; COBRA, Combined Bisulfite Restriction Analysis; CST9L, cystatin 9-like gene; CT, childhood trauma; CTI, Childhood Trauma Interview; CTQ(-SF), Childhood Trauma Questionnaire (Short Form); DIGS, Diagnostic Interview for Genetic Studies; DIP-R, Revised Diagnostic Interview for Borderlines; DRD2, dopamine receptor D2 gene; EA, emotional abuse; EDE, Eating Disorder Examination Interview; EFNB1, Ephrin B1 gene; ELA, early life adversity; ELISA, enzyme-linked immunosorbent assay; EN, emotional neglect; EP400, E1A binding protein P400 gene; FAM163A, family with sequence similarity 163 member A gene; GATA4, GATA binding protein 4 gene; GWA, genome-wide methylation analysis; HC, healthy control; HPLC, high performance liquid chromatography; HTR2A, serotonin receptor 2A gene; HTR3A, serotonin receptor 3A gene; I-DBT, Intensive Dialectical Behavioural Therapy; IAS, Iowa Adoptee Study; KCNQ1, potassium voltage-gated channel subfamily Q member 1 gene; MAOA(-B), monoamine oxidase A(B) gene; MDD, major depressive disorder; MFAP2, microfibrillar associated protein 2 gene; miR137, microRNA 137 gene; miR124-3, microRNA 124-3 gene; NE, no eating disorder; NINJ2, ninjurin 2 gene; NR3C1, nuclear receptor subfamily 3 group C member 1 gene (glucocorticoid receptor gene); NT5DC2, 5′-nucleotidase domain containing 2 gene; OCA2, oculocutaneous albinism II gene; PA, physical abuse; PBC, peripheral whole blood cells; PCR, polymerase chain reaction; PN, physical neglect; PRIMA1, proline rich membrane anchor 1 gene; PTSD, posttraumatic stress disorder; RPH3L, rabphilin 3A-like gene; SA, sexual abuse; SCID-I/-II, Structured Clinical Interview I/II for DSM-IV Personality Disorders; SPSB2, splA/ryanodine receptor domain and SOCS box containing 2 gene; STAXI, State-Trait Anger Expression Inventory; TCI, Temperament and Character Inventory; VTNR, variable number tandem repeats; WDR60, WD repeat domain 60 gene; WURS, Wender Utah ADHD Rating Scale.

compared PBC DNA methylation levels of eight CpG sites within the 5HT3A gene in subjects with BPD ($n = 116$), attention deficit hyperactivity disorder (ADHD) ($n = 111$) and bipolar disorder (BD) ($n = 122$). They also considered single nucleotide variants (SNP) of the gene and CT history as additional factors and explored associations with methylation levels of the particular CpG sites.

Methylation levels between the patient groups differed significantly in most of the CpG sites and showed a distinct pattern of hyper- and hypomethylation in the several disorders in selected CpG sites. For BPD, subjects showed the highest scores in the CTQ and the highest methylation level between the patient groups. CT was associated with mean methylation status, and CTQ total score and physical abuse each with different selected CpG sites. CT was further associated with higher severity of disease. Carrying the CC-allele was significantly associated with methylation at one specific CpG site independent of CT (in all disorders).

Dammann et al. (26) analyzed five neuropsychiatric genes assumed to be of significance for psychopathological phenotype, in particular genes coding for soluble catechol-O-methyltransferase (*s-COMT*), serotonin receptor 2A (*HTR2A*), *NR3C1*, and X-chromosomal *MAOA* and *MAOB*. Methylation levels of each gene promoter were quantified in PBC DNA of individuals with BPD ($n = 26$, 24 female) and in healthy controls ($n = 11$, all female). In comparison to healthy controls, quantitative DNA methylation analysis showed significant elevated overall methylation levels in BPD subjects within *HTR2A*, *NR3C1*, and *s-COMT*. Gene methylation of *MAOA* and *MAOB* could only be analyzed in female subjects, and methylation of *MAOA* was significantly higher in BPD (of *MAOB* only by trend). Considering all 27 individual CpG sites, across the five genes that were investigated, average methylation level across all quantified regions was significantly higher in BPD patients compared to controls. Implications of attendant data as trauma history of the subjects weren't presented as part of the study, but it was noted that aberrant methylation had not been associated with traumatic experience in appropriate statistical tests.

Meanwhile epigenetic assays include genome-wide association studies (GWA) that indicate specific CpG sites of aberrant methylation levels across the whole genomic DNA and facilitate comprehensive aspects within epigenetic evaluations.

In extension to the aforementioned study, Teschler et al. (27) performed a GWA in PBC DNA between female BPD ($n = 24$) and HC ($n = 11$) subjects. Results showed a total of 256 significantly hypermethylated CpG sites in BPD, but significance of any of each didn't persist post Bonferroni correction. The research group selected seven hypermethylated genes for validation analyses and could endorse increased methylation in five of the genes, with specified CpG sites related to the amyloid beta (A4) precursor protein-binding family A member 2 (*APBA2*) and member 3 (*APBA3*) genes, potassium voltage-gated channel KQT-like subfamily member 1 gene (*KCNQ1*), MCF2 cell line derived transforming sequence gene (*MCF2*) and the ninjurin 2 gene (*NINJ2*). GATA binding protein 4 (*GATA4*) and holocarboxylase synthetase (*HLCS*) genes showed increased methylation in BPD in the GWA, but not in the validation analysis.

Methylation studies of the ribosomal RNA gene (*rDNA*) promoter, 5′ external transcribed spacer gene (*5′ETS*) and of the proline rich membrane anchor 1 gene (*PRIMA1*) promoter in PBC DNA of female subjects with BPD ($n = 24$) and HC ($n = 11$) revealed significantly *less* methylation of the *rDNA* promoter region in BPD compared with HC subjects, and hypomethylation of the *5′ETS* in BPD by trend. *PRIMA1* showed a *higher* methylation in BPD subjects (28).

Another GWA with PBC DNA was performed by Prados et al. (29) on BPD subjects affected with high levels of childhood adversity ($n = 96$) and subjects with MDD and a history of low levels of childhood adversity ($n = 93$). Uni- and multivariate analyses revealed significant methylation differences in a significant number of particular CpG sites associated with BPD compared with MDD subjects or related to childhood maltreatment, respectively. Contrasting BPD with MDD subjects, most significant results of multivariate analyses resulted in significantly different methylated CpG sites located e.g., within the gene coding for a ligand of Eph-related receptor tyrosine kinases (*EFBN1*), closely to the gene coding for a suppressor of cytokine signaling (SOCS) family member (*SPSB2*) and near the gene coding for a protein similar to mouse cystatin 9 (*CST9L*). Univariate analyses detected hypomethylated CpG sites in BPD i.e., near the encoding region of microRNA 124 (*miR124-3*), which targets several genes that have been described to be correlated with BPD (including *NR3C1*), near the gene coding for the WD repeat domain 60 (*WD60*), and a CpG site within the gene of the family with sequence similarity 163 member A (*FAM163A*). Many of the significantly hypermethylated sites were found on chromosome X. Targeting on CT, results of multivariate analyses with the CTQ revealed strong associations with loci within or near the genes of human homolog of the mouse p (pink-eyes dilution) (*OCA2*), microfibrillar-associated protein 2 (*MFAP2*), *CST9L*, E1A binding protein p400 (*EP400*), *KCNQ2*, alpha-2-macroglobulin-like 1 (*A2ML1*), 5′-nucleotide domain containing 2 (*NT5DC2*) and rabphilin 3A-like (*RPH3AL*). Univariate analyses yielded most significant alterations located within the gene coding for the interleukin 17 receptor A (*IL17RA*), in an intergenic region on chromosome 6p22.1, and closed by *miR124-3* and *miR137*. Methylation of *miR124-3* was associated with both severity of childhood adversity (higher methylation) and with BPD (lower methylation).

In summary, large part of the studies in PD focused on single genes, including *MAOA* in ASPD, and *BDNF*, *NR3C1*, *DRD2*, and *HTR3A* in BPD, or on a set of theory-driven suggestive genes (26). They revealed significant methylation differences in blood cell DNA of subjects with the respective PD. Within all independent gene-targeted studies, *NR3C1* hypermethylation was most frequently and consistently found to be associated with BPD; therefore, current results most strongly indicate *NR3C1* to be implicated in BPD. *NR3C1* further was the only gene that was as well affected in one of the GWA (29), however this was mediated by methylation differences of *miR124-3* which targets, among other genes, on *NR3C1*. In contrast, GWA studies, as performed by Teschler and Prados, found large number of genes that were differentially methylated in BPD, indicating a system-wide involvement in PD including genes associated with immune-response, cell-signaling or transcription control (27–29). The transcriptional relevance of the respective methylation differences was only verified by two authors. Thus, Checknita et al. found an indirect negative association of *MAOA* promoter hypermethylation with 5-HT serum level *in vitro* (20). Otherwise, Perroud et al. (21) didn't found an association of *BDNF* promoter methylation and the peripheral protein serum level of BDNF. All studies were based on DNA extracted from PBC, in most cases from whole blood cells, partly from only leucocytes (21–23), or selective from lymphocytes (19). However, the studies particularly differ in their design of study subjects and controls, and at least in the consideration of environmental factors that have impact on epigenetic modulation like early childhood adversity, which impedes a well-defined interpretation in most of the studies (**Table 1**, col. "Limitations").

Personality Traits

Most original publications on methylation and personality traits were found with antisocial or aggressive features in connection with epigenetic alterations associated with the functionality of the serotonergic system or the hypothalamic–pituitary–adrenal (HPA-) axis functionality, which is the main neuroendocrine system for regulation of stress reaction and adaptation. Accordingly, theory-driven studies examined genes associated with these systems, such as the serotonin transporter gene (*SLC6A4*), dopamine and serotonin receptor genes (*DRD1, HTR1B, HTR1D, HTR3A*), *MAOA*, and *NR3C1* promoter exon 1F. With respect to its role in socio-affective perception and processing, some studies exist that pertain to antisocial behavior and oxytocin and oxytocin receptor genes (*OXT, OXTR*). Further, the role of cytokines and other factors were considered.

Antisocial Traits

Consistent with a large body of literature that implicates the serotonergic system in the regulation of anxiety, aggression, and stress response, epigenetic alterations in the serotonin transporter gene (*SLC6A4*) were found to be related to a history of child sexual abuse as well as to antisocial behavior in adulthood by Beach et al. (30). The authors performed methylation analyses on the participant's peripheral blood lymphocyte DNA that was EBV transformed into lymphoblast cell lines. Participants (n = 155, all female) were gradually diagnosed by means of symptom score of ASPD. Child sexual abuse was highly associated with mean methylation level and methylation was highly significantly associated with symptoms of ASPD, thereby playing a modulating role to develop antisocial traits after childhood sexual abuse. Interestingly, influence of *SLC6A4* methylation on ASPD severity was impacted by genotype, since association of methylation with the ss and the sl genotype of *SLC6A4* was significant, but not with the ll genotype. These results suggest an aggravating effect of methylation in *SLC6A4* risk (s) alleles for ASPD, further, methylation was increasingly associated with ASPD in carriers with greater number of s alleles.

Moul et al. found antisocial traits being associated with genetic and epigenetic modulation of the rs11568817 SNP in the *HTR1B* promoter region (31). In an investigation with boys (n = 117) exhibiting callous-unemotional (CU) traits and antisocial behavior problems, and grouped by high and less strong CU traits, they found lower methylation levels of *HTTR1B* in saliva cell DNA in the high CU trait group. In turn, methylation was decisively moderated by rs11568817 SNP genotype and carried by two exclusive CpG sites (CpG12 and CpG14), which individual methylation levels were negatively associated with overall methylation levels in this gene region. The authors assume two ways of risk for high CU traits, first, carrier of the risk (minor) allele (s) with low levels of methylation at CpG sites 12 and 14 (what was associated with high overall promoter methylation) and second, carrier without risk allele but with high methylation at CpG 12 and CpG14 (what was associated with low overall methylation) and high expression of *HTR1B* (31).

In the same sample of participants stratified by CU score level and by age, the aforementioned research group analyzed methylation characteristics of the ocytocin receptor gene (*OXTR*) in PBC DNA. They revealed high CU traits being associated with increased methylation at two of the six analyzed CpG loci within the *OXTR* promoter and being correlated with decreased oxytocin blood levels. Yet, when divided in age group, these findings reached significance only in the older group (age 9–16 years), not in the prepubertal children (age 4–8 years) (here only by trend). Similarly, oxytocin serum levels significantly were negatively correlated with gene methylation level in the older boys (32).

Further, in a prospective, longitudinal study, Cecil et al. (18) studied 84 youth with early-onset and persistent conduct problems with regard to early life risks and to methylation changes of *OXTR* in PBC DNA. Clinical surveys took place at birth, age 7, 9, and 13 years, and collected an environmental risk score (kind and time of risk factor), diagnosis of conduct problems, CU traits and internalizing problems. Equally, methylation analyses were performed longitudinally with sampling at birth (cord blood), and at age 7 and 9 years (peripheral blood). Finally, for evaluation subjects were divided by severity of internalizing problems, collected by maternal reports at each study time.

Results for youth with *low* internalizing problems revealed that *OXTR* hypermethylation at birth was significant related to higher CU traits at age 13. *OXTR* methylation at birth further was associated with decreased experience of victimization during early childhood, specifically direct victimization. The only environmental risk factor associated with *OXTR* methylation at birth was a prenatal parental risk i.e., maternal psychopathology, criminal behaviors, and substance use. Within the youth with *high* internalizing problems, CU traits showed no significant association with *OXTR* gene methylation, but were positively correlated with prenatal, specifically interpersonal, risks like intimate partner violence or family conflicts. Interestingly, CU traits were negatively correlated with postnatal risks, specifically life events as the death of a relative, an accident or illness. These different correlation results are suggestive for discriminative pathways in the development of CU traits, the one epigenetically co-determined, and the other influenced by different environmental factors. If associated with *OXTR* hypermethylation at birth, CU traits may protect for internalizing problems and for experienced victimization, as discussed by the authors as a possible evocative correlation (18).

In view of ASPD symptoms, Philibert et al. (33) explored the *MAOA* VTNR polymorphism genotype and methylation status in EBV transformed lymphoblast cell lines with respect to lifetime symptom severity of ASPD and substance use disorder as defined as alcohol or nicotine dependence in a collective of 191 subjects (96 female). Methylation level was consistently higher in the female subjects than in males at each analyzed CpG site. There was only a statistical trend for women homozygous for the 3,3 allele showing higher average methylation than for the 4,4 allele. The research revealed no association between symptom counts for ASPD and methylation levels in neither men nor women (33).

With attention to multifaceted features in subjects with early-onset behavior problems as i.e., higher irritability, anxiety, impulsivity, possibly associated with an impaired hypothalamic-pituitary-adrenal (HPA) function, Dadds et al. (34) examined the methylation patterns of the *NR3C1* promoter exon 1F in whole blood and saliva cell DNA and the morning plasma cortisol levels within a study collective (n = 241, 51 female) with full criteria or features of conduct disorder (CD) or oppositional defiant disorder (ODD) in contrast to an Australian normative sample as control (35). Psychopathologic symptoms were scaled into more internalizing disorders in contrast to features of externalizing disorders like CU traits or conduct problems. Overall methylation levels of *NR3C1* exon 1 in blood and saliva DNA probes were associated with higher levels of internalizing disorders. Distinctly, CpG10 showed an association of increased methylation with higher scores of internalizing symptoms. In contrast, methylation levels of CpG3 and CpG4 in saliva DNA probes predicted externalizing severity (34). Peripheral morning cortisol plasma levels were associated with hypermethylation of CpG9 in PBC DNA only.

Additionally, Radtke et al. (36) investigated the mutual influences of childhood maltreatment history, methylation of the *NR3C1* promoter in peripheral blood lymphocytes and psychopathological load in subjects of a convenience sample (n = 46, 28 female). Their findings didn't indicate a significant correlation between average methylation of the *NR3C1* promoter region with childhood maltreatment severity or with scores of the collected psychometric data. Though, by single analyses they depicted two of 41 selected CpG sites that interacted with childhood maltreatment and vulnerability to psychopathology. One of the two mentioned CpG site was located in exon 1F promoter and its methylation was highly significantly correlated with the number of experienced childhood adversities according to the CTQ as well as with BPD symptoms. With performing a linear model the authors revealed an independently strong effect of both childhood maltreatment and methylation status of this CpG site on the development of BPD-associated symptoms, and they found an additive effect of both of these factors (36).

In summary, studies on epigenetic associations with antisocial traits all focused on single genes. Each one study revealed significant methylation modifications in the *SLC6A4* promoter (30) and in *HTR1B* (31), both in interaction with genotype variants of the concerned gene. Two studies focused on *OXTR*, with different results. In the first study, high CU traits were associated with *OXTR* hypermethylation, which was correlated with lower serum OXT level (32). In another, longitudinally performed study, *OXTR* hypermethylation at birth was associated with higher CU traits at prepubertal age in youth with low internalizing problems, but *OXTR* methylation was not associated with CU traits in youth with high internalizing problems, in which they were positively correlated with prenatal interpersonal risks and negatively with negative life events (18). This suggests a different (epi-)genetic pathogenesis of CU traits. In contrast, mean methylation of *MAOA* was not associated with ASPD symptom scores (33), nor was it significantly related to the *MAOA* VTNR genotypes. However, differentiated results exist in the two independent studies with *NR3C1*. Therefore, hypermethylation of distinct CpG-Sites within *NR3C1* promoter exon 1F, but not overall methylation, was associated with externalizing symptoms (34). This is consistent with the results of another study, in which *NR3C1* promoter exon 1F methylation showed no correlation with psychometric scores, but in consideration with childhood maltreatment both factors interacted in predicting vulnerability to psychopathology (36). Interestingly, *NR3C1* was most investigated in BPD (-> Borderline Personality Disorder). Only two studies considered ELA as an independent factor (30, 36). All studies fail to provide a healthy control group; most of the studies are restricted to only male or female study subjects. Only one study analyzed the transcriptional relevance of the detected methylation alterations by means of the protein level (32). Hence, the represented studies in antisocial and BPD-associated personality traits yet cannot provide a base for general conclusions.

Aggression

Within a 21 year longitudinal study on early onset aggression the research group Wang et al. specified children by severity and persistence of aggressive behavior during their age of 6–15 years and established four states of childhood aggression trajectories: the first consisted in subjects with no physical aggression at any time points (no physical aggression, NPA), a second in subjects with low to moderate aggression that declined between age 10–15 (low physical aggression, LPA), the third in subjects with high rates of aggression that subsequently declined (childhood-limited high physical aggression, CLHPA) and finally in subjects with consistently high physical aggression until age 15 (chronic high physical aggression, CPA).

Among the described study cohort, Wang et al. (37) studied *SLC6A4* methylation in comparison of healthy male young adult subjects with childhood-limited high physical aggression (CLHPA, $n = 7$) and those with no and low physical aggression in childhood, combining the latter as a control group ($n = 18$). They analyzed DNA extracted from isolated peripheral monocytes and in T cells. Not in T cells but in monocytes the authors found a significantly higher average methylation level across all CpG sites and the authors suggest monocytes to be more reliably in their association study. However, functional analysis in a luciferase assay showed significantly decreased

SLC6A4 gene transcriptional activity for both T cells and monocytes in the CLHPA group. Regarding particular CpG sites individually, methylation at CpG11 and CpG12 were highly positively correlated and significantly higher in the CLHPA group. Individual methylation at CpG5 and CpG6 were highly correlated and higher in the CLHPA subjects. No association was found between mean methylation levels of *SLC6A4* with mRNA level, and with the existing serotonin-transporter-linked polymorphic region (5-HTTLPR) genotype. Amendatory, in a cranial PET scan, the authors observed a significant negative association between methylation levels at CpG 11 and CpG12 in T cells or at CpG5 and CpG6 in monocytes, respectively, and *in vivo* 5-HT synthesis in the lateral left and right orbitofrontal cortex (OBFC), indicating long-term functional effects *in vivo*. The authors discuss their results with caution due to the small sample size (37). In connection with the aforementioned study, Provençal et al. (38) compared male adult subjects with chronic high physical aggression (CPA, $n = 8$) with subjects of a conjoint cohort of the other three above defined aggression groups (37) which had developed normal aggression trajectories in adulthood ($n = 12$). They surveyed the methylation status in extracted DNA from peripheral monocytes and T cells with a comprehensive microarray encompassing the entire genomic region including the cytokines IL1A, IL6, IL8, IL4, and IL10 and the transcription factors nuclear factor kappa B subunit 1 (*NFkB1*), nuclear factor of activated T cells 5 (*NFAT5*), signal transducer and activator of transcription 6 (*STAT6*) in both study groups. The results showed significant methylation differences concerning each of the analyzed cytokine gene loci. In CPA subjects overall methylation levels were significantly decreased in *IL1A*, *IL4*, *IL6*, and *IL8*, and were significantly increased in *IL10*. Methylation was positively correlated with serum protein levels of IL1A (significant), IL4, and IL-6, and was negatively correlated for IL-8 and IL-10, respectively. In regard to the transcription factors, two regions closely located to the TSS of each *STAT6* isoform were significantly higher methylated in the CPA group, which was significantly associated with lower transcription of IL4. Next, Provençal et al. conducted a GWA (39) in connection with CPA by comparing male young adult subjects with early development of CPA ($n = 8$) with subjects without any history of high physical aggression in childhood (NPA, $n = 16$) according to the former study definition (37, 38). They analyzed DNA from peripheral T cells and found early onset CPA being associated with clustered and genome-wide methylation differences at 900 sites within 448 distinct gene promoters. The detected genes comprised several that have been associated with aggression earlier: arginine vasopressin receptor 1A (*AVPR1A*), serotonin receptor 1D (*HTR1D*) and glutamate metabotropic receptor 5 (*GRM5*) genes with less methylation in the CPA group, and the dopamine receptor D1 gene (*DRD1*) and *SLC6A3* with higher methylation in the CPA group. In total, most functional categories of genes with different methylation in CPA included behavior (hyperactivity), metabolic and neurological diseases, inflammatory response (chemotaxis and phagocytes), cellular growth and proliferation, and gene expression (transcription factors, signal transducer as *STAT6*). Concerned specific canonical pathways included cytokine signaling and G-protein coupled receptor signaling.

In a further GWA Guillemin et al. studied methylation aberrancies in DNA from isolated peripheral T-cells in female subjects with CPA trajectories since childhood ($n = 5$) compared to women without any aggression history ($n = 16$) (40). A total of 917 probes corresponding to 430 distinct gene promoters were differentially methylated, of which many are involved in immune and inflammatory responses such as *FOS*, *GATA1*, *GATA3*, hepatocyte growth factor (*HGF*), *TNF*, *IFNG*, *IL1A*, *IL1B*, *IL10*, *IL13*, *IL17R*, and *IL18*. Thereof, some had previously been shown to be associated with aggressive behavior, including Tryptophan hydroxylase 2 (*TPH2*), *NR3C1*, and Corticotrophin-releasing hormone-binding protein (*CRHBP*), all of them were significantly less methylated in the CPA subjects.

In a second step, the researchers compared their results with their previous data of a GWA in male subjects out of the same underlying longitudinal study by Provençal et al. (39). Methylation levels of 31 gene promoters emerged to associate with physical aggression in both women and men and therewith constituted a significant overlap, including *TPH2*, *CRHBP*, and *NR3C1*. In the region within the zinc finger protein 366 gene (*ZNF366*) promoter, aggression-associated methylation was differentially directed in both women and men (40).

Van Dongen et al. (41) studied methylation differences with respect to aggressive behavior in 40 monozygotic twins (20 pairs) highly discordant for aggressive traits. They performed a GWA with PBC DNA and received about 24 methylation sites with high methylation difference, yet differences were generally twin pair-specific; thus, statistically no genome-wide significant methylation differences were identified in this sample.

Subsuming the main results of studies on aggressive traits, four of the five studies derived from the same study group. Two studies were theory-driven and gene-targeted. Their results indicate increased methylation of *SLC6A4* in healthy men with a history of CLHPA with implications for the transcriptional activity *in vitro*, and showed associations with brain 5-HT in the left lateral OBFC (37). A more comprehensive genome region analysis including *IL1A*, *IL4*, *IL6*, *IL8*, *IL10*, and transcription factors *NFkB1*, *NFAT5*, and *STAT6* revealed significant methylation differences in men with CPA in transcriptional relevant sites near or within each of the investigated genes. However, correlations with interleukin serum plasma levels only were significant for *IL1A*. Many of the identified methylation aberrances concerned sites outlying the intrinsic gene sequences, underlining the relevancy of methylation analyses that are not restricted to targeted gene sequences (38). A complementary study in women with CPA revealed similar results for immune and inflammatory genes (40). GWA results confirmed genome-wide involvement of methylation differences with respect to aggressive traits in men (39). The mentioned studies were performed in a small sample size of 8 (men) and 5 (women) subjects, respectively, in the aggression group. None of the studies considered the experience of childhood trauma.

Overall, the depicted studies confirm the need of genome-wide methylation assays, or at least a focus on a comprehensive set of functional associated genes. Future studies should consider childhood trauma, and specify an applicable control group.

Impulsiveness

By performing a GWA Ruggeri et al. (42) studied methylation aberrancies in PBC DNA of monozygotic twin pairs ($n = 18$) discordant for alcohol use disorder. The authors received 77 differentially methylated regions associated with 62 genes. Replication of these findings in a microarray only revealed significant methylation changings at one CpG site in the 3′UTR of 3′-protein-phosphatase-1G gene (*PPM1G*). Hypermethylation in *PPM1G* was positively correlated with lower mRNA levels of *PPM1G* and significantly associated with early escalation of alcohol use, as well as with increased impulsiveness. Further analyses evidenced that *PPM1G* hypermethylation was independently associated with both trait impulsiveness and right subthalamic nucleus activation, presumptively due to an increased effort to carry out control inhibition. Since *PPM1G* is assembled with five SNP's, the authors performed regression analyses which could rule out significant influences of genotype variations on *PPM1G* methylation. Further, no correlation was found for the SNP's with the trait impulsiveness (42).

Studies on personality traits are summarized in **Table 2**.

DISCUSSION

The objective of this review was to summarize the first complete number of current original publications on human personality disorders and personality traits in connection with epigenetic modifications and to discuss the results as to pathogenetic impact and treatment-relevant insights. Remarkably, literature search yielded no single study of epigenetic evaluations in narcissistic, histrionic, anankastic, avoidant, dependent, eccentric, paranoid, schizoid and schizotypal personality aspects. Neither there was any result with any keyword on histone modification, nor results with studies on microRNA, but only on methylation aberrancies. Aggression and antisocial traits were prevalently explored, possibly preferred since these behavioral characteristics have a high genetic loading [e.g., (43)].

Most of the theory-driven studies focussed on gene loci involved in the serotonergic, dopaminergic or noradrenergic neurotransmitter system, e.g., serotonin receptor and transporter, dopamine receptor, and MAOA. Further crucial interest was in epigenetic modulation of the functionality of neurotrophic factors, the HPA-axis circuit, and the oxytocinergic system. This seems consequent, since these gene products are constitutive for brain function. Thusly, MAOA, a X-chromosomal encoded enzyme, is responsible for the oxidative breakdown of monoamine neurotransmitters, that is in the brain specifically serotonin, epinephrine, norepinephrine, and dopamine. Mutations in the MAOA gene with impaired gene activity lead to excess of serotonin and norepinephrine which is associated with disturbed control of an affected subject's impulsivity and aggression (NIH, Genetics Home Reference). BDNF is involved in growth, maturation and maintenance of nerve cells and plays a crucial role in building up synapses and in synaptic plasticity. Polymorphisms in the BDNF gene are associated with an increased risk of psychiatric disorders like bipolar disorder, anxiety, and eating disorders. However, results from genome-wide association studies refer to epigenetic alterations of genes that, besides neurofunctional genes, include genomic regions affecting genes involved in inflammation, cell-signaling, metabolism, and genes coding for proteins of the transcriptional machinery themselves (27, 29, 39–42). Methylation differences therefore represent a complex pattern that precludes feasible functional verification tests of the concerned gene loci, as it complicates a conclusive interpretation. The here reviewed GWA studies all, except for Prados et al., lack the consideration of additional factors possibly influencing the epigenetic configuration, especially early childhood experiences, which is also of main interest in understanding the development of a PD. For example, early life adversity was associated with methylation of *SLC6A4* that in turn showed association to brain structure and function (44). In contrast, most of the studies on PD and single gene analyses respected childhood trauma as a confounding factor in their epigenetic analyses. According to previous data, these gene targeted studies confirmed the relevance of the serotonergic system for affective regulation and revealed methylation aberrances of the serotonin transporter (*SLC6A4*) and receptor genes (*5HTR1B*, *5HTR2A*, and *5HTR3A*) to be linked with antisocial traits (30, 31) and BPD (25, 26). As well for *DRD2*, methylation status was shown to be associated with BPD (24). Based on its effect on the pathway of each serotonin, dopamine and norepinephrine, epigenetic changes of *MAOA* congruently were found to be associated with antisocial personality traits, ASPD and BPD (19, 20, 26, 33). Studies also indicate a significant role of *NR3C1* promoter exon 1 methylation status in antisocial traits, as well as, in combination with early life adversity, in BPD (22, 26). Indeed, with the insight in a genome-wide involvement of epigenetic modified gene loci, the validity of the studies on particular genes today seems to be restricted.

Aside from a general association of epigenetic changes in personality disorders and traits, the study results highly differ regarding the particular gene sites of epigenetic differences. One major reason could be the lack or the incomparability of the respective control group in each study. Another methodical deficit is the inconstant consideration of environmental factors, particularly early child adversity. Epigenetically vulnerable influences further include exposure to intimate partner violence during pregnancy as well as mood, smoking or diet habits of the mother during pregnancy, and stress of the subject as a fetus or in its early life (45–49). Notably, in many studies, the sample size is very small and might impact the results.

All studies used extracted DNA from peripheral blood cells for methylation analyses, albeit different cell fractions, preferably whole blood cells, leucocytes, lymphocytes, T cells. There is evidence that peripheral mononuclear cells, particularly lymphocytes, show similar epigenetic pattern with brain tissue [i.e., (9)], and the use of peripheral blood cells has gained acceptance for epigenetic studies of neuropsychiatric disorders. But results also indicate differences of epigenetic patterns between blood leucocyte lines (37, 38) which also could account for discrepancies within the studies. Future studies should

TABLE 2 | Studies on epigenetics in personality traits.

Author	Year	Trait	Gene	Co-factors	Results	Sample	Tissue/DNA	Limitations
Beach et al. (30)	2011	Antisocial	*SLC6A4*	5-HTLPR genotype, SA	No significant association of child SA on ASPD symptom score (only by trend). Significant association of *SLC6A4* methylation level with child SA and with ASPD symptom score, resp. Impact of genotype: significant correlation between *SLC6A4* promoter methylation and ASPD in subjects with ss genotype, and with sl genotype, but not with ll genotype. Methylation potentiated the effect of *SLC6A4* risk alleles.	*Subjects:* adult female participants of the IAS (n = 155). *Diagnostics:* Retrospective clinical interview on childhood sexual abuse, ASPD symptoms: SSAGA-II (consistent with DSM-IV). *Methods:* DNA bisulfite treatment, selected methylation analysis of 71 CpG sites within the *SLC6A4* promoter by quantitative mass spectroscopy DNA sequencing for genotyping.	EBV-transformed lymphoblast cell lines	Only female subjects. No HC.
Moul et al. (31)	2015	Antisocial	*HTR1B*	SNP genotype	*Genotype and CU traits:* high CU subjects were significantly more likely to be heterozygous for the minor (risk) allele. *Genotype and methylation:* genotype was significantly associated with overall methylation level of *HTR1B*. Significantly lower methylation levels in minor homozygotes compared to heterozygotes or major homozygotes. *Methylation and CU traits:* No main effect of genotype or *HTR1B* methylation on CU traits, but genotype by methylation was a significant predictor of CU traits. In heterozygotes CU traits were significantly positively correlated with *HTR1B* methylation. In major homozygotes CU traits were significantly negatively correlated with *HTR1B* methylation. Individual CpG sites: 2 of 19 CpG sites (CpG 12 and 14) interacted with the genotype as significant predictors for CU traits, and correlated negatively with overall *HTR1B* methylation. CpG12: significant negative correlation between methylation and CU traits in heterozygotes, significant positive correlation in major homozygotes.	*Subjects:* male children (n = 117) with CU traits, aged 3–16 years. Subjects were grouped by CU traits (see text). Comorbidity: ODD/CD n = 57), ADHD (n = 33), anxiety/depression (n = 11), ASD (n = 15). *Diagnostic:* DSM-IV, DISCAP, APSD, SDQ, QFE. *Methods:* DNA sequencing of *HTR1B* SNP rs11568817genotype by PCR and mass spectrometry analysis. Selected methylation quantification by quantitative mass spectroscopy of three CpG rich regions surrounding the SNP (19 CpG).	Saliva	Only male subjects. No HC. No consideration of ELA.
Dadds et al. (32)	2014	Antisocial	*OXTR*		In the whole sample, higher CU traits were associated with higher methylation levels at two particular CpG sites of *OXTR* and with lower OXT blood levels. Methylation level and OXT blood level were inversely correlated. If grouped by CU severity and by age, in the older group methylation was significantly higher and OXT serum levels significant lower in the high-CU subjects. In the prepubertal group methylation and OXT blood levels varied similar but only by trend.	*Subjects:* male children (n = 156), aged 4–16 years with conduct problems (full or symptoms of ODD or CD according to DSM-IV) with a severity >3 (scale 0–6) in to the DISCAP. Prepubertal group (age 4–8 years), pubertal group (age 9–16 years). Subjects were grouped by CU traits (see text). *Diagnostics:* DSM-IV, DISCAP, APSD (level of CU), SDQ, QFE. *Methods:* genotyping by PCR and mass spectrometry analysis. Selected methylation analysis of 11 CpG sites within an *OXTR* CpG island (Chr3: 8810680- 8810890) by quantitative mass spectroscopy (subsample n = 98). OXT plasma levels (subsample n = 37), OXT extraction by cold acetone ether, quantification by radioimmunoassay.	PBC	Only male subjects. No HC. No consideration of ELA.

(Continued)

TABLE 2 | Continued

Author	Year	Trait	Gene	Co-factors	Results	Sample	Tissue/DNA	Limitations
Cecil et al. (18)	2014	Antisocial	*OXTR*		*Youth with low internalizing problems:* OXTR methylation at birth was related to higher CU traits at age 13 and to decreased experience of direct victimization during early childhood. OXTR methylation at birth was positively associated with prenatal parental risks (maternal psychopathology, criminal behaviors, substance use) and was temporal more stable than in youth with high internalizing problems. *Youth with high internalizing problems:* CU traits showed no association with OXTR methylation, but were positively correlated with prenatal, especially interpersonal risks (intimate partner violence, family conflict). CU traits were negatively associated with postnatal risks, specifically life events (death of relative, accidents, illness).	*Subjects:* youth (n =84), aged 0–13 years with early-onset and persistent conduct problems, divided in groups with low (n = 39) and high level (n = 45) of internalizing problems. *Diagnostics at birth, age 7, age 9, age 13:* Strengths and Difficulties Questionnaire (subscale "conduct problem"), Environmental risk score (by maternal reports), Development and Well-being Assessment (internalizing problems, by maternal reports), CU traits questionnaire oriented on Antisocial Process Screening Device (by mothers report). *Methods:* cord blood (at birth) and peripheral blood (at age 7+9). DNA bisulfite treatment, BeadChip technology for methylation quantification. Selected methylation analysis of 12 CpG sites within an *OXTR* CpG island (hg19; chr3:8808962–8811280).	PBC	No HC. No consideration of ELA.
Philibert et al. (33)	2008	Antisocial	*MAOA*	VTNR genotype	No significant association of overall methylation of *MAOA* and symptom counts for ASPD in women or men. Each particular CpG site showed higher methylation in female subjects. By statistical trend women homozygous for the 3,3 allele have higher average methylation of *MAOA* than 4,4 allele subjects.	*Subjects:* adult participants of the IAS (s.a.) (n = 191, 96 female). *Diagnostics:* DSM-IV. *Methods:* DNA bisulfite treatment, PCR amplification and selected methylation analysis of two CpG-rich regions (10 and 70 CpG-sites) of *MAOA* by quantitative mass spectroscopy. DNA Sequencing of *MAOA* VTNR genotype.	EBV-transformed lymphoblast cell lines	No consideration of ELA.
Dadds et al. (34)	2015	Antisocial	*NR3C1*		*NR3C1* overall methylation level (blood and saliva) was associated with higher levels of internalizing disorders. Hypermethylation (blood and saliva) of CpG10 was associated with higher internalizing symptoms. CpG3 and CpG4 hypermethylation (saliva) predicted externalizing severity. Elevated morning cortisol plasma levels were associated with increased methylation of CpG9 (blood).	*Subjects:* children (n = 241, 51 female), aged 4–16 years with conduct problems (full or symptoms of ODD or CD according DSM-IV), referred to the Australian Normative Sample as control (19). *Diagnostics:* DSM-IV, SDQ, DISCAP. Comorbidity: ODD/CD 66%, ADHD 26%, anxiety/depression 6%, ASD 5%. *Methods:* Genotyping and selective methylation analysis of *NR3C1* promoter exon 1F (12 CpG sites) by mass spectroscopy. Morning cortisol plasma levels were quantified by chemiluminescent enzyme immunoassay.	PBC (n = 90), saliva (n = 151)	HC only for diagnostic data. No consideration of ELA.

(Continued)

TABLE 2 | Continued

Author	Year	Trait	Gene	Co-factors	Results	Sample	Tissue/DNA	Limitations
Radtke et al. (36)	2015	Antisocial	*NR3C1*	CM	CM and *NR3C1* promoter methylation was strongly correlated with an increased vulnerability to psychopathology. No significant correlation of *NR3C1* methylation neither with CM nor with applied psychometric measurements. Individual CpG sites: methylation at CpG cg17860381 (located in exon 1F) was significantly associated with the number of experienced CM and with severity of BPD symptoms (nearly significantly with depression). It was positively (not significant) correlated with ODD-associated symptoms and behavioral strength and difficulties. Interaction of CM and *NR3C1* methylation: CM and *NR3C1* mean methylation significantly interacted in predicting psychological health. CM and methylation of CpG cg17860381 showed an additive, but no interactive impact on the development of BPD-associated symptoms.	*Subjects:* convenience sample from the local community ($n = 46$, 28 female), aged 11–21 years. *Diagnostics:* KERF-I (specifies CM in 8 dimensions: parental PA, parental EA, SA, witnessed physical violence toward parents/siblings, peer physical violence, PN and EN), BPD: BSC-23, HSC-25 (depression, anxiety), MINI (ODD/OD). KIDSCREEN-53, SDQ. *Methods:* DNA bisulfite treatment, GWA by Human Methylation 450K Array, covering 41 CpG sites within the *NR3C1* promoter.	Lymphocytes (isolated by Ficoll gradient)	No group design.
Wang et al. (37)	2012	Aggression	*SLC6A4*	5-HTLPR genotype	*T-cells:* no significant differences in *SLC64A* average methylation level of CLHPA subjects and controls, but high variability in methylation status at individual CpG sites. Methylation at CpG11 and CpG12 was significantly higher in CLHPA subjects. *Monocytes:* average methylation level was higher in CLHPA. In particular methylation at CpG5 and CpG6 was significantly increased in CLHPA subjects. No association of methylation levels and 5-HTTLPR genotype. *Functional analysis:* Hypermethylation of SLC6A4 significantly decreased gene transcriptional activity in the luciferase assay. *5-HT synthesis:* methylation of CpG11 and CpG12 in T-cells, and of CpG5 and CpG6 in monocytes, respectively, was significantly negatively correlated with 5-HT synthesis in the lateral left OBFC.	*Subjects:* healthy male young adults with none or low aggression (LPA) in childhood (controls, $n = 18$) and CLHPA ($n = 7$). Tissue: T-cells, monocytes. *Diagnostics:* based on longitudinal observation data collected annually between age 6 and 15, clinical diagnostic, SDQ. *Methods:* DNA bisulfite treatment, PCR amplification, quantitative pyrosequencing of *SLC6A4* promoter (24 CpG sites). Genotyping of *5-HTLPR*. *In vitro* functional analysis (luciferase assay). PET: tracer alpha-[(11)C]methyl-L-tryptophan ((11)C-AMT) for 5-HT synthesis analysis. Voxel of interest: hippocampus, lateral and medial OBFC, ncl. caudate.	Monocytes, CD3+ T cells (density centrifugation)	Only clinically healthy subjects, only men. No consideration of ELA.

(Continued)

TABLE 2 | Continued

Author	Year	Trait	Gene	Co factors	Results	Sample	Tissue/DNA	Limitations
Provençal et al. (38)	2013	Aggression	*IL1A, IL4, IL6, IL8, IL10, NFkB1, NFAT5, STAT6*		Methylation status of the 5 cytokine and 3 transcription factor gene loci was different in each analyzed CpG site in either T-cells (20 loci) or monocytes (28). In CPA subjects mean methylation levels were significantly decreased in *IL1A*, *IL4*, *IL6*, and *IL8*, and increased in *IL10*. Methylation levels were positively correlated with Plasma protein level for IL1a, IL-4, IL-6, and negatively correlated for IL-8 and IL10. Two regions closed to the TSS of each *STAT6* isoform were significantly hypermethylated in the CPA group. Many of the revealed methylation deviant loci were associated with DNAse clusters.	*Subjects:* male young adults with CPA ($n = 8$), controls ($n = 12$) recruited from all the trajectory groups NPA, LPA, CLHPA. *Diagnostics* and definitions as described earlier (22). *Methods:* Methylated DNA immunoprecipitation with microarray hybridization for *IL1A*, *IL4*, *IL6*, *IL8*, *IL10*, *NFkB1*, *NFAT5*, *STAT6*. Microarray validation: DNA bisulfite treatment, PCR amplification, quantitative pyrosequencing (48 CpG sites).	Monocytes, CD3+ T cells (density centrifugation)	Only men. No consideration of ELA.
Provençal et al. (39)	2014	Aggression	genome-wide		High physical aggression was associated with clustered and genome-wide variations in promoter methylation. Within the plenty, 227 gene loci were significantly more methylated in the control group (including 10 micro RNA promoters) and 171 were significantly more methylated in the CPA group (including 2 microRNA promoters). Five of the genes were already described to be linked with aggression: *AVPR1A*, *HTR1D*, *GRM5* were less methylated in the CPA group and *DRD1* and *SLC6A3* were hypermethylated.	*Subjects:* male young adults with CPA ($n = 8$), controls with no (never) history of high physical aggression from age 6–15 ($n = 12$). *Diagnostics* and definitions as described earlier (22). *Methods:* GWA: Methylated DNA immunoprecipitation with microarray hybridization. Microarray validation: by quantitative real-time PCR on immunoprecipitated DNA and by pyrosequencing of bisulfite treated DNA.	Monocytes, CD3+ T cells (density centrifugation)	Only men. No consideration of ELA.
Guilleminet al. (40)	2014	Aggression	genome-wide		Significant association of CPA with methylation aberrances in a plenty of genes, many involved in immune and inflammatory responses such as *FOS*, *GATA1*, *GATA3*, *HGF*, *TNF*, *IFNG*, *IL1A*, *IL1B*, *IL17R*, *IL10*, *IL13*, and *IL18*. Methylation differences were aggression-associated in 31 promoter sites in both woman and men, i.a. *TPH2*, *CRHBP*, *NR3C1* (less methylated in the CPA group). One CpG site was significantly associated with aggression in both women and men, but was differentially deviant methylated (*ZNF366* promoter region).	*Subjects:* female young adults with CPA ($n = 5$), controls without any aggression history ($n = 16$). *Diagnostics* as described earlier (22). *Methods:* GWA: Methylated DNA immunoprecipitation with microarray hybridization. Microarray validation: gene-specific by quantitative real-time PCR on immunoprecipitated DNA and genome-wide by using BeadChip technology. Retrospective comparison with results in male young adults (28)	CD3+ T cells (density centrifugation)	Only women. No consideration of ELA.
van Dongen et al. (41)	2015	Aggression	genome-wide		Large number of differently methylated loci, none resisting Bonferroni correction. In the subsample of 20 MZ twin pairs discordant for aggressive traits, methylation differed at 24 sites which were twin pair-specific and without statistically relevance in the whole assay. Suggestive CpG sites were i.e. gene loci near *RAB39*, *SIGLEC10*, *PREP*.	*Subjects:* subjects from the Netherlands Twin Register. First GWA: 2029 subjects (1247 MZ, 663 DZ, parents and other siblings). Second GWA: 20 MZ pairs, highly discordant for aggression. *Diagnostics:* ASR. *Methods:* DNA bisulfite treatment, GWA BeadChip technology*.	PBC	No consideration of ELA.

(Continued)

TABLE 2 | Continued

Author	Year	Trait	Gene	Co-factors	Results	Sample	Tissue/DNA	Limitations
Ruggeri et al. (42)	2015	Impulsiveness	genome-wide, *PPM1G*		GWA resulted in 77 differently methylated sites. In the replication array, only methylation of *PPM1G* was significantly different and was positively associated with increased impulsiveness. PPM1G hypermethylation was significantly associated with lower mRNA levels. *PPM1G* hypermethylation was independently associated with both trait impulsiveness and right subthalamic nucleus activation.	*Subjects:* MZ twin pairs ($n = 18$), aged 24y. *Diagnostics:* DSM-III-R, RAPI, SURPS, PDS. *Methods:* GWA. Validation assay: bisulfite PCR for genes *PPMG1*, *INS-IGF2*, *FMN1*, *SEPHS2*, *SLC6A3*, *AIM1*, *OPRL1*, and *PIPOX*. Functional analysis: mRNA quantification by hybridizing labeled cRNA on BeadChip technology. fMRI: BOLD brain analysis during an inhibitory control task	PBC	No consideration of ELA.

*5-HT, 5-hydroxytryptophane (serotonin); 5-HTTLPR, serotonin-transporter-linked polymorphic region; ADHD, attention deficit hyperactivity disorder; APSD, Antisocial Process Screening Device; ASD, Autism spectrum disorder; ASPD, Antisocial personality disorder; ASR, ASEBA Adult Self Report; AVPR1A, arginine vasopressin receptor 1A gene; BOLD, blood-oxygen-level-dependent response; BPD, borderline personality disorder; BSC-23, Borderline Symptoms Checklist-23; CD, conduct disorder; CLHPA, childhood-limited high physical aggression; CM, childhood maltreatment; CPA, chronic high physical aggression; CRHBP, CREB binding protein gene; CU, callous-unemotional; DISCAP, Diagnostic Interview Schedule for Children, Adolescents and Parents; DRD1, dopamine receptor D1 gene; DZ, dizygotic; EA, emotional abuse; ELA, early life adversity; EN, emotional neglect; FOS, fos proto-oncogene AP-1, transcription factor subunit; GATA1/GATA3, GATA binding protein 1/3; GRM5, glutamate metabotropic receptor 5 gene; GWA, genome-wide methylation analysis; HC, healthy control; HGF, hepatocyte growth factor gene; HSC-25, Hopkins Symptoms Checklint-25; HTR1B/HTR1D, serotonin receptor 1B/1D gene; HTR3A, serotonin receptor 3A gene; IAS, Iowa Adoptee Study; IFNG, interferon gamma gene; IL1A, (1B/4/6/8/10/13/17A/18) interleukin 1A (1B/4/6/8/10/13/17A/18) gene; IL17RA, interleukin 17 receptor A gene; IPV, interpersonal violence; KERF-I, German version of MACE (Maltreatment and Abuse Chronology of Exposure); KIDSCREEN-53, children questionnaire of health-related quality of life; LPA, low physical aggression (subjects); MAOA, monoamine oxidase A gene; MINI, Mini-International Neuropsychiatric Interview; MZ, monozygotic; NR3C1, glucocorticoid receptor gene; OBFC, orbital frontal cortex; ODD, oppositional-defiant disorder; OXT, oxytocin; OXTR, oxytocin receptor gene; PA, physical abuse; PBC, peripheral whole blood cells; PDS, Pubertal Development Scale; PN, physical neglect; PPM1G, 3'-protein-phosphatase-1G gene; PREP, prolyl endopeptidase gene; PTSD, posttraumatic stress disorder; QFE, Quality of the Family Environment questionnaire; RAB39, RAS oncogene family 39 gene; RAPI, Rudgers Alcohol Problem Index; SA, sexual abuse; SDQ, Strengths and Difficulties Questionnaire; SIGLEC10, Sialic Acid Binding Ig Like Lectin 10 gene; SLC6A3, dopamine transporter gene; SLC6A4, serotonin transporter gene; SNP, single nucleotide polymorphism; SSAGA-II, Semi-Structured Assessment for the Genetics of Alcoholism; STAT6, signal transducer and activator of transcription 6; SURPS, Substance Use Risk Profile Scale; TPH2, tryptophan hydroxylase 2 gene; VTNR, variable number tandem repeats; ZNF366, zinc finger protein 366. *Results were corrected for white cell counts.*

consider cell type and preparation from whole blood, since cell stress can cause epigenetic changes in the cells (50).

High requirements in the technical methods and in an expedient study design make the disentangling of personality-specific methylation patterns a sensitive challenge, especially since there might be more than one way to (epi-)genetically forward the development of a PD. This also might be a reason for the diversity of the final clinical epiphenotypes of these disorders. Conversely, the variety of pathogenesis and of the individually developed clinical shapes impedes the attribution of possibly identified genetic or epigenetic aberrances to a specific personality trait or disorder.

If the functional attribution of epigenetic aberrations to personality disorders is so highly impeded, which benefit can we gain in doing so?

The possibility of epigenetic subtyping helps to assess the individual pathophysiologic condition as well as to improve deductive therapeutic approaches. The identification of someone's epigenetic risk profile could initiate efforts to establish standards for intensified clinical watching in afflicted children, and methods for early parental coaching or for premature intervention in order to prevent further development of a full-blown clinical picture of a PD. As impressively shown by Cecil et al., divergent epigenetic conditions within psychopathologically similar subjects can elicit different implications for the individual treatment requirements (18).

As in other mental disorders, epigenetic patterns can help to predict medical response. Thus, in depression, selected methylation aberrations could predict different therapy response to escitalopram and between escitalopram and nortriptyline (51, 52). In BPD, methylation levels of *APBA3* and *MCF2* were predictive for psychotherapy outcome (53).

In cancer, advanced therapy today comprises epigenetic drugs targeting i.e., on silenced tumor suppressing genes. Due to the plurality and individual diversity of involved genes in psychiatric disorders, the use of demethylating drugs cannot be targeted to distinct genes. Adverse effects with general hypomethylation might conflict with the aimed benefits. But there is evidence that methyldonor components as valproic or folic acid have positive therapeutic effects in mental disorders by themselves as well as by increasing the effect of fluoxetine (54–57).

Aside from their primary neurobiological effect, psychotropic drugs can further exert direct epigenetic effects. Studies on antidepressants and antipsychotic drugs i.e., evidenced their possibility to modulate the epigenome by acetylation of gene-associated histones, by methylation changes in dopamine pathways (58), by increasing expression of DNA-methyltransferases, and by inducing chromatin remodeling (58, 59). Methylation aberrations also can be remodulated by psychopharmacological treatment or psychotherapy (60, 61).

These merely exemplary findings suggest a high dynamic in epigenetic processes in mental disorders and their course. The interaction of psychotropic drugs and other therapeutic interventions with epigenetic remodeling seems still understudied. Finally, the fact of this interaction then could be utilized as an intraindividual control of lasting therapy response.

IMPLICATIONS AND FUTURE OPTIONS

The pathophysiological principle of gene-environment-interaction not only explains the obvious differences in the severity or combination of a person's personality traits but further implicates the existence of genetic and epigenetic risk and protective factors during the formation of the ultimate personality structure. Hitherto epigenetic studies underline the impact of early life adversity on the multifactorial pathway to PD. They reveal several relevant gene loci that are epigenetically affected in PD but differ in between the studies. This can partially be explained by the multifactorial and multi-step genesis of each PD, leading to different pathogenetic subtypes.

Epigenetic analyses in connection with PD represent a complex, but suitable amendment in the elucidation of personality development, and pose as valuable diagnostic step in the specification of an individual's premorbid risks, and for the development of individually tailored therapeutic strategies. They might play a valuable role in the future design and observation of early and personalized therapeutic intervention and thus could help to prevent the unfolding in severe dysfunctional conduct or personality disorder in risk subjects.

AUTHOR CONTRIBUTIONS

DG conducted the full literature search process, read all found articles, wrote the manuscript. KK critically overworked focus and manuscript. TH and HF provided expert advice in epigenetics. JK and TF reviewed the manuscript and collaborated in the interpretation of the results and for the discussion.

REFERENCES

1. Szyf M, McGowan P, Meaney M. The social environment and the epigenome. *Environ Mol Mutagen.* (2008) 49:46–60. doi: 10.1002/em.20357
2. Szyf M, Bick J. DNA methylation: a mechanism for embedding early life experiences in the genome. *Child Dev.* (2013) 84:49–57. doi: 10.1111/j.1467-8624.2012.01793.x
3. Weaver IC, Cervoni N, Champagne FA, D'Alessio AC, Sharma S, Seckl JR, et al. Epigenetic programming by maternal behavior. *Nat Neurosci.* (2004) 7:847–54. doi: 10.1038/nn1276
4. Roth TL, Lubin FD, Funk AJ, Sweatt JD. Lasting epigenetic influence of early-life adversity on the BDNF gene. *Biol Psychiatry* (2009) 65:760–9. doi: 10.1016/j.biopsych.2008.11.028
5. Murgatroyd C, Patchev AV, Wu Y, Micale V, Bockmuhl Y, Fischer D, et al. Dynamic DNA methylation programs persistent adverse effects of early-life stress. *Nat Neurosci.* (2009) 12:1559–66. doi: 10.1038/nn.2436
6. McGowan PO, Sasaki A, D'Alessio AC, Dymov S, Labonte B, Szyf M, et al. Epigenetic regulation of the glucocorticoid receptor in human brain associates with childhood abuse. *Nat Neurosci.* (2009) 12:342–8. doi: 10.1038/nn.2270
7. McGowan PO, Suderman M, Sasaki A, Huang TC, Hallett M, Meaney MJ, et al. Broad epigenetic signature of maternal care in the brain of adult rats. *PLoS ONE* (2011) 6:e14739. doi: 10.1371/journal.pone.0014739
8. Suderman M, McGowan PO, Sasaki A, Huang TC, Hallett M, Meaney MJ, et al. Conserved epigenetic sensitivity to early life experience in the rat and human hippocampus. *Proc Natl Acad Sci USA.* (2012) 109(Suppl. 2):17266–72. doi: 10.1073/pnas.1121260109
9. Provençal N, Suderman MJ, Guillemin C, Massart R, Ruggiero A, Wang D, et al. The signature of maternal rearing in the methylome in rhesus macaque prefrontal cortex and T cells. *J Neurosci.* (2012) 32:15626–42. doi: 10.1523/JNEUROSCI.1470-12.2012
10. Klengel T, Mehta D, Anacker C, Rex-Haffner M, Pruessner JC, Pariante CM, et al. Allele-specific FKBP5 DNA demethylation mediates gene-childhood trauma interactions. *Nat Neurosci.* (2013) 16:33–41. doi: 10.1038/nn.3275
11. Auta J1, Smith RC, Dong E, Tueting P, Sershen H, Boules S, et al. DNA-methylation gene network dysregulation in peripheral blood lymphocytes of schizophrenia patients. *Schizophr Res.* (2013) 150:312–8. doi: 10.1016/j.schres.2013.07.030
12. Yuan LW, Gambee JE. Histone acetylation by p300 is involved in CREB-mediated transcription on chromatin. *Biochim Biophys Acta* (2001) 1541:161–9. doi: 10.1016/S0167-4889(01)00141-0
13. Weaver IC, Hellstrom IC, Brown SE, Andrews SD, Dymov S, Diorio J, et al. The methylated-DNA binding protein MBD2 enhances NGFI-A (egr-1)-mediated transcriptional activation of the glucocorticoid receptor. *Philos Trans R Soc Lond B Biol Sci.* (2014) 369:20130513. doi: 10.1098/rstb.2013.0513
14. Weaver IC, D'Alessio AC, Brown SE, Hellstrom IC, Dymov S, Sharma S, et al. The transcription factor nerve growth factor-inducible protein a mediates epigenetic programming: altering epigenetic marks by immediate-early genes. *J Neurosci.* (2007) 27:1756–68. doi: 10.1523/JNEUROSCI.4164-06.2007
15. Zhou Z, Hong EJ, Cohen S, Zhao WN, Ho HY, Schmidt L, et al. Brain-specific phosphorylation of MeCP2 regulates activity-dependent Bdnf transcription, dendritic growth, and spine maturation. *Neuron* (2006) 52:255–69. doi: 10.1016/j.neuron.2006.09.037
16. Chen WG, Chang Q, Lin Y, Meissner A, West AE, Griffith EC, et al. Derepression of BDNF transcription involves calcium-dependent phosphorylation of MeCP2. *Science* (2003) 302:885–9. doi: 10.1126/science.1086446
17. Shamseer L, Moher D, Clarke M, Ghersi D, Liberati A, Petticrew M, et al. Preferred reporting items for systematic review and meta-analysis protocols (PRISMA-P) 2015: elaboration and explanation. *BMJ* (2015) 349:g7647. doi: 10.1136/bmj.g7647
18. Cecil CA, Lysenko LJ, Jaffee SR, Pingault JB, Smith RG, Relton CL, et al. Environmental risk, oxytocin receptor gene (OXTR) methylation and youth callous-unemotional traits: a 13-year longitudinal study. *Mol Psychiatry* (2014) 19:1071–7. doi: 10.1038/mp.2014.95
19. Philibert RA, Wernett P, Plume J, Packer H, Brody GH, Beach SR. Gene environment interactions with a novel variable monoamine oxidase A transcriptional enhancer are associated with antisocial personality disorder. *Biol Psychol.* (2011) 87:366–71. doi: 10.1016/j.biopsycho.2011.04.007
20. Checknita D, Maussion G, Labonté B, Comai S, Tremblay RE, Vitaro F, et al. Monoamine oxidase A gene promoter methylation and transcriptional downregulation in an offender population with antisocial personality disorder. *Br J Psychiatry* (2015) 206:216–22. doi: 10.1192/bjp.bp.114.144964
21. Perroud N, Salzmann A, Prada P, Nicastro R, Hoeppli ME, Furrer S, et al. Response to psychotherapy in borderline personality disorder and methylation status of the BDNF gene. *Transl Psychiatry* (2013) 3:e207. doi: 10.1038/tp.2012.140
22. Martín-Blanco A, Ferrer M, Soler J, Salazar J, Vega D, Andión O, et al. Association between methylation of the glucocorticoid receptor gene, childhood maltreatment, and clinical severity in borderline personality disorder. *J Psychiatr Res.* (2014) 57:34–40. doi: 10.1016/j.jpsychires.2014.06.011
23. Perroud N, Paoloni-Giacobino A, Prada P, Olié E, Salzmann A, Nicastro R, et al. Increased methylation of glucocorticoid receptor gene (NR3C1) in adults with a history of childhood maltreatment: a link with the severity and type of trauma. *Transl Psychiatry* (2011) 1:e59. doi: 10.1038/tp.2011.60
24. Groleau P, Joober R, Israel M, Zeramdini N, DeGuzman R, Steiger H. Methylation of the dopamine D2 receptor (DRD2) gene promoter in women with a bulimia-spectrum disorder: associations with borderline personality disorder and exposure to childhood abuse. *J Psychiatr Res.* (2014) 48:121–7. doi: 10.1016/j.jpsychires.2013.10.003
25. Perroud N, Zewdie S, Stenz L, Adouan W, Bavamian S, Prada P, et al. Methylation of serotonin receptor 3A in ADHD, Borderline Personality,

and bipolar disorders: link with severity of the disorders and childhood maltreatment. *Depress Anxiety* (2016) 33:45–55. doi: 10.1002/da.22406
26. Dammann G, Teschler S, Haag T, Altmüller F, Tuczek F, Dammann RH. Increased DNA methylation of neuropsychiatric genes occurs in borderline personality disorder. *Epigenetics* (2011) 6:1454–62. doi: 10.4161/epi.6.12.18363
27. Teschler S, Bartkuhn M, Künzel N, Schmidt C, Kiehl S, Dammann G, et al. Aberrant methylation of gene associated CpG sites occurs in borderline personality disorder. *PLoS ONE* (2013) 8:e84180. doi: 10.1371/journal.pone.0084180
28. Teschler S, Gotthardt J, Dammann G, Dammann RH. Aberrant DNA Methylation of rDNA and PRIMA1 in borderline personality Disorder. *Int J Mol Sci.* (2016) 17:E67. doi: 10.3390/ijms17010067
29. Prados J, Stenz L, Courtet P, Prada P, Nicastro R, Adouan W, et al. Borderline personality disorder and childhood maltreatment: a genome-wide methylation analysis. *Genes Brain Behav.* (2015) 14:177–88. doi: 10.1111/gbb.12197
30. Beach SR, Brody GH, Todorov AA, Gunter TD, Philibert RA. Methylation at 5HTT mediates the impact of child sex abuse on women's antisocial behavior: an examination of the Iowa adoptee sample. *Psychosom Med.* (2011) 73:83–7. doi: 10.1097/PSY.0b013e3181fdd074
31. Moul C, Dobson-Stone C, Brennan J, Hawes DJ, Dadds MR. Serotonin 1B receptor gene (HTR1B) methylation as a risk factor for callous-unemotional traits in antisocial boys. *PLoS ONE* (2015) 10:e0126903. doi: 10.1371/journal.pone.0126903
32. Dadds MR, Moul C, Cauchi A, Dobson-Stone C, Hawes DJ, Brennan J, et al. Methylation of the oxytocin receptor gene and oxytocin blood levels in the development of psychopathy. *Dev Psychopathol.* (2014) 26:33–40. doi: 10.1017/S0954579413000497
33. Philibert RA, Gunter TD, Beach SR, Brody GH, Madan A. MAOA methylation is associated with nicotine and alcohol dependence in women. *Neuropsychiatr Genet.* (2008) 147B:565–70. doi: 10.1002/ajmg.b.30778
34. Dadds MR, Moul C, Hawes DJ, Mendoza Diaz A, Brennan J. Individual differences in childhood behavior disorders associated with epigenetic modulation of the cortisol receptor gene. *Child Dev.* (2015) 86:1311–20. doi: 10.1111/cdev.12391
35. Mellor, D. Normative data for the strengths and difficulties questionnaire in Australia. *Aust Psychol.* (2005) 40:215–22. doi: 10.1080/00050060500243475
36. Radtke KM, Schauer M, Gunter HM, Ruf-Leuschner M, Sill J, Meyer A, et al. Epigenetic modifications of the glucocorticoid receptor gene are associated with the vulnerability to psychopathology in childhood maltreatment. *Transl Psychiatry* (2015) 5:e571. doi: 10.1038/tp.2015.63
37. Wang D, Szyf M, Benkelfat C, Provençal N, Turecki G, Caramaschi D, et al. Peripheral SLC6A4 DNA methylation is associated with *in vivo* measures of human brain serotonin synthesis and childhood physical aggression. *PLoS ONE* (2012) 7:e39501. doi: 10.1371/journal.pone.0039501
38. Provençal N, Suderman MJ, Caramaschi D, Wang D, Hallett M, Vitaro F, et al. Differential DNA methylation regions in cytokine and transcription factor genomic loci associate with childhood physical aggression. *PLoS ONE* (2013) 8:e71691. doi: 10.1371/journal.pone.0071691
39. Provençal N, Suderman MJ, Guillemin C, Vitaro F, Côté SM, Hallett M, et al. Association of childhood chronic physical aggression with a DNA methylation signature in adult human T cells. *PLoS ONE* (2014) 9:e89839. doi: 10.1371/journal.pone.0089839
40. Guillemin C, Provençal N, Suderman M, Côté SM, Vitaro F, Hallett M, et al. DNA methylation signature of childhood chronic physical aggression in T cells of both men and women. *PLoS ONE* (2014) 9:e86822. doi: 10.1371/journal.pone.0086822
41. Van Dongen J, Nivard MG, Baselmans BM, Zilhão NR, Ligthart L, BIOS Consortium, et al. Epigenome-wide association study of aggressive behavior. *Twin Res Hum Genet.* (2015) 18:686–98. doi: 10.1017/thg.2015.74
42. Ruggeri B, Nymberg C, Vuoksimaa E, Lourdusamy A, Wong CP, Carvalho FM, et al. Association of protein phosphatase PPM1G with alcohol use disorder and brain activity during behavioral control in a genome-wide methylation analysis. *Am J Psychiatry* (2015) 172:543–52. doi: 10.1176/appi.ajp.2014.14030382
43. Viding E, Blair RJR, Moffitt TE, Plomin R. Evidence for substantial genetic risk for psychopathy in 7-years-olds. *J Child Psychol Psychiatry* (2005) 46:592–7. doi: 10.1111/j.1469-7610.2004.00393.x
44. Frodl T, Szyf M, Carballedo A, Ly V, Dymov S, Vaisheva F, et al. DNA methylation of the serotonin transporter gene (SLC6A4) is associated with brain function involved in processing emotional stimuli. *J Psychiatry Neurosci.* (2015) 40:296–305. doi: 10.1503/jpn.140180
45. Reik W. Stability and flexibility of epigenetic gene regulation in mammalian development. *Nature* (2007) 447:425–32. doi: 10.1038/nature05918
46. Feil R, Fraga MF. Epigenetics and the environment: emerging patterns and implications. *Nat Rev Genet* (2012) 13:97–109. doi: 10.1038/nrg3142
47. Radtke KM, Ruf M, Gunter HM, Dohrmann K, Schauer M, Meyer A, et al. Transgenerational impact of intimate partner violence on methylation in the promoter of the glucocorticoid receptor. *Transl Psychiatry* (2011) 1:e21. doi: 10.1038/tp.2011.21
48. Zeilinger S, Kühnel B, Klopp N, Baurecht H, Kleinschmidt A, Gieger C, et al. Tobacco smoking leads to extensive genome-wide changes in DNA methylation. *PLoS ONE* (2013) 8:e63812. doi: 10.1371/journal.pone.0063812
49. McGowan PO, Meaney MJ, Szyf M. Diet and the epigenetic (re)programming of phenotypic differences in behavior. *Brain Res.* (2008) 1237:12–24. doi: 10.1016/j.brainres.2008.07.074
50. Philibert R, Caspers K, Beach SRH, Bakermans-Kranenburg MJ, van Ijzendoorn MH. Reply to: epstein-barr virus transformed DNA as a source of false positive findings in methylation studies of psychiatric conditions. *Biol Psychiatry* (2011) 70:e27–8. doi: 10.1016/j.biopsych.2011.02.029
51. Domschke K, Tidow N, Schwarte K, Deckert J, Lesch KP, Arolt V, et al. Serotonin transporter gene hypomethylation predicts impaired antidepressant treatment response. *Int J Neuropsychopharmacol.* (2014) 17:1167–76. doi: 10.1017/S146114571400039X
52. Uher R, Huezo-Diaz P, Perroud N, Smith R, Rietschel M, Mors O, et al. Genetic predictors of response to antidepressants in the GENDEP project. *Pharmacogenomics J.* (2009) 9:225–33. doi: 10.1038/tpj.2009.12
53. Knoblich N, Gundel F, Brückmann C, Becker-Sadzio J, Frischholz C, Nieratschker V. DNA methylation of APBA3 and MCF2 in borderline personality disorder: potential biomarkers for response to psychotherapy. *Eur Neuropsychopharmacol.* (2018) 28:252–63. doi: 10.1016/j.euroneuro.2017.12.010
54. Morris DW, Trivedi MH, Rush AJ. Folate and unipolar depression. *J Altern Complement Med.* (2008)14:277–85. doi: 10.1016/j.jad.2011.04.032
55. Farah A. The role of L-methylfolate in depressive disorders. *CNS Spectr.* (2009) 14:2–7. doi: 10.1017/S1092852900003473
56. Coppen A, Bailey J. Enhancement of the antidepressant action of fluoxetine by folic acid: a randomised, placebo controlled trial. *J Affect Disord.* (2000) 60:121–30. doi: 10.1016/S0165-0327(00)00153-1
57. Godfrey PS, Toone BK, Carney MW, Flynn TG, Bottiglieri T, Laundy M, et al. Enhancement of recovery from psychiatric illness by methylfolate. *Lancet* (1990) 336:392–5. doi: 10.1016/0140-6736(90)91942-4
58. Swathy B, Banerjee M. Understanding epigenetics of schizophrenia in the backdrop of its antipsychotic drug therapy. *Epigenomics* (2017) 9:721–36. doi: 10.2217/epi-2016-0106
59. Zimmermann N, Zschocke J, Perisic T, Yu S, Holsboer F, Rein T. Antidepressants inhibit DNA methyltransferase 1 through reducing G9a levels. *Biochem J.* (2012) 448:93–102. doi: 10.1042/BJ20120674
60. Vialou V, Feng J, Robison AJ, Nestler EJ. Epigenetic mechanisms of depression and antidepressants action. *Ann Rev Pharmacol Toxicol.* (2013) 53:59–87. doi: 10.1146/annurev-pharmtox-010611-134540
61. Yehuda R, Daskalakis NP, Desarnaud F, Makotkine I, Lehrner AL, Koch E, et al. Epigenetic biomarkers as predictors and correlates of symptom improvement following psychotherapy in combat veterans with PTSD. *Front Psychiatry* (2013) 4:118. doi: 10.3389/fpsyt.2013.00118

16

Association of the Polygenic Scores for Personality Traits and Response to Selective Serotonin Reuptake Inhibitors in Patients with Major Depressive Disorder

*Azmeraw T. Amare[1], Klaus Oliver Schubert[1,2], Fasil Tekola-Ayele[3], Yi-Hsiang Hsu[4,5,6], Katrin Sangkuhl[7], Gregory Jenkins[8], Ryan M. Whaley[7], Poulami Barman[8], Anthony Batzler[8], Russ B. Altman[9], Volker Arolt[10], Jürgen Brockmöller[11], Chia-Hui Chen[12], Katharina Domschke[13], Daniel K. Hall-Flavin[14], Chen-Jee Hong[15,16], Ari Illi[17], Yuan Ji[18], Olli Kampman[17,19], Toshihiko Kinoshita[20], Esa Leinonen[17,21], Ying-Jay Liou[15,16], Taisei Mushiroda[22], Shinpei Nonen[23], Michelle K. Skime[14], Liewei Wang[18], Masaki Kato[20], Yu-Li Liu[24], Verayuth Praphanphoj[25], Julia C. Stingl[26], William V. Bobo[14], Shih-Jen Tsai[15,16], Michiaki Kubo[22], Teri E. Klein[7], Richard M. Weinshilboum[18], Joanna M. Biernacka[8,14] and Bernhard T. Baune[1]**

Correspondence:
Bernhard T. Baune
bernhard.baune@adelaide.edu.au

[1] Discipline of Psychiatry, School of Medicine, University of Adelaide, Adelaide, SA, Australia, [2] Northern Adelaide Local Health Network, Mental Health Services, Adelaide, SA, Australia, [3] Epidemiology Branch, Division of Intramural Population Health Research, National Institute of Child Health and Human Development, National Institutes of Health, Bethesda, MD, United States, [4] HSL Institute for Aging Research, Harvard Medical School, Boston, MA, United States, [5] Program for Quantitative Genomics, Harvard School of Public Health, Boston, MA, United States, [6] Broad Institute of MIT and Harvard, Cambridge, MA, United States, [7] Biomedical Data Science, Stanford University, Stanford, CA, United States, [8] Department of Health Sciences Research, Mayo Clinic, Rochester, NY, United States, [9] Department of Bioengineering, Stanford University, Stanford, CA, United States, [10] Department of Psychiatry and Psychotherapy, University of Muenster, Muenster, Germany, [11] Department of Clinical Pharmacology, University Göttingen, Göttingen, Germany, [12] Department of Psychiatry, Taipei Medical University-Shuangho Hospital, New Taipei City, Taiwan, [13] Department of Psychiatry and Psychotherapy, Faculty of Medicine, University of Freiburg, Freiburg, Germany, [14] Department of Psychiatry and Psychology, Mayo Clinic, Rochester, NY, United States, [15] Department of Psychiatry, Taipei Veterans General Hospital, Taipei, Taiwan, [16] Division of Psychiatry, School of Medicine, National Yang-Ming University, Taipei, Taiwan, [17] Department of Psychiatry, Faculty of Medicine and Life Sciences, University of Tampere, Tampere, Finland, [18] Department of Molecular Pharmacology and Experimental Therapeutics, Mayo Clinic Rochester, Rochester, MN, United States, [19] Department of Psychiatry, Seinäjoki Hospital District, Seinäjoki, Finland, [20] Department of Neuropsychiatry, Kansai Medical University, Osaka, Japan, [21] Department of Psychiatry, Tampere University Hospital, Tampere, Finland, [22] RIKEN Center for Integrative Medical Sciences, Kanagawa, Japan, [23] Department of Pharmacy, Hyogo University of Health Sciences, Hyogo, Japan, [24] Center for Neuropsychiatric Research, National Health Research Institutes, Miaoli, Taiwan, [25] Center for Medical Genetics Research, Rajanukul Institute, Department of Mental Health, Ministry of Public Health Bangkok, Bangkok, Thailand, [26] Research Division Federal Institute for Drugs and Medical Devices, Bonn, Germany

Studies reported a strong genetic correlation between the Big Five personality traits and major depressive disorder (MDD). Moreover, personality traits are thought to be associated with response to antidepressants treatment that might partly be mediated by genetic factors. In this study, we examined whether polygenic scores (PGSs) derived from the Big Five personality traits predict treatment response and remission in patients with MDD who were prescribed selective serotonin reuptake inhibitors (SSRIs). In addition, we performed meta-analyses of genome-wide association studies (GWASs) on these traits to identify genetic variants underpinning the cross-trait polygenic association. The

PGS analysis was performed using data from two cohorts: the Pharmacogenomics Research Network Antidepressant Medication Pharmacogenomic Study (PGRN-AMPS, $n = 529$) and the International SSRI Pharmacogenomics Consortium (ISPC, $n = 865$). The cross-trait GWAS meta-analyses were conducted by combining GWAS summary statistics on SSRIs treatment outcome and on the personality traits. The results showed that the PGS for openness and neuroticism were associated with SSRIs treatment outcomes at $p < 0.05$ across P_T thresholds in both cohorts. A significant association was also found between the PGS for conscientiousness and SSRIs treatment response in the PGRN-AMPS sample. In the cross-trait GWAS meta-analyses, we identified eight loci associated with (a) SSRIs response and conscientiousness near *YEATS4* gene and (b) SSRI remission and neuroticism eight loci near *PRAG1*, *MSRA*, *XKR6*, *ELAVL2*, *PLXNC1*, *PLEKHM1*, and *BRUNOL4* genes. An assessment of a polygenic load for personality traits may assist in conjunction with clinical data to predict whether MDD patients might respond favorably to SSRIs.

Keywords: pharmacogenomics, polygenic score, personality traits, major depression, antidepressants, selective serotonin reuptake inhibitors

INTRODUCTION

A major depressive disorder (MDD) is the most common and disabling mental health diseases worldwide (1, 2) with a lifetime prevalence of ~12% (3). Studies estimated a 61.6 million years of life lived with disability caused by MDD accounting for 2.5% of the total disability-adjusted life years and for 8.1% of the total years lived with disability resulted from all diseases (2, 4).

Selective serotonin reuptake inhibitors (SSRIs) are commonly used as the first-line pharmacological treatment for MDD (5). However, treatment efficacy with SSRIs varies widely between individual patients and is inadequate in many cases. Clinical response rates range from 48 to 64% (6, 7) and reported remission rates are as low as 23.5% (7, 8). To improve this situation, an investigation of the biological and psychosocial factors that drive heterogeneity in treatment outcomes is necessary.

There is growing evidence from genetic studies that antidepressant treatment response is substantially influenced by genes (7, 9–17). A study involving nearly 3,000 MDD patients estimated that genetic factors explain 42% of the differences in the level of treatment response (18). A number of genes and single nucleotide polymorphisms (SNPs) that could influence antidepressant treatment outcomes have been reported, including polymorphisms within the *COMT* (9), *HTR2A* (10), *HTR1A* (11), *CNR1* (11), *SLC6A4* (12), *NPY* (13), *MAOA* (14), and *IL1B* (15) genes. A pharmacogenomic study on SSRIs response by the International SSRIs Pharmacogenomics Consortium (ISPC) identified several SNPs with suggestive association after 4 weeks of treatment, including the neuregulin-1 gene, which is involved in many aspects of brain development, such as neuronal maturation (7).

In addition to genetic factors, multiple demographic, clinical, and psychological predictors of SSRI response in MDD have been identified, collectively explaining 5–15% of the variance in treatment outcomes (19–23). Among the psychological predictors, personality traits defined by the Five-Factor Model of Personality ("Big Five": extraversion, agreeableness, conscientiousness, neuroticism, openness) (24) have previously been reported to influence antidepressant treatment response and remission (25–29). Of these, neuroticism is a frequently reported predisposing factor for depression and was shown to negatively affect antidepressants treatment response (30, 31). In a recent study, MDD patients resistant to antidepressants were more likely to report high clinical scores for neuroticism, but low scores for openness, conscientiousness, and extraversion (26). In a large study of patients with MDD ($n = 8{,}229$), pre-existing personality dysfunction was associated with poor response to antidepressants (27). Further, some studies have suggested that SSRIs have a direct positive impact on scores for neuroticism or extraversion in MDD patients, and that part of the antidepressant effect might be explained through these adjustments (28, 29, 32, 33). Moreover, shared genes are thought to play a key role in the association between personality factors and MDD (34). For example, studies have estimated the genetic correlation between MDD and neuroticism at 55–75% (35, 36). However, no previous work has directly addressed the question whether there is a genetic relationship between the Big Five personality traits and SSRI treatment response and remission in MDD. It has been shown that the genetic architecture of personality traits is highly polygenic, in which several genes of small effect contribute to the overall phenotype (35, 37). Thus, a polygenic score (PGS) analysis approach proposed by the schizophrenia consortium (38) and later applied in several studies (16, 39), is potentially powerful to investigate the genetic influence of each of the Big Five personality traits on antidepressant treatment outcomes. A PGS for each of the Big five personality traits quantifies the combined effects of genetic variants across the whole genome, computed as a weighted summation of effect sizes obtained from genome-wide association studies (GWASs). A successful multi-trait polygenic model may assist for an early screening of diseases risk, clinical diagnosis, and the prediction of treatment response and prognosis (38, 39).

Implicitly, one could also interpret a polygenic association as a biological relationship partly explained by the role of shared genes and common molecular mechanisms. With this in mind, we conducted GWAS meta-analyses by combining GWAS summary statistics on the Big Five personality traits and SSRIs treatment outcome to identify shared genes involved in the cross-trait association.

MATERIALS AND METHODS

The characteristics of the clinical and genetic data, as well as the sources of the GWAS summary statistics used in our analysis are described below.

Study Samples

Pharmacogenomics Research Network Antidepressant Medication Pharmacogenomic Study (PGRN-AMPS)

The PGRN-AMPS is a clinical trial on the response to escitalopram or citalopram of 529 MDD patients over 8 weeks of treatment. The baseline and follow-up assessment of depression severity were performed using the 16-item Quick Inventory of Depressive Symptomatology (QIDS-C16) (40).

ISPC Study

The ISPC is an International Consortium established to discover genes that are responsible for SSRIs treatment response in patients with MDD. For our study, we used data from 865 MDD patients recruited in the USA, Germany, Thailand, Taiwan, and Japan who received SSRI treatment. The 17-item Hamilton Depression Rating Scale was used as a measurement tool to assess and follow-up the treatment progress (7).

Genotyping and Quality Control

The genotype and clinical data for the PGRN-AMPS were available *via* a controlled access system at the database of Genotypes and Phenotypes: dbGaP[1] and the ISPC data were obtained from the ISPC consortium (7).

For the genotype data of both samples, we implemented quality control (QC) steps using PLINK (41) and samples with low genotype rates <95%, sex inconsistencies (X-chromosome heterozygosity) and genetically related individuals were excluded. We also excluded SNPs that had poor genotyping rate <95%, an ambiguity (A/T and C/G SNPs), a minor allele frequency (MAF $\leq$ 1%), or showed deviation from Hardy–Weinberg Equilibrium ($p < 10^{-6}$).

Imputations

Genotype data passing QC criteria were imputed in the Michigan server[2] (42) separately for each study samples using 1000 Genomes project reference panel.

After excluding the low-frequency SNPs (MAF < 10%), poor-quality variants (imputation INFO <0.9 and indels), the imputed dosages were converted to best guess genotypes. The subsequent PGS analyses were performed using the best guess genotypes.

GWAS Summary Statistics Data

The PGSs were calculated using the approach previously described by the International Schizophrenia Consortium (38). This method requires an estimated effect size for each SNP to compute weighted PGS. The effect estimates (betas) for this study were the summary statistics obtained from previously published GWASs on extraversion, openness, agreeableness, conscientiousness (37), and on neuroticism (35). The data were publicly available for download at http://www.tweelingenregister.org/GPC/ and http://www.thessgac.org/data, respectively. The effect size estimates for each SNP—quantified as beta was extracted from the download file and used to compute weighted PGS in the PGRN-AMPS and ISPC cohorts.

Definition of SSRI Treatment Outcomes

Treatment response and remission to SSRIs were defined after 4 weeks of treatment follow-up of MDD patients in both cohorts. In addition, PGS associations were evaluated at 8 weeks in PGRN-AMPS. While treatment response was determined as a ≥50% reduction from baseline in the HRSD-17 or QIDS-C16 total scores, SSRI treatment remission was defined as achieving a HRSD-17 score ≤7 or a QIDS-C16 score ≤5 at 4 or 8 weeks of treatment.

Data on the covariates—age, gender, and type of SSRIs medications were also collected and the details can be found in earlier publications (7, 40, 43).

Statistical Analyses

PGS Computation and Association Analyses

The PGSs were computed for each of the Big Five personality traits using imputed genetic data weighted by GWAS summary statistics of the respective personality traits, separately for the two cohorts: PGRN-AMPS (n = 529) and ISPC (n = 865) (**Table 1**; **Figure 1**). First, quality-controlled SNPs were clumped for linkage disequilibrium (LD) using genome-wide association p-value informed clumping with $r^2 = 0.1$ in a 250-kb window to create an independent SNP-set using PLINK software run on Linux. Next, weighted PGSs were calculated for each individual at a range of p-value thresholds (P_T) as a weighted sum of allele dosages (0, 1, or 2). The P_T refers to the p-values associated

TABLE 1 | Baseline characteristics of major depressive disorder patients and their treatment outcomes with selective serotonin reuptake inhibitors after 4 weeks of follow-up.

Patient characteristics	PGRN-AMPS N = 529	ISPC N = 865	Total N = 1,394
Responders, N (%)	206 (44.4)	416 (48.1)	622 (46.8)
Remitters, N (%)	128 (27.6)	226 (26.1)	354 (26.7)
Age, mean (SD)	39.6 (13.7)	43.7 (14.7)	42.2 (14.5)
Sex, female, N (%)	335 (63.3)	561 (64.9)	896 (64.3)

PGRN-AMPS, the Pharmacogenomics Research Network Antidepressant Medication Pharmacogenomics Study; ISPC, the International SSRI Pharmacogenomics Consortium study.

[1] http://www.ncbi.nlm.nih.gov/gap.

[2] https://imputationserver.sph.umich.edu

with the effect size of each of the SNPs, as listed in the GWAS summary statistics (35, 37). The weighting was performed by multiplying the dosage of each effect increasing allele by its effect size derived from the GWAS summary statistics (β-coefficient), then divided by the total number of SNPs in each threshold. The PGS was computed at a range of P_T ($<1 \times 10^{-2}$, $<5 \times 10^{-2}$, <0.1, <0.2, <0.3, <0.4, <0.5, and <1.0) separately for each of the two cohorts. Performing the PGS at different P_T provides a range of alternative scores to choose the most significantly associated (optimal) PGS that will be used for prediction modeling. At each P_T, a logistic regression modeling was applied to response/remission to SSRIs (dependent variables) using the PGS for each of the Big Five personality traits as the main predictor variable and adjusting for common covariates, such as age, sex, and cohort-specific covariates including four principal components in the PGRN-AMPS and "study sites" in the ISPC. A statistically significant association between the PGSs for the Big Five personality traits and response/remission to SSRIs was determined at $p < 0.05$, across the P_T in both study samples. The prediction accuracy, the percentage of variance explained, Nagelkerke R^2, by the PGSs were calculated as the Nagelkerke R^2 of the full model with PGS and covariates minus the Nagelkerke R^2 of the model with only covariates. To determine the effect of high or low polygenic load on treatment outcomes, the study subjects were grouped into PGS quartiles (Q_1–Q_4) at the optimal P_T. Then, we estimated the odds of treatment response/remission to SSRIs for MDD patients within the group with a high polygenic load for the Big Five personality traits (Q_2, Q_3, Q_4) compared to patients in the lowest PGS quartile (Q_1).

Cross-Trait Meta-Analyses of GWASs

In the cross-trait meta-analyses, we applied the O'Brien's (OB) method and the direct Linear Combination of dependent test statistics (dLC) approach (39, 44, 45), which are implemented in the C++ eLX package. Briefly, the OB method and the dLC approach help to combine GWAS effect estimates of genome-wide SNPs, obtained from univariate GWASs and generated two test statistics and associated *p*-values—one for the OB method and one for the dLC method. More details can be found elsewhere (44, 45). The eLX package is available at https://sites.google.com/site/multivariateyihsianghsu/.

Here, GWAS on personality traits that have shown a significant association in the PGS analysis were combined with GWAS on SSRIs treatment outcome. The GWAS summary statistics on SSRIs treatment response (7) were combined with those on (i) conscientiousness (34) and (ii) openness personality (34). Similarly, the GWAS summary statistics on SSRIs treatment remission (7) was meta-analyzed with (i) openness personality (34) and (ii) neuroticism (35).

Statistical significance was determined based on the smaller of the OB or the dLC *p*-values. A significant association was determined if (1) the *p*-value for the cross-trait meta-analysis reached genome-wide significance ($p < 5 \times 10^{-8}$) and (2) the univariate GWAS effects were at least nominally significant ($p < 0.05$). For each cross-trait meta-analysis, only one lead SNP per locus was reported. Nearby SNPs in LD ($r^2 > 0.1$) with the lead SNP were considered dependent and belonging to the same locus.

RESULTS

Patient Characteristics and Treatment Outcomes

In this study, we analyzed data from 1,394 MDD patients who had SSRI treatment divided into PGRN-AMPS ($n = 529$) and ISPC ($n = 865$) samples. The average age of the patients was 42.2 years and the majority of them (64.3%) were females (**Table 1**).

Of all patients, 622 (46.8%) were classified as treatment responders with a slight variation across the study samples 44.4% in the PGRN-AMPS and 48.1% in the ISPC. Remission rates were 27.6 and 26.1% in the PGRN-AMPS and ISPC samples, respectively. The rate of remission combined across the two studies was 26.7% (**Table 1**).

Association of the PGS for the Big Five Personality Traits with SSRIs Treatment Outcomes

Polygenic scores were computed for each of the Big Five personality traits, and we investigated their association with two SSRI treatment outcomes—response and remission, after 4 weeks (PGRN-AMPS and ISPC) and 8 weeks (PGRN-AMPS) of treatment.

After 4 weeks of treatment, genetic predisposition to openness, conscientiousness, and neuroticism were associated with SSRIs treatment response and/or remission at $p < 0.05$ across PT thresholds, in at least one of the two assessed cohorts (**Figures 1A–C**). Genetic loading for openness was associated with response and remission in both cohorts (**Figure 1A**1,2). An elevated PGS for conscientiousness was associated with treatment response, but not remission, in the PGRN-AMPS sample only (**Figure 1B**). A PGS association for neuroticism with remission, but not treatment response, was shown in both cohorts (**Figure 1C**). The PGSs for extraversion and agreeableness were associated with neither response nor remission.

We also assessed the level of observed variation in SSRI treatment outcomes accounted for by these personality traits, and found that personality traits at the most significant thresholds explained a considerable amount of variance in treatment outcomes. For example, the PGS for openness accounted for ~1.5% of the observed variation in SSRIs treatment response and ~2.8% of the variance in remission. The PGS for neuroticism explained ~1.5% of the variance in remission and the PGS for conscientiousness contributed to ~1.5% of the variability in SSRI treatment response.

The status of treatment response and remission for patients in personality trait quartiles (Q2–Q4) was compared with those in the lowest personality trait PGS quartile (Q1) (**Figure 2**). Our analysis revealed that MDD patients with a high polygenic load for openness personality had initially poorer remission and response rates at 4 weeks of treatment, with Q4 versus Q1 odds ratios (ORs) ranging from 0.30 [ISPC: 95%CI, 0.15–0.59] to 0.52 [PGRN-AMPS: 95%CI, 0.29–0.90] (**Figure 2A**1,2, green and brown graphs). After longer treatment duration, we observed a reverse effect. Here, a higher polygenic load for openness was associated with a better SSRIs treatment response at 8 weeks

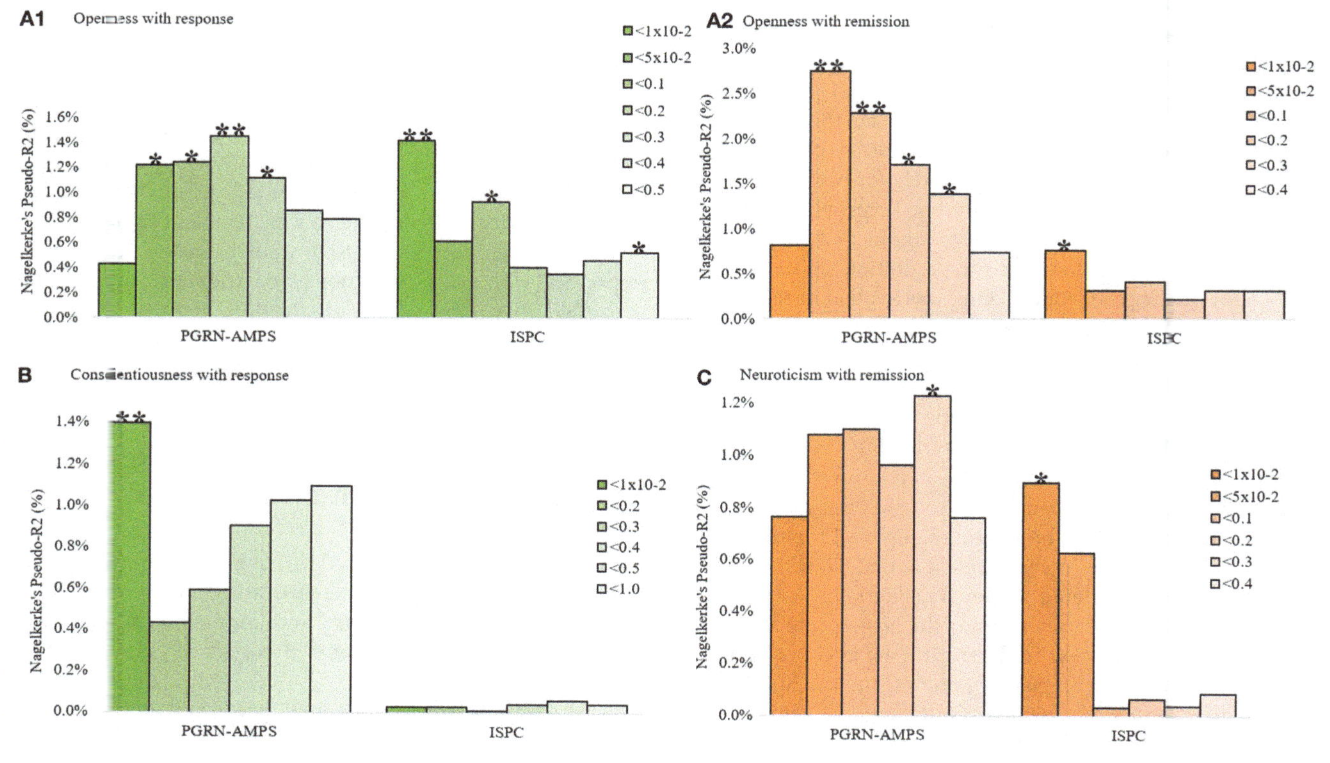

FIGURE 1 | The bar graphs **(A–C)** show the association of the PGSs for the Big Five personality traits with SSRIs response or remission at different p-value thresholds (P_T) after 4 weeks of treatment in the PGRN-AMPS (n = 529) and ISPC (n = 865) samples. The y-axis (Nagelkerke's Pseudo-R^2) refers to the percentage of variance in SSRIs treatment response/remission accounted for the PGSs of the Big Five personality traits at a particular P_T in each sample. On the x-axis, plotted from left to right, are the GWAS P_T for personality traits used to group the SNPs for the PGSs. The *sign on the top of each bar signify the statistical significance of the PGS association as *p < 0.05, **p < 0.01, ***p < 0.001. Abbreviations: PGRN-AMPS, the Pharmacogenomics Research Network Antidepressant Medication Pharmacogenomic Study; ISPC, the International SSRI Pharmacogenomics Consortium study; SNP, single nucleotide polymorphism; PGS, polygenic score; SSRIs, selective serotonin reuptake inhibitors.

in the PGRN-AMPS, with OR of 1.58 [95%CI, 1.10–2.90] (**Figure 2A**.2, blue graphs).

Major depressive disorder patients with a higher polygenic load for conscientiousness personality had 1.95 [95% CI, 1.13–3.36] times better SSRIs treatment response compared to those patients in the lowest PGS, although this association was only significant in the PGRN-AMPS sample at 4 weeks of treatment (**Figure 2B**).

Conversely, MDD patients with a higher polygenic load for neuroticism personality had poorer treatment outcomes with SSRIs. After 4 weeks of treatment, patients in Q4 based on the PGS for neurotic personality had about 50% lower odds of remission compared to patients in Q1 with OR ranging from 0.50 [PGRN-AMPS: 95%CI, 0.28–0.90] to 0.54 [ISPC: 95%CI, 0.33–0.89] (**Figure 2C**). Constantly, results after 8 weeks of treatment showed a trend inverse association between the PGS for neurotic personality and SSRIs treatment remission, although this was not statistically significant (**Figure 2C**).

To assess the potential effect of false-positive findings, the association p-values were corrected for multiple testing at each P_T for SSRIs treatment response and remission using the Benjamini and Hochberg (BH) method. Each of the p-values was adjusted assuming a conventionally accepted level of 5% false discovery rate (FDR) (46). After FDR adjustment, the associations of the PGS for openness personality with SSRIs treatment response remained statistically significant (in the ISPC sample: FDR adjusted p-value = 0.02 at $P_T < 1 \times 10^{-2}$) and with remission (in the PGRN-AMPS sample: FDR adjusted p-value = 0.04 at $P_T < 5 \times 10^{-2}$). The PGSs for conscientiousness and neuroticism were not associated with SSRIs treatment outcome after implementing the FDR adjusted p-value <0.05.

Cross-Trait Meta-Analyses of GWASs

For personality traits that showed a significantly associated PGS, cross-trait GWAS meta-analyses was performed by combining summary GWAS data on SSRIs treatment outcomes and personality traits. **Table 2** and **Figure 3** summarize the cross-trait meta-analyses findings, including the list of genetic loci and nearest genes that are potentially overlapping between the traits. At a p-value of $<5 \times 10^{-8}$, we identified eight genetic loci located within or near to protein-coding genes with possible overlapping effects on SSRIs treatment outcomes and personality traits. We found (i) one locus associated with conscientiousness and SSRI response near the *YEATS4* gene (**Table 2; Figure 3A**) and (ii) seven loci associated with remission and neuroticism located at

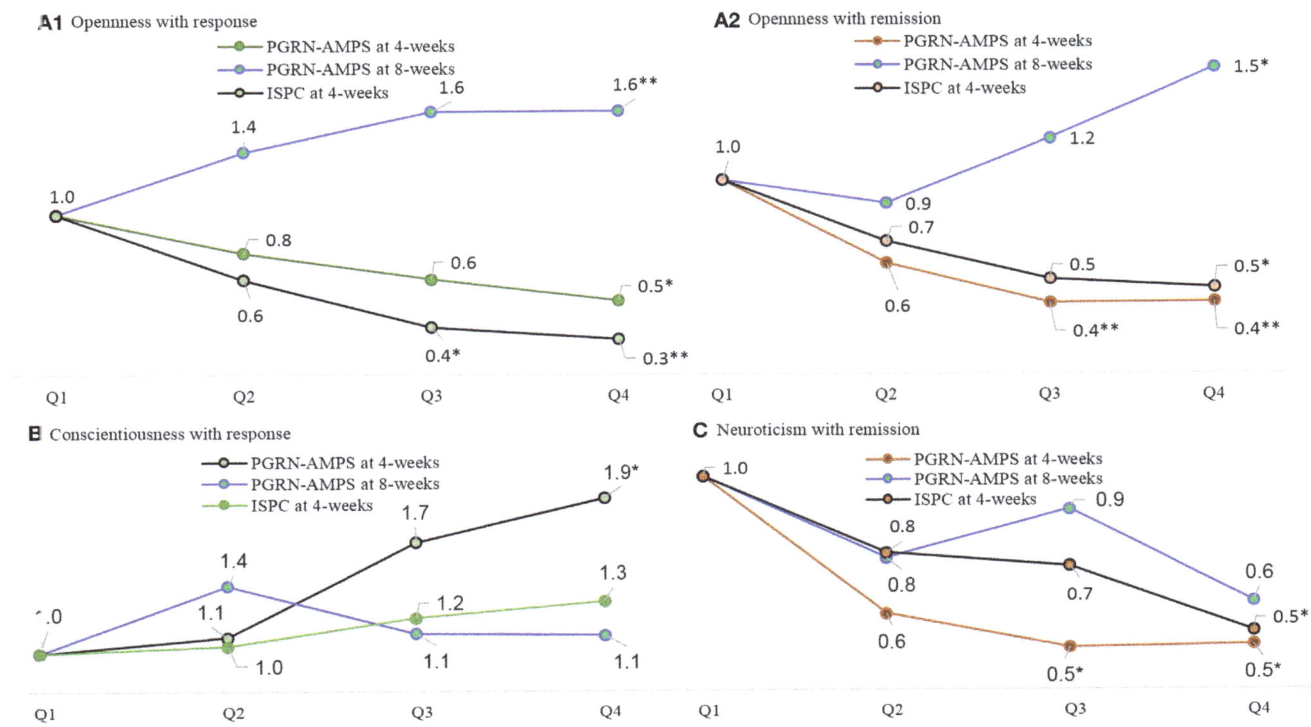

FIGURE 2 | The line plots represent the ORs for favorable response or remission to selective serotonin reuptake inhibitors treatment in patients with MDD with a high personality traits polygenic load (Q2, Q3, and Q4) compared to patients with the lowest polygenic load (Q1), estimated at the most significant *p*-value thresholds. The quartile-based polygenic scores analyses were performed using data at 4 weeks in the ISPC and at 4 and 8 weeks in the PGRN-AMPS. A polygenic loading for openness personality trait was initially associated with poor response and remission to selective serotonin reuptake inhibitors (SSRIs) in the first 4 weeks of treatment (ISPC, PGRN-AMPS at 4 weeks). After a longer (8 weeks) treatment follow-up, the genetic loading for openness had shown a favorable effect to SSRIs response and remission (PGRN-AMPS at 8 weeks). The polygenic loading for conscientiousness personality was favorably associated with response to SSRIs treatment. However, a polygenic loading for neuroticism personality had shown a negative impact on SSRIs remission. The ORs are reported on the lines and the *sign indicates the statistical significance of the ORs as $^{*}p < 0.05$, $^{**}p < 0.01$, $^{***}p < 0.001$. Abbreviations: PGRN-AMPS, the Pharmacogenomics Research Network Antidepressant Medication Pharmacogenomic Study; ISPC, the International SSRI Pharmacogenomics Consortium study. OR, odds ratio; Q1, quartiles 1; Q2, quartiles 2; Q3, quartiles 3; Q4, quartiles 4; MDD, major depressive disorder.

or near *PRAG1*, *MSRA*, *XKR6*, *ELAVL2*, *PLXNC1*, *PLEKHM1*, and *BRUNOL4* genes (**Table 2**; **Figure 3B**). From the meta-analyses of SSRIs treatment outcomes with openness personality, we identified only suggestive evidence at significance $p < 1 \times 10^{-6}$ (**Table 2**).

DISCUSSION

In this study, we analyzed data from 1,394 MDD patients who had been treated with SSRIs and assessed whether it is possible to predict antidepressants treatment outcomes—response and remission, using PGS for the Big Five personality traits. To further validate the PGS association findings and provide additional evidence, cross-trait meta-analyses of GWASs on SSRIs treatment outcomes versus GWASs on the Big Five personality traits were performed. Our findings from both analyses found complementary evidence that the association of the Big Five personality traits with SSRIs treatment outcomes is partly genetic.

Among the Big Five personality traits, the PGS for openness, conscientiousness, and neuroticism were significantly associated with SSRI treatment outcomes in patients with MDD. A high polygenic load for openness predicted poorer odds of response and remission to SSRIs after 4 weeks of treatment. However, after 8 weeks of treatment, the odds of response and remission was reversed and high loading for openness was associated with favorable outcomes. Patients with a high polygenic load for conscientiousness had a better odd of response to SSRIs after 4 weeks of treatment, but were neither more nor less likely to have good outcomes after 8 weeks. In contrast, patients who possessed a higher polygenic load for neuroticism risk genetic variants responded poorer to SSRIs treatment at both time points.

The discrepancy between short-term and intermediate-term treatment outcomes in patients with high polygenic loading for openness was unexpected in the context of the previous literature (26, 27), and raises the question whether statements about personality impact on SSRI treatment outcomes can be reliably reached on the basis of assessments conducted within the first month. While longitudinal studies of treatment outcomes in MDD suggest that treatment response within the first month occurs for a majority of patients who will eventually remit (47),

TABLE 2 | Significant loci resulting from the cross-trait meta-analyses of genome-wide association studies (GWASs) on selective serotonin reuptake inhibitors (SSRIs) treatment response/remission and GWAS on the Big Five personality traits at univariate GWAS *p*-value $<5 \times 10^{-2}$ and Cross-trait meta-analysis *p*-value $<5 \times 10^{-8}$.

SNP	Chr	Position Ch37	A1	A2	GWAS *p*-value for		Cross-trait GWAS *p*-value	Nearest gene	Effect direction
					SSRIs response (*N* = 865) (7)	Openness (*N* = 260,861) (34)			
rs7555693	1	106838539	A	G	6.46×10^{-3}	4.485×10^{-5}	1.37×10^{-6}	*PRMT6*	−−
rs9321987	6	145030284	A	G	7.49×10^{-3}	1.056×10^{-5}	5.05×10^{-7}	*UTRN*	−−
rs352759	8	15599714	T	A	6.16×10^{-4}	2.820×10^{-4}	5.52×10^{-7}	*TUSC3*	+−
rs7828021	8	50640014	C	G	3.68×10^{-3}	2.913×10^{-6}	7.43×10^{-8}	*SNTG1*	−−
rs11591827	10	82887882	A	G	1.87×10^{-2}	4.643×10^{-6}	8.70×10^{-7}	*SH2D4B*	−−
rs7189979	16	12630187	C	A	2.28×10^{-3}	1.659×10^{-5}	1.77×10^{-7}	*SNX29*	+−
					SSRIs response (*N* = 865) (7)	Conscientiousness (*N* = 260,861) (34)			
rs3825243	12	69750839	A	G	5.78×10^{-4}	1.41×10^{-5}	4.04×10^{-8}	*YEATS4*	−−
					SSRIs remission (*N* = 865) (7)	Neuroticism (*N* = 170,911) (35)			
rs2979204	8	8298857	T	C	3.24×10^{-3}	5.48×10^{-10}	8×10^{-11}	*PRAG1*	++
rs11990063	8	10165195	T	C	4.00×10^{-2}	6.77×10^{-9}	9×10^{-9}	*MSRA*	−−
rs35792458	8	10822431	C	G	1.00×10^{-2}	5.25×10^{-10}	1×10^{-12}	*XKR6*	−+
rs12555870	9	23347724	G	A	4.00×10^{-2}	1.25×10^{-6}	1×10^{-8}	*ELAVL2*	+−
rs4761545	12	94426468	G	T	2.00×10^{-2}	3.54×10^{-7}	8×10^{-10}	*PLXNC1*	++
rs144733372	17	43564222	G	T	1.00×10^{-2}	1.23×10^{-9}	3×10^{-11}	*PLEKHM1*	−+
rs11082011	18	35145122	C	T	1.00×10^{-2}	8.60×10^{-9}	4×10^{-8}	*BRUNOL4*	−+
					SSRIs remission (*N* = 865) (7)	Openness (*N* = 260,861) (34)			
rs55679149	1	89534338	T	C	2.77×10^{-3}	6.31×10^{-5}	8.25×10^{-7}	*G3BP1*	+−
rs11728985	4	130036435	T	C	1.93×10^{-2}	1.24×10^{-6}	4.03×10^{-7}	*C4orf33*	−+
rs11155372	6	145019738	T	G	5.11×10^{-4}	5.85×10^{-5}	1.28×10^{-7}	*UTRN*	−+
rs7828021	8	50640014	C	G	1.23×10^{-2}	2.91×10^{-6}	4.18×10^{-7}	*SNTG1*	−−
rs1411216	9	24520194	A	G	7.81×10^{-3}	6.88×10^{-6}	4.53×10^{-7}	*CRIPAK*	++
rs7189979	16	12630187	C	A	2.82×10^{-3}	1.66×10^{-5}	2.73×10^{-7}	*SNX29*	+−

A1, effect allele; A2, another allele; SNP, single nucleotide polymorphism.
The effect direction represents the SNPs effect on SSRIs treatment response or remission for the effect allele based on the ISPC GWAS (7) versus its effect on the GWASs of personality traits listed in the table.

they also indicate that there is a considerable proportion of patients who achieve response and remission after much longer treatment periods (48, 49). In this context, our finding raises the possibility that the different Big Five personality traits could have differential effects on early- versus delayed responses to treatment in MDD.

Moreover, the inconsistences in the direction of the relationship between the Big Five personality traits and response to long-term versus short-term treatment to SSRIs might be explained by a psychological theory (50–52). Studies suggested that antidepressants have a primary effect on emotional processing, providing a platform for long-term cognitive and psychological recovery (50), and the clinical effects of antidepressant treatment may be mediated by early changes in emotional processing (51, 52).

In our data, consistency between the outcome parameters—treatment response and remission was variable. Only the PGS for openness showed a significant association with both treatment response and remission. The PGS for conscientiousness was associated with better treatment response, but not with remission. The PGS for neuroticism predicted lower odds of treatment remission, but not poorer treatment response. At face value, these findings suggest that openness and neuroticism could play more important roles in predicting ultimate remission from depressive episodes, whereas conscientiousness might drive early treatment effects rather than longer term outcomes. However, another explanation is that our cohorts might have been underpowered to detect more consistent effects, or that some of the observed associations were chance findings, perhaps driven by multiple testing. Indeed, only the associations of the PGS for openness personality with SSRIs treatment response remained statistically significant after FDR adjustment. Therefore, future genetic studies with higher patients' numbers are required to confirm our findings.

In all, our genetic findings are in line with previous clinical investigations of the influence of personality characteristics on antidepressant treatment response in MDD. A study in Japan revealed as depressed patients who were resistant to treatment had a higher neuroticism score and lower scores for openness, conscientiousness, and extraversion than patients who remitted and healthy controls (26). In another study higher clinical scores for openness at baseline were associated with improved treatment response to antidepressants, whereas a higher score for neuroticism was associated with poor treatment outcomes (53). More generally, poor treatment response was associated with personality dysfunction in a large sample study of more than 8,000 antidepressant-treated adults with MDD (27). Similarly, a meta-analysis of 34 clinical studies concluded that MDD patients with a comorbid personality disorder had double the risk of overall poor clinical and treatment outcomes, compared to patients no co-occurring personality disorder (54).

Additionally, previous studies have shown genetic correlations between Big Five personality traits and psychiatric disorders and

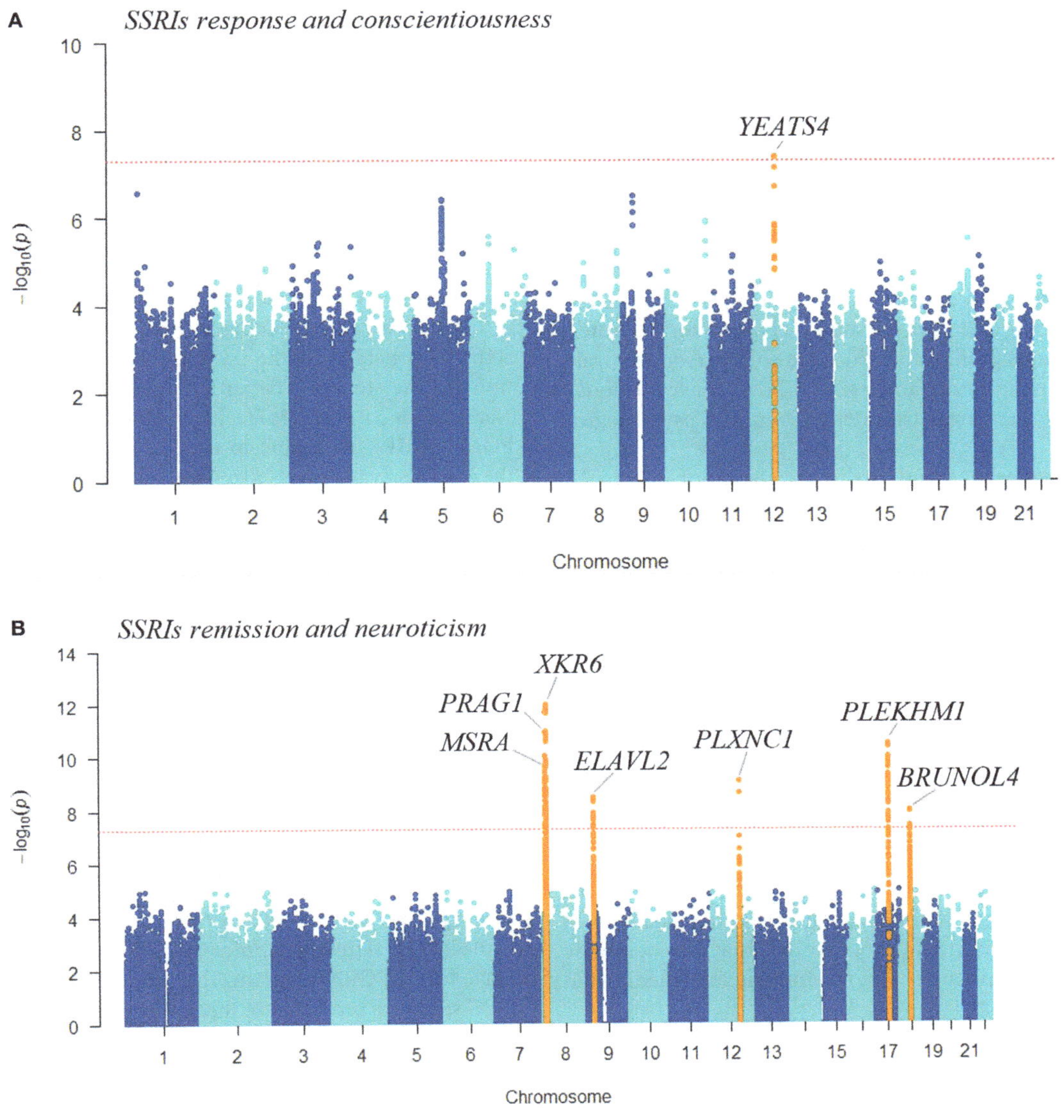

FIGURE 3 | The Manhattan plots show the results of the cross-trait meta-analysis of genome-wide association studies (GWASs) on selective serotonin reuptake inhibitors treatment outcomes (response or remission) with GWASs on: **(A)** conscientiousness personality trait; **(B)** neuroticism personality, highlighting the loci that showed genome-wide significance (orange), and the nearest genes. The −log10 (cross-trait *p*-value) is plotted against the physical position of each SNP on each chromosome. The threshold for genome-wide significance (cross-trait *p*-value <5 × 10^{-8}) is indicated by the red dotted horizontal line.

the PGS for neuroticism was significantly associated with MDD (55).

Since the PGS association reflects a shared genetic etiology, we applied cross-trait GWAS meta-analyses by combining summary statistics on SSRI treatment outcomes with personality traits, and identified eight overlapping genetic loci. The *YEATS4* gene locus was associated with treatment response to SSRIs and conscientiousness. Previously, a gene expression analysis in depressed patients further replicated in mice found lower levels of *YEATS4* in depressed patients compared to healthy controls. Moreover, the expression level of this gene was correlated with the dose of imipramine (a tricyclic antidepressant) (56).

The second gene locus (rs144733372) in *PLEKHM*, which was found in the cross-trait meta-analysis of neuroticism and SSRIs treatment remission, is highly linked (LD: $r^2 > 0.8$) with several other SNPs located within the *CRHR1* gene. The *CRHR1* gene encodes a G-protein coupled receptor that binds with the neuropeptides of the corticotrophin-releasing hormone family, a major regulator of the hypothalamic–pituitary–adrenal pathway (57). Functional gene polymorphisms in the *CRHR1* gene have been associated with SSRIs treatment response (58), and it moderates the association of maltreatment with neuroticism (59). Corticotrophin-releasing hormone signaling has previously been implicated in mood disorders and treatment response to antidepressants (60).

Another gene showing shared associations with SSRI treatment response and neurotic personality is *MSRA*, which has shown the highest levels of expression in brain tissue (61). Previous studies reported that genetic variants within the *MSRA* gene could be associated with schizophrenia, bipolar disorder (62, 63), executive cognitive function (64), fluid intelligence (63), and self-reported irritable temperament (65).

Further, loci within the *PRAG1* and *PLXNC1* genes have shown overlapping influence on SSRI treatment and neuroticism personality. A genetic polymorphism rs706895C/T within the *FYN* gene belonging to the same family of genes (tyrosine protein kinase family) was significantly associated with personality traits (66). SNPs within the plexin family gene *PLXNA2* have previously been implicated in neuroticism, depression, and psychological distress (67).

Overall, these findings lend further weight to our PGS analyses and reinforce the idea that certain gene polymorphisms have a dual impact on personality structure and antidepressant treatment outcomes in MDD. Studying the individual mechanism of each significant genetic locus in relation to antidepressants in the future studies might lead to novel insights in the molecular underpinnings of these drugs. In conclusion, our study provides evidence in the potential ability of the PGS for the Big Five personality traits to elucidate shared biological mechanisms and to predict SSRI treatment outcomes. Whether these PGSs could be applied to everyday clinical practice in the future relies on their ability to stratify MDD patients into categories of good treatment responders versus nonresponders. Further research is required to determine if this is the case. However, the small effect sizes found in our study give rise to cautious interpretation. In our view, their full clinical value likely lies in their contribution to multi-variable models that also comprise clinical and environmental factors influencing medication response.

AUTHOR CONTRIBUTIONS

AA, KS, and BB developed the study concept and design, performed the statistical analysis, and drafted the manuscript. Other authors contributed data, resources and were involved in critical revision of the manuscript, obtained funding, and contributed to cohort and genetic data and study supervision.

ACKNOWLEDGMENTS

The authors are grateful to the study subjects who participated in the studies, and we appreciate the contributions of research staffs who helped in the patient recruitment and data collection for the studies. The authors also would like to thank the National Institutes of Health (NIH), USA for making the PGRN-AMPS accessible to us. The complete clinical data for the ISPC is available at http://www.pharmgkb.org/downloads/. The PGRN-AMPS data were obtained through controlled access distributed from the NIH in the dbGaP (https://www.ncbi.nlm.nih.gov/gap). The analysis of this study was carried out using the high-performance computational capabilities of the University of Adelaide, Phoenix supercomputer (https://www.adelaide.edu.au/phoenix/).

FUNDING

AA received a Postgraduate Research Scholarship support from the University of Adelaide through the Adelaide Scholarship International program. Funding support for the PGRN-AMPS was provided by the National Institute of General Medical Sciences, National Institutes of Health, through the PGRN grant to Principal Investigators RW and LW (U19 GM61388). Dr. D. Mrazek served as the Principal Investigator for the PGRN-AMPS study within the Mayo Clinic PGRN program. The main sources of funding for the ISPC study are presented in the earlier publication (7).

REFERENCES

1. Whiteford HA, Degenhardt L, Rehm J, Baxter AJ, Ferrari AJ, Erskine HE, et al. Global burden of disease attributable to mental and substance use disorders: findings from the global burden of disease study 2010. *Lancet* (2013) 382(9904):1575–86. doi:10.1016/S0140-6736(13)61611-6
2. Global Burden of Disease Study 2013 Collaborators. Global, regional, and national incidence, prevalence, and years lived with disability for 301 acute and chronic diseases and injuries in 188 countries, 1990-2013: a systematic analysis for the global burden of disease study 2013. *Lancet* (2015) 386(9995):743–800. doi:10.1016/S0140-6736(15)60692-4
3. Andrade L, Caraveo-Anduaga JJ, Berglund P, Bijl RV, De Graaf R, Vollebergh W, et al. The epidemiology of major depressive episodes: results from the International Consortium of Psychiatric Epidemiology (ICPE) surveys. *Int J Methods Psychiatr Res* (2003) 12(1):3–21. doi:10.1002/mpr.138
4. Ferrari AJ, Charlson FJ, Norman RE, Patten SB, Freedman G, Murray CJ, et al. Burden of depressive disorders by country, sex, age, and year: findings from the global burden of disease study 2010. *PLoS Med* (2013) 10(11):e1001547. doi:10.1371/journal.pmed.1001547
5. Hieronymus F, Emilsson JF, Nilsson S, Eriksson E. Consistent superiority of selective serotonin reuptake inhibitors over placebo in reducing depressed mood in patients with major depression. *Mol Psychiatry* (2016) 21(4):523–30. doi:10.1038/mp.2015.53
6. Hirschfeld RM. Efficacy of SSRIs and newer antidepressants in severe depression: comparison with TCAs. *J Clin Psychiatry* (1999) 60(5):326–35. doi:10.4088/JCP.v60n0511
7. Biernacka JM, Sangkuhl K, Jenkins G, Whaley RM, Barman P, Batzler A, et al. The International SSRI Pharmacogenomics Consortium (ISPC): a genome-wide association study of antidepressant treatment response. *Transl Psychiatry* (2015) 5:e553. doi:10.1038/tp.2015.47
8. Papakostas GI, Fava M, Thase ME. Treatment of SSRI-resistant depression: a meta-analysis comparing within- versus across-class switches. *Biol Psychiatry* (2008) 63(7):699–704. doi:10.1016/j.biopsych.2007.08.010
9. Baune BT, Hohoff C, Berger K, Neumann A, Mortensen S, Roehrs T, et al. Association of the COMT val158met variant with antidepressant treatment response in major depression. *Neuropsychopharmacology* (2008) 33(4):924–32. doi:10.1038/sj.npp.1301462
10. Horstmann S, Lucae S, Menke A, Hennings JM, Ising M, Roeske D, et al. Polymorphisms in GRIK4, HTR2A, and FKBP5 show interactive effects in predicting remission to antidepressant treatment. *Neuropsychopharmacology* (2010) 35(3):727–40. doi:10.1038/npp.2009.180
11. Domschke K, Dannlowski U, Ohrmann P, Lawford B, Bauer J, Kugel H, et al. Cannabinoid receptor 1 (CNR1) gene: impact on antidepressant treatment response and emotion processing in major depression. *Eur Neuropsychopharmacol* (2008) 18(10):751–9. doi:10.1016/j.euroneuro.2008.05.003
12. Baune BT, Hohoff C, Mortensen LS, Deckert J, Arolt V, Domschke K. Serotonin transporter polymorphism (5-HTTLPR) association with melancholic depression: a female specific effect? *Depress Anxiety* (2008) 25(11):920–5. doi:10.1002/da.20433
13. Baffa A, Hohoff C, Baune BT, Muller-Tidow C, Tidow N, Freitag C, et al. Norepinephrine and serotonin transporter genes: impact on

treatment response in depression. *Neuropsychobiology* (2010) 62(2):121–31. doi:10.1159/000317285

14. Domschke K, Hohoff C, Mortensen LS, Roehrs T, Deckert J, Arolt V, et al. Monoamine oxidase A variant influences antidepressant treatment response in female patients with major depression. *Prog Neuropsychopharmacol Biol Psychiatry* (2008) 32(1):224–8. doi:10.1016/j.pnpbp.2007.08.011
15. Baune BT, Dannlowski U, Domschke K, Janssen DG, Jordan MA, Ohrmann P, et al. The interleukin 1 beta (IL1B) gene is associated with failure to achieve remission and impaired emotion processing in major depression. *Biol Psychiatry* (2010) 67(6):543–9. doi:10.1016/j.biopsych.2009.11.004
16. Amare AT, Schubert KO, Baune BT. Pharmacogenomics in the treatment of mood disorders: strategies and opportunities for personalized psychiatry. *EPMA J* (2017) 8(3):211–27. doi:10.1007/s13167-017-0112-8
17. Direk N, Williams S, Smith JA, Ripke S, Air T, Amare AT, et al. An analysis of two genome-wide association meta-analyses identifies a new locus for broad depression phenotype. *Biol Psychiatry* (2017) 82(5):322–9. doi:10.1016/j.biopsych.2016.11.013
18. Tansey KE, Guipponi M, Hu X, Domenici E, Lewis G, Malafosse A, et al. Contribution of common genetic variants to antidepressant response. *Biol Psychiatry* (2013) 73(7):679–82. doi:10.1016/j.biopsych.2012.10.030
19. Iniesta R, Malki K, Maier W, Rietschel M, Mors O, Hauser J, et al. Combining clinical variables to optimize prediction of antidepressant treatment outcomes. *J Psychiatr Res* (2016) 78:94–102. doi:10.1016/j.jpsychires.2016.03.016
20. Smagula SF, Butters MA, Anderson SJ, Lenze EJ, Dew MA, Mulsant BH, et al. Antidepressant response trajectories and associated clinical prognostic factors among older adults. *JAMA Psychiatry* (2015) 72(10):1021–8. doi:10.1001/jamapsychiatry.2015.1324
21. Dodd S, Berk M. Predictors of antidepressant response: a selective review. *Int J Psychiatry Clin Pract* (2004) 8(2):91–100. doi:10.1080/13651500410005423
22. Caudill MM, Hunter AM, Cook IA, Leuchter AF. The antidepressant treatment response index as a predictor of reboxetine treatment outcome in major depressive disorder. *Clin EEG Neurosci* (2015) 46(4):277–84. doi:10.1177/1550059414532443
23. De Carlo V, Calati R, Serretti A. Socio-demographic and clinical predictors of non-response/non-remission in treatment resistant depressed patients: a systematic review. *Psychiatry Res* (2016) 240:421–30. doi:10.1016/j.psychres.2016.04.034
24. Digman JM. Personality structure: emergence of the five-factor model. *Annu Rev Psychol* (1990) 41(1):417–40. doi:10.1146/annurev.ps.41.020190.002221
25. Quilty LC, De Fruyt F, Rolland JP, Kennedy SH, Rouillon PF, Bagby RM. Dimensional personality traits and treatment outcome in patients with major depressive disorder. *J Affect Disord* (2008) 108(3):241–50. doi:10.1016/j.jad.2007.10.022
26. Takahashi M, Shirayama Y, Muneoka K, Suzuki M, Sato K, Hashimoto K. Low openness on the revised NEO personality inventory as a risk factor for treatment-resistant depression. *PLoS One* (2013) 8(9):e71964. doi:10.1371/journal.pone.0071964
27. Gorwood P, Rouillon F, Even C, Falissard B, Corruble E, Moran P. Treatment response in major depression: effects of personality dysfunction and prior depression. *Br J Psychiatry* (2010) 196(2):139–42. doi:10.1192/bjp.bp.109.067058
28. Quilty LC, Meusel LA, Bagby RM. Neuroticism as a mediator of treatment response to SSRIs in major depressive disorder. *J Affect Disord* (2008) 111(1):67–73. doi:10.1016/j.jad.2008.02.006
29. Tang TZ, DeRubeis RJ, Hollon SD, Amsterdam J, Shelton R, Schalet B. Personality change during depression treatment: a placebo-controlled trial. *Arch Gen Psychiatry* (2009) 66(12):1322–30. doi:10.1001/archgenpsychiatry.2009.166
30. Bagby RM, Joffe RT, Parker JDA, Kalemba V, Harkness KL. Major depression and the five-factor model of personality. *J Pers Disord* (1995) 9(3):224–34. doi:10.1521/pedi.1995.9.3.224
31. Mulder RT. Personality pathology and treatment outcome in major depression: a review. *Am J Psychiatry* (2002) 159(3):359–71. doi:10.1176/appi.ajp.159.3.359
32. Du L, Bakish D, Ravindran AV, Hrdina PD. Does fluoxetine influence major depression by modifying five-factor personality traits? *J Affect Disord* (2002) 71(1–3):235–41. doi:10.1016/S0165-0327(01)00370-6
33. Jylhä P, Ketokivi M, Mantere O, Melartin T, Holma M, Rytsälä H, et al. Do antidepressants change personality?—A five-year observational study. *J Affect Disord* (2012) 142(1):200–7. doi:10.1016/j.jad.2012.04.026
34. Lo M-T, Hinds DA, Tung JY, Franz C, Fan C-C, Wang Y, et al. Genome-wide analyses for personality traits identify six genomic loci and show correlations with psychiatric disorders. *Nat Genet* (2017) 49(1):152–6. doi:10.1038/ng.3736
35. Okbay A, Baselmans BML, De Neve J-E, Turley P, Nivard MG, Fontana MA, et al. Genetic variants associated with subjective well-being, depressive symptoms, and neuroticism identified through genome-wide analyses. *Nat Genet* (2016) 48(6):624–33. doi:10.1038/ng.3552
36. Kendler KS, Neale MC, Kessler RC, Heath AC, Eaves LJ. A longitudinal twin study of personality and major depression in women. *Arch Gen Psychiatry* (1993) 50(11):853–62. doi:10.1001/archpsyc.1993.01820230009001
37. de Moor MH, Costa PT, Terracciano A, Krueger RF, de Geus EJ, Toshiko T, et al. Meta-analysis of genome-wide association studies for personality. *Mol Psychiatry* (2012) 17(3):337–49. doi:10.1038/mp.2010.128
38. International Schizophrenia Consortium, Purcell SM, Wray NR, Stone JL, Visscher PM, O'Donovan MC, et al. Common polygenic variation contributes to risk of schizophrenia that overlaps with bipolar disorder. *Nature* (2009) 460(7256):748–52. doi:10.1038/nature08185
39. Amare AT, Schubert KO, Hou L, Clark SR, Papiol S, Heilbronner U, et al. Association of polygenic score for schizophrenia and HLA antigen and inflammation genes with response to lithium in bipolar affective disorder: a genome-wide association study. *JAMA Psychiatry* (2018) 75(1):65–74. doi:10.1001/jamapsychiatry.2017.3433
40. Mrazek DA, Biernacka JM, McAlpine DE, Benitez J, Karpyak VM, Williams MD, et al. Treatment outcomes of depression: the pharmacogenomic research network antidepressant medication pharmacogenomic study. *J Clin Psychopharmacol* (2014) 34(3):313–7. doi:10.1097/JCP.0000000000000099
41. Purcell S, Neale B, Todd-Brown K, Thomas L, Ferreira MA, Bender D, et al. PLINK: a tool set for whole-genome association and population-based linkage analyses. *Am J Hum Genet* (2007) 81(3):559–75. doi:10.1086/519795
42. Das S, Forer L, Schonherr S, Sidore C, Locke AE, Kwong A, et al. Next-generation genotype imputation service and methods. *Nat Genet* (2016) 48(10):1284–7. doi:10.1038/ng.3656
43. Fava M, Rush AJ, Trivedi MH, Nierenberg AA, Thase ME, Sackeim HA, et al. Background and rationale for the sequenced treatment alternatives to relieve depression (STAR*D) study. *Psychiatr Clin North Am* (2003) 26(2):457–94,x. doi:10.1016/S0193-953X(02)00107-7
44. Yang Q, Wu H, Guo CY, Fox CS. Analyze multivariate phenotypes in genetic association studies by combining univariate association tests. *Genet Epidemiol* (2010) 34(5):444–54. doi:10.1002/gepi.20497
45. Yang Q, Wang Y. Methods for analyzing multivariate phenotypes in genetic association studies. *J Probab Stat* (2012) 2012:652569. doi:10.1155/2012/652569
46. Benjamini Y, Hochberg Y. Controlling the false discovery rate: a practical and powerful approach to multiple testing. *J R Stat Soc Ser B (Methodol)* (1995) 57(1):289–300.
47. Henkel V, Seemuller F, Obermeier M, Adli M, Bauer M, Mundt C, et al. Does early improvement triggered by antidepressants predict response/remission? Analysis of data from a naturalistic study on a large sample of inpatients with major depression. *J Affect Disord* (2009) 115(3):439–49. doi:10.1016/j.jad.2008.10.011
48. Seemuller F, Riedel M, Obermeier M, Bauer M, Adli M, Kronmuller K, et al. Outcomes of 1014 naturalistically treated inpatients with major depressive episode. *Eur Neuropsychopharmacol* (2010) 20(5):346–55. doi:10.1016/j.euroneuro.2009.11.011
49. Uher R, Mors O, Rietschel M, Rajewska-Rager A, Petrovic A, Zobel A, et al. Early and delayed onset of response to antidepressants in individual trajectories of change during treatment of major depression: a secondary analysis of data from the Genome-Based Therapeutic Drugs for Depression (GENDEP) study. *J Clin Psychiatry* (2011) 72(11):1478–84. doi:10.4088/JCP.10m06419
50. Harmer CJ, Goodwin GM, Cowen PJ. Why do antidepressants take so long to work? A cognitive neuropsychological model of antidepressant drug action. *Br J Psychiatry* (2009) 195(2):102–8. doi:10.1192/bjp.bp.108.051193
51. Godlewska BR, Norbury R, Selvaraj S, Cowen PJ, Harmer CJ. Short-term SSRI treatment normalises amygdala hyperactivity in depressed patients. *Psychol Med* (2012) 42(12):2609–17. doi:10.1017/S0033291712000591
52. Di Simplicio M, Norbury R, Reinecke A, Harmer CJ. Paradoxical effects of short-term antidepressant treatment in fMRI emotional processing models in volunteers with high neuroticism. *Psychol Med* (2014) 44(2):241–52. doi:10.1017/S0033291713000731

53. Bagby RM, Quilty LC, Segal ZV, McBride CC, Kennedy SH, Costa PT. Personality and differential treatment response in major depression: a randomized controlled trial comparing cognitive-behavioural therapy and pharmacotherapy. *Can J Psychiatry* (2008) 53(6):361–70. doi:10.1177/070674370805300605
54. NEWTON-HOWES G, TYRER P, JOHNSON T. Personality disorder and the outcome of depression: meta-analysis of published studies. *Br J Psychiatry* (2006) 188(1):13–20. doi:10.1192/bjp.188.1.13
55. de Moor MH, van den Berg SM, Verweij KJ, Krueger RF, Luciano M, Arias Vasquez A, et al. Meta-analysis of genome-wide association studies for neuroticism, and the polygenic association with major depressive disorder. *JAMA Psychiatry* (2015) 72(7):642–50. doi:10.1001/jamapsychiatry.2015.0554
56. Yamagata H, Uchida S, Matsuo K, Harada K, Kobayashi A, Nakashima M, et al. Identification of commonly altered genes between in major depressive disorder and a mouse model of depression. *Sci Rep* (2017) 7(1):3044. doi:10.1038/s41598-017-03291-x
57. O'Leary NA, Wright MW, Brister JR, Ciufo S, Haddad D, McVeigh R, et al. Reference sequence (RefSeq) database at NCBI: current status, taxonomic expansion, and functional annotation. *Nucleic Acids Res* (2016) 44(D1):D733–45. doi:10.1093/nar/gkv1189
58. Dong C, Wong ML, Licinio J. Sequence variations of ABCB1, SLC6A2, SLC6A3, SLC6A4, CREB1, CRHR1 and NTRK2: association with major depression and antidepressant response in Mexican-Americans. *Mol Psychiatry* (2009) 14(12):1105–18. doi:10.1038/mp.2009.92
59. DeYoung CG, Cicchetti D, Rogosch FA. Moderation of the association between childhood maltreatment and neuroticism by the corticotropin-releasing hormone receptor 1 gene. *J Child Psychol Psychiatry* (2011) 52(8):898–906. doi:10.1111/j.1469-7610.2011.02404.x
60. Amare AT, Schubert KO, Klingler-Hoffmann M, Cohen-Woods S, Baune BT. The genetic overlap between mood disorders and cardiometabolic diseases: a systematic review of genome wide and candidate gene studies. *Transl Psychiatry* (2017) 7:e1007. doi:10.1038/tp.2016.261
61. Pruitt KD, Brown GR, Hiatt SM, Thibaud-Nissen F, Astashyn A, Ermolaeva O, et al. RefSeq: an update on mammalian reference sequences. *Nucleic Acids Res* (2014) 42(Database issue):D756–63. doi:10.1093/nar/gkt1114
62. Walss-Bass C, Soto-Bernardini MC, Johnson-Pais T, Leach RJ, Ontiveros A, Nicolini H, et al. Methionine sulfoxide reductase: a novel schizophrenia candidate gene. *Am J Med Genet B Neuropsychiatr Genet* (2009) 150b(2):219–25. doi:10.1002/ajmg.b.30791
63. Ma X, Deng W, Liu X, Li M, Chen Z, He Z, et al. A genome-wide association study for quantitative traits in schizophrenia in China. *Genes Brain Behav* (2011) 10(7):734–9. doi:10.1111/j.1601-183X.2011.00712.x
64. Ni P, Ma X, Lin Y, Lao G, Hao X, Guan L, et al. Methionine sulfoxide reductase A (MsrA) associated with bipolar I disorder and executive functions in A Han Chinese population. *J Affect Disord* (2015) 184:235–8. doi:10.1016/j.jad.2015.06.004
65. Day FR, Helgason H, Chasman DI, Rose LM, Loh P-R, Scott RA, et al. Physical and neuro-behavioural determinants of reproductive onset and success. *Nat Genet* (2016) 48(6):617–23. doi:10.1038/ng.3551
66. Li J, Ma H, Deng S, Wu L, Huang Y, Zhu G. Fyn polymorphisms are associated with distinct personality traits in healthy Chinese-Han subjects. *J Mol Neurosci* (2011) 44(1):1–5. doi:10.1007/s12031-010-9485-z
67. Wray NR, James MR, Mah SP, Nelson M, Andrews G, Sullivan PF, et al. Anxiety and comorbid measures associated with PLXNA2. *Arch Gen Psychiatry* (2007) 64(3):318–26. doi:10.1001/archpsyc.64.3.318

17

Efficacy and Acceptability of Interventions for Attenuated Positive Psychotic Symptoms in Individuals at Clinical High Risk of Psychosis

Cathy Davies[1], Joaquim Radua[1,2,3], Andrea Cipriani[4,5], Daniel Stahl[6], Umberto Provenzani[1,7], Philip McGuire[8,9,10] and Paolo Fusar-Poli[1,7,9,10]*

[1] Early Psychosis: Interventions and Clinical-Detection Lab, Department of Psychosis Studies, Institute of Psychiatry, Psychology and Neuroscience, King's College London, London, United Kingdom, [2] FIDMAG Germanes Hospitalàries, CIBERSAM, Barcelona, Spain, [3] Department of Clinical Neuroscience, Centre for Psychiatry Research, Karolinska Institutet, Stockholm, Sweden, [4] Department of Psychiatry, University of Oxford, Oxford, United Kingdom, [5] Oxford Health NHS Foundation Trust, Oxford, United Kingdom, [6] Department of Biostatistics, Institute of Psychiatry, Psychology and Neuroscience, King's College London, London, United Kingdom, [7] Department of Brain and Behavioral Sciences, University of Pavia, Pavia, Italy, [8] Department of Psychosis Studies, Institute of Psychiatry, Psychology and Neuroscience, King's College London, London, United Kingdom, [9] National Institute for Health Research Maudsley Biomedical Research Centre, London, United Kingdom, [10] OASIS Service, South London and Maudsley NHS Foundation Trust, London, United Kingdom

***Correspondence:**
Cathy Davies
cathy.davies@kcl.ac.uk*

Background: Attenuated positive psychotic symptoms represent the defining features of the clinical high-risk for psychosis (CHR-P) criteria. The effectiveness of each available treatment for reducing attenuated positive psychotic symptoms remains undetermined. This network meta-analysis (NMA) investigates the consistency and magnitude of the effects of treatments on attenuated positive psychotic symptoms in CHR-P individuals, weighting the findings for acceptability.

Methods: Web of Science (MEDLINE), PsycInfo, CENTRAL and unpublished/gray literature were searched up to July 18, 2017. Randomized controlled trials in CHR-P individuals, comparing at least two interventions and reporting on attenuated positive psychotic symptoms at follow-up were included, following PRISMA guidelines. The primary outcome (efficacy) was level of attenuated positive psychotic symptoms at 6 and 12 months; effect sizes reported as standardized mean difference (SMD) and 95% CIs in mean follow-up scores between two compared interventions. The secondary outcome was treatment acceptability [reported as odds ratio (OR)]. NMAs were conducted for both primary and secondary outcomes. Treatments were cluster-ranked by surface under the cumulative ranking curve values for efficacy and acceptability. Assessments of biases, assumptions, sensitivity analyses and complementary pairwise meta-analyses for the primary outcome were also conducted.

Results: Overall, 1,707 patients from 14 studies (57% male, mean age = 20) were included, representing the largest evidence synthesis of the effect of preventive treatments on attenuated positive psychotic symptoms to date. In the NMA for efficacy, ziprasidone + Needs-Based Intervention (NBI) was found to be superior to

NBI (SMD = −1.10, 95% CI −2.04 to −0.15), Cognitive Behavioral Therapy-French and Morrison protocol (CBT-F) + NBI (SMD = −1.03, 95% CI −2.05 to −0.01), and risperidone + CBT-F + NBI (SMD = −1.18, 95% CI −2.29 to −0.07) at 6 months. However, these findings did not survive sensitivity analyses. For acceptability, aripiprazole + NBI was significantly more acceptable than olanzapine + NBI (*OR* = 3.73; 95% CI 1.01 to 13.81) at 12 months only. No further significant NMA effects were observed at 6 or 12 months. The results were not affected by inconsistency or evident small-study effects, but only two studies had an overall low risk of bias.

Conclusion: On the basis of the current literature, there is no robust evidence to favor any specific intervention for improving attenuated positive psychotic symptoms in CHR-P individuals.

Keywords: psychosis, risk, interventions, symptoms, network meta-analysis, treatments

INTRODUCTION

Indicated prevention in people at Clinical High Risk for Psychosis (hereafter CHR-P) (1) represents one of the first attempts to alter the course of the most severe psychiatric disorder and thereby improve the lives of many young people (2, 3). Recent meta-analytical evidence has suggested that it is potentially the only effective way to reduce the duration of untreated psychosis, which is a key factor determining outcomes (4). CHR-P individuals accumulate several risk factors for psychosis (5), leading to subtle symptoms (6) and functional impairments (7) that trigger help-seeking behaviors (8). CHR-P individuals have around 20% risk [eTable 4 from Fusar-Poli et al. (9)] of developing psychosis [but not any other non-psychotic disorder (10, 11)] at 2 years. After two decades of CHR-P research, the paradigm is at standstill (12). The principal limitations of knowledge are: (i) poor penetrance of detection strategies for identifying at-risk individuals (13, 14), (ii) the prognostic accuracy of CHR-P tools in clinical use (15) being substantially dependent on idiosyncratic sampling and recruitment strategies (16–20), and (iii) an unclear effect of preventive treatments. Our research group has previously addressed the first two limitations, and only more recently have we completed a meta-analysis that has investigated the consistency and magnitude of the effects of treatments to prevent psychosis in CHR-P individuals. We used a network meta-analytic approach, which allows head-to-head comparisons to be performed across different preventive treatments, and which is the recommended evidence synthesis method for informing treatment guidelines (21). The key result of our analysis was that there is no evidence to favor any specific preventive treatment for CHR-P individuals over any others (22). This finding is not completely surprising, given that all of the most recent trials in this area were negative (23–31). Therefore, currently, there is no convincing evidence that indicated interventions implemented in CHR-P individuals can effectively prevent the onset of psychosis. The impact of available preventive interventions on the underlying neurobiology that characterizes the CHR-P state and the onset of psychosis is similarly unclear (3). We have fully discussed these findings and the limitations of our analysis in our previous report (22). Here, we complement our previous meta-analysis by focusing on outcomes other than the onset of new psychotic disorders. It is indeed apparent that CHR-P individuals may present with problems other than the development of psychosis at follow-up, such as the persistence of subthreshold psychotic symptoms (32). In particular, attenuated positive psychotic symptoms represent the defining features of the core CHR-P criteria. Meta-analytical evidence indicates that around 85% (95% CI 79% to 90%) of CHR-P individuals meet the intake criteria because of attenuated positive psychotic symptoms [see eFigure 1 in Fusar-Poli et al. (9)]. The severity and frequency of attenuated positive psychotic symptoms are carefully measured by experienced clinicians using specific semi-structured [and not self-administered (33)] CHR-P instruments (34). Investigating the effect of treatments on attenuated positive psychotic symptoms may also be associated with empirical research benefits. For example, it has been suggested that using continuous outcomes -such as attenuated positive psychotic symptoms- rather than the binary transition to psychosis may overcome the problems of arbitrary thresholds defining a categorical onset of psychosis (35). Investigating the impact of interventions on attenuated positive psychotic symptoms is also relevant for informing clinical guidelines. For example, the National Institute for Health and Care Excellence (NICE) guidelines recommend cognitive behavioral therapies (CBT) for presenting symptoms (36), but there is no clear evidence which can reliably support this recommendation. The other relevant outcome for CHR-P individuals is the acceptability of treatments. Given the relatively high proportion of false positives with respect to transition to psychosis, it is essential that treatments have a benign side effect profile, are well tolerated and acceptable to this patient group.

To address these gaps in knowledge, we present here a network meta-analysis investigating the consistency and magnitude of the effects of preventive treatments for reducing attenuated positive psychotic symptoms in CHR-P individuals, weighting the findings for acceptability. We focus on randomized controlled trials (RCTs) to avoid the selection biases associated with observational studies. Our primary aim was to test whether any specific treatments are any more or less effective (compared to any others) in improving attenuated positive psychotic symptoms in CHR-P individuals, and to provide an evidence-based ranking of treatments on the basis of efficacy and acceptability. We intended that this work would contribute to the rigorous evidence-based assessment of the strengths and limitations of the CHR-P paradigm (12). Our overarching vision is that by understanding the limitations of current knowledge—which is an essential prerequisite to finding ways of overcoming them—the CHR-P field can advance with the development of refined approaches that may ultimately achieve an effective prevention of psychosis.

METHODS

Included Interventions

In a first step we listed the preventive interventions of interest. The current study included all RCTs involving non-pharmacological and/or pharmacological interventions administered to CHR-P individuals. We focused on the following types of treatments: CBT (different protocols), integrated psychological therapies, psychoeducational interventions, supportive counseling, family therapy, needs-based interventions (NBI), antipsychotic molecules (aripiprazole, ziprasidone, risperidone, olanzapine) and any novel/experimental therapeutics (D-serine and omega-3 fatty acids). Although these interventions had been defined *a priori*, we also allowed the inclusion of additional treatments that were emerging from the most recent literature search. In a second step, we carefully reviewed the available systematic reviews and meta-analyses to operationalize specific definitions of the preventive treatments in CHR-P individuals. This is an essential step to address heterogeneity across different types of interventions and to characterize the specific nodes that were composing our network. We defined each treatment component as indicated in the following paragraphs.

Needs-Based Interventions (NBI)

CHR-P individuals enrolled in clinical trials are traditionally young people who are experiencing subtle symptoms and functional impairment (7) and who are therefore seeking help for their problems (8). Accordingly, it is felt unethical to randomize them to a pure placebo or "no treatment" condition (37). In this scenario it is also difficult to provide an exact definition of "treatment as usual," because although treatment guidelines do exist (36), in reality treatment implementation is determined by local health service priorities, resources and configurations as well as availability of specialist training. We therefore decided on a pragmatic approach and adopted the operationalization of NBI provided by the founders of the CHR-P paradigm (38). This definition focuses on the symptoms and problems already presented by the help-seeking individual (39), and may encompass any of the following components: (a) needs-based supportive psychotherapy for problems with, for example, relationships, work or family; (b) case management for resolving issues with education, housing or employment; (c) brief family psychoeducation and general advice; (d) different types of medications other than antipsychotics; and (e) clinical monitoring alone or coupled with crisis management (38, 40).

Cognitive Behavioral Therapy, French and Morrison Protocol (CBT-F)

The CBT-F protocol (41), like the majority of CBT protocols, is grounded on the principles established by Beck (42). The intervention is problem-focused and time-limited, with treatment strategies selected based on the formulation of each patient's presenting problems but from a range of permissible, manualized strategies. Although each person's therapy will be tailored to their presenting needs, the core components include building engagement, collaborative goal-setting and formulation, normalizing psychotic-like experiences, evaluating core beliefs, and different types of behavioral experiments (41, 43).

Cognitive Behavioral Therapy, van der Gaag Protocol (CBT-V)

The protocol developed by van der Gaag et al. (44) is based on the French and Morrison protocol (41), which is then expanded by the addition of two novel components that target cognitive biases. The first additional component is education on dopamine system super-sensitivity and its relation to attenuated psychotic symptoms and exaggeration of cognitive biases, with the aim of normalizing aberrant perceptual experiences and reducing associated distress. The individual is taught how biases in cognition, such as selective attention, confirmation bias and jumping-to-conclusions contribute to the formation of delusions and paranoia (44). The second component involves exercises/behavioral experiments to correct these biases through examination of initial appraisals and testing of alternative explanations (45). Further aims of CBT-V include supporting school attendance and employment, improving relationships with friends and relatives, and if applicable, reducing cannabis use (44).

Integrated Psychological Interventions, Bechdolf Protocol (IPI)

The protocol developed by Bechdolf et al. (46) is a multi-component package of care. In addition to manualized and time-limited individual CBT-F (41), IPI also includes manualized group skills training, which focuses on scheduling and monitoring leisure activities, training in social skills, problem-solving and mastery of difficult situations, and developing "keeping well" strategies (46). The third component was computerized cognitive remediation to address thought and perception deficits (basic symptoms), and a final component included multi-family psychoeducation group sessions, which aimed to reduce interpersonal conflict and associated stress by helping family members better understand the CHR-P state (46, 47).

Family-Focused Therapy, Miklowitz Protocol (FFT)

The family-focused therapy (FFT) protocol by Miklowitz et al. (28) was originally developed for individuals with or at risk of bipolar disorder. The FFT was then adapted for CHR-P individuals, which has three broad stages. The first stage of FFT encompasses psychoeducation and the development of a patient-family prevention plan, which helps to increase understanding of the stressors contributing to attenuated positive and negative symptoms, while also detailing coping strategies and behavioral activation goals. The second stage focuses on enhancing constructive patient-family communication, and the third stage consists of improving problem-solving skills (28).

Psychopharmacological Interventions

Pharmacological interventions included licensed medications, experimental pharmacotherapies as well as nutritional supplements.

Placebo

The placebo component was reserved for pharmacological placebos administered in the control arms of randomized controlled trials.

Node Composition

We carefully identified the specific interventions (as listed above) for each arm of every study, which were then linearly combined to compose the precise treatment "nodes" of our network. As discussed above, this definition of nodes is an essential prerequisite for performing a robust NMA that can be of clinical relevance. Each pharmacological treatment was assigned to its own node, but different dosages of the same molecule were categorized within the same node. While placebo was initially considered as a separate node from NBI, after performing sensitivity analyses to explore the effect of pooling them together, we decided to combine them in the same node (see below for details).

Search Strategy and Selection Criteria

The first step of our literature search involved systematic electronic searches in the Web of Science (which includes Web of Science Core Collection, BIOSIS Citation Index, KCI-Korean Journal Database, MEDLINE, Russian Science Citation Index and SciELO Citation Index) and Ovid/ PsychINFO databases, the Cochrane Central Register of Controlled Trials and the NHS Centre for Reviews and Dissemination (CRD), using the following keywords: (risk OR prodromal OR prodrom* OR ultra-high risk OR clinical high risk OR high risk OR genetic high risk OR at risk mental state OR risk of progression OR progression to first-episode OR prodromally symptomatic OR basic symptoms) AND (psychosis) AND (RCT OR randomized controlled trial OR placebo controlled trial OR trial). The searches were conducted up to 18th July 2017 and no language restrictions were applied. In a second step, we used Scopus/Web of Science to screen the reference lists of articles identified in the previous step and those of existing systematic reviews and meta-analyses. For comprehensiveness, we also searched the reference lists of relevant clinical guidelines. In a third step, we looked for published and unpublished material in relevant conference proceedings, trial registries (e.g., https://clinicaltrials.gov) or regulatory agencies. The OpenGrey database (http://www.opengrey.eu) was used to identify unpublished material from the gray literature.

The above search strategies led us to identifying potential abstracts of interest. The abstracts were then screened for potential inclusion and those that survived this initial filter were downloaded as full-text articles. These were then carefully inspected against the full inclusion and exclusion criteria which are described below.

In line with the PRISMA guidance, two independent researchers conducted the literature search, study selection and data extraction (48). During the above steps, disagreement between extractors was addressed through discussion with a third researcher until consensus was obtained. We defined the specific inclusion and exclusion criteria to ensure that the population represented in the final database would be broadly representative of the target CHR-P population as a whole (49).

Our inclusion criteria were (a) being an original article, abstract or pilot study; (b) being a randomized controlled trial (including cluster randomized trials, but excluding cross-over studies); (c) being designed as blinded (either single- or double-blind); (d) being conducted in CHR-P individuals with CHR-P criteria ascertained through the use of internationally validated psychometric assessments, i.e., the Comprehensive Assessment of At-Risk Mental States (CAARMS) (6), the Structured Interview for Psychosis-risk Syndromes (SIPS) (50), the Positive and Negative Syndrome Scale (PANSS) (51), the Brief Psychiatric Rating Scale (BPRS) (52), or the Early Recognition Inventory (ERIraos) (53); (e) comparing specific preventive interventions as defined in the sections above; (f) providing sufficient data to perform meta-analytic computation; (g) providing a sample size of 10 or greater (54).

Our exclusion criteria were defined as (a) being a review or reporting non-original data; (b) lacking at least two compared groups, such as open-label trials in a single group of CHR-P patients exposed to treatment; (c) investigating patient samples affected with an established first-episode psychosis or any at-risk group other than CHR-P samples; (d) lacking sufficient data needed to perform the essential meta-analytical computations; (e) design lacking proper randomization, such as quasi-randomization or observational naturalistic studies - however, studies that were initially conceived and designed as blinded but could not maintain blinding during follow-up (e.g., for psychological interventions) were not excluded; (f) including a sample size smaller than 10 (i.e., $N = 9$ or less); (g) presenting overlapping data (i.e., for the same outcome at the same time point as data that was already included)-in the case of overlapping data/samples, we preferred the data relating to the largest sample size.

Outcome Measures and Data Extraction

Due to the variable effect of time on clinical outcomes in these samples (9, 55), analyses for time-dependent outcomes were conducted. The primary outcome (efficacy) was the level of attenuated positive psychotic symptoms at follow-up, indexed by the relevant subscales of validated assessments, such as the PANSS, CAARMS, BPRS and SIPS. For each arm of every study, we extracted the mean and standard deviation (SD) of these scores at 6 and 12 month follow-up time points. Where studies did not report sufficient data to extract the primary outcome, we used DigitizeIt software (http://www.digitizeit.de/) to extract data presented graphically (means and 95% confidence intervals (CIs) for each follow-up time point). When necessary,

SDs were back-calculated using standard formulae. If none of the aforementioned were available, we estimated follow-up data using information available from the published paper and using assumptions established in previous literature. Sample sizes were based on the numbers randomized to each arm.

A high benefit-to-harm ratio is essential when adopting preventive strategies that may lead to the unnecessary treatment of false positives. We therefore selected the acceptability of interventions (discontinuation due to any cause) as our secondary outcome measure. In line with previous authoritative publications, we defined the acceptability of interventions as the number of participants who dropped out of each arm for any reason following randomization, over those randomized at baseline (56–58).

In order to describe our population, assess the transitivity assumption (see below), address the risk of bias and conduct meta-regression analyses, we also extracted details on the first author and year of publication of each trial, country where the trial was conducted, types of outcomes reported, definitions of intervention and control arms (in line with the treatment components described above), trial design, risk of bias assessment, duration of each intervention and follow-up, sample size, mean age, percent male, and the psychometric CHR-P instrument used to ascertain attenuated positive psychotic symptoms.

Risk of Bias

The assessment of bias is of paramount importance for rigorously interpreting the results of evidence synthesis studies and for testing their robustness. We used the Cochrane Risk of Bias tool (59) to classify the risk of bias in each study using *a priori* defined criteria. Using these standardized criteria, we evaluated whether each trial was at high, low or unclear risk of bias across six specific domains. These included random sequence generation, allocation concealment, blinding of participants and study personnel, blinding of outcome assessments, incomplete outcome data, and selective outcome reporting. Once these domains were assessed, the Cochrane Risk of Bias tool allowed production of an overall risk of bias classification of high, low or unclear. The overall rating of low risk was assigned when none of the six domains were found to be at high risk and if three or less domains were found to be at unclear risk. The overall rating of moderate risk was assigned when one domain was found to be at high risk; or no domains were found to be at high risk but four or more were found to be at unclear risk. In all other cases, the trial was classified as having an overall high risk of bias (60).

Statistical Analysis

Network Meta-Analysis

Frequentist NMAs were conducted for both primary (attenuated positive psychotic symptoms) and secondary (acceptability) outcomes at 6 and 12 months using the *network* package in STATA (version SE 14.2). Effect sizes for the primary outcome were calculated and reported as the standardized mean difference Hedges' adjusted *g* (SMD) and 95% CIs in mean follow-up scores between two compared interventions, using the pooled SD at follow-up (61). Follow-up data are considered preferable when measuring continuous outcomes that are difficult to measure (62). Effect sizes for the secondary outcome were reported as odds ratio (OR) and 95% CIs. We first constructed network plots - for each outcome- to ensure that the geometry of the networks were sufficiently connected (63, 64). We then performed a NMA assuming consistency and a common heterogeneity across all comparisons in the network. This allowed us to derive a single summary treatment effect (SMD for attenuated positive psychotic symptoms; OR for acceptability) for every possible pairwise comparison of treatments. This summary effect draws on all evidence from the network of trials, including direct and indirect evidence. Correlations in effect sizes induced by multi-arm trials were accounted for (63, 65). The resulting relative SMDs or ORs with 95% CIs for each pair of treatments were reported in league tables (66). Statistical significance was set at $p < 0.05$.

When performing NMA it is possible to rank an outcome of interest using the Surface Under the Cumulative RAnking curve (SUCRA) procedure. Such an approach allows integration of both the location and the variance of any relative effect on the outcome of interest (67). In simple terms, the SUCRA procedure summarizes the overall ranking of each intervention through a single number ranging from 0 to 100% (68). In this manuscript, the higher the SUCRA value, the higher the likelihood that an intervention will be in the top rank, and vice versa (68). In line with our objective, we performed cluster ranking (63, 67) of the SUCRA values for attenuated positive psychotic symptoms and acceptability (at 6 and 12 months, separately) and presented the results in two-dimensional plots (64). These plots aid visualization of the relative balance between a treatment's ranking across different outcomes, and show the clustering of treatments into meaningful groups as determined by hierarchical cluster analysis (63, 64).

Consistency in a network refers to the equivalence of direct and indirect estimates of the same treatment comparison pairs, and can be investigated in each closed loop of evidence (66). We assessed this assumption by calculating an inconsistency factor along with 95% CIs (truncated at 0) and associated *p*-values for each closed loop of the primary outcome (63). Inconsistency was defined as disagreement between direct and indirect evidence, with 95% CIs for inconsistency factors excluding zero. Because the loop-specific approach focuses on local inconsistency and has low power, we also tested a full design-by-treatment model (69) for the primary outcome to evaluate global inconsistency. This entailed performing a NMA under the inconsistency model and using the χ^2-test to estimate the statistical significance of all possible inconsistencies in the networks (70).

Transitivity was examined by assessing the distributions of potential effect modifiers across comparisons in the networks. These effect modifiers encompassed the following items: percent male, age, percent exposed to antipsychotic medications at baseline, type of blinding and publication year.

The presence of small-study effects was assessed by visual inspection of comparison-adjusted funnel plots (71). In this analysis we used NBI (or when not available, CBT-F + NBI) as the reference. We assumed that small-study effects, if present, would be expected to exaggerate the effectiveness of the "active" (or newer/experimental) treatment, rather than NBI or CBT-F

+ NBI, which currently represent the most widely implemented interventions for this patient group.

Complementary Analyses

Sensitivity analyses were performed to address the impact of study quality and our data analysis strategy. Specifically, we repeated the NMA analyses on attenuated positive psychotic symptoms using only: (a) studies with a low risk of bias for the blinding of attenuated positive psychotic symptom assessments; (b) studies whose meta-analytical data (i.e., mean and SD of attenuated positive psychotic symptoms) were not estimated using assumptions established in previous literature; and (c) published trials only (i.e., excluding conference proceedings). In addition, we repeated the NMA after pooling NBI and placebo nodes and after pooling different types of antipsychotic molecules. To ensure that the use of follow-up scores did not unduly influence our results, we repeated the analyses using SMD calculated from change score and pooled baseline SD, which is recommended when a full ANCOVA model is not feasible (62). Furthermore, we complemented the sensitivity analyses through network meta-regression analyses. These were planned only when substantial heterogeneity was observed and when at least 10 independent trials were available (72) for each outcome of interest. These meta-regressions were planned to investigate the potential impact of the different CHR-P psychometric instruments used for measuring attenuated positive psychotic symptoms (34).

For the primary outcome, we also conducted conventional pairwise meta-analyses (random effects model) of every direct treatment comparison using the *metan* package in STATA. The random effects meta-analyses were stratified by (a) follow-up time (6 or 12 months), and (b) pairwise intervention comparisons (i.e., each type of treatment vs. its control was treated as a meta-analysis, no overall summary effect computed across comparisons of different treatments). The resulting meta-analytic SMDs together with 95% CIs and measures of heterogeneity (I^2) were calculated and presented in tables. When pairwise groups had more than three contributing studies, we performed leave-one-out sensitivity analyses to explore the robustness of the results to influential individual studies.

RESULTS

Characteristics of Trials and Patients

Our initial literature search identified 1,556 references. However, most of them did not report on RCTs in CHR-P individuals. As indicated in **Figure 1**, 49 of them were eventually downloaded and fully inspected against the inclusion and exclusion criteria, which resulted in a final sample of 14 studies. We found only three, three two and two trials reporting the outcome data of interest at 18, 24, 36, and >36 month time points, respectively. Consequently, the current meta-analysis focuses only on the 6 and 12 month time points. The 14 studies used in the analyses contributed data on a total of 1707 patients, with a mean age of 20.1 ± 2.9 years, and of whom 57% were male (**Table 1**). The mean sample size was 122 (range 44–304). Five studies were conducted in North America, five in Europe, three in Australia and one was multi-national. Two trials adopted a three-arm design while all of the others employed a two-arm design. Two of the included studies were identified from conference proceedings and gray literature/clinical trial databases (24, 30). Two studies had a treatment duration of <6 months, eight of 6 months, and four of 12 months. Three of the 12 trials that reported enough information to identify the source of sponsorship or funding acknowledged pharmaceutical company involvement. The SIPS was the most common assessment used for measuring attenuated positive psychotic symptoms ($N = 6$). Only two studies had an overall low risk of bias (30, 40), four had unclear risk (24, 26, 27, 73) and the remaining eight had high risk; the full risk of bias assessment is presented in **Figure 2**.

For the primary outcome, eight studies provided data for both 6 and 12 month networks, three only provided data for 6 months, and another 3 only for 12 months, resulting in 11 studies contributing data for the 6 month analysis, and 11 to the 12 month analysis. For the 6 month analysis, 11 studies ($N = 1459$) provided data on 15 direct comparisons between 8 different treatment nodes (**Figure 3A**). For the 12 month analysis, 11 studies ($N = 1483$) provided data on 15 direct comparisons between 7 different treatment nodes (**Figure 3B**).

At 6 months, seven studies provided the required follow-up symptom data directly or indirectly, two provided means and SD graphically (28, 40), and for two studies symptom data were estimated on the basis of available data and assumptions established in previous literature (27, 30). At 12 months, nine studies provided the required data directly or indirectly, one provided data graphically (40), and for one study symptom data were estimated on the basis of available data and assumptions established in previous literature (27).

All studies, except one (38), provided data for the secondary outcome (acceptability) at both 6 and 12 months. Network plots for the acceptability outcome were the same as those for the primary outcome (**Figure 3**).

Pairwise Meta-Analysis

Pairwise meta-analysis results for the primary outcome are presented in **Table 2**. Only three pairwise intervention vs. control groups had two or more studies: CBT-F + NBI vs. NBI; omega-3 + NBI vs. NBI; and risperidone + CBT-F + NBI vs. NBI. The remaining pairwise intervention vs. control groups were composed of single studies.

At 6 months, there was no significant difference between CBT-F + NBI vs. NBI alone (SMD = −0.06, 95% CI −0.26 to 0.13; 5 studies, $N = 652$). However, there was meta-analytical evidence of a greater reduction in attenuated positive psychotic symptoms in CBT-F + NBI vs. NBI alone at 12 months (SMD = −0.22, 95% CI −0.37 to −0.07; 6 studies, $N = 712$). Leave-one-out sensitivity analyses showed that this effect was dependent on the presence of one study (74). When this study was removed, the combined effect at 12 months became non-significant (SMD = −0.12, 95% CI −0.32 to 0.08; 5 studies, $N = 424$). The non-significant summary effect at 6 months did not become significant throughout any iteration of the leave-one-out analyses.

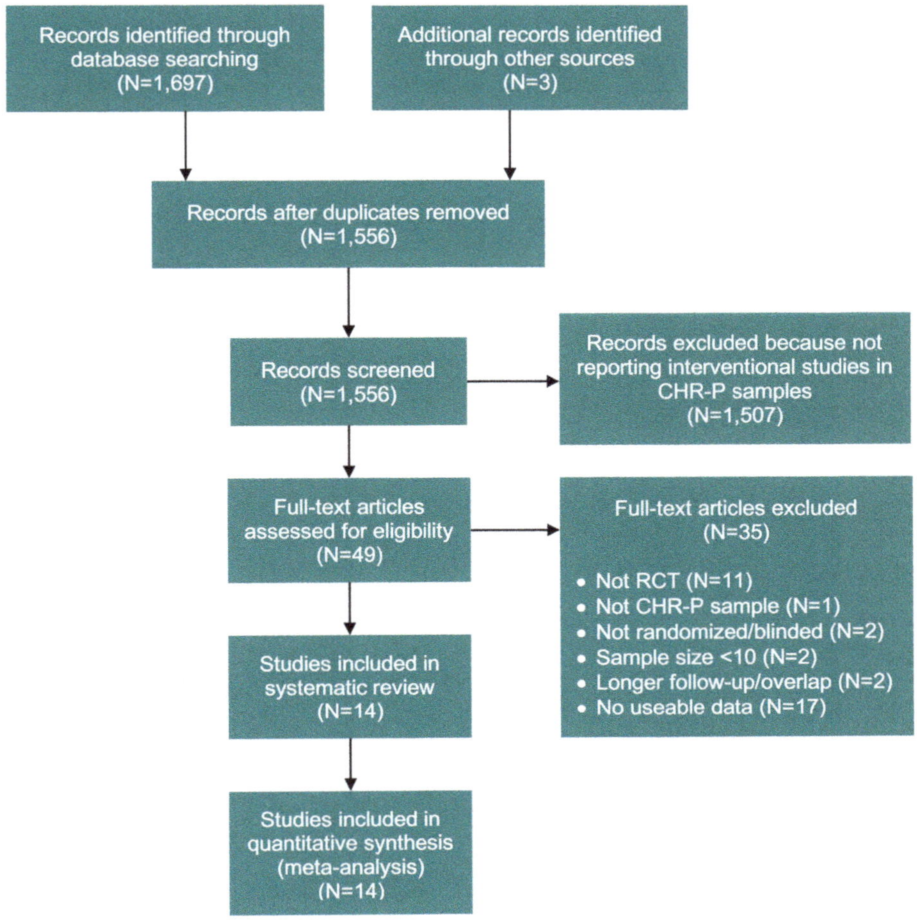

FIGURE 1 | PRISMA flow chart of the study selection process. CHR-P, clinical high risk for psychosis; RCT, randomized controlled trial.

Two studies compared omega-3 + NBI to NBI alone, but both 6 and 12 month summary effect estimates were not significant (6 month SMD = −0.48, 95% CI −1.62 to 0.67, 2 studies, $N = 385$; 12 month SMD = −0.38, 95% CI −1.38 to 0.63, 2 studies, $N = 385$). Significant heterogeneity was detected between these two studies at both 6 ($I^2 = 95\%$, $p < 0.001$) and 12 ($I^2 = 94\%$, $p < 0.001$) month time points. Statistical investigation of potential sources of heterogeneity using meta-regression was precluded by the limited number of studies.

Combined therapy with risperidone + CBT-F + NBI was not significantly different from NBI alone at either 6 (SMD = 0.02, 95% CI −0.33 to 0.37, 2 studies, $N = 130$) or 12 months (SMD = 0.00, 95% CI −0.38 to 0.38, 2 studies, $N = 130$). While available data on all further pairwise treatments vs. controls are listed in **Table 2** for completeness, they represent single studies and thus cannot be considered meta-analytic results.

Network Meta-Analysis – Effect on Attenuated Positive Psychotic Symptoms

Results of the NMA are presented in **Tables 3**, **4**. At 6 months, ziprasidone + NBI was found to be significantly more effective at reducing attenuated positive psychotic symptoms compared to NBI alone (SMD = −1.10, 95% CI −2.04 to −0.15); compared to CBT-F + NBI (SMD = −1.03, 95% CI −2.05 to −0.01); and compared to risperidone + CBT-F + NBI (SMD = −1.18, 95% CI −2.29 to −0.07). There were no other significant effects of any one intervention over any others (**Table 3**). Using NBI as a comparator, the relative treatment effect estimates (all SMD < 0 favor the given treatment) at 6 months were: ziprasidone + NBI (SMD = −1.10, 95% CI −2.04 to −0.15); omega-3 + NBI (SMD = −0.42, 95% CI −1.01 to 0.16); aripiprazole + NBI (SMD = −0.18, 95% CI −0.90 to 0.53); family-focused therapy + NBI (SMD = −0.41, 95% CI −1.22 to 0.41); CBT-F + NBI (SMD = −0.07, 95% CI −0.44 to 0.31); D-serine + NBI (SMD = −0.10, 95% CI −1.05 to 0.84); and risperidone + CBT-F + NBI (SMD = 0.08, 95% CI −0.50 to 0.67).

At 12 months, there was no evidence that any one intervention was superior over any others, with all 95% CIs crossing zero (**Table 4**). Using NBI as a comparator, the relative treatment effect estimates (all SMD < 0 favor the given treatment) at 12 months were: olanzapine + NBI (SMD = −0.53, 95% CI −1.28 to 0.22); omega-3 + NBI (SMD = −0.30, 95% CI −0.77 to 0.17);

TABLE 1 | Characteristics of included studies.

Study	Study arms (N)	Total N	Network inclusion	Treatment duration (months)	Follow-up time points (months)	% male	Mean age	Measure of symptoms	Study design	Country	% exposed to antipsychotics at baseline
Addington et al. (37)	CBT-F + NBI [27] NBI [24]	51	6, 12	6	6, 12, 18	71	20.9	SIPS	SB-RCT	Canada	0
Amminger et al. (40)	Omega-3 + NBI [41] NBI [40]	81	6, 12	3	6, 12, 84	33	16.4	PANSS	DB-RCT	Austria	0
Bechdolf et al. (46, 75)	IPI [63] NBI [65]	128	12	12	6, 12, 18, 24	63	26.0	PANSS	SB-RCT	Germany	0
Bechdolf et al. (24)	ARI + NBI [96] NBI [55] CBT-F + NBI [129]	280	6, 12	12	6, 12	66	24.4	SIPS	SB-RCT	Germany	3.4
Kantrowitz et al. (26)	D-serine + NBI [20] NBI [24]	44	6	4	4	66	19.4	SIPS	DB-RCT	US	11.4
McGlashan et al. (73)	OLA + NBI [31] NBI [29]	60	12	12	12, 24	65	17.7	SIPS	DB-RCT	US, Canada	10
McGorry et al. (38)	RIS + CBT-F + NBI [31] NBI [28]	59	6, 12	6	6, 12, 36–48	58	20.0	BPRS	SB-RCT	Australia	0
McGorry et al. (27)	Omega-3 + NBI [153] NBI [151]	304	6, 12	6	6, 12	46	19.2	BPRS	DB-RCT	Multi-national	0
Miklowitz et al. (28)	FFT + NBI [66] NBI [63]	129	6	6	6	57	17.4	SIPS	SB-RCT	US, Canada	20.9
Morrison et al. (43)	CBT-F + NBI [37] NBI [23]	60	12	6	6, 12, 36	69	22.0	PANSS	SB-RCT	UK	0
Morrison et al. (74)	CBT-F + NBI [144] NBI [144]	288	6, 12	6	6, 12, 18, 24	63	20.7	CAARMS	SB-RCT	UK	0
Stain et al. (29)	CBT-F + NBI [30] NBI [27]	57	6, 12	6	6, 12	40	16.3	CAARMS	SB-RCT	Australia	0
Woods et al. (30, 31)	ZIP + NBI [24] NBI [27]	51	6	6	6	64	22.3	SIPS	DB-RCT	US	0
Yung et al. (76) and McGorry et al. (77)	CBT-F + NBI [44] RIS + CBT-F + NBI [43] NBI [28]	115	6, 12	12	6, 12	39	18.1	BPRS	SB-RCT	Australia	0

CBT-F, cognitive-behavioral therapy (French and Morrison protocol); NBI, needs-based interventions (including placebo); IPI, integrated psychological interventions; ARI, aripiprazole; OLA, olanzapine; RIS, risperidone; FFT, family-focused therapy; ZIP, ziprasidone; SIPS, Structured Interview for Psychosis-risk Syndromes; PANSS, Positive and Negative Syndrome Scale; BPRS, Brief Psychiatric Rating Scale; CAARMS, Comprehensive Assessment of At-Risk Mental States; SB-RCT, single-blind randomized controlled trial; DB-RCT, double-blind randomized controlled trial.

aripiprazole + NBI (SMD = −0.23, 95% CI −0.78 to 0.33); CBT-F + NBI (SMD = −0.15, 95% CI −0.43 to 0.13); risperidone + CBT-F + NBI (SMD = −0.04, 95% CI −0.52 to 0.44); and integrated psychological interventions (SMD = 0.20, 95% CI −0.45 to 0.84).

Inconsistency and Small-Study Effects

There was no statistically significant inconsistency in the 6 or 12 month networks. The 95% CIs for all inconsistency factors were compatible with zero inconsistency. However, it is important to note that only two loops were available at both 6 and 12 months, which may have limited our ability to detect inconsistency. When we used the design-by-treatment interaction model, there was no evidence for significant inconsistency in the 6 ($p = 0.92$) or 12 month ($p = 0.92$) networks.

Visual inspection of comparison-adjusted funnel plots suggested no clear small-study effects (publication biases), with a regression line almost flat at 6 months (Figure S1A in Supplementary Material) and completely flat at 12 months (Figure S1B in Supplementary Material).

Sensitivity Analyses for NMA of Primary Outcome

We tested the robustness of the core NMA findings (that ziprasidone + NBI is superior to NBI alone, CBT-F + NBI, and risperidone + CBT-F + NBI at 6 months) through various sensitivity analyses. At 6 months, two studies (27, 30) were based on estimated follow-up data, one of which was the single ziprasidone + NBI vs. NBI study (30). Repeating the analyses after removal of the latter study (30) inherently meant that there was now no ziprasidone + NBI node and all estimates were non-significant. Removal of the other study -by McGorry et al (27)- did not affect the current results at 6 or 12 months; however, one change of note is that at 12 months, CBT-F + NBI became significantly more effective than NBI, which is interesting in light of the pairwise significance of CBT-F + NBI vs. NBI at 12 months, and lack thereof in the main NMA analyses.

	Random sequence generation (selection bias)	Allocation concealment (selection bias)	Blinding of participants and personnel (performance bias)	Blinding of outcome assessment (detection bias)	Incomplete outcome data (attrition bias)	Selective reporting (reporting bias)	Overall bias level
Addington, 2011	+	+	-	+	-	+	-
Amminger, 2010	+	+	+	+	+	?	+
Bechdolf, 2012	+	?	-	?	-	?	-
Bechdolf, 2016	?	?	?	+	-	?	?
Kantrowitz, 2015	+	+	+	+	-	?	?
McGlashan, 2006	?	+	+	+	-	?	?
McGorry, 2002	?	?	-	-	?	?	-
McGorry, 2017	+	+	+	+	-	+	?
Miklowitz, 2014	+	+	-	+	-	?	-
Morrison, 2004	+	+	-	-	-	+	-
Morrison, 2012	+	+	-	+	-	+	-
Stain, 2016	+	+	-	+	-	+	-
Woods, 2017	+	+	+	+	?	?	+
Yung, 2011; McGorry, 2013	?	?	-	?	-	?	-

FIGURE 2 | Risk of bias summary. Review authors' judgements about each risk of bias item for each included study. Green circles (+) indicate low risk of bias; yellow circles (?) indicate unclear risk; red circles (–) indicate high risk of bias.

The ziprasidone + NBI results were not robust to the removal of two studies (38, 76) at high or unclear risk of bias for the blinding of outcome assessments, which resulted in only the ziprasidone + NBI vs. NBI comparison remaining significant. Repeating the analyses after removing unpublished studies (24, 30), pooling together different antipsychotic molecules, and using change scores instead of follow-up scores all abolished the ziprasidone + NBI results. Repeating the analyses treating NBI + placebo as a separate node to NBI had some effect on the NMA estimates at 6 months (ziprasidone + NBI was now superior only to NBI + placebo) and had no effect at 12 months; we therefore used the pooled NBI + placebo in the main analysis (**Tables 1–4**, **Figures 3**, **4**). There were too few studies to allow robust meta-regression analyses on the type of instruments used to measure attenuated positive psychotic symptoms.

Network Meta-Analysis – Effect on Acceptability

There were no significant differences in acceptability between any treatments at 6 months (**Table 3**). At 12 months, aripiprazole + NBI was significantly more acceptable than olanzapine + NBI (*OR* = 3.73; 95% CI 1.01 to 13.81). There were no further significant differences at 12 months (**Table 4**). However, at both time points, the 95% CIs for the comparisons were often very wide, indicating substantial imprecision in the estimates.

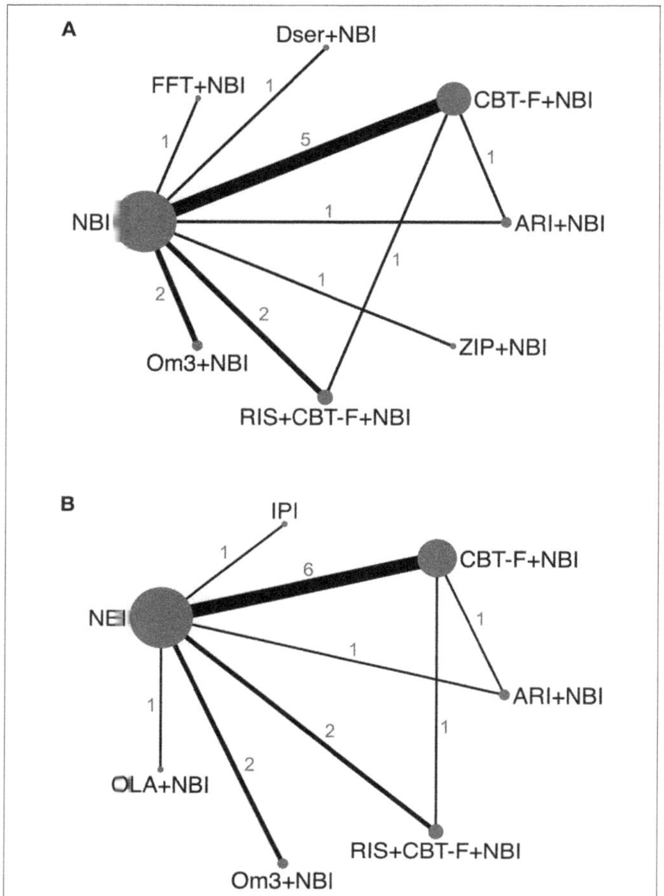

FIGURE 3 | Network plots of direct comparisons at 6 **(A)** and 12 **(B)** months. The width of the lines is proportional to the number of trials comparing each pair of treatments and the size of each node is proportional to the number of studies testing the specific treatment. Numbers represent the number of studies contributing data to each comparison. ARI, aripiprazole; NBI, needs-based interventions (including placebo); CBT-F, cognitive behavioral therapy (French and Morrison protocol); Dser, D-serine; FFT, family-focused therapy; Om3, omega-3 fatty acids; RIS, risperidone; ZIP, ziprasidone; IPI, integrated psychological interventions; OLA, olanzapine.

Network Meta-Analysis – Cluster Ranking for Attenuated Positive Psychotic Symptoms and Acceptability

The cluster ranking plots of SUCRA values for attenuated positive psychotic symptoms (efficacy) and acceptability are illustrated in **Figure 4A** (for 6 months) and **Figure 4B** (for 12 months). However, it should be noted that although the treatments were cluster ranked, there was no statistically significant difference between any treatments (with the exception of ziprasidone + NBI) in the main network meta-analysis results (see **Tables 3, 4** for details).

Three distinct clusters were found in the cluster ranking at 6 months (**Figure 4A**). Notably, while ziprasidone + NBI had the highest SUCRA for efficacy (94%), it was also the most poorly tolerated, having the lowest SUCRA value for acceptability (23%). In a second cluster, omega-3 + NBI and family-focused therapy + NBI had similar SUCRA scores for efficacy (67% and 63%, respectively), however, they differed markedly in their SUCRA for acceptability; family-focused therapy + NBI had the highest acceptability SUCRA of all treatments (70%), while that of omega-3 + NBI was mid-range (49%). The third cluster comprised the remaining treatments, whose SUCRA values for efficacy were all below 50%, but whose acceptability SUCRAs varied from 62% for aripiprazole + NBI, to 37% (the worst) for NBI.

At 12 months, four distinct clusters were found (**Figure 4B**). Similar to above, while olanzapine + NBI was ranked highest of all treatments for efficacy SUCRA (82%), it also scored worst for acceptability (13%). A second cluster, with a more balanced profile of efficacy and acceptability SUCRA values, comprised aripiprazole + NBI, omega-3 + NBI and CBT-F + NBI. Of these, omega-3 + NBI had the highest SUCRA value in terms of efficacy (70%) but lower acceptability (57%), aripiprazole + NBI had slightly lower efficacy (60%) but the highest acceptability of all treatments (91%), and CBT-F + NBI had mid-range values for both outcomes. NBI and risperidone + CBT-F + NBI were found in a third, intermediate cluster with low mid-range SUCRA values. The final cluster was composed of integrated psychological interventions, with SUCRA values of 19% and 26% for efficacy and acceptability, respectively.

DISCUSSION

To the best of our knowledge, this is the first network meta-analysis to have explored the effect of preventive treatments on attenuated positive psychotic symptoms in CHR-P individuals. Focusing exclusively on RCTs to minimize selection biases, we included a total of 14 non-overlapping studies, for a total database of 1,707 CHR-P individuals, representing the largest evidence synthesis of this topic to date. By using the most updated evidence we defined two networks at 6 and 12 months, on which we performed the core analyses. These two networks included 8 and 7 nodes, respectively. There were not enough studies to generate networks beyond these time points. Overall, our network meta-analyses indicated no robust evidence of superior efficacy for any specific intervention on attenuated positive psychotic symptoms at any time point, with the exception of ziprasidone + NBI, which was superior to NBI alone, CBT-F + NBI, and risperidone + CBT-F + NBI. However, the evidence specifically relating to ziprasidone + NBI was based on a single study only and did not survive sensitivity analyses. The results were not affected by inconsistency or evident small-study effects (publication biases).

The main finding of the current study is that there is a lack of evidence to favor specific effective interventions for reducing attenuated positive psychotic symptoms in CHR-P individuals. While ziprasidone + NBI demonstrated some superiority in the 6 month network meta-analyses, these results are not robust. First, the efficacy of ziprasidone + NBI comes from only one as-yet unpublished study. Second, the results did not survive most of the sensitivity analyses. Finally, in the cluster ranking, it was clear that while ziprasidone + NBI was the most efficacious in reducing

TABLE 2 | Pairwise meta-analytic results for attenuated psychotic symptoms at 6 and 12 months.

Time point; months	Treatment condition	Control condition	Number of studies (references)	Total N		SMD (*g*)	Lower 95%CI	Upper 95%CI	Heterogeneity		
				Treatment	Control				I^2	Q	P
6	ARI + NBI	NBI	1 (24)	96	55	−0.22	−0.56	0.11	–	0.00	–
	ARI + NBI	CBT-F+NBI	1 (24)	96	129	−0.06	−0.33	0.20	–	0.00	–
	CBT-F + NBI	NBI	5 (24, 29, 37, 74, 76)	374	278	−0.06	−0.26	0.13	24.2	5.27	0.26
	Dser + NBI	NBI	1 (26)	20	24	−0.10	−0.70	0.49	–	0.00	–
	FFT + NBI	NBI	1 (28)	66	63	−0.41	−0.76	−0.06	–	0.00	–
	Om3 + NBI	NBI	2 (27, 40)	194	191	−0.48	−1.62	0.67	94.8	19.4	<0.001
	RIS + CBT-F + NBI	CBT-F+NBI	1 (76)	43	44	0.37	−0.05	0.80	–	0.00	–
	RIS + CBT-F + NBI	NBI	2 (38, 76)	74	56	0.02	−0.33	0.37	0.00	0.72	0.40
	ZIP + NBI	NBI	1 (30)	24	27	−1.10	−1.69	−0.50	–	0.00	–
12	ARI + NBI	NBI	1 (24)	96	55	−0.22	−0.55	0.12	–	0.00	–
	ARI + NBI	CBT-F+NBI	1 (24)	96	129	−0.08	−0.34	0.18	–	0.00	–
	CBT-F + NBI	NBI	6 (24, 29, 37, 43, 74, 77)	411	301	<u>**−0.22**</u>	<u>**−0.37**</u>	<u>**−0.07**</u>	0.00	3.27	0.66
	IPI	NBI	1 (46)	63	65	0.20	−0.15	0.54	–	0.00	–
	OLA + NBI	NBI	1 (73)	31	29	−0.53	−1.05	−0.02	–	0.00	–
	Om3 + NBI	NBI	2 (27, 40)	194	191	−0.38	−1.38	0.63	93.5	15.49	<0.001
	RIS + CBT-F + NBI	CBT-F+NBI	1 (77)	43	44	−0.07	−0.49	0.35	–	0.00	–
	RIS + CBT-F + NBI	NBI	2 (38, 77)	74	56	0.00	−0.38	0.38	16.2	1.19	0.28

Underlined bold text within the SMD and 95% CI columns indicates statistically significant meta-analytic treatment effect. SMD below 0 favors the given treatment condition. ARI, aripiprazole; NBI, needs-based interventions (including placebo); CBT-F, cognitive behavioral therapy (French & Morrison protocol); Dser, D-serine; FFT, family-focused therapy; Om3, omega-3 fatty acids; RIS, risperidone; ZIP, ziprasidone; IPI, integrated psychological interventions; OLA, olanzapine. Dashes (–) indicate no heterogeneity estimate due to having only one contributing study (and thus cannot be considered a true meta-analytic result).

attenuated positive symptoms, it was poorly tolerated with the lowest ranking for acceptability. Similarly, the only significant result in pairwise analyses was for CBT-F + NBI vs. NBI at 12 months. Again, this was found to be reliant on the inclusion of one particular study (74) in sensitivity analyses. Given that the data relating to the CBT-F + NBI element are identical in both the pairwise and network meta-analyses, the driving factor for the disparity (in significance of CBT-F + NBI vs. NBI in pairwise vs. network meta-analyses) likely emerges from the additional data about NBI that the NMA had gained from the rest of the network (i.e., the relative effectiveness of NBI as derived indirectly from the other -direct- comparisons). Support for this explanation comes from the finding that, when one particular study (27) was removed from the 12 month network (in sensitivity analyses), the CBT-F + NBI vs. NBI comparison became significant. Inspection of the data for this removed study (27) showed that it had the largest NBI arm ($N = 151$) of all trials, and although the study-specific SMD was not significant, the SMD was favoring NBI over the comparative intervention (omega-3 + NBI). This suggests that the relative effectiveness of NBI may have been underestimated by the direct (pairwise) CBT-F + NBI vs. NBI estimates compared to the NMA-derived estimates.

Overall, our negative results are concordant with several lines of evidence pointing toward ineffective treatments for CHR-P individuals. Beyond the lack of evidence for specific treatments reducing the risk of developing psychosis -as determined by our earlier study (22)-, another recently published network meta-analysis found no evidence that any treatments were better than any others in improving attenuated negative symptoms in CHR-P individuals (78, 79). The lack of impact on attenuated negative symptoms is in line with meta-analytical evidence showing that full-blown negative symptoms are refractory to any kind of treatment (72). More to the point, there is not even evidence that current preventive treatments can ameliorate clinical outcomes such as functional level (80–83), depressive comorbidities (83), distress (81) and quality of life (81, 83) in CHR-P individuals. It is possible that the lack of evidence for effective treatments to reduce transition to psychosis may be secondary to low statistical power for testing this outcome. In turn, this can be caused by the recruitment strategies adopted by recent RCTs that have focused on individuals that were poorly risk enriched, causing a dilution of the final risk for psychosis (23). On the contrary, the lack of evidence for effects on attenuated positive psychotic symptoms cannot simply be attributed to low statistical power. Rather, it is possible that the available treatments are not disease-modifying because they are not targeting the core pathophysiological processes underlying the onset of psychosis in CHR-P individuals (3). It is also possible that effective preventive treatments do exist, but we are currently unable to detect them because of the large noise and between-subject heterogeneity that is observed. For example, the level of attenuated positive psychotic symptoms varies considerably across different CHR-P subgroups. We have previously found that CHR-P individuals meeting the short-lived psychotic episode subgroup have the highest risk of developing psychosis (about 40–50% at 2 years) (9, 84), those meeting the attenuated psychotic symptoms subgroup have an intermediate risk (about 20% at 2 years) (9), and those meeting the genetic risk subgroup have a low risk (about

TABLE 3 | Network meta-analytic relative treatment effects for efficacy and acceptability at 6 months.

ZIP + NBI	1.77 (0.32,9.79)	2.63 (0.42,16.68)	2.22 (0.39,12.75)	1.83 (0.24,13.78)	1.79 (0.40,8.07)	1.55 (0.38,6.27)	2.28 (0.34,15.09)
−0.67 (−1.78,0.44)	**Om3 + NBI**	1.49 (0.31,7.07)	1.26 (0.30,5.30)	1.04 (0.18,6.01)	1.01 (0.33,3.13)	0.88 (0.33,2.35)	1.29 (0.26,6.44)
−0.69 (−1.94,0.56)	−0.01 (−1.02,0.99)	**FFT + NBI**	0.84 (0.17,4.15)	0.69 (0.11,4.59)	0.68 (0.18,2.56)	0.59 (0.18,1.96)	0.87 (0.15,4.98)
−0.91 (−2.10,0.27)	−0.24 (−1.16,0.68)	−0.23 (−1.31,0.86)	**ARI + NBI**	0.82 (0.14,4.93)	0.80 (0.28,2.28)	0.70 (0.25,1.98)	1.03 (0.21,5.02)
−0.99 (−2.33,0.35)	−0.32 (−1.43,0.79)	−0.30 (−1.55,0.94)	−0.08 (−1.26,1.11)	**Dser + NBI**	0.98 (0.21,4.65)	0.85 (0.20,3.63)	1.25 (0.18,8.60)
−1.03 (−2.05,−0.01)	−0.36 (−1.05,0.34)	−0.34 (−1.24,0.56)	−0.11 (−0.82,0.59)	−0.04 (−1.05,0.98)	**CBT-F + NBI**	0.87 (0.50,1.51)	1.27 (0.36,4.46)
−1.10 (−2.04,−0.15)	−0.42 (−1.01,0.16)	−0.41 (−1.22,0.41)	−0.18 (−0.90,0.53)	−0.10 (−1.05,0.84)	−0.07 (−0.44,0.31)	**NBI**	1.47 (0.41,5.25)
−1.18 (−2.29,−0.07)	−0.50 (−1.33,0.32)	−0.49 (−1.49,0.51)	−0.26 (−1.16,0.63)	−0.18 (−1.30,0.93)	−0.15 (−0.78,0.48)	−0.08 (−0.67,0.50)	**RIS + CBT-F + NBI**

Comparisons between treatments should be read from left to right, and the estimate is in the cell in common between the column-defining treatment and the row-defining treatment. For the primary outcome (attenuated positive psychotic symptoms) estimates, results are SMD (95% CI), where SMD below 0 favors the column-defined treatment. For acceptability, results are OR (95% CI), where OR < 1 favors the row-defined treatment. Significant results are in bold. The order of treatments in the diagonal is arbitrary and does not reflect ranking. ZIP, ziprasidone; NBI, needs-based interventions (including placebo); Om3, omega-3 fatty acids; FFT, family-focused therapy; ARI, aripiprazole; Dser, D-serine; CBT-F, cognitive behavioral therapy (French & Morrison protocol); RIS, risperidone.

Comparison.

Efficacy (attenuated psychotic symptoms; SMD [95% CI]).

Acceptability (dropout; OR [95% CI]).

TABLE 4 | Network meta-analytic relative treatment effects for efficacy and acceptability at 12 months.

OLA + NBI	2.31 (0.64,8.32)	**3.73 (1.01,13.81)**	2.39 (0.73,7.83)	1.98 (0.47,8.32)	2.31 (0.75,7.05)	1.38 (0.30,6.38)
−0.23 (−1.12,0.65)	**Om3 + NBI**	1.61 (0.64,4.07)	1.03 (0.50,2.12)	0.86 (0.29,2.53)	1.00 (0.53,1.86)	0.59 (0.18,2.02)
−0.31 (−1.24,0.63)	−0.07 (−0.80,0.66)	**ARI + NBI**	0.64 (0.32,1.26)	0.53 (0.18,1.57)	0.62 (0.31,1.22)	0.37 (0.11,1.29)
−0.38 (−1.19,0.42)	−0.15 (−0.70,0.40)	−0.08 (−0.63,0.47)	**CBT-F + NBI**	0.83 (0.35,2.00)	0.97 (0.64,1.45)	0.58 (0.19,1.78)
−0.49 (−1.39,0.40)	−0.26 (−0.93,0.41)	−0.19 (−0.90,0.53)	−0.11 (−0.62,0.40)	**RIS + CBT-F + NBI**	1.16 (0.47,2.86)	0.69 (0.17,2.76)
−0.53 (−1.28,0.22)	−0.30 (−0.77,0.17)	−0.23 (−0.78,0.33)	−0.15 (−0.43,0.13)	−0.04 (−0.52,0.44)	**NBI**	0.60 (0.21,1.71)
−0.73 (−1.72,0.26)	−0.50 (−1.30,0.30)	−0.42 (−1.28,0.43)	−0.35 (−1.05,0.36)	−0.24 (−1.04,0.57)	−0.20 (−0.84,0.45)	**IPI**

Comparisons between treatments should be read from left to right, and the estimate is in the cell in common between the column-defining treatment and the row-defining treatment. For the primary outcome (attenuated positive psychotic symptoms) estimates, results are SMD (95% CI), where SMD below 0 favors the column-defined treatment. For acceptability, results are OR (95% CI), where OR < 1 favors the row-defined treatment. Significant results are in bold. The order of treatments in the diagonal is arbitrary and does not reflect ranking. OLA, olanzapine; NBI, needs-based interventions (including placebo); Om3, omega-3 fatty acids; ARI, aripiprazole; CBT-F, cognitive behavioral therapy (French & Morrison protocol); RIS, risperidone; IPI, integrated psychological interventions.

Comparison.

Efficacy (attenuated psychotic symptoms; SMD [95% CI]).

Acceptability (dropout; OR [95% CI]).

3% at 2 years) (9). In a subsequent prospective cohort study, we confirmed that CHR-P individuals meeting the short-lived psychotic episode subgroup criteria have a very high risk of developing persistent psychotic episodes (85). Additional ongoing analyses revealed that these three subgroups are associated with different clinical needs and use of mental health services. These results led us to propose clinical stratification of the CHR-P population across different subgroups (1), which has been endorsed by other leading researchers in this area (2, 86). However, because most trials were conducted before such knowledge emerged, response to preventive treatment was not stratified across these different subgroups and we have been unable to control for this variable in meta-regression analyses. The clinical heterogeneity of this population is further amplified by the heterogeneous accumulation of risk factors for psychosis (5), which is reflected in a variable enrichment

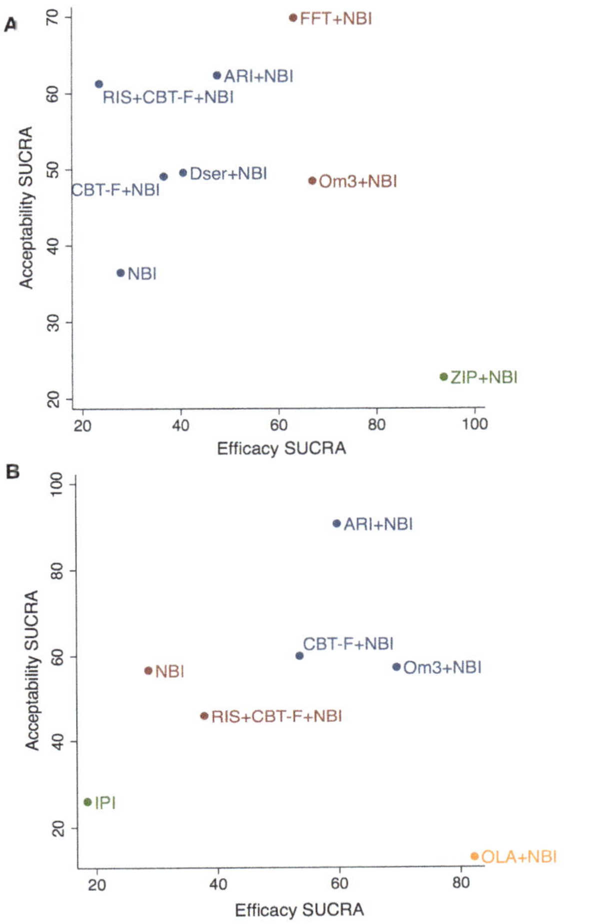

FIGURE 4 | Cluster-ranking of treatments according to SUCRA values for efficacy and acceptability at 6 **(A)** and 12 **(B)** months. Colors reflect treatments belonging to the same cluster. Please note that although the treatments have been ranked, there is no statistical difference between them -with the exception of ziprasidone+NBI for efficacy- (see **Tables 3,4** for further details). ARI, aripiprazole; NBI, needs-based interventions (including placebo); CBT-F, cognitive behavioral therapy (French and Morrison protocol); Dser, D-serine; FFT, family-focused therapy; Om3, omega-3 fatty acids; RIS, risperidone; ZIP, ziprasidone; IPI, integrated psychological interventions; OLA, olanzapine.

of risk to psychosis (17) and different clinical outcomes. The latter may include the development of psychosis, persistence of symptoms and comorbidities, or recovery (32). Overall, the above considerations indicate that the "one-size-fits-all" approach to offering preventative strategies to CHR-P individuals is unlikely to work, namely due to the heterogeneity of the CHR-P state. This raises the possibility that the available treatments have been ineffective because they were applied to all CHR-P subjects, rather than to stratified subgroups. For example, a true preventive effect may be difficult to detect in those at low risk or in those who are responding to placebo or low-level needs-based interventions.

These findings may be informative for future research. For example, they suggest that a stratified precision medicine approach may improve the apparent effectiveness of available treatments. Identifying specific factors that predict response to preventive treatments at the individual subject level may substantially advance clinical care for CHR-P individuals by personalizing their preventive interventions. This could be achieved using the existing RCT data under an individual participant data network meta-analytic approach. These advanced meta-analytical approaches allow the stratification of treatment response through the development of predictive risk estimation tools (87) and could potentially produce a breakthrough advancement of clinical knowledge in this area. Our research group has recently completed the protocol for an individual participant data network meta-analyses (PROSPERO 2018 CRD42018089161) which is due to start imminently. At the same time, the lack of convincing evidence for effective treatments should foster refreshed collaborative efforts to test innovative novel treatments for CHR-P individuals. It is important to note that challenges in developing effective preventive treatments are not specific to the CHR-P field but are common across other branches of clinical medicine, such as in the prevention of dementia. Promising compounds are on the horizon. For example, the first ever industry-funded RCT for CHR-P individuals will be investigating the efficacy of a phosphodiesterase inhibitor to prevent psychosis (88). Of relevance, to partially reduce the clinical heterogeneity discussed above, this RCT will focus only on CHR-P individuals presenting with attenuated positive psychotic symptoms and who are enriched in risk as determined by a specific risk stratification algorithm (89). Another promising candidate treatment is cannabidiol, which was found to be well tolerated and reduced symptoms in an early-phase trial in CHR-P individuals, although the full report is not yet available (90, 91). A larger-scale RCT of cannabidiol is due to start at our institute in the near future. The discovery and development of more effective treatments for attenuated positive psychotic symptoms also requires an improved regulatory platform to reliably sustain the next generation of research. For example, while the DSM-5 includes a newly introduced diagnostic category for attenuated psychosis syndrome (92), there will be no similar diagnostic category in the ICD-11. Diagnostic controversies, as well as different methods of ascertainment of attenuated psychotic symptoms [for a comparative analysis of different CHR-P instruments see (34)] are unlikely to facilitate the large-scale collaborations that are necessary to overcome the current limitations.

There are some important limitations to our work. First, the interpretation of negative findings is always challenging. In fact, as noted by leading authors, absence of evidence is not evidence of absence (93). Such an observation is particularly relevant in the case of large CIs, such as those that have been observed in the current analyses (see **Tables 3, 4**). Therefore, some sizeable effects may still have been missed by our analyses. Furthermore, only 14 RCTs were included, reflecting the scarcity of studies available in this field. Although network meta-analyses are characterized by increased power and precision (94), the geometry of the networks in the current study limited our ability to test for inconsistency, and potentially resulted in more imprecise estimates and wide 95% CIs. An additional limitation is that the overall quality of our network meta-analysis is dependent on the quality of each included study, most of which were at high or unclear risk of bias. We partially controlled for this problem through assessment of biases and sensitivity analyses. The final limitation concerns the use of dropout for any reason as a proxy measure for acceptability. While this measure is generally accepted in network meta-analyses of RCTs (56–58), it is a rather crude and spurious outcome measure. The use of a more specific side effect outcome could have revealed more subtle differences in acceptability across the available treatments. We have been unable to analyse any specific side effects because these were infrequently reported in the available literature.

CONCLUSIONS

In conclusion, on the basis of the most comprehensive evidence synthesis to date, there is currently no robust evidence to favor specific interventions for improving attenuated positive psychotic symptoms in CHR-P individuals.

AUTHOR CONTRIBUTIONS

All authors made substantial contributions to the conception or design of the work, or the acquisition, analysis or interpretation of data. PF-P designed the study; AC optimized the study; CD and UP conducted the literature search and data extraction; JR extracted the digital data; CD and PF-P conducted the analyses under the supervision of AC and DS; CD and PF-P wrote the first draft of the manuscript; PM reviewed the draft of the manuscript.

ACKNOWLEDGMENTS

This work was supported in part by the UK National Institute for Health Research (NIHR) Biomedical Research Centre (BRC) at South London and Maudsley NHS Foundation Trust and King's College London, a King's College London Confidence in Concept award (MC_PC_16048) from the Medical Research Council (MRC) to PFP, and by the Department of Psychosis Studies, Institute of Psychiatry, Psychology and Neuroscience, King's College London. AC is supported by the NIHR Oxford Cognitive Health Clinical Research Facility. DS was part funded by NIHR BRC at South London and Maudsley NHS Foundation Trust and King's College London. The funders had no influence on the design, collection, analysis and interpretation of the data, writing of the report and decision to submit this article for publication. The views expressed are those of the authors and not necessarily those of the NHS, the NIHR or the Department of Health and Social Care.

REFERENCES

1. Fusar-Poli P. The clinical high-risk state for psychosis (CHR-P), Version II. *Schizophr Bull.* (2017) **43**:44–7. doi: 10.1093/schbul/sbw158
2. Fusar-Poli P, McGorry PD, Kane JM. Improving outcomes of first-episode psychosis: an overview. *World Psychiatry* (2017) **16**:251–65. doi: 10.1002/wps.20446
3. Millan MJ, Andrieux A, Bartzokis G, Cadenhead K, Dazzan P, Fusar-Poli P, et al. Altering the course of schizophrenia: progress and perspectives. *Nat Rev Drug Discov.* (2016) **5**:485–51. doi: 10.1038/nrd.2016.28
4. Oliver D, Davies C, Crossland G, Lim S, Gifford G, McGuire P, et al. Can we reduce the duration of untreated psychosis? A meta-analysis of controlled interventional studies. *Schizophr Bull.* (2018). doi: 10.1093/schbul/sbx166. [Epub ahead of print].
5. Fusar-Poli P, Tantardini M, De Simone S, Ramella-Cravaro V, Oliver D, Kingdon J, et al. Deconstructing vulnerability for psychosis: Meta-analysis of environmental risk factors for psychosis in subjects at ultra high-risk. *Eur Psychiatry* (2017) **40**:65–75. doi: 10.1016/j.eurpsy.2016.09.003
6. Yung A, Yuen H, McGorry P, Phillips L, Kelly D, Dell'Olio M, et al. Mapping the onset of psychosis: the Comprehensive Assessment of At-Risk Mental States. *Aust N Z J Psychiatry* (2005) **39**:964–71. doi: 10.1080/j.1440-1614.2005.01714.x
7. Fusar-Poli P, Rocchetti M, Sardella A, Avila A, Brandizzi M, Caverzasi E, et al. Disorder, not just a state of risk: meta-analysis of functioning and quality of life in subjects at high clinical risk for psychosis. *Br J Psychiatry* (2015) **207**:198–206. doi: 10.1192/bjp.bp.114.157115
8. Falkenberg I, Valmaggia L, Byrnes M, Frascarelli M, Jones C, Rocchetti M, et al. Why are help-seeking subjects at ultra-high risk for psychosis help-seeking? *Psychiatry Res.* (2015) **228**:808–15. doi: 10.1016/j.psychres.2015.05.018
9. Fusar-Poli P, Cappucciati M, Borgwardt S, Woods SW, Addington J, Nelson B, et al. Heterogeneity of psychosis risk within individuals at clinical high risk. *JAMA Psychiatry* (2016) **73**:113. doi: 10.1001/jamapsychiatry.2015.2324
10. Webb JR, Addington J, Perkins DO, Bearden CE, Cadenhead KS, Cannon TD, et al. Specificity of incident diagnostic outcomes in patients at clinical high risk for psychosis. *Schizophr Bull.* (2015) **41**:1066–75. doi: 10.1093/schbul/sbv091
11. Fusar-Poli P, Rutigliano G, Stahl D, Davies C, De Micheli A, Ramella-Cravaro V, et al. Long-term validity of the at risk mental state (ARMS) for predicting psychotic and non-psychotic mental disorders. *Eur Psychiatry* **2017**:49–54. doi: 10.1016/j.eurpsy.2016.11.010
12. Fusar-Poli P. The hype cycle of the clinical high risk state for psychosis: the need of a refined approach. *Schizophr Bull.* (2018) **44**:250–53. doi: 10.1093/schbul/sbx181
13. Fusar-Poli P, Rutigliano G, Stahl D, Davies C, Bonoldi I, Reilly T, et al. Development and validation of a clinically based risk calculator for the transdiagnostic prediction of psychosis. *JAMA Psychiatry* (2017) **74**:493–500. doi: 10.1001/jamapsychiatry.2017.0284
14. Fusar-Poli P. Extending the benefits of indicated prevention to improve outcomes of first-episode psychosis. *JAMA Psychiatry* (2017) **74**:667–8. doi: 10.1001/jamapsychiatry.2017.1009
15. Oliver D, Kotlicka-Antczak M, Minichino A, Spada G, McGuire P, Fusar-Poli P. Meta-analytical prognostic accuracy of the Comprehensive Assessment of At Risk Mental States (CAARMS): the need for a refined prediction. *Eur Psychiatry* (2018) **49**:62–8. doi: 10.1016/j.eurpsy.2017.10.001
16. Fusar-Poli P, Palombini E, Davies C, Oliver D, Bonoldi I, Ramella-Cravaro V, et al. Why transition risk to psychosis is not declining at the OASIS ultra high risk service: the hidden role of stable pretest risk enrichment. *Schizophr Res* . (2017) **92**:385–90. doi: 10.1016/j.schres.2017.06.015
17. Fusar-Poli P, Rutigliano G, Stahl D, Schmidt A, Ramella-Cravaro V, Shetty H, et al. Deconstructing pretest risk enrichment to optimize prediction of psychosis in individuals at clinical high risk. *JAMA Psychiatry* (2016) **73**:1260–7. doi: 10.1001/jamapsychiatry.2016.2707

18. Fusar-Poli P, Schultze-Lutter F, Cappucciati M, Rutigliano G, Bonoldi I, Stahl D, et al. The dark side of the moon: meta-analytical impact of recruitment strategies on risk enrichment in the clinical high risk state for psychosis. *Schizophr Bull.* (2016) **42**:732–43. doi: 10.1093/schbul/sbv162
19. Fusar-Poli P. Why ultra high risk criteria for psychosis prediction do not work well outside clinical samples and what to do about it. *World Psychiatry* (2017) **16**:212–3. doi: 10.1002/wps.20405
20. Fusar-Poli P, Schultze-Lutter F. Predicting the onset of psychosis in patients at clinical high risk: practical guide to probabilistic prognostic reasoning. *Evid Based Ment Health* (2016) **19**:10–5. doi: 10.1136/eb-2015-102295
21. Leucht S, Chaimani A, Cipriani AS, Davis JM, Furukawa TA, Salanti G. Network meta-analyses should be the highest level of evidence in treatment guidelines. *Eur Arch Psychiatry Clin Neurosci.* (2016) **266**:477–80. doi: 10.1007/s00406-016-0715-4
22. Davies C, Cipriani A, Ioannidis JP, Radua J, Stahl D, Provenzani U, et al. Lack of evidence to favor specific preventive interventions in psychosis: a network meta-analysis. *World Psychiatry* (2018) **17**:196–209. doi: 10.1002/wps.20526
23. Fusar-Poli P. Negative psychosis prevention trials. *JAMA Psychiatry* (2017) **74**:651. doi: 10.1001/jamapsychiatry.2017.0185
24. Bechdolf A, Müller H, Stützer H, Lambert M, Karow A, Zink M, et al. 108. PREVENT: a randomized controlled trial for the prevention of first-episode psychosis comparing cognitive-behavior therapy (CBT), clinical management, and aripiprazole combined and clinical management and placebo combined. *Schizophr Bull.* (2016) **43**:S56. doi: 10.1093/schbul/sbx021.146
25. Cadenhead K, Addington J, Cannon T, Cornblatt B, Mathalon D, McGlashan T, et al. 23. Omega-3 fatty acid versus placebo in a clinical high-risk sample from the north american prodrome longitudinal studies (NAPLS) consortium. *Schizophr Bull.* (2017) **43**:S16. doi: 10.1093/schbul/sbx021.042
26. Kantrowitz JT, Woods SW, Petkova E, Cornblatt B, Corcoran CM, Chen H et al. D-serine for the treatment of negative symptoms in individuals at clinical high risk of schizophrenia: a pilot, double-blind, placebo-controlled, randomised parallel group mechanistic proof-of-concept trial. *Lancet Psychiatry* (2015) **2**:403–12. doi: 10.1016/S2215-0366(15)00098-X
27. McGorry PD, Nelson B, Markulev C, Yuen HP, Schäfer MR, Mossaheb N et al. Effect of ω-3 polyunsaturated fatty acids in young people at ultrahigh risk for psychotic disorders. *JAMA Psychiatry* (2017) **74**:19. doi: 10.1001/jamapsychiatry.2016.2902
28. Miklowitz DJ, O'Brien MP, Schlosser DA, Addington J, Candan KA, Marshall C et al. Family-focused treatment for adolescents and young adults at high risk for psychosis: results of a randomized trial. *J Am Acad Child Adolesc Psychiatry* (2014) **53**:848–58. doi: 10.1016/j.jaac.2014.04.020
29. Stain HJ, Bucci S, Baker AL, Carr V, Emsley R, Halpin S, et al. A randomised controlled trial of cognitive behaviour therapy versus non-directive reflective listening for young people at ultra high risk of developing psychosis: the detection and evaluation of psychological therapy (DEPTh) trial. *Schizophr Res.* (2016) **176**:212–9. doi: 10.1016/j.schres.2016.08.008
30. Woods S, Saksa J, Compton M, Daley M, Rajarethinam R, Graham K, et al. 112. Effects of ziprasidone versus placebo in patients at clinical high risk for psychosis. *Schizophr Bull.* (2017) **43**:S58.doi: 10.1093/schbul/sbx021.150
31. Woods SW. *Ziprasidone in the Psychosis Prodrome (ZIP) ClinicalTrials.gov Identifier: NCT00635700 [Last updated: September 6, 2016].* (2016).
32. Rutigliano G, Valmaggia L, Landi P, Frascarelli M, Cappucciati M, Sear V, et al. Persistence or recurrence of non-psychotic comorbid mental disorders associated with 6-year poor functional outcomes in patients at ultra high risk for psychosis. *J Affect Disord.* (2016) **203**:101–10. doi: 10.1016/j.jad.2016.05.053
33. Fusar-Poli P, Raballo A, Parnas J. What is an attenuated psychotic symptom? on the importance of the context. *Schizophr Bull.* (2017) **43**:687–92. doi: 10.1093/schbul/sbw182
34. Fusar-Poli P, Cappucciati M, Rutigliano G, Lee TY, Beverly Q, Bonoldi I, et al. Towards a standard psychometric diagnostic interview for subjects at ultra high risk of psychosis: CAARMS versus SIPS. *Psychiatry J.* (2016) **2016**:7146341. doi: 10.1155/2016/7146341
35. Fusar-Poli P, Van Os J. Lost in transition: setting the psychosis threshold in prodromal research. *Acta Psychiatr Scand.* (2013) **127**:248–52. doi: 10.1111/acps.12028
36. NICE. *Psychosis and Schizophrenia in Adults: Prevention and Management.* (2014). Available online at: https://www.nice.org.uk/guidance/cg178/chapter/1-Recommendations#preventing-psychosis-2.
37. Addington J, Epstein I, Liu L, French P, Boydell KM, Zipursky RB. A randomized controlled trial of cognitive behavioral therapy for individuals at clinical high risk of psychosis. *Schizophr Res.* (2011) **125**:54–61. doi: 10.1016/j.schres.2010.10.015
38. McGorry PD, Yung AR, Phillips LJ, Yuen HP, Francey S, Cosgrave EM, et al. Randomized controlled trial of interventions designed to reduce the risk of progression to first-episode psychosis in a clinical sample with subthreshold symptoms. *Arch Gen Psychiatry* (2002) **59**:921. doi: 10.1001/archpsyc.59.10.921
39. Yung AR, McGorry PD, Francey SM, Nelson B, Baker K, Phillips LJ, et al. PACE: a specialised service for young people at risk of psychotic disorders. *Med J Aust.* (2007) **187**:S43–6.
40. Amminger GP, Schäfer MR, Papageorgiou K, Klier MC, Cotton MS, Harrigan MS, et al. Long-chain omega-3 fatty acids for indicated prevention of psychotic disorders. *Arch Gen Psychiatry* (2010) **67**:146–54. doi: 10.1001/archgenpsychiatry.2009.192
41. French P, Morrison A. *Early Detection and Cognitive Therapy for People at High Risk of Developing Psychosis.* Chichester: Wiley (2004) p.117–20.
42. Beck AT. *Cognitive Therapy and the Emotional Disorders.* Madison: International University Press (1976).
43. Morrison AP, French P, Walford L, Lewis SW, Kilcommons A, Green J, et al. Cognitive therapy for the prevention of psychosis in people at ultra-high risk: randomised controlled trial. *Br J Psychiatry* (2004) **185**:291–7. doi: 10.1192/bjp.185.4.291
44. van der Gaag M, Nieman DH, Rietdijk J, Dragt S, Ising HK, Klaassen RMC, et al. Cognitive behavioral therapy for subjects at ultrahigh risk for developing psychosis: a randomized controlled clinical trial. *Schizophr Bull.* (2012) **38**:1180–8. doi: 10.1093/schbul/sbs105
45. Rietdijk J, Dragt S, Klaassen R, Ising H, Nieman D, Wunderink L, et al. A single blind randomized controlled trial of cognitive behavioural therapy in a help-seeking population with an At Risk Mental State for psychosis: the Dutch Early Detection and Intervention Evaluation (EDIE-NL) trial. *Trials* (2010) **11**:30. doi: 10.1186/1745-6215-11-30
46. Bechdolf A, Wagner M, Ruhrmann S, Harrigan S, Putzfeld V, Pukrop R, et al. Preventing progression to first-episode psychosis in early initial prodromal states. *Br J Psychiatry* (2012) **200**:22–9. doi: 10.1192/bjp.bp.109.066357
47. Bechdolf A, Puetzfeld V, Gross S, Guettgemanns J. Cognitive behaviour therapy for people at-risk of psychosis. *A Treatment Manual.* Bern: Huber. (2010).
48. Hutton B, Salanti G, Caldwell DM, Chaimani A, Schmid CH, Cameron C, et al. The PRISMA extension statement for reporting of systematic reviews incorporating network meta-analyses of health care interventions: checklist and explanations. *Ann Intern Med.* (2015) **162**:777. doi: 10.7326/M14-2385
49. Fusar-Poli P, Borgwardt S, Bechdolf A, Addington J, Riecher-Rossler A, Schultze-Lutter F, et al. The psychosis high-risk state a comprehensive state-of-the-art review. *JAMA Psychiatry* (2013) **70**:107–20. doi: 10.1001/jamapsychiatry.2013.269
50. McGlashan T, Walsh B, Woods S. *The Psychosis-Risk Syndrome: Handbook for Diagnosis and Follow-Up.* Oxford: Oxford University Press (2010).
51. Kay SR, Fiszbein A, Opler LA. The positive and negative syndrome scale (PANSS) for schizophrenia. *Schizophr Bull.* (1987) **13**:261–76. doi: 10.1093/schbul/13.2.261
52. Overall J, Gorham D. The brief psychiatric rating scale (BPRS): recent developments in ascertainment and scaling. *Psychopharmacol Bull.* (1988) **24**:97–9.
53. Haefner H, Bechdolf A, Klosterkotter J, Maurer K. *Early Detection and Intervention in Psychosis. A Practise Handbook.* Stuttgart: Schattauer (2011).

54. Cipriani A, Zhou X, Del Giovane C, Hetrick SE, Qin B, Whittington C, et al. Comparative efficacy and tolerability of antidepressants for major depressive disorder in children and adolescents: a network meta-analysis. *Lancet* (2016) **388**:881–90. doi: 10.1016/S0140-6736(16)30385-3
55. Kempton MJ, Bonoldi I, Valmaggia L, McGuire P, Fusar-Poli P. Speed of psychosis progression in people at ultra-high clinical risk. *JAMA Psychiatry* (2015) **72**:622. doi: 10.1001/jamapsychiatry.2015.0094
56. Cipriani A, Furukawa TA, Salanti G, Geddes JR, Higgins JP, Churchill R, et al. Comparative efficacy and acceptability of 12 new-generation antidepressants: a multiple-treatments meta-analysis. *Lancet* (2009) **373**:746–58. doi: 10.1016/S0140-6736(09)60046-5
57. Cipriani A, Barbui C, Salanti G, Rendell J, Brown R, Stockton S, et al. Comparative efficacy and acceptability of antimanic drugs in acute mania: a multiple-treatments meta-analysis. *Lancet* (2011) **378**:1306–15. doi: 10.1016/S0140-6736(11)60873-8
58. Miura T, Noma H, Furukawa TA, Mitsuyasu H, Tanaka S, Stockton S, et al. Comparative efficacy and tolerability of pharmacological treatments in the maintenance treatment of bipolar disorder: a systematic review and network meta-analysis. *Lancet Psychiatry* (2014) **1**:351–9. doi: 10.1016/S2215-0366(14)70314-1. [Epub ahead of print].
59. Higgins JPT, Altman DG, Gotzsche PC, Juni P, Moher D, Oxman AD, et al. The Cochrane Collaboration's tool for assessing risk of bias in randomised trials. *BMJ* (2011) **343**:d5928. doi: 10.1136/bmj.d5928
60. Furukawa TA, Salanti G, Atkinson LZ, Leucht S, Ruhe HG, Turner EH, et al. Comparative efficacy and acceptability of first-generation and second-generation antidepressants in the acute treatment of major depression: protocol for a network meta-analysis. *BMJ Open* (2016) **6**:e010919. doi: 10.1136/bmjopen-2015-010919
61. Borenstein M, Hedges LV, Higgins JPT, Rothstein HR. *Introduction to Meta-Analysis*. Chichester: John Wiley & Sons, Ltd. (2009).
62. Higgins JPT, Green S. (eds). *Cochrane Handbook for Systematic Reviews of Interventions Version 5.1.0 [updated March 2011]*. The Cochrane Collaboration (2011). Available online at: http://handbook.cochrane.org
63. Chaimani A, Higgins JPT, Mavridis D, Spyridonos P, Salanti G. Graphical tools for network meta-analysis in STATA. *PLoS ONE* (2013) **8**:e76654. doi: 10.1371/journal.pone.0076654
64. Chaimani A, Salanti G. Visualizing assumptions and results in network meta-analysis: the network graphs package. *Stata J.* (2015) **15**:905–50.
65. White IR. Multivariate random-effects meta-regression: updates to mvmeta. *Stata J.* (2011) **11**:255–70.
66. Mavridis D, Giannatsi M, Cipriani A, Salanti G. A primer on network meta-analysis with emphasis on mental health. *Evid Based Mental Health* (2015) **18**:40–6. doi: 10.1136/eb-2015-102088
67. Salanti G, Ades AE, Ioannidis JPA. Graphical methods and numerical summaries for presenting results from multiple-treatment meta-analysis: an overview and tutorial. *J Clin Epidemiol.* (2011) **64**:163–71. doi: 10.1016/j.jclinepi.2010.03.016
68. Mbuagbaw L, Rochwerg B, Jaeschke R, Heels-Andsell D, Alhazzani W, Thabane L, et al. Approaches to interpreting and choosing the best treatments in network meta-analyses. *Syst Rev.* (2017) **6**:79. doi: 10.1186/s13643-017-0473-z
69. Higgins JPT, Jackson D, Barrett JK, Lu G, Ades AE, White IR. Consistency and inconsistency in network meta-analysis: concepts and models for multi-arm studies. *Res Synth Methods* (2012) **3**:98–110. doi: 10.1002/jrsm.1044
70. Chaimani A, Salanti G, Leucht S, Geddes JR, Cipriani A. Common pitfalls and mistakes in the set-up, analysis and interpretation of results in network meta-analysis: what clinicians should look for in a published article. *Evid Based Ment Health.* (2017) **20**:88–94. doi: 10.1136/eb-2017-102753
71. Chaimani A, Salanti G. Using network meta-analysis to evaluate the existence of small-study effects in a network of interventions. *Res Synth Methods* (2012) **3**:161–76. doi: 10.1002/jrsm.57
72. Fusar-Poli P, Papanastasiou E, Stahl D, Rocchetti M, Carpenter W, Shergill S, et al. Treatments of negative symptoms in schizophrenia: meta-analysis of 168 randomized placebo-controlled trials. *Schizophr Bull.* (2015) **41**:892–9. doi: 10.1093/schbul/sbu170
73. McGlashan TH, Zipursky RB, Perkins D, Addington J, Miller T, Woods SW, et al. Randomized, double-blind trial of olanzapine versus placebo in patients prodromally symptomatic for psychosis. *Am J Psychiatry* (2006) **163**:790–9. doi: 10.1176/ajp.2006.163.5.790
74. Morrison AP, French P, Stewart SL, Birchwood M, Fowler D, Gumley AI, et al. Early detection and intervention evaluation for people at risk of psychosis: multisite randomised controlled trial. *BMJ* (2012) **344**:e2233. doi: 10.1136/bmj.e2233
75. Wessels H, Wagner M, Frommann I, Berning J, Pützfeld V, Janssen B, et al. Neuropsychological functioning as a predictor of treatment response to psychoeducational, cognitive behavioral therapy in people at clinical high risk of first episode psychosis. *Psychiatr Prax.* (2015) **42**:313–9. doi: 10.1055/s-0035-1552713
76. Yung AR, Phillips LJ, Nelson B, Francey SM, PanYuen H, Simmons MB, et al. Randomized controlled trial of interventions for young people at ultra high risk for psychosis. *J Clin Psychiatry* (2011) **72**:430–40. doi: 10.4088/JCP.08m04979ora
77. McGorry PD, Nelson B, Phillips LJ, Yuen HP, Francey SM, Thampi A, et al. Randomized controlled trial of interventions for young people at ultra-high risk of psychosis: twelve-month outcome. *J Clin Psychiatry* (2013) **74**:349–56. doi: 10.4088/JCP.12m07785
78. Devoe J, Peterson A, Addington J. Negative symptom interventions in youth at risk of psychosis: a systematic review and network meta-analysis. *Schizophr Bull.* (2018). doi: 10.1093/schbul/sbx139
79. Devoe J, Peterson A, Addington J. Erratum to: Negative symptom interventions in youth at risk of psychosis: a systematic review and network meta-analysis. *Schizophr Bull.* (2018) **44**:463. doi: 10.1093/schbul/sbx193
80. Schmidt SJ, Schultze-Lutter F, Schimmelmann BG, Maric NP, Salokangas RKR, Riecher-Rössler a, et al. EPA guidance on the early intervention in clinical high risk states of psychoses. *Eur Psychiatry* (2015) **30**:388–404. doi: 10.1016/j.eurpsy.2015.01.013
81. Hutton P, Taylor PJ. Cognitive behavioural therapy for psychosis prevention: a systematic review and meta-analysis. *Psychol Med.* (2014) **44**:449–68. doi: 10.1017/S0033291713000354
82. van der Gaag M, Smit F, Bechdolf A, French P, Linszen DH, Yung AR, et al. Preventing a first episode of psychosis: meta-analysis of randomized controlled prevention trials of 12 month and longer-term follow-ups. *Schizophr Res.* (2013) **149**:56–62. doi: 10.1016/j.schres.2013.07.004
83. Stafford MR, Jackson H, Mayo-Wilson E, Morrison AP, Kendall T. Early interventions to prevent psychosis: systematic review and meta-analysis. *BMJ* (2013) **346**:f185. doi: 10.1136/bmj.f185
84. Fusar-Poli P, Cappucciati M, Bonoldi I, Hui C, Rutigliano G, Stahl D, et al. Prognosis of brief psychotic episodes: a meta-analysis. *JAMA Psychiatry* (2016) **73**:211–20. doi: 10.1001/jamapsychiatry.2015.2313
85. Fusar-Poli P, Cappucciati M, De Micheli A, Rutigliano G, Bonoldi I, Tognin S, et al. Diagnostic and prognostic significance of brief limited intermittent psychotic symptoms (BLIPS) in individuals at ultra high risk. *Schizophr Bull.* (2017) **43**:48–56. doi: 10.1093/schbul/sbw151
86. Carrion RE, Correll CU, Auther AM, Cornblatt BA. A severity-based clinical staging model for the psychosis prodrome: longitudinal findings from the new york recognition and prevention program. *Schizophr Bull.* (2017) **43**:64–74. doi: 10.1093/schbul/sbw155
87. Ahmed I, Debray TP, Moons KG, Riley RD. Developing and validating risk prediction models in an individual participant data meta-analysis. *BMC Med Res Methodol.* (2014) **14**:3. doi: 10.1186/1471-2288-14-3
88. Keefe R, Woods S, Cannon T, Ruhrmann S, Mathalon D, McGuire P, et al. 868. Early intervention in attenuated psychosis syndrome: a phase II Study evaluating efficacy, safety, and tolerability of Oral BI 409306. *Biological Psychiatry* (2017) **81**:S351. doi: 10.1016/j.biopsych.2017.02.593
89. Cannon TD, Yu C, Addington J, Bearden CE, Cadenhead KS, Cornblatt BA, et al. An individualized risk calculator for research in prodromal psychosis. *Am J Psychiatry* (2016) **173**:980–8. doi: 10.1176/appi.ajp.2016.15070890
90. McGuire P, Englund A, Bhattacharyya S. Commentary on "The Potential of Cannabidiol Treatment for Cannabis Users With Recent-Onset Psychosis." *Schizophr Bull.* (2018) **44**:18–9. doi: 10.1093/schbul/sbx124
91. *Cannabidiol as a Novel Therapeutic Agent for Patients at Ultra High-Risk of Psychosis: An Experimental Medicine Approach*. Available online at: http://gtr.rcuk.ac.uk/project/0C8EE617-3E76-48A8-A5BE-C726FCE0428A.

92. Fusar-Poli P, Carpenter WT, Woods SW, McGlashan TH. Attenuated psychosis syndrome: ready for DSM-5.1? *Ann Rev Clin Psychol.* (2014) **10**:155–92. doi: 10.1146/annurev-clinpsy-032813-153645
93. Altman DG, Bland JM. Statistics notes: absence of evidence is not evidence of absence. *BMJ* (1995) **311**:485. doi: 10.1136/bmj.311.7003.485
94. Thorlund K, Mills EJ. Sample size and power considerations in network meta-analysis. *Syst Rev.* (2012) **1**:41. doi: 10.1186/2046-4053-1-41

18

Using EEG-Guided Basket and Umbrella Trials in Psychiatry: A Precision Medicine Approach for Cognitive Impairment in Schizophrenia

*Yash B. Joshi[1] and Gregory A. Light[1,2]**

[1] Department of Psychiatry, University of California, San Diego, La Jolla, CA, United States, [2] VISN-22 Mental Illness, Research, Education and Clinical Center (MIRECC), VA San Diego Health Care System, San Diego, CA, United States

***Correspondence:**
Gregory A. Light
glight@ucsd.edu

Due to advances over the last several decades, many fields of medicine are moving toward a precision medicine approach where treatments are tailored to nuanced patient factors. While in some disciplines these innovations are commonplace leading to unique biomarker-guided experimental medicine trials, there are no such analogs in psychiatry. In this brief review, we will overview two unique biomarker-guided trial designs for future use in psychiatry: basket and umbrella trials. We will illustrate how such trials could be useful in psychiatry using schizophrenia as a candidate illness, the EEG measure mismatch negativity as the candidate biomarker, and cognitive impairment as the target disease dimension.

Keywords: schizophrenia, mismatch negativity, biomarker, clinical trial, cognitive impairment

INTRODUCTION

In stark contrast to our growing understanding of mental illnesses, diagnoses and treatments heavily rely on the clinical interview rather than direct, reliable assays of brain function. The results are hardly surprising: we have not meaningfully improved clinically relevant endpoints for many serious mental illnesses in the last several decades (1). Recent advances in biomarker development, however, hold promise for ushering in a new era of precision medicine-style trials for treating psychiatric illnesses.

Biomarker-informed clinical trial approaches are becoming common in other fields of medicine [(2); for reviews see (3), (4)]. As one example, anti-neoplastic agents are currently selected not only based on what type of cancer a patient has and its stage, but also on the molecular phenotype and genetic aberrations unique to the cancer. Such biomarker-informed approaches are best exemplified by two conceptually related clinical trial designs: "basket" and "umbrella" trials (5, 6). Basket trials assess the effectiveness of a candidate drug based on the mechanism rather than the underlying cancer type. For example, a neoplastic drug which targets a specific genetic mutation would be given to cohorts, or "baskets," of patients with cancers of different origin (i.e., prostate, breast, lung, etc.) who share molecular signatures, vastly expanding the number of patients that could benefit from such a precision intervention (7). Umbrella trials take patients with the same type of cancer, and assign them to treatment arms based on unique mutations—thus, every single arm is one spoke of the large "umbrella" of therapeutic interventions. As the prototypical example, the National Cancer Institute's MATCH trial recruits patients with advanced solid tumors, lymphomas and myelomas, performs extensive genotyping and molecular stratification, and places participants into one of over a dozen different treatment arms (8).

While psychiatry currently has no candidate biomarkers which have graduated from academic laboratories to guide treatments in real-world settings, the stage is being set for a future which successfully leverages a precision psychiatry approach. In this brief review, we provide an overview of what a precision psychiatry approach could look like using a well-validated translational electroencephalography (EEG) measure called mismatch negativity (MMN) as a candidate biomarker, and neurocognitive impairment in schizophrenia as a target disease dimension.

SCHIZOPHRENIA AND NEUROCOGNITIVE IMPAIRMENT

Schizophrenia (SZ) is characterized by positive (e.g., hallucinations, delusions, etc.) and negative (e.g., avolition, diminished emotional expressivity etc.) symptoms which contribute to functional impairment. Beyond these defining symptoms of SZ, hundreds of studies have suggested that neurocognitive impairments are both core features of the illness and robust determinants of psychosocial disability (9–12). Neurocognitive deficits in SZ are broad, and include abnormalities in perceptual functioning, attention, verbal and non-verbal memory, language, and executive functioning (13). The severity of deficits on these neuropsychological domains are directly linked to diminished community functioning and impaired activities of daily living (14, 15).

Indeed, recent analyses of over 1,400 patients with chronic psychoses recruited for the multi-site Consortium on the Genetics of Schizophrenia (COGS) provided strong empirical support for a hierarchical model linking cognition with functional outcome in SZ (16). In this study, structural equation modeling was used to better understand how functional outcome in SZ could be better understood in relation to symptoms, cognition and early auditory information processing (EAIP). Interestingly, abnormalities in EAIP, as indexed by EEG biomarkers, had a direct and causal effect on cognition, which in turn directly affected negative symptoms, impacting overall functional outcome. Particularly noteworthy was the finding that abnormalities in EEG biomarkers linked to EAIP also independently affected functional outcome in SZ patients.

Neurophysiological indicators have indexed abnormalities in EAIP in SZ for several decades, and differences in EAIP in patients are prominently featured as endophenotypes in genomic studies. The above analyses confirmed that the neurocognitive impairments in SZ appear to be a core disease component, reliably able to be measured and directly-linked to the symptoms and functional outcomes. Despite this advance, decades of clinical trials testing the effectiveness of currently approved antipsychotic medications and other novel therapeutics as putative pro-cognitive agents have failed to improve cognitive symptoms in SZ in any durable, meaningful way (17, 18). The development of novel pro-cognitive treatment strategies is therefore of paramount importance but remains a critical unmet need (19). These elements provide the ground on which biomarkers can be used to guide research and clinical implementation of novel precision-medicine therapeutic strategies in SZ.

MISMATCH NEGATIVITY: A NEUROPHYSIOLOGICAL BIOMARKER FOR EARLY AUDITORY INFORMATION PROCESSING

The usefulness of EEG measures in guiding new treatments depends on their ability to serve as biomarkers. Useful biomarkers must be accessible and measurable in preclinical models of disease; should be sufficiently well-characterized such that those biomarkers are linked to relevant underlying neural circuits and known mechanisms of dysfunction in psychiatric disease; and are able to be assessed in both healthy subjects and affected individuals. For usefulness in human trials biomarkers must be insensitive to practice or order effects, reliable, and responsive to interventions. To succeed in real-world settings, biomarker acquisition should also be scalable, low-cost, and suitable for use in multi-center studies.

All of the above criteria have been identified for biomarker development for neurocognitive impairment in SZ by a variety of expert consensus panels (20–23). The first panel, the Measurement and Treatment Research to Improve Cognition in Schizophrenia (MATRICS) initiative, agreed that there was a lack of consensus on a well-accepted instrument for measuring neurocognition in clinical trials (20), on the best molecular targets for drug development, on the optimal trial design for studies of those targets, and how regulatory agencies ought to approve and label novel agents. The outcome of this initiative identified the following criteria as desirable in an FDA-approved battery for use in clinical outcome measures: high test-retest reliability, utility as a repeated measure, relationship to functional outcome, tolerability and practicality, and responsivity to pro-cognitive therapeutics. The Cognitive Neuroscience Treatment Research to Improve Cognition in Schizophrenia (CNTRICS) initiative, launched after MATRICS, further expanded on the MATRICS criteria by adding that measures should have construct validity, be mechanistically related to relevant neural circuitry, and be measurable in animal models (21, 22).

At the time of CNTRICS, mismatch negativity (MMN) was already considered a mature neurophysiologic biomarker based on meeting the above criteria, and generally believed to be ready for widespread implementation in clinical trial studies (21, 23). In fact, as a real-world readiness demonstration, MMN has been extensively characterized in multi-center trials without the use of highly-trained specialists or centers (16, 24).

MMN is an event-related potential and a neurophysiological measure of EAIP that is evoked when a train of "standard" auditory stimuli is interrupted by an oddball or "deviant" stimulus that differs from standards as shown in **Figure 1** (25–27). Differences from standard stimuli in pitch, duration, intensity, or spatial location can elicit a deviant MMN response.

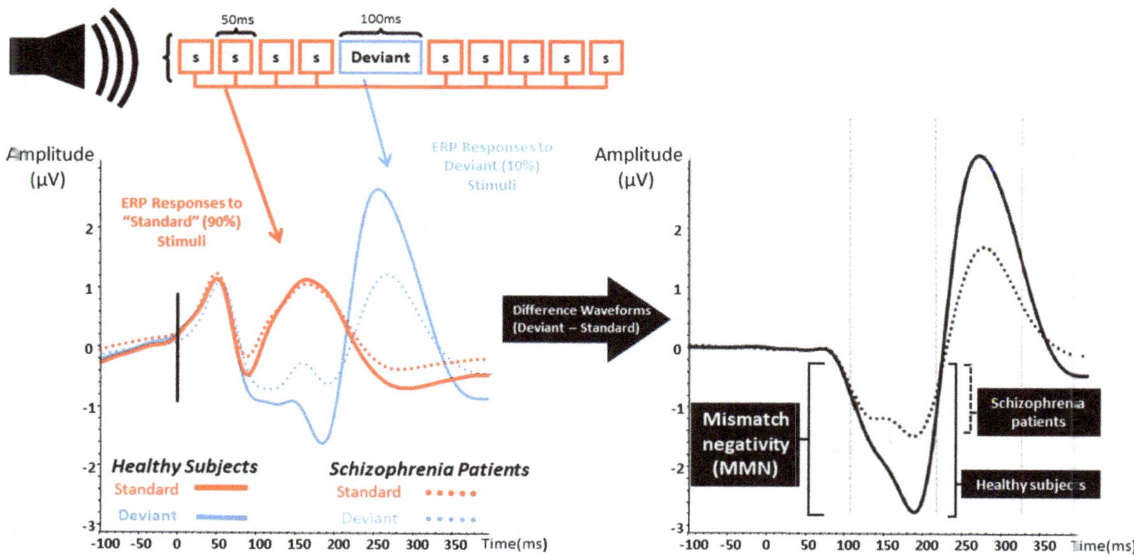

FIGURE 1 | Mismatch negativity. The left graph represents the event related potentials evoked by trains of standard stimuli (S; in red) with interposed rare deviant stimuli (blue) in both healthy subject (solid lines) and patients with schizophrenia (dashed lines). The right graph represents the difference waveform a negative inflection 100–200 ms after stimulus onset which is called mismatch negativity (MMN). Patients with schizophrenia show a reduction in the amplitude of MMN when compared to healthy subjects.

MMN is pre-attentive, primarily reflects an automatic response to sensory stimuli, and is able to be evoked without effort, behavioral response, or conscious awareness (26–31). After auditory deviant stimuli presentation, MMN onset begins after ~50 ms and peaks after an additional 100–150 ms (32, 33). Localization studies have consistently revealed cortical sources located in broadly distributed temporal, frontal, and parietal brain regions (34–36).

Reduction of auditory MMN amplitude was reported over two decades ago in SZ and has been replicated numerous times (37). MMN deficits are found in those with chronic psychosis (27, 37–50), in unmedicated SZ patients (29, 40, 46, 47, 51, 52), and are shown to be resistant to antipsychotics (46, 53–58). Abnormal MMN is also found in recent-onset psychosis as well as prodromal illness (30, 51, 59–66). Baseline MMN amplitude appears to be smaller in clinically high risk populations who eventually develop psychosis at follow up, and MMN in those who do not convert appears to be similar to age-matched controls (30, 51, 63). Strikingly, MMN amplitude seems to anticipate time-to-convert to psychosis—more severe MMN deficits relate to shorter time for psychosis to declare (51, 63).

Mechanistically, auditory MMN is thought to be an index of N-methyl-D aspartate receptor (NMDA) functioning (67, 68). NMDA receptor antagonists diminish MMN in non-human primates, and ketamine, an NMDA antagonist, reduces MMN in healthy control human subjects (69–75). Lower baseline MMN is also associated with psychotic-like behavioral effects experienced by healthy subjects when exposed to ketamine (72). Furthermore, MMN has shown to be highly heritable with amplitude reductions present in asymptomatic first-degree relatives of those with SZ (76–80). MMN deficits are also found in patients with chromosome 22q deletion, which result in congenital syndromes associated with SZ-like psychoses (81).

Arguably, the most important metric of biomarker applicability in psychiatric illnesses is the ability to track functional outcome. In patients with SZ, several studies have detailed that MMN deficits are able to account for a large degree of variance in cognitive and psychosocial functioning, as well as the ability to achieve or maintain independent living (17, 34, 46, 64, 82–86).

BIOMARKER-INFORMED INSIGHTS FOR A PRECISION MEDICINE APPROACH: MMN AND COGNITIVE ENHANCEMENT STRATEGIES IN SCHIZOPHRENIA

Given the cognitive deficits observed in SZ, many studies have attempted to use pro-cognitive drugs to help attenuate this dimension of illness (87). In particular, there has been great interest in the NMDA receptor antagonist, memantine, which has been approved for use in Alzheimer's disease (88, 89).

Memantine is a non-competitive moderate affinity NMDAR antagonist (90, 91). It is thought to bind the same site as magnesium, an endogenous blocker of the NMDA receptor channel, and impedes current flow only if the NMDA receptor channel is open. Upon depolarization, memantine rapidly leaves the NMDA receptor channel. Thus, functionally, memantine is thought to block sustained and pathological activation of NMDA receptors, but not affect physiological activity. In this sense, memantine is unique from other NMDA receptor antagonists which have slower un-blocking kinetics, (i.e., ketamine, phencyclidine). Interestingly, ketamine and phencyclidine are well-known to produce psychotogenic effects but memantine does not exacerbate psychosis or cognitive deficits in antipsychotic medicated patients (92–96). This discrepancy remains an area of active investigation.

In clinical trials with Alzheimer's disease patients, memantine has been found to have a modest pro-cognitive impact (97, 98). However, clinical trials using memantine in SZ targeting cognitive impairment have been inconsistent. Meta-analyses have suggested that memantine is associated with improvement in cognitive tests such as the Mini-Mental State Exam (94). While some double blind randomized clinical trials where memantine has been added on to antipsychotic medications also report reduction in cognitive deficits, others have not, including a study which showed cognitive improvement reported at 12 weeks was lost at 52 weeks (99–101). Given these discrepancies, it has been speculated that patient factors may be obscuring signals of memantine effects on cognition in SZ. Indeed, there is evidence that suggests that within the spectrum of illnesses in chronic psychotic disorders like SZ there exist separable cognitive "biotypes" which have different profiles of cognitive impairment (102, 103). Thus, without a clearer understanding of knowing which patients with SZ are able to experience benefits of memantine, results from clinical trials using such a pro-cognitive intervention—and more broadly, all pro-cognitive interventions in SZ—are difficult to interpret.

However, recent work assessing the effect of memantine on MMN could provide insights into a precision-medicine approach (94, 96, 103, 104). For example, our group has used a double blind single-dose placebo-controlled trial assessing the effects of memantine on MMN in patients with SZ (95, 96). This study employed a within-subject cross-over design such that all participants were randomized to receive either placebo or memantine, and 7 days later, receive the other intervention, thus allowing for each subject to serve as his or her own baseline. MMN was assessed $\sim$ 6 h after placebo or memantine ingestion, which is the approximate T_{max} of memantine, on both testing days. We found that memantine enhanced MMN in patients with SZ; since improved MMN is associated with less cognitive impairment and greater psychosocial success, this type of signal suggests that MMN could be a biomarker of treatment engagement in pro-cognitive interventions. While only a single dose of memantine would not be expected to durably improve cognition, the ability of memantine to alter MMN in a patient could signify that such an individual has the neural plasticity to benefit from pro-cognitive interventions (96, 103, 105). Indeed, not all patients in the cohort showed MMN enhancement—but, these results suggest that for future trials which aim to test the effectiveness of pro-cognitive medications, MMN malleability in response to early exposure to a putative pharmacologic agent could be important for enriching trials to maximize a therapeutic signal.

Beyond medication interventions, MMN also has the potential to predict gains in non-pharmacologic pro-cognitive interventions in SZ. For example, there has been significant interest in using targeted cognitive training (TCT) for enhancing cognition in patients with chronic psychoses (106, 107). TCT is an emerging computerized, auditory-based intervention which aims to improve EAIP through adaptive exercises with participants (105, 108). TCT is typically delivered in 1 h sessions 3–5 h a week for ~20–40 h. At the group level patients with SZ show reduction in cognitive deficits which are linked to improved functional outcomes. However, 20–40% of subjects with SZ fail to show benefit, even in some cases, after 100 h of training (108–111). A biomarker measure that would identify which patients could benefit (or, conversely, which patients have a high likelihood of not benefitting) would be critical in scaling such a pro-cognitive intervention as part of a comprehensive neurorehabilitation strategy (112). As with malleability of MMN following initial exposure to memantine, MMN also appears to be a sensitive index of the neural systems engaged by the first "dose" of TCT exercises. In this context, Perez et al. found that MMN was a sensitive index of the perceptual learning that takes place in the first hour of training, with amplitude of MMN correlating with gains in auditory perceptual learning (113). More work has better elaborated this relationship, finding that on an individual level MMN changes in the direction of normalization after 1 h of TCT predict benefit from TCT after a full course (114).

UMBRELLAS AND BASKETS IN PSYCHIATRY: A POSSIBLE FUTURE FOR CLINICAL TRIALS IN PSYCHIATRY

With what is currently known about MMN and neurocognitive impairment in SZ, we can consider how EEG biomarkers can be used in the service of a precision medicine approach to clinical trials in psychiatry.

While pro-cognitive interventions for psychotic illnesses tend to focus on single diseases like SZ, cognitive impairment has been noted in related illnesses, including schizoaffective disorder and bipolar disorder with psychotic features. This parallels genetic evidence which supports a link between SZ, schizoaffective disorder and bipolar disorder. Despite this link, in traditional drug development pro-cognitive interventions are generally assessed in one population first (i.e., SZ), and then subsequent trials assess if such an intervention is useful in other related conditions. However, a basket-style precision medicine approach using EEG biomarkers could offer a more streamlined way to discover drugs targeted at transdiagnostically-related illness domains like cognitive impairment. For example, as shown in **Figure 2A**, a novel pro-cognitive trial testing a new Drug X could recruit patients with SZ, schizoaffective disorder and bipolar disorder and include only those who have MMN malleability. Since MMN malleability is a strong indicator of target engagement and neural plasticity, such an approach would enrich the study population to benefit from a pro-cognitive intervention. Furthermore, such a trial would test the effectiveness of a new intervention and would not necessarily be limited by traditional criteria, and have relevance across multiple illnesses (115).

Similarly, using EEG-guided umbrella designs in psychiatry would better improve pragmatic trials matching interventions to patient strengths. For example, in a SZ trial comparing different

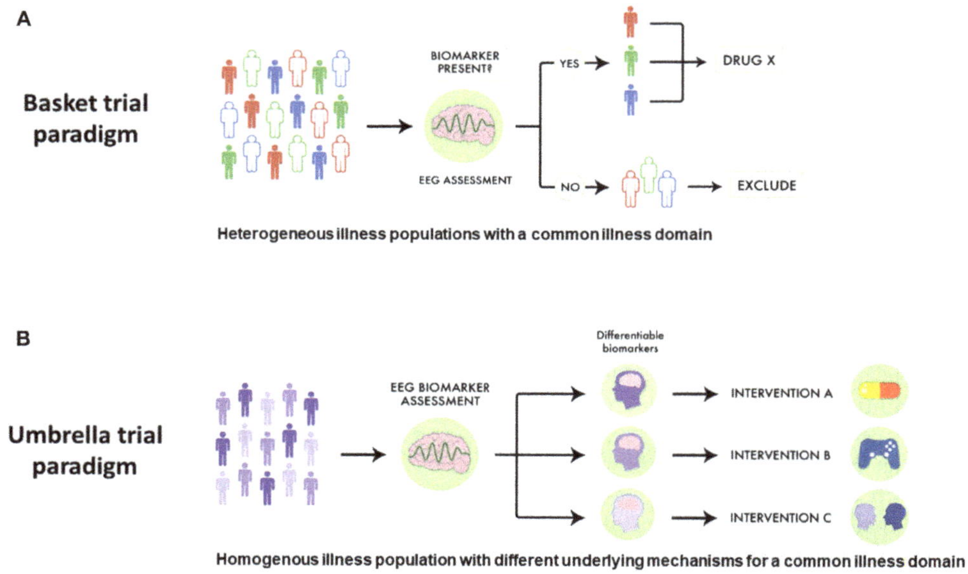

FIGURE 2 | Using EEG biomarkers to design basket and umbrella trials. **(A)** Using EEG-guided basket trials could allow for different psychiatric populations who share the same disease dimension to be given a therapeutic intervention, allowing more patients to potentially benefit. In this scheme subjects are separated by different colors to denote different diseases. Those who have favorable EEG biomarker profiles are indicated by solid coloring while those are not responsive are in outline. EEG-guided basket trials have the potential to select subjects for clinical trials assessing novel drugs for optimal response. **(B)** Similarly, using EEG-guided umbrella trials could allow for patients with the same illness to be assigned to different treatments, allowing for a more specific intervention strategy. In this scheme, subjects with different biological mechanisms underlying a particular illness domain are indicated by different gradations in coloring. EEG biomarkers can be used to assess which patients may be suitable for which intervention. EEG-guided umbrella trials have the potential to improve pragmatic clinical trials assessing treatment effectiveness.

pro-cognitive interventions, positive response to particular EEG biomarkers would help stratify different treatment strategies (see **Figure 2B**). In such a trial, SZ patients with favorable auditory MMN malleability could receive TCT aimed to improve auditory sensory processing, while those with equivocal or poor MMN malleability could respectively receive pro-cognitive medications or specialized behavioral therapy.

These new trial designs are not without limitations. First, due to their relative novelty such designs have not yet been attempted in psychiatry, and thus there is little precedent for how these trials would be staged. Such trials require greater logistical burdens, require larger cohorts of patients, and are costlier to run. Furthermore, such trials may face barriers in recruiting enough patients with specific biomarker profiles, and experience challenges in balancing treatment arms. Both basket and umbrella trials would require new collaborative frameworks, and require nuanced statistical and administrative support.

Despite these potential limitations, using biomarkers to inform clinical trials in psychiatry holds the potential to improve our current understanding of psychiatric illness, and creates an additional way to determine the effectiveness of novel therapeutic strategies. Just as how various cancers are currently molecularly phenotyped, neurophysiologically-guided basket and umbrella trials could help "EEG-phenotype" cognitive impairment in illnesses like SZ. This precision-medicine approach would enhance the development of not only novel drugs, but also other comprehensive rehabilitation strategies in SZ like TCT.

While this mini-review has focused on neurophysiological biomarkers in SZ, the rationale described could broadly apply to other psychiatric illnesses and other types of biomarkers, including genetic and imaging biomarkers. We anticipate that as the tools of neuroscience allow us to understand complex diseases in a more nuanced way, further development of biomarker-informed precision medicine approaches to clinical trials will help further optimize matching the right treatment to the right patient.

AUTHOR CONTRIBUTIONS

Both authors have made a substantial, direct and intellectual contribution to the work, and approved it for publication.

FUNDING

This work was supported by grants by the Sidney R. Baer, Jr. Foundation, Brain and Behavior Research Foundation, and Department of Veteran Affairs VISN-22 Mental Illness Research, Education, and Clinical Center (MIRECC).

ACKNOWLEDGMENTS

The authors thank Rebecca Eliscu for assistance in creating **Figure 2**.

REFERENCES

1. Insel TR. The NIMH experimental medicine initiative. *World Psychiatry* (2015) 14:151–3. doi: 10.1002/wps.20227
2. Friedman AA, Letai A, Fisher DE, Flaherty KT. Precision medicine for cancer with next-generation functional diagnostics. *Nat Rev Cancer* (2015) 15:747–56. doi: 10.1038/nrc4015
3. Kramer F, Sabbah HN, Januzzi JJ, Zannad F, Peter van Tintelen J, Schelbert EB, et al. Redefining the role of biomarkers in heart failure trials: expert consensus document. *Hear Fail Rev.* (2017) 22:263–77. doi: 10.1007/s10741-017-9608-5
4. Ritter A, Cummings J. Fluid biomarkers in clinical trials in Alzheimer's disease therapeutics. *Front Neurol.* (2015) 31:186. doi: 10.3389/fneur.2015.00186
5. Menis J, Hasan B, Besse B. New clinical research strategies in thoracic oncology: clinical trial design, adaptive, basket and umbrella trials, new end-points and new evaluations of response. *Eur Respir Rev.* (2015) 23:367–78. doi: 10.1183/09059180.00004214
6. Simon R. Critical review of umbrella, basket, and platform designs for oncology clinical trials. *Clin Pharmacol Ther.* (2017) 102:934–41. doi: 10.1002/cpt.814
7. Tao JJ, Schram AM, Hyman DM. Basket studies: redefining clinical trials in the era of genome-driven oncology. *Annu Rev Med.* (2018) 69:319–31. doi: 10.1146/annurev-med-062016-050343
8. Coyne GO, Takebe N, Chen AP. Defining precision: the precision medicine initiative trials NCI-MPACT and NCI-MATCH. *Curr Probl Cancer* (2017) 41:182–93. doi: 10.1016/j.currproblcancer.2017.02.001
9. Bora E, Binnur Akdede B, Alptekin K. Neurocognitive impairment in deficit and non-deficit schizophrenia: a meta-analysis. *Psychol Med.* (2017) 47:2401–13. doi: 10.1017/S0033291717000952
10. Fioravanti M, Bianchi V, Cinti ME. Cognitive deficits in schizophrenia: an updated metanalysis of the scientific evidence. *BMC Psychiatry* (2012) 12:64. doi: 10.1186/1471-244X-12-64
11. Sitskoorn MM, Aleman A, Ebisch SJ, Appels MC, Kahn RS. Cognitive deficits in relatives of patients with schizophrenia: a meta-analysis. *Schizophr Res.* (2004) 71:285–95. doi: 10.1016/j.schres.2004.03.007
12. Heinrichs RW, Zakzanis KK. Neurocognitive deficits in schizophrenia: a quantitative review of the evidence. *Neuropsychology* (1998) 12:426–45. doi: 10.1037/0894-4105.12.3.426
13. Green MF, Kern RS, Braff DL, Mintz J. Neurocognitive deficits and functional outcome in schizophrenia: are we measuring the "right stuff"? *Schizophr Bull.* (2000) 26:119–36. doi: 10.1093/oxfordjournals.schbul.a033430
14. Zipursky RB. Why are the outcomes in patients with schizophrenia so poor? *J Clin Psychiatry* (2014) 74:20–4. doi: 10.4088/JCP.13065su1.05
15. Matza LS, Buchanan R, Purdon S, Brewster-Jordan J, Zhao Y, Revicki DA. Measuring changes in functional status among patients with schizophrenia: the link with cognitive impairment. *Schizophr Bull.* (2006) 32:666–78. doi: 10.1093/schbul/sbl004
16. Thomas ML, Green MF, Hellemann G, Sugar CA, Tarasenko M, Calkins ME, et al. Modeling deficits from early auditory information processing to psychosocial functioning in schizophrenia. *JAMA Psychiatry* (2017) 74:37–46. doi: 10.1001/jamapsychiatry.2016.2980
17. Brown D, Nkagome K, Cordes J, Brenner R, Grunder G, Keefe RSE, et al. Evaluation of the efficacy, safety, and tolerability of BI 409306, a novel phosphodiesterase 9 inhibitor, in cognitive impairment in schizophrenia: a randomized, double-blind, placebo-controlled, phase II trial. *Schizophr Bull.* (2018). doi: 10.1093/schbul/sby049. [Epub ahead of print].
18. Talpos JC. Symptomatic thinking: the current state of Phase III and IV clinical trials for cognition in schizophrenia. *Drug Discov Today* (2017) 22:1017–26. doi: 10.1016/j.drudis.2017.04.014
19. Girgis RR, Zoghbi AW, Javitt DC, Lieberman JA. The past and future of novel, non-dopamine-2 receptor therapeutics for schizophrenia: a critical and comprehensive review. *J Psychiatr Res.* (2018). doi: 10.1016/j.jpsychires.2018.07.006. [Epub ahead of print].
20. Green MF, Nueichterlein KH, Gold JM, Barch DM, Cohen J, Essock S, et al. Approaching a consensus cognitive battery for clinical trials in schizophrenia: the NIMH-MATRICS conference to select cognitive domains and test criteria. *Biol Psychiatry* (2004) 56:301–7. doi: 10.1016/j.biopsych.2004.06.023
21. Green, MF, Butler PD, Chen Y, Geyer MA, Silverstein S, Wynn JK, et al. Perception measurement in clinical trials of schizophrenia: promising paradigms from CNTRICS. *Schizophr Bull.* (2009) 35:163–81. doi: 10.1093/schbul/sbn156
22. Carter CS, Barch DM, Buchanan RW, Bullmore E, Krystal JH, Cohen J, et al. Identifying cognitive mechanisms targeted for treatment development in schizophrenia: an overview of the first meeting of the Cognitive Neuroscience Treatment Research to Improve Cognition in Schizophrenia Initiative. *Biol Psychiatry* (2008) 64:4–10. doi: 10.1016/j.biopsych.2008.03.020
23. Butler PD, Chen Y, Ford JM, Geyer MA, Silverstein SM, Green MF. Perceptual measurement in schizophrenia: promising electrophysiology and neuroimaging paradigms from CNTRICS. *Schizophr Bull.* (2012) 38:81–91. doi: 10.1093/schbul/sbr106
24. Light GA, Naatanen R. Mismatch negativity is a breakthrough biomarker for understanding and treating psychotic disorders. *Proc Natl Acad Sci USA.* (2013) 110:15175–6. doi: 10.1073/pnas.1313287110
25. Näätänen R, Giallard AW, Mantysalo S. Early selective-attention effect on evoked potential reinterpreted. *Acta Psychol.* (1978) 42:313–29. doi: 10.1016/0001-6918(78)90006-9
26. Näätänen R, Tederm W, Alho K, Lavikainen J. Auditory attention and selective input modulation: a topographical ERP study. *Neuroreport* (1992) 3:493–6. doi: 10.1097/00001756-199206000-00009
27. Näätänen R. *Attention and Brain Function.* Hillsdale, NJ: Lawrence Erlbaum Associates, Inc (1992).
28. Näätänen R. The mismatch negativity: a powerful tool for cognitive neuroscience. *Ear Hear.* (1995) 16:6–18. doi: 10.1097/00003446-199502000-00002
29. Light GA, Swerdlow NR, Rissling AJ, Radant A, Sugar CA, Sprock J, et al. Characterization of neurophysiologic and neurocognitive biomarkers for use in genomic and clinical outcomes studies of schizophrenia. *PLoS ONE* (2012) 7:e39434. doi: 10.1371/journal.pone.0039434
30. Nagai T, Tada M, Kirihara K, Araki T, Jinde S, Kasai K. Mismatch negativity as a "translatable" brain marker toward early intervention for psychosis: a review. *Front Psychiatry* (2013) 4:115. doi: 10.3389/fpsyt.2013.00115
31. Rissling AJ, Park SH, Young JW, Rissling MB, Sugar CA, Sprock J, et al. Demand and modality of directed attention modulate "pre-attentive" sensory processes in schizophrenia patients and nonpsychiatric controls. *Schizophr Res.* (2013) 146:326–35. doi: 10.1016/j.schres.2013.01.035
32. Todd J, Michie PT, Schall U, Ward PB, Catts, SV. Mismatch negativity (MMN) reduction in schizophrenia—impaired prediction-error generation, estimation or salience? *Int J Psychophysiol.* (2012) 83:222–31. doi: 10.1016/j.ijpsycho.2011.10.003
33. Näätänen R, Paavilainen P, Rinne T, Alho K. The mismatch negativity (MMN) in basic research of central auditory processing: a review. *Clin Neurophysiol.* (2007): 118:2544–90. doi: 10.1016/j.clinph.2007.04.026
34. Alho K. Cerebral generators of mismatch negativity (MMN) and its magnetic counterpart (MMNm) elicited by sound changes. *Ear Hear.* (1995) 16:38–51. doi: 10.1097/00003446-199502000-00004
35. Takahashi H, Rissling AJ, Pascual-Marqui R, Kirihara K, Pela M, Sprock J, et al. Neural substrates of normal and impaired preattentive sensory discrimination in large cohorts of nonpsychiatric subjects and schizophrenia patients as indexed by MMN and P3a change detection response. *Neuroimage* (2013) 66:594–603. doi: 10.1016/j.neuroimage.2012.09.074
36. Rissling AJ, Miyakoshi M, Sugar CA, Braff DL, Makeig S, Light GA. Cortical substrates and functional correlates of auditory deviance processing deficits in schizophrenia. *NeuroImage Clin.* (2014) 6:424–37. doi: 10.1016/j.nicl.2014.09.006
37. Shelley AM, Ward PB, Catts SV, Michie PT, Andrews S, McConaghy N. Mismatch negativity: an index of a preattentive processing deficit in schizophrenia. *Biol Psychiatry* (1991) 30:1059–62. doi: 10.1016/0006-3223(91)90126-7
38. Umbricht D, Krljes S. Mismatch negativity in schizophrenia: a meta-analysis. *Schizophr Res.* (2005) 76:1–23. doi: 10.1016/j.schres.2004.12.002
39. Javitt DC, Steinschneider M, Schroeder CE, Vaughan HG Jr, Arezzo JC. Detection of stimulus deviance within primate primary auditory cortex:

intracortical mechanisms of mismatch negativity (MMN) generation. *Brain Res.* (1994): 667:192–200. doi: 10.1016/0006-8993(94)91496-6
40. Catts SV, Shelley AM, Ward PB, Liebert B, McConaghy N, Andrews S, et al. Brain potential evidence for an auditory sensory memory deficit in schizophrenia. *Am J Psychiatry* (1995) 152:213–9. doi: 10.1176/ajp.152.2.213
41. Javitt, DC, Shelley AM, Silipo G, Lieberman JA. Deficits in auditory and visual context-dependent processing in schizophrenia: defining the pattern. *Arch Gen Psychiatry* (2000) 57: 1131–7. doi: 10.1001/archpsyc.57.12.1131
42. Michie PT. What has MMN revealed about the auditory system in schizophrenia? *Int J Psychophysiol.* (2001) 42:177–94. doi: 10.1016/S0167-8760(01)00166-0
43. Umbricht D, Koller R, Schmid L, Skrabo A, Grubel C, Huber T, et al. How specific are deficits in mismatch negativity generation to schizophrenia? *Biol Psychiatry* (2003) 53:1120–31. doi: 10.1016/S0006-3223(02)01642-6
44. Salisbury DF, Kuroki N, Kasai K, Shenton ME, McCarley RW. Progressive and interrelated functional and structural evidence of post-onset brain reduction in schizophrenia. *Arch Gen Psychiatry* (2007) 64:521–9. doi: 10.1001/archpsyc.64.5.521
45. Salisbury DF, Shenton ME, Griggs CB, Bonner-Jackson A, McCarley RW. Mismatch negativity in chronic schizophrenia and first-episode schizophrenia. *Arch Gen Psychiatry* (2002) 59:686–94. doi: 10.1001/archpsyc.59.8.686
46. Light GA, Swerdlow NR, Thomas ML, Calkins ME, Green MF, Greenwood TA, et al. Validation of mismatch negativity and P3a for use in multi-site studies of schizophrenia: characterization of demographic, clinical, cognitive, and functional correlates in COGS-2. *Schizophr Res.* (2015) 163:63–72. doi: 10.1016/j.schres.2014.09.042
47. Brockhaus-Dumke A, Tendolkar I, Pukrop R, Schultze-Lutter F, Klosterkötter J, Ruhrmann S. Impaired mismatch negativity generation in prodromal subjects and patients with schizophrenia. *Schizophr Res.* (2005) 73:297–310. doi: 10.1016/j.schres.2004.05.016
48. Oknina LB, Wild-Wall N, Oades RD, Juran SA, Ropcke B, Pfueller U, et al. Frontal and temporal sources of mismatch negativity in healthy controls, patients at onset of schizophrenia in adolescence and others at 15 years after onset. *Schizophr Res.* (2005) 76:25–41. doi: 10.1016/j.schres.2004.10.003
49. Oades, RD, Wild-Wall N, Juran, SA, Sachsse J, Oknina LB, Röpcke B. Auditory change detection in schizophrenia: sources of activity, related neuropsychological function and symptoms in patients with a first episode in adolescence, and patients 14 years after an adolescent illness-onset. *BMC Psychiatry* (2006) 6:7. doi: 10.1186/1471-244X-6-7
50. Joshi YB, Breitenstein B, Tarasenko M, Thomas ML, Chang WL, Sprock J, et al. Mismatch negativity impairment is associated with deficits in identifying real-world environmental sounds in schizophrenia. *Schizophr Res.* (2018) 191:5–9. doi: 10.1016/j.schres.2017.05.020
51. Bodatsch M, Ruhrmann S, Wagner M, Müller R, Schultze-Lutter F, Frommann I, et al. Prediction of psychosis by mismatch negativity. *Biol Psychiatry* (2011) 69:959–66. doi: 10.1016/j.biopsych.2010.09.057
52. Kirino E, Inoue R. The relationship of mismatch negativity to quantitative EEG and morphological findings in schizophrenia. *J Psych Res.* (1999) 33:445–56. doi: 10.1016/S0022-3956(99)00012-6
53. Fawzy N, Gado O, Abdalla AM, Ibrahim WM. Auditory mismatch negativity, P300, and disability among first-episode schizophrenia patients without auditory hallucinations. *Egypt J Psychiatry* (2015) 36:112. doi: 10.4103/1110-1105.158120
54. Düring S, Glenthøj BY, Oranje B. Effects of blocking D2/D3 receptors on mismatch negativity and P3a amplitude of initially antipsychotic naïve, first episode schizophrenia patients. *Int J Neuropsychopharmacol.* (2016) 19:pyv109. doi: 10.1093/ijnp/pyv109
55. Umbricht D, Javitt D, Novak G, Bates J, Pollack S, Lieberman J, et al. Effects of clozapine on auditory event-related potentials in schizophrenia. *Biol Psychiatry* (1998) 44:716–25. doi: 10.1016/S0006-3223(97)00524-6
56. Umbricht D, Javitt D, Novak G, Bates J, Pollack S, Lieberman J, et al. Effects of risperidone on auditory event-related potentials in schizophrenia. *Int J Neuropsychopharmacol.* (1999) 2:299–304. doi: 10.1017/S1461145799001595
57. Schall U, Catts SV, Karayanidis F, Ward PB. Auditory event-related potential indices of fronto-temporal information processing in schizophrenia syndromes: valid outcome prediction of clozapine therapy in a three-year follow-up. *Int J Neuropsychopharmacol.* (1999) 2:83–93. doi: 10.1017/S1461145799001418
58. Rissling AJ, Braff DL, Swerdlow NR, Hellemann G, Rassovsky Y, Sprock J, et al. Disentangling early sensory information processing deficits in schizophrenia. *Clin Neurophysiol.* (2012) 123:1942–9. doi: 10.1016/j.clinph.2012.02.079
59. Jahshan C, Cadenhead KS, Rissling AJ, Kirihara K, Braff DL, Light GA. Automatic sensory information processing abnormalities across the illness course of schizophrenia. *Psychol Med.* (2012) 42:85–97. doi: 10.1017/S0033291711001061
60. Atkinson RJ, Michie PT, Schall U. Duration mismatch negativity and P3a in first-episode psychosis and individuals at ultra-high risk of psychosis. *Biol Psychiatry* (2012) 71:98–104. doi: 10.1016/j.biopsych.2011.08.023
61. Shaikh M, Valmaggia L, Broome MR, Dutt A, Lappin J, Day F, et al. Reduced mismatch negativity predates the onset of psychosis. *Schizophr Res.* (2012) 134:42–8. doi: 10.1016/j.schres.2011.09.022
62. Higuchi Y, Sumiyoshi T, Seo T, Miyanishi T, Kawasaki Y, Suzuki M. Mismatch negativity and cognitive performance for the prediction of psychosis in subjects with at-risk mental state. *PLoS ONE* (2013) 8:e54080. doi: 10.1371/journal.pone.0054080
63. Perez VB, Woods SW, Roach BJ, Ford JM, McGlashan TH, Srihari VH, et al. Automatic auditory processing deficits in schizophrenia and clinical high-risk patients: forecasting psychosis risk with mismatch negativity. *Biol Psychiatry* (2014) 75:459–69. doi: 10.1016/j.biopsych.2013.07.038
64. Koshiyama D, Kirihara K, Tada M, Nagai T, Fujioka M, Koike S, et al. Association between mismatch negativity and global functioning is specific to duration deviance in early stages of psychosis. *Schizophr Res.* (2018) 195:378–84. doi: 10.1016/j.schres.2017.09.045
65. Fusar-Poli P, Bonoldi I, Yung AR, Borgwardt S, Kempton MJ, Valmaggia L, et al. Predicting psychosis: meta-analysis of transition outcomes in individuals at high clinical risk. *Arch Gen Psychiatry* (2012) 69:220–9. doi: 10.1001/archgenpsychiatry.2011.1472
66. Cannon TD, Cadenhead K, Cornblatt B, Woods SW, Addington J, Walker E, et al. Prediction of psychosis in youth at high clinical risk: a multisite longitudinal study in North America. *Arch Gen Psychiatry* (2008) 65:28–37. doi: 10.1001/archgenpsychiatry.2007.3
67. Catts VS, Lai YL, Weickert CS, Weickert TW, Catts SV. A quantitative review of the postmortem evidence for decreased cortical N-methyl-d-aspartate receptor expression levels in schizophrenia: how can we link molecular abnormalities to mismatch negativity deficits? *Biol Psychol.* (2016) 116:57–67. doi: 10.1016/j.biopsycho.2015.10.013
68. Michie PT, Malmierca MS, Harms L, Todd J. The neurobiology of MMN and implications for schizophrenia. *Biol Psychol.* (2016):116:90–97. doi: 10.1016/j.biopsycho.2016.01.011
69. Javitt DC, Zukin SR, Heresco-Levy U, Umbricht D. Has an angel shown the way? Etiological and therapeutic implications of the PCP/NMDA model of schizophrenia. *Schizophr Bull.* (2012) 38:958–66. doi: 10.1093/schbul/sbs069
70. Rosburg T, Kreitschmann-Andermahr I. The effects of ketamine on the mismatch negativity (MMN) in humans–a meta-analysis. *Clin Neurophysiol.* (2016) 127:1387–94. doi: 10.1016/j.clinph.2015.10.062
71. Gil-da-Costa R, Stoner GR, Fung R, Albright TD. Nonhuman primate model of schizophrenia using a noninvasive EEG method. *Proc Natl Acad Sci USA.* (2013) 110:15425–30. doi: 10.1073/pnas.1312264110
72. Umbricht D, Koller R, Vollenweider FX, Schmid L. Mismatch negativity predicts psychotic experiences induced by NMDA receptor antagonist in healthy volunteers. *Biol Psychiatry* (2002) 51:400–6. doi: 10.1016/S0006-3223(01)01242-2
73. Kreitschmann-Andermahr I, Rosburg T, Demme U, Gaser E, Nowak H, Sauer H. Effect of ketamine on the neuromagnetic mismatch field in healthy humans. *Brain Res Cogn Brain Res.* (2001) 12:109–16. doi: 10.1016/S0926-6410(01)00043-X
74. Nagai T, Kirihara K, Tada M, Koshiyama D, Koike S, Suga M, et al. Reduced mismatch negativity is associated with increased plasma

level of glutamate in first-episode psychosis. *Sci Rep.* (2017) 7:2258. doi: 10.1038/s41598-017-02267-1
75. Rowland LM, Summerfelt A, Wijtenburg SA, Du X, Chiappelli JJ, Krishna N, et al. Frontal glutamate and gamma-aminobutyric acid level and their associations with mismatch negativity and digit sequencing task performance in schizophrenia. *JAMA Psychiatry* (2016) 73:466–74. doi: 10.1001/jamapsychiatry.2015.2680
76. Hall MH, Schulze K, Rijsdijk F, Picchioni M, Ettinger U, Bramon E, et al. Heritability and reliability of p300, P50 and duration mismatch negativity. *Behav Genet.* (2006) 36:845–57. doi: 10.1007/s10519-006-9091-6
77. Hong LE, Moran LV, Du X, O'Donnell P, Summerfelt A. Mismatch negativity and low frequency oscillations in schizophrenia families. *Clin Neurophysiol.* (2012) 123:1980–8. doi: 10.1016/j.clinph.2012.03.011
78. Earls HA, Curran T, Mittal V. A meta-analytic review of auditory event-related potential components as endophenotypes for schizophrenia: perspectives from first-degree relatives. *Schizophr Bull.* (2016) 42:1504–16. doi: 10.1093/schbul/sbw047
79. Erickson MA, Ruffle A, Gold JM. A meta-analysis of mismatch negativity in schizophrenia: from clinical risk to disease specificity and progression. *Biol Psychiatry* (2016) 79:980–7. doi: 10.1016/j.biopsych.2015.08.025
80. Ranlund S, Adams RA, Diez A, Constante M, Dutt A, Hall MH, et al. Impaired prefrontal synaptic gain in people with psychosis and their relatives during the mismatch negativity. *Hum Brain Mapp.* (2016) 37:351–65. doi: 10.1002/hbm.23035
81. Zarchi O, Carmel M, Avni C, Attias J, Frisch A, Michaelovsky E, et al. Schizophrenia-like neurophysiological abnormalities in 22q11.2 deletion syndrome and their association to COMT and PRODH genotypes. *J Psychiatr Res.* (2013) 47:1623–9. doi: 10.1016/j.jpsychires.2013.07.004
82. Light GA, Braff DL. Stability of mismatch negativity deficits and their relationship to functional impairments in chronic schizophrenia. *Am J Psychiatry* (2003) 162:1741–3. doi: 10.1176/appi.ajp.162.9.1741
83. Wynn JK, Sugar C, Horan WP, Kern R, Green MF. Mismatch negativity, social cognition, and functioning in schizophrenia patients. *Biol Psychiatry* (2010) 67:940–7. doi: 10.1016/j.biopsych.2009.11.024
84. Rasser PE, Schall U, Todd J, Michie, PT, Ward, PB, Johnston P, et al. Gray matter deficits, mismatch negativity, and outcomes in schizophrenia. *Schizophr Bull.* (2011) 37:131–40. doi: 10.1093/schbul/sbp060
85. Kawakubo Y, Kasai K. Support for an association between mismatch negativity and social functioning in schizophrenia. *Prog Neuropsychopharmacol Biol Psychiatry* (2006) 30:1367–8. doi: 10.1016/j.pnpbp.2006.03.003
86. Lee SH, Sung K, Lee KS, Moon E, Kim CG. Mismatch negativity is a stronger indicator of functional outcomes than neurocognition or theory of mind in patients with schizophrenia. *Prog Neuropsychopharmacol Biol Psychiatry* (2014) 48:213–9. doi: 10.1016/j.pnpbp.2013.10.010
87. Kishi T, Ikuta T, Oya K, Matsunaga S, Matsuda Y, Iwata N. Anti-dementia drugs for psychopathology and cognitive impairment in schizophrenia: a systematic review and meta-analysis. *Int J Neuropsychopharmacol.* (2018) 21:748-57. doi: 10.1093/ijnp/pyy045
88. Di Iorio, Baroni G, Lorusso M, Montemitro C, Spano MC, di Giannanotonio M. Efficacy of memantine in schizophrenia patients: a systematic review. *J Amino Acids* (2017) 2017:7021071. doi: 10.1155/2017/7021071
89. Zdanys K, Tampi RR. A systematic review of off-label uses of memantine for psychaitric disorder. *Prog Neuropsychopharmacol Biol Psychiatry* (2008) 32:1362–74. doi: 10.1016/j.pnpbp.2008.01.008
90. Johnson JW, Kotermanski SE. Mechanism of action of memantine. *Curr Opin Pharmacol.* (2006) 6:61–7. doi: 10.1016/j.coph.2005.09.007
91. Lipton SA. The molecular basis of memantine action in Alzheimer's disease and other neurological disorder: low-affinity, uncompetitive antagonism. *Curr Alzheimer Res.* (2005) 2:155–65. doi: 10.2174/1567205053585846
92. Swerdlow NR, van Bergeijk DP, Bergsma F, Weber E, Talledo J. The effects of memantine on prepulse inhibition. *Neuropsychopharmacology* (2009). 34:1854–64. doi: 10.1038/npp.2009.7
93. Kishi T, Matsuda Y, Iwata N. Memantine add-on to antipsychotic treatment for residual negative and cognitive symptoms of schizophrenia: a meta-analysis. *Psychopharmacology* (2017) 234:2113–25. doi: 10.1007/s00213-017-4616-7
94. Zheng W, Li XH, Yang XH, Cai DB, Ungvari GS, Ng CH, et al. Adjunctive use of memantine for schizophrenia: a meta-analysis of randomized, double-blind, placebo-controlled trials. *Psychol Med.* (2018) 48:72–81. doi: 10.1017/S0033291717001271
95. Swerdlow NR, Bhakta S, Chou HH, Telledo JA, Balvaneda B, Light GA. Memantine effects on sensorimotor gating and mismatch negativity in patients with chronic psychosis. *Neuropsychopharmacology* (2016) 41:419–30. doi: 10.1038/npp.2015.162
96. Bhakta SG, Chou HH, Rana B, Telledo JA, Balvaneda B, Gaddis L, et al. Effects of acute memantine administration on MATRICS Consensus Cognitive Battery performance in psychosis: testing an experimental medicine strategy. *Psychopharmacology* (2016) 233:2399–410. doi: 10.1007/s00213-016-4291-0
97. Kirby J, Green C, Loveman E, Clegg A, Picot J, Takeda A, et al. A systematic review of the clinical and cost-effectiveness of memantine in patients with moderately severe to severe Alzheimer's disease. *Drugs Aging* (2006) 23:227–40. doi: 10.2165/00002512-200623030-00005
98. Areosa SA, Sherriff F, McShane R. Memantine for dementia. *Cochrane Database Syst Rev.* (2005) CD003154.
99. Veerman SR, Schulte PF, Smith JD, de Haan L. Memantine augmentation in clozapine-refractory schizophrenia: a randomized, double-blind placebo-controlled crossover study. *Psychol Med.* (2017) 46:1909–21. doi: 10.1017/S00332917160 00398
100. Veerman SR, Schulte PF, Deijen JB, de Haan L. Adjunctive memantine in clozapine-treated refractory schizophrenia: an open-label 1-year extension study. *Psychol Med.* (2017) 47:363–75. doi: 10.1017/S00332917160 02476
101. Mazinani R, Nejati S, Khodaei M. Effects of memantine added to risperidone on the symptoms of schizophrenia: a randomized dobule-blind placebo-controlled clinical trial. *Psychiatry Res.* (2017) 247:291–5. doi: 10.1016/j.psychres.2016.09.028
102. Ivleva EI, Clementz BA, Dutcher AM, Arnold SJM, Jeon-Slaughter H, Aslan S, et al. Brain structure biomarkers in the psychosis biotypes: findings from the bipolar-schizophrenia network for intermediate phenotypes. *Biol Psychiatry* (2017) 82:26–39. doi: 10.1016/j.biopsych.2016. 08.030
103. Swerdlow NR, Bhakta SG, Light GA. Room to move: plasticity in early auditory information processing and auditory learning in schizophrenia revealed by acute pharmacological challenge. *Schizophr Res.* (2018) 199:285–91. doi: 10.1016/j.schres.2018.03.037
104. Light GA, Zhang W, Joshi YB, Bhakta S, Talledo JA, Swerdlow NR. Single-dose memantine improves cortical oscillatory response dynamics in patients with schizophrenia. *Neuropsychopharmacology* (2017) 42:2633–9. doi: 10.1038/npp.2017.81
105. Kantrowitz JT, Swerdlow NR, Dunn W, Vinogradov S. Auditory system target engagement during plasticity-based interventions in schizophrenia: a focus on modulation of N-methyl-D-aspartate-type glutamate receptor function. *Biol Psychiatry Cogn Neurosci Neuroimaging* (2018) 3:581–90. doi: 10.1016/j.bpsc.2018.02.002
106. Fisher M, Harman A, Stephens DB, Vinogradov S. Neuroscience-informed computer-assisted cognitive training in schizophrenia. *Ann NY Acad Sci.* (2016) 1366:90–114. doi: 10.1111/nyas.13042
107. Genevsky A, Garrett CT, Alexander PP, Vinogradov S. Cognitive training in schizophrenia: a neuroscience-based approach. *Dialogues Clin Neurosci.* (2010) 12:416–21.
108. Loewy R, Fisher M, Schlosser DA, Biagianti B, Stuart B, Mathalon DH, et al. Intensive auditory cognitive training improves verbal memory in adolescents and young adults at clinical high risk for psychosis. *Schiophr Bull.* (2016) 42 (Suppl. 1):S118–26. doi: 10.1093/schbul/sbw009
109. Fisher M, Mellon SH, Wolkowitz O, Vinogradov S. Neuroscience-informed auditory training in schizophrenia: a final report of the effects on cognition and serum brain-derived neurotrophic factor. *Schizophr Res Cogn.* (2016) 3:1–7. doi: 10.1016/j.scog.2015.10.006

110. Dale CL, Brown EG, Fisher M, Herman AB, Dowling AF, Hinkley LB, et al. Auditory cortical plasticity drives training-induced cognitive changes in schizophrenia. *Schizophr Bull.* (2016) 42:220–8. doi: 10.1093/schbul/sbv087

111. Fisher M, Loewy R, Carter C, Lee A, Ragland JD, Niendam T, et al. Neuroplasticity-based auditory training via laptop computer improves cognition in young individuals with recent onset schizophrenia. *Schizophr Bull.* (2015) 41:250–8. doi: 10.1093/schbul/sbt232

112. Vinogradov S, Fisher M, Nagarajan S. Cognitive training in schizophrenia: golden age or wild west? *Biol Psychiatry* (2013) 73:935–7. doi: 10.1016/j.biopsych.2013.03.015

113. Perez VB, Tarasenko M, Miyakoshi M, Pianka ST, Makeig SD, Braff DL, et al. Mismatch negativity is a sensitive and predictive biomarker of perceptual learning during auditory cognitive training in schizophrenia. *Neuropsychopharmacology* (2017) 42:2206–13. doi: 10.1038/npp.2017.25

114. Hochberger WC, Joshi YB, Thomas ML, Zhang W, Bismark AW, Treichler EBH, et al. Neurophysiologic measures of target engagement predict response to auditory-based cognitive training in treatment refractory schizophrenia. *Neuropsychopharmacology* (in press).

115. Braff DL, Light GA. Preattentional and attentional cognitive deficits as targets for treating schizophrenia. *Psychopharmacology* (2004) 174:75–85. doi: 10.1007/s00213-004-1848-0

19

Lipidomics in Major Depressive Disorder

Andreas Walther[1], Carlo Vittorio Cannistraci[2,3], Kai Simons[4], Claudio Durán[2], Mathias J. Gerl[4], Susanne Wehrli[1] and Clemens Kirschbaum[1]*

[1] Biological Psychology, TU Dresden, Dresden, Germany, [2] Biomedical Cybernetics Group, Biotechnology Center (BIOTEC), Center for Molecular and Cellular Bioengineering (CMCB), Center for Systems Biology Dresden (CSBD), Department of Physics, TU Dresden, Dresden, Germany, [3] Brain Bio-Inspired Computing (BBC) Lab, IRCCS Centro Neurolesi "Bonino Pulejo", Messina, Italy, [4] Lipotype GmbH, Dresden, Germany

***Correspondence:**
Andreas Walther
andreas.walther@tu-dresden.de

Omic sciences coupled with novel computational approaches such as machine intelligence offer completely new approaches to major depressive disorder (MDD) research. The complexity of MDD's pathophysiology is being integrated into studies examining MDD's biology within the omic fields. Lipidomics, as a late-comer among other omic fields, is increasingly being recognized in psychiatric research because it has allowed the investigation of global lipid perturbations in patients suffering from MDD and indicated a crucial role of specific patterns of lipid alterations in the development and progression of MDD. Combinatorial lipid-markers with high classification power are being developed in order to assist MDD diagnosis, while rodent models of depression reveal lipidome changes and thereby unveil novel treatment targets for depression. In this systematic review, we provide an overview of current breakthroughs and future trends in the field of lipidomics in MDD research and thereby paving the way for precision medicine in MDD.

Keywords: major depressive disorder, depression, lipidomics, machine learning, computational psychiatry, cortisol, inflammation, prostaglandin

INTRODUCTION

Major depressive disorder (MDD) is a psychiatric illness with devastating consequences with regard to personal and social functioning as well as physical health (1, 2). According to the Diagnostic and Statistical Manual of Mental Disorders (DSM-5), MDD is a heterogeneous disorder, defined and diagnosed on the basis of its core symptoms of a depressed mood or anhedonia and a combination of four of nine other symptoms, such as changes in appetite, sleep, fatigue, concentration, feelings of worthlessness and suicidal ideations persisting for the majority of the day over at least a 2 week period (3). The World Health Organization has declared MDD the leading cause of disability with over 300 million people being affected worldwide (4). Regrettably, no sizeable improvement in population mental health for MDD has been achieved during the last decade (5). Diagnosing and treating MDD is complicated due to its heterogeneous illness presentation exemplified by anhedonia, considered a cardinal feature of MDD, but is truly present in only up to 50% of patients (6). The subjective nature of the patients' report of symptoms makes clinical judgment based on a person's history and cultural norms a difficult task. The high non-responder rates to standard antidepressant treatment present further challenges to clinical practice (7, 8). These factors contribute to low diagnostic reliability and the potential for misdiagnosis (9, 10).

Therefore, during the last few decades, tremendous efforts have been undertaken in order to identify a diagnostic biomarker for MDD, enabling a reliable diagnosis and potentially identifying treatment targets for novel therapeutic approaches. Although advancements in elucidating the pathophysiology of MDD have been achieved (11), one needs to acknowledge that the reductionis single biomarker approach employed during the last decades has been a failure (12). It has become increasingly clear that the pathophysiology of MDD depends on a wide array of biological parameters that cannot be measured by a single biomarker and that only a systems approach might be successful in identifying diagnostic bio-signatures for MDD.

Newly developed high-throughput screening technologies, which facilitate the quantification of omics data, offer new approaches for systems analyses with regard to MDD (13). New computational methods are currently revolutionizing biomarker research by using unsupervised data driven approaches such as machine intelligence or deep learning; these provide increased analytical power in order to come to grips with the complex pathophysiology of MDD (14–16). These computational approaches are capable of delivering multi-parametric disease signatures based on different omics data sets that can be used to identify functional networks (17).

Although studies using omics approaches (e.g., genomic, proteomic, brain connectomics, metabolomics) have increased exponentially during the last 18 years, achieving breakthroughs for example in the field of genome-wide or neurophysiological classification of MDD (18, 19), reproducibility has proved challenging the field. Lipidomics is no exception (12). However, this situation is now improving with the developments of new lipidomics platforms (20) that provide reliable absolute quantitation and inter-site reproducibility (21), which are the basis for clinical applications (12). In this systematic review we will provide an up-to-date overview of existing studies in lipidomics and MDD or rodent models of depression.

THE LIPIDOME IN MDD

The lipidome—the complete lipid profile of an organism—has central roles in most aspects of cell biology (22). The human organism invests substantial resources for the production of thousands of molecular species attributable to eight different lipid categories with multiple classes and sub-classes (23). These classes are strongly interconnected and perturbations in a lipid species often result in global lipidome changes (23, 24). An enormous variety of different functions is carried out by lipids, such as energy storage by triacylglycerol (TAG) in lipid droplets or membrane formation and trafficking by amphipathic lipids such as glycerophospholipids (e.g., phosphatidylcholines [PC], phosphatidylethanolamines [PE], and phosphatidylinositols [PI]) (25). Lipids also determine the localization and function of proteins in the cell membranes of neurons and may further act as neurotransmitters (26). Many lipid structures have been shown to be essential for neuronal signaling and survival (27–29), and thereby critically influence an individuals' mood and behavior (26). Lipids also function to sub-compartmentalize cell membranes, forming functional platforms (lipid rafts) that operate in signaling and many other membrane activities (30). Finally, lipids act as second messengers in signal transduction, also regulating glucocorticoid action as well as inflammatory processes (25). Therefore, there is a plethora of lipid markers potentially related to MDD. Reviews and meta-analyses investigating the action of single lipids in MDD suggest that polyunsaturated fatty acids (e.g., omega-3 and omega-6) (31), cholesterol (32), as well as lipids of the sphingomyelin-ceramide (SM-Cer) pathway could be crucially related to mood disorders (33, 34). However, as outlined above, lipids are strongly interconnected and hierarchically organized so that a systems approach based on networks will be an indispensable tool to reveal the role and mechanisms of the lipidome in MDD. Since lipid nomenclature is not yet standardized, in the following, we will report lipid species as in original reports (35).

We will describe the systematic search process for studies applying lipidomic approaches in MDD or rodent models of depression (see **Figure 1**). Subsequently, we will review the identified studies with regard to their biological interpretation and discriminative power for MDD classification (see **Table 1**) and compare identified lipid species between studies (see **Supplementary Table 1**). Finally, we will integrate the findings into a model in which the relationship between the lipidome and MDD is mediated via dysregulated processes in the hypothalamus-pituitary-adrenal (HPA) axis and the immune system (see **Figure 2**).

SEARCH STRATEGY AND STUDY SELECTION

Candidate studies were identified via PubMed/Medline, EMBASE and PsycINFO using the following search strategy, whereby separate searches were performed for human and rodent studies respectively. The applied key terms for human studies were [(depressive mood OR depressed mood OR depression OR major depression) AND (lipidomics OR lipidome)], whereas for rodent studies the key terms [(depression OR depressive behavior OR depressive-like behavior OR depressed mood OR depressive mood OR antidepressant OR chronic unpredictable stress OR chronic unpredictable mild stress OR learned helplessness OR inescapable foot shock OR pain-induced depression OR social defeat) AND (rodents OR rats OR mice) AND (lipidomics OR lipidome)] were used for searching in the title, abstract and/or any other field registered in the database. The search was restricted to English language journal articles published between database inception and 25th April 2018. The final set of articles was cross-validated and further completed based on prior reviews. In sum, 123 records were extracted. The set was refined by removing (i) duplicate entries ($n = 46$). Titles and abstracts were then screened for relevance, removing (ii) reviews, meta-analyses, case studies, meeting abstracts, study protocols, practical guidelines and books ($n = 27$). In a next step, the full text of the remaining 50 articles was assessed for eligibility, subsequently excluding all studies that did not deal with (iii) lipidomics ($n = 6$) or (iv) MDD or behavioral mouse models

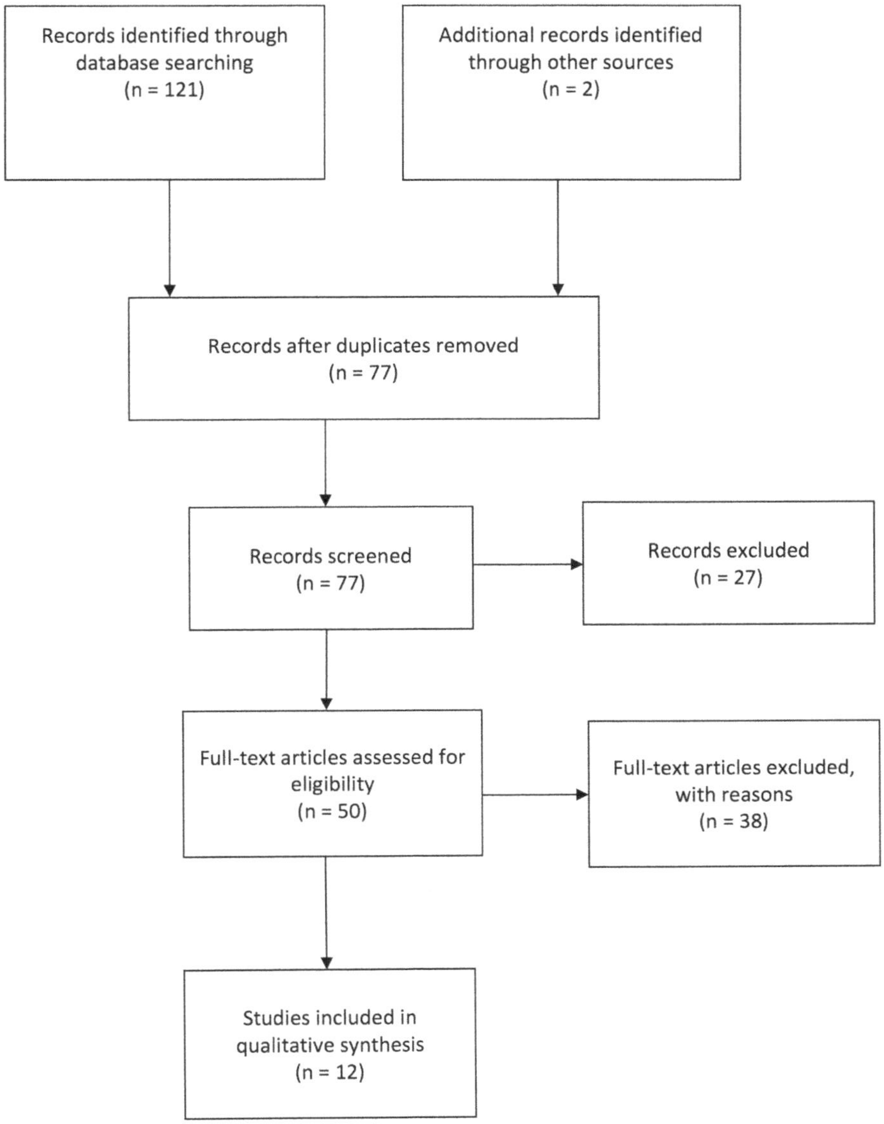

FIGURE 1 | Flow chart visualization of systematic search process according to PRISMA guidelines.

of depression (n = 29). In a final step, studies (v) with a special focus on bio-technologies (n = 3) were eliminated. **Figure 1** shows the sample development throughout the selection process, reaching the final set of 12 studies for review including 7 human and 5 rodent studies (see **Table 1**). The study selection and eligibility screening were conducted according to the PRISMA guidelines (47).

LIPIDOMIC STUDIES IN MDD AND RODENT MODELS OF DEPRESSION

Human Studies

In humans, a pioneering study by Demirkan et al. using unsupervised lipidomic analysis of 148 plasma phospho- and sphingolipid species in a sample of 742 individuals identified significant associations with a psychometric depression measure (Center for Epidemiological Studies-Depression Scale: CES-D) for the ratio sphingomyelin (SM) 23:1 to SM 16:0 and the absolute amount of PC (alkyl subclass) O 36:4, as well as the ratio of PC O 36:4 to Cer 20:0 (37). However, subsequent analysis of an independent replication dataset (N = 753) only revealed absolute levels of PC O 36:4 to be robustly inversely related to depressive symptoms. Though being robustly associated to the CES-D in this study, this lipid structure alone did not provide sufficient discriminating power to adequately differentiate between individuals suffering from MDD and healthy controls. The authors of the study further highlighted that PC O 36:4 is a potential target of phospholipase A2 (PLA2),

TABLE 1 | Summary of included studies on lipidomics in MDD or rodent models of depression.

Reference	Population	Depression status categorization	Behavioral assessment	Sample	Quantification method	Study design	Finding
HUMAN STUDIES							
Chan et al. (36)	Human, patients with coronary artery disease (CAD), North America	Dimensional depression scale (CES-D: equal/above vs. below cut off for depression = 16)	–	Patients with CAD and elevated depressive symptoms $N = 37$, mean age: 60.4, Control patients with CAD but not elevated depressive symptoms $N = 49$, mean age: 62.8 Total $N = 86$	Targeted gas chromatography	Discovery	Phospholipid bio-signature including 10 species discriminated between groups with AUC 84%. Findings indicate phospholipid-proinflammatory dependent pathway in patients suffering from CAD and MDD.
Demirkan et al. (37)	Human, general population, Europe	Dimensional depression scales (HADS-D, CES-D)	–	Erasmus Rucphen Family (ERF; genetically isolated population located in Netherlands), mean age discovery: 53.09, mean age validation: 48.13, discovery $N = 742$, validation $N = 753$, Total $N = 1{,}495$	Targeted electrospray ionization tandem mass spectrometry	Discovery / Validation	In the discovery set SM 23:1 and PC O 36:4 emerged as significantly correlated to depression measures. In a second, independent validation set the association for PC O 36:4 was replicated.
Hennebelle et al. (38)	Human, patients with seasonal affective disorders (SAD), North America	MDD diagnosis by structured clinical interview (DSM-V)	–	unmedicated participants euthymic at baseline, who met depression criteria in winter, mean age: 46.7, $N = 9$	Targeted liquid chromatography tandem mass-spectrometry	Discovery	No differential lipids were identified. In SAD patients, 4 increased oxylipins were identified in winter pointing toward inflammatory states in SAD patients. Potential association between winter depression and changes in cytochrome p450- and sEH-derived oxylipins were suggested.
Kim et al. (39)	Human, female MDD patients (current-MDD & remitted-MDD) vs. HCs, Korea	MDD diagnosis by Mini-International Neuropsychiatric Interview (MINI) according to DSM-IV criteria	–	Korean population, female MDD patients with a current major depressive episode: $N = 25$, MDD with current remission: $N = 25$, controls: N = 25, Total $N = 75$	Targeted liquid chromatography–mass spectrometry	Discovery	Lipid species of the LPA and TAG classes were differential between current, remitted, and non-depressed individuals. Discrimination power for different comparisons ranged between 60% (remitted vs. controls) and 76% (current vs. controls).
Knowles et al. (40)	Human, general population, North America	Continuous index of MDD based on Mini-International Neuropsychiatric Interview (MINI)	–	Participant data stems from randomly selected participants of the San Antonio Family Study (SAFS) mean age: 49.47, $N = 567$	Targeted liquid chromatography electrospray ionization-tandem mass spectrometry	Discovery	PC O and PC P species were associated to a genetic risk for MDD. PCO and PC P species containing AA exhibited the greatest degree of genetic overlap with MDD.
Kuwano et al. (41)	Human, general population, Japan	MDD diagnosis by structured clinical interview (DSM-IV TR)	–	Drug-naïve MDD patients, $N = 15$, healthy controls $N = 19$	Targeted liquid chromatography-mass spectrometry	Discovery	No differences between the plasma lipidome of MDD patients and HCs was identified. Depressive symptoms correlated with plasma tryptophan-kynurenine and lipid related metabolites.

(Continued)

TABLE 1 | Continued

Reference	Population	Depression status categorization	Behavioral assessment	Sample	Quantification method	Study design	Finding
Liu et al. (42)	Human, general population, China	MDD diagnosis according to DSM-IV	–	Discovery *N*: drug-naïve MDD = 60, HC = 59. Validation N: drug-naïve/drug-treated MDD= 75, HC = 52 Mean age discovery, HC: 43.98, mean age discovery MDD: 42.42, mean age validation HC: 33.67, mean age validation MDD: 36.04.	Non-targeted, ultra-performance liquid chromatography coupled with quadrupole time-of-flight mass spectrometry	Discovery / Validation	A diagnostic biomarker consisting of five differential lipids (LPE 20:4, PC 34:1, PI 40:4, SM 39:1, and TAG 44:2) was suggested with an AUC of 0.855 (moderately depressed vs. HC) and 0.931 (severely depressed vs. HC). Total levels of LPC, LPE, PC, PE, PI, DAG, TAG lipid classes were elevated in depressed individuals, while total PE O and several SM species were decreased
Rodent studies	**Population**	**Phenotype**	**Behavioral assessment**	**Sample**	**Quantification method**	**Study design**	**Finding**
Chen et al. (43)	Rodents	Chronic restraint stress for 6 weeks	Tail suspension test	Male Wistar rats, experimental *N* = 12, Allium macrostemon treated depression group = 11, control group = 12, total *N* = 35	Liquid chromatography/ion trap-time of flight mass spectrometry. Liquid chromatography/triple quadrupole mass spectrometry.	Experimental	Chronic restraint stress was associated with increased LPCs and reduced PCs
Faria et al. (44)	Rodents	Chronic unpredictable stress	Forced swimming test	Male, C57/BL6 mice with mice myocardium control (CTL), age: 9 weeks old, experimental *N* = 5 and Control *N* = 5, *N* = 3 for independent experiments	Targeted liquid chromatography–mass spectrometry, phosphorous assay, tissue samples of brain and myocardium	Experimental	An increases on brain lipid class level in the relative content of PC and PE levels and a decrease in the relative content of PI levels in the stressed mice could also be observed
Lee et al. (45)	Rodents	Injections of 10 mg/kg of the antidepressants maprotiline, fluoxetine and paroxetine for 4 weeks	-	male Balb/C mice, weighing 20–30 g each, aged 6–8 weeks, *N* = 16	Targeted, high-performance liquid chromatography/mass spectrometry, tissue samples of prefrontal cortex, hippocampus, striatum, cerebellum	Experimental	Decreased PC and increased LPC species due to maprotiline and paroxetine were observed in the prefrontal cortex indicating increased PLA2 activity due to treatment.
Lee et al. (46)	Rodents	Injection of the antidepressant maprotiline 10 mg/kg for 4 weeks or maprotiline plus bilateral prefrontal cortical injections of antisense oligonucleotide to iPLA2	Forced swimming test	Balb/C mice weighing 20–30 g each, aged 6–8 weeks, *N* = 20	Targeted, high-performance liquid chromatography (HPLC)/mass spectrometry, tissue samples of prefrontal cortex	Experimental	Decreased levels in PCs containing PUFAs and increased LPC levels were identified after maprotiline treatment indicating increased PLA2 activity due to treatment.
Oliveira et al. (34)	Rodents	Chronic unpredictable stress for 4 weeks or subcutaneous injections with 40 mg synthetic CORT 40 mg/kg for 4 weeks	Elevated plus maze	Adult male Wistar rats, aged 2 months, different conditions: Control *N* = 10, CUS Paradigm N = 10, CORT injections *N* = 10, Vehicle control group (sesame oil injections) *N* = 10,	Targeted, liquid chromatography mass spectrometry, tissue samples of prefrontal cortex, amygdala, hippocampus, cerebellum	Experimental	Due to the CUS paradigm relative levels of LPC, PA, PG, Cer species were increased, while relative levels of PC, PC E and PE species were decreased. After exogeneous CORT administration several brain lipid alterations were observed: decrease in PCs and PEs; increase in LPCs, Cers, PAs, PGs

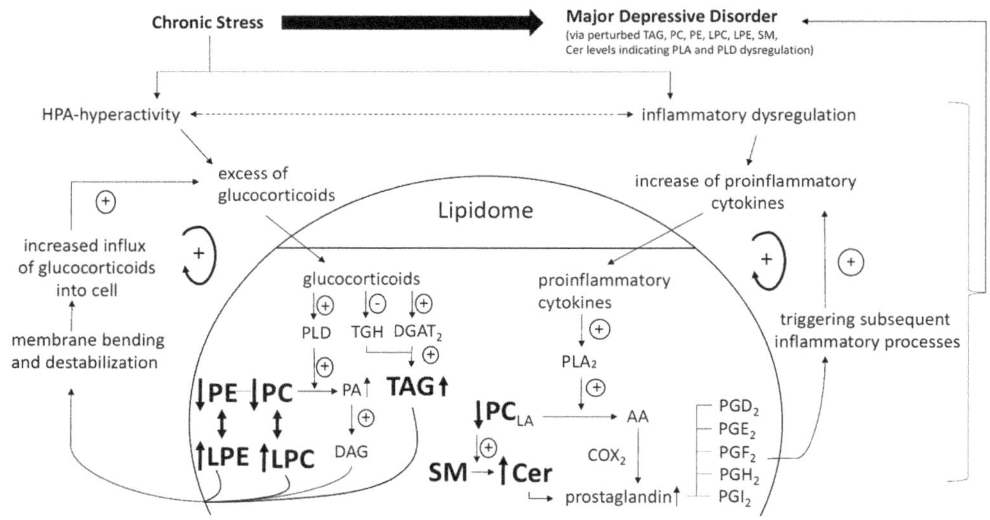

FIGURE 2 | Pathway linking chronic stress, HPA hyperactivity, increased inflammation, lipidomic dysregulation, and development of MDD. *Glucocorticoid positive spiral pathway A:* Chronic stress leads to HPA hyperactivity. Increased levels of glucocorticoids increase PLD activity (48). Increased PLD activity leads to increased turnover of phosphatidylcholines (PC) and phosphatidylethanolamine (PE) to phosphatidic acid (PA) and also lysophosphatidylcholine (LPC) and lysophosphatidylethanolamine (LPE). Due to is chemical properties, PA is swiftly converted to diacylglycerol (DAG). DAG, LPC, and LPE cause membrane bending and destabilization allowing more influx of glucocorticoids into the cell. *Glucocorticoid positive spiral pathway B:* Increased levels of glucocorticoids decrease triacylglycerol hydrolase (TGH) expression. Increased levels of glucocorticoids increase triacylglycerol (TAG) biosynthesis via increase of (diacylglycerol acyltransferase 2) DGAT2. Reduced TGH expression and increased TAG biosynthesis lead to increased levels of TAG (49). TAG in turn is related to increased levels of glucocorticoids. *Inflammatory positive spiral pathway:* Chronic stress leads to inflammatory dysregulation. An excess of proinflammatory cytokines and phase reactants increase phospholipase A2 (PLA2) (50). Increased PLA2 activity leads to increased turnover of linoleic acid (LA) containing phosphatidylcholines (PC_{LA}) to arachidonic acid (AA). AA is subsequently converted to prostaglandins (PG) of which the series 2 is proinflammatory (e.g., PGA2, PGD2, PGE2, PGF2, PGH2, PGI2). PG further increase inflammatory reactions (40). PC degradation is associated with SM-Cer turn over further increasing PG levels (22). *Lipid Nomenclature:* following annotations are used: Lipid class <sum of carbon atoms>:<sum of double bonds>; < sum of hydroxyl groups>, e.g., SM 34:1;2 signifies a SM species with 34 carbon atoms, 1 double bond and 2 hydroxyl groups in the ceramide backbone. Lipid molecular subspecies annotation (35) contains additional information about the exact identity of their fatty acids, the exact position of which cannot be discriminated in relation to the glycerol backbone (*sn*-1 or *sn*-2). This is indicated by a dash: "-." For example, PC 18:1;0-16:0;0 denotes a phosphatidylcholine with a 18:1;0 (18 carbon atoms, 1 double bond, 0 hydroxylation) and a 16:0;0 fatty acid. CE 18:1;0 denotes a cholesteryl ester with a 18:1;0 fatty acid.

which converts PC O 36:4 to lysophosphatidylcholines (LPCs). When PC O 36:4 is hydrolyzed by PLA2, arachidonic acid (AA) is produced, which is subsequently rapidly converted into inflammatory mediators (prostaglandins), potentially leading to increased neuro-inflammation, which has consistently been related to MDD (51). AA itself, however, is known to directly modulate neural cell function via different processes (e.g., membrane fluidity and polarization) and thereby AA could negatively affect brain function and contribute directly to depressive symptomatology (37) [see also the study by Knowles et al. section Lipidome associations with glucocorticoids and inflammatory markers. for lipid-inflammation dependent pathways in MDD (40)].

Liu et al. based on prior work (52), conducted a non-targeted lipidomic approach comparing 60 patients with diagnosed MDD with 60 healthy controls (HCs) in a discovery set and a validation set of a similar size (42). The authors reported that several differential lipid species were significantly correlated with depression severity measured by the Hamilton Depression Scale (HAMD) (42). Total levels of the following lipid classes were elevated in depressed individuals LPC, lysophosphatidylethanolamine (LPE), PC, PE, phosphatidylinositol (PI), DAG, and TAG, while total PE O and several SM species were decreased in depressed individuals. The authors, however, did not elaborate on the molecular mechanisms linking these lipid classes with MDD. Yet, negative associations between specific SM species and depressive symptoms were also reported by Demirkan et al. (37). An experimental study further investigated the effects of acid sphingomyelinase (Asm), which releases ceramides (Cer) from SMs (33). In this study, it was shown that therapeutic concentrations of two different antidepressants reduced Asm activity and Cer levels, while increased neuroplasticity and non-depressive behavior was observed (33). This suggests that SM levels and the turnover to Cer are dysregulated in MDD and restored with antidepressant medication. Furthermore, using unsupervised statistical approaches, Liu et al. extracted a combinatorial lipid marker including five lipids as diagnostic biomarker with an area under the curve (AUC) between 0.855 and 0.931 suggesting a good discriminative power for MDD and HCs. However, the identified five lipids LPE 20:4, PC 34:1, PI 40:4, SM 39:1, and TAG 44:2 were not further validated in subsequent lipidomic studies on MDD. Unfortunately, the authors did not provide values for the area under the precision/recall curve (AUPR), although unbalanced analysis was performed when comparing HCs ($N = 111$) to either moderately depressed ($N = 78$) or severely depressed individuals ($N = 57$). Here, it is important to note that AUC alone is not a good measure of performance in unbalanced data sets as represented by the comparison of moderately or severely depressed vs. HCs. Thus, combined reporting of AUC and AUPR is required. AUC alone can present an overly optimistic view of the algorithm's performance when there is a skew in the class distribution (53). Comparing these results, a metabolomics/lipidomic study reports an accuracy for their extracted combinatorial biomarker of 72.2% for the discrimination of MDD and HCs, which is significantly lower (54). The authors subsequently sub-classified MDD individuals into anxious depressed ($N = 58$) and melancholic depressed ($N = 21$) and compared these groups to HC ($N = 97$). Using this approach, an accuracy of 83.8% for melancholic depressed individuals (72% for anxious depressed individuals) was achieved. However, the authors neither reported AUC nor AUPR levels (54). This might therefore still overestimate the actual discriminative power since the false positive rate was not considered within the accuracy measure. In this study, of the lipids, PC and SM levels were decreased and Cer levels were increased, again indicating increased SM to Cer turnover by Asm hyperactivity (54).

A study by Kim et al. including 25 currently affected MDD cases, 25 remitted MDD cases, and 25 HCs, identified a lipid marker consisting of lysophosphatidic acid (LPA) 16:1, TAG 44:0, and TAG 54:8, discriminating between HCs and MDD cases with 76% accuracy (HCs vs remitted with 60% accuracy; LPA16:1, TAG52:6, TAG54:8, TAG58:10) (39). With regard to differentially elevated lipids in the three groups, an inconsistent picture emerged with no differential PC and PE species, while TAG and DAG species showed the most differentiating power and were significantly increased in MDD patients compared to controls (39). TAGs are the most abundant lipid species in the human organism and constitute a major source of energy, while lipoprotein lipase (LPL) enzymes such as adipose triglyceride lipase (ATGL) and hormone sensitive lipase (HSL) are responsible for the breakdown of TAG into DAG and free fatty acids (FFA) (55). In the brain, TAG degradation by LPL informs neurons and astrocytes about energy expenditure (56), while a dysfunction of these enzymes leading to increased TAG levels may underlie the increased fatigue observed in depressive disorders.

Chan et al. further investigated the lipidome in patients with coronary artery disease (CAD) and identified 10 phospholipids, which showed good discriminative power (84%) to differentiate between CAD patients with substantial depressive burden (CES-D $\geq$ 16) and those without (36). The identified phospholipids contained several proinflammatory compounds (e.g., linoleic acid [LA] or AA), which are released by PLA2 and are crucially implicated in proinflammatory processes (57, 58). This finding further underlines a lipid-inflammation-dependent pathway in MDD. In line with this, Hennebelle et al. report that in seasonal affective disorders (SAD), four oxylipins, which are oxidation products of polyunsaturated fatty acids, were increased in winter (38). Since oxylipins are involved in regulating proinflammatory processes, this suggests that season-dependent changes in omega-3/-6 metabolism underlie inflammatory states in SAD. However, it is important to mention that a smaller study by Kuwano et al. failed to identify any significant differences in the plasma lipidome of first-episode drug-naïve MDD patients ($N = 15$) compared to HCs ($N = 19$), but identifed two metabolites (tryptophan and kynurenine) that were significantly reduced in patients (41).

Therefore, due to the plethora of potential lipid species and inconsistent results of lipidomic studies in MDD, uncertainty prevails about which lipids are implicated in MDD pathophysiology and which lipids best segregate between MDD and HCs. Furthermore, no data on the time course of these processes exist in humans, while rodent studies provide some insight into the causal relation between the lipidome and depression models.

Rodent Studies

Important insights emerged from recent rodent studies investigating the lipidome in models of depression. One of the first rodent studies examining the lipidome in rodents used a 4 week antidepressant treatment and compared the prefrontal cortex of the rats with regard to changes in the lipidome (45). In the prefrontal cortex, robust significant reduction in the relative abundance of PC species (PC36:1, PC38:3, PC40:2, PC40:6, PC40:5, PC42:7, PC42:6, and PC42:5) and increases of LPC species (LPC16:0, LPC18:0, and LPC18:2) were identified in response to maprotiline and paroxetine, but not fluoxetine treatment indicating an increase in PLA2 activity and possible release of long-chain fatty acids on the rat brain lipidome (45). For maprotiline and paroxetine, an increase in Cer levels (Cer18:1/18:0, Cer18:1/20:0, Cer18:1/22:0,) was also observed, as well as a decrease in PE levels (PE36:4, PE36:5) and mixed changes with regard to the direction of change in SM levels (increase: SM18/16:0; decrease: SM18/24:0, SM18/24:1). PCs are the major lipids distributed in the cell membrane, while LPCs directly exert effects on membrane permeability, and SMs and Cers are also critically integrated in the membrane formation process. These results indicate that antidepressant treatments influence membrane formation, structure and permeability. Here, it is important to mention that the authors did not experimentally induce depression in the rodents and then treat them with antidepressant medication, but instead directly treated the rodents with antidepressant medication. Although this might be beneficial on a behavioral level, altering an organism's homeostasis might be related to adverse consequences with regard to its lipidome. However, the same group added behavioral testing to the reported lipidome changes for maprotiline and showed increased non-depressive behavior for maprotiline treatment (46). Interestingly, when rodents concomitantly experienced PLA2 suppression, increased depressive behavior could be observed indicating a crucial role of PLA2 activity with regard to antidepressant treatment (46). PLA2 hydrolyses the fatty acid from the sn-2 position of PCs, rendering the cleavage products available for subsequent biological actions increasing LPC, DAG, and TAG levels (59). Contrasting these results in a study using chronic restraint stress, the depressed rodents exhibited increased plasma levels of LPC (LPC18:1, LPC20:1, LPC-O16:2, LPC-O18:3) and decreased levels of PC (PC32:1, PC36:4, PC37:4, PC38:4, PC40:6, PC-O36:4, PC-O38:5) compared to control animals (43). However, a rodent study of chronic unpredictable stress (CUS; a commonly used paradigm in preclinical depression research) showed significant increases on brain lipid class level in the relative content of PC and PE levels in the stressed mice. A significant decrease in the relative content of PI levels could also be observed indicating membrane structure and function change due to chronic stress (44). Another study which used the CUS model revealed somewhat opposing changes in the rat brain lipidome and mainly in the prefrontal cortex, with increased LPC, LPE, and Cer levels and decreased PE, ether phosphatidylcholines (PC E), and SM levels (34). Interestingly, with regard to serotonin deficiency investigated in a genetic knockout model TPH2-/-, serotonin-deficient mice expressed corresponding differences in the lipid profile, with reduced levels in several PC, PE, PI species and increased levels in several LPC, LPE, and Cer species (60). Taken together, the rodent studies, unlike the human studies, form a more consistent picture, showing that experimentally induced depressive states reduced PC, PE, PI, and increased LPC, LPE, Cer, DAG and TAG levels.

LIPIDOME ASSOCIATIONS WITH GLUCOCORTICOIDS AND INFLAMMATORY MARKERS

After more than 30 years of biomarker research in MDD, hypercortisolism and chronic low grade inflammation are considered to be the two most consistent findings and the most salient biomarkers in MDD research (11). In the following, we provide an overview of the functional cross-talk between glucocorticoid secretion, inflammatory processes and the lipidome.

Studies by Mocking and colleagues have shown that in patients with recurrent MDD, salivary cortisol was negatively associated to fatty acid-metabolism in three fatty acids (arachidonic acid (AA), eicosapentaenoic acid (EPA), docosahexaenoic acid (DHA) (61). Furthermore, in a longitudinal study including 70 MDD patients and 51 matched controls, fatty acid-metabolism showed a significantly stronger negative relationship to salivary cortisol in patients than in the controls, while a stronger negative relationship between fatty acid-metabolism and cortisol levels was predictive for non-response to antidepressants in patients (62). Importantly, a rodent study examined the lipidome after exogeneous-corticosterone administration and several brain lipid alterations were observed [decrease in: PCs, PE; increase in: LPC, Cer, PA, phosphatidylglycerol (PG)], revealing a tight interconnectedness between glucocorticoids and brain lipids (34). However, other studies reported contradictory results with regard to chronic stress (44), or found that there was no effect of corticosterone administration on Cer levels or acid sphingomyelinase (Asm), which metabolizes SM to Cer (33). However, in these contradictory studies, differing forms of application and dosages were used (oral 0.25 mg mL^{-1} via drinking water vs. subcutaneous injections of 40 mg kg^{-1}) suggesting that higher doses of corticosterone administration reveal stronger changes in the rat brain lipidome. *In vitro* examinations further showed that dexamethasone-treated M-1 cells (a mammalian cell line from the cortical collecting duct) express higher phospholipase D (PLD) activity, which hydrolyzes PC to PA, subsequently leading to vesicle formation, budding, and fission from neurons (48). Increased PLD activity has also been related to neuro-inflammatory states via astrogliosis (63).

In line with this, a recently conducted lipidomic and genetic analysis in patients with MDD identified a shared genetic etiology between MDD and PC indicating markers of the PC-inflammation pathway as diagnostic markers for MDD (40). In addition, MDD patients were shown to demonstrate higher levels of AA and C-reactive protein (CRP; a marker for systemic inflammation) than those in HCs. In patients, AA correlates positively with CRP levels (64). Pro-inflammatory markers such as CRP have been shown to feature upstream in the inflammatory process, triggering PCs containing AA, which is subsequently released from the cell membrane via PLA2. This leaves necessary fatty acids available for prostaglandin production and further triggers subsequent pro-inflammatory processes (65). Pro-inflammatory markers were shown to increase PLA2 activity up to 14-fold (50). Recently, it has been shown that linoleic acid administration causes an increase in CRP secretion providing further evidence for a lipid-inflammation dependent pathway for MDD (57).

Therefore, it is suggested that lipidomic risk-profiles seem to predispose individuals to MDD and that these at-risk individuals subsequently become ill and show intensified glucocorticoid and inflammatory dysregulations. Thus, a testable model of the pathophysiology of MDD, as presented in **Figure 2**, emerges, suggesting that dysregulated candidate lipid networks increase the risk of MDD via direct effects on neurosignaling and their causal influence on hyper-cortisolism and systemic low grade inflammation (64).

CONCLUSION

Due to the clear integration of multiple identified lipids in the pathophysiology of MDD based on our systematic review, lipidomics emerges as a powerful approach to identify a diagnostic biomarker for MDD, with promising results stemming from pioneering studies. However, prediction power is currently insufficient to extract clinically applicable lipid biomarkers for MDD. Furthermore, several differential lipid species were identified for MDD, although somewhat inconsistent between studies (see **Supplementary Table 2**). However, the emerging pattern of reduced PC, PE, PI, and increased LPC, LPE, Cer, TAG, and DAG levels in response to depressed states needs to be replicated in independent studies using lipidomics analysis (20). Recent advances in the field of computational psychiatry may further increase the predictive power of lipidomics for MDD (66), while quantitative analyses of identified lipid species and sub-species are needed to evaluate the most predictive lipids. However, potential pathways linking the lipidome to MDD highlight the inflammatory system as well as the glucocorticoid system as important mediators (see **Figure 2**). Furthermore, the one problem that all of the presented human lipidomic studies in MDD have in common is their cross-sectional nature. Not a single longitudinal lipidomic study in patients with MDD has been carried out so far. Thus, no data on possible alterations of lipid profiles with regard to changes of the disease state are available to date. Although potential molecular pathways linking MDD with lipid profiles via inflammatory and steroidal dysregulations have been suggested (34, 44), only longitudinal lipidomic studies in large human samples including classical inflammatory markers as well as glucocorticoids will provide clarification as to whether the proposed pathophysiologic model can be validated o r not. Finally, lipid pathway enrichment analyses of the identified lipids such as provided by LIPEA (67) will further shed light on the underlying mechanisms of how perturbed lipid pathways are contributing to MDD paving the way to precision medicine and thus providing novel drug targets for more effective treatments in MDD.

AUTHOR CONTRIBUTIONS

AW designed and supported the systematic review and wrote the first draft of the manuscript. CC, KS, MG, CD, and CK contributed with important intellectual content and edited subsequent versions of the manuscript. SW supported the systematic review and created the art work.

FUNDING

We acknowledge support by the German Research Foundation and the Open Access Publication Funds of the TU Dresden.

ACKNOWLEDGMENTS

We would like to thank B.Sc. Johannes Steffen for supporting and conducting the systematic search of lipidomic studies in MDD/rodent models of depression. We would also like to thank Laura Mugford for language editing.

REFERENCES

1. Kessler RC. The costs of depression. *Psychiatr Clin N Am.* (2012) 35:1–14. doi: 10.1016/j.psc.2011.11.005
2. Merikangas K, Ames M, Cui L, Stang P, Ustun T, Von Korff M, et al. The impact of comorbidity of mental and physical conditions on role disability in the us adult household population. *Arch Gen Psychiatry* (2007) 64:1180–8. doi: 10.1001/archpsyc.64.10.1180
3. American Psychiatric Association. *Diagnostic and Statistical Manual of Mental Disorders (DSM-5®), 5th Edn.* Arlington, VA: American Psychiatric Pub (2013).
4. World Health Organisation (WHO). *Depression and Other Common Mental Disorders Global Health Estimates.* Geneva: World Health Organisation (2017).
5. Vos T, Abajobir AA, Abbafati C, Abbas KM, Abate KH, Abd-Allah F, et al. Global, regional, and national incidence, prevalence, and years lived with disability for 328 diseases and injuries for 195 countries, 1990-2016: a systematic analysis for the Global Burden of Disease Study 2016. *Lancet* (2017) 390:1211–59. doi: 10.1016/S0140-6736(17) 32154-2
6. Bogdan R, Nikolova YS, Pizzagalli DA. Neurogenetics of depression: a focus on reward processing and stress sensitivity. *Neurobiol Dis.* (2013) 52:12–23. doi: 10.1016/j.nbd.2012.05.007
7. Akil H, Gordon J, Hen R, Javitch J, Mayberg H, Mcewen B, et al. Treatment resistant depression: a multi-scale, systems biology approach. *Neurosci Biobehav Rev.* (2017) 84:272–88. doi: 10.1016/j.neubiorev.2017.08.019
8. Wager TD, Woo CW. Imaging biomarkers and biotypes for depression. *Nat Med.* (2017) 23:16–7. doi: 10.1038/nm.4264
9. Sanislow CA, Pine DS, Quinn KJ, Kozak MJ, Garvey MA, Heinssen RK, et al. Developing constructs for psychopathology research: research domain criteria. *J Abnorm Psychol.* (2010) 119:631–9. doi: 10.1037/a0020909
10. Regier DA, Kupfer DJ, Kuhl EA, Greiner L, Kraemer HC. DSM-5 field trials in the United States and Canada, part i: study design, sampling strategy, implementation, and analytic approaches. *Am J Psychiatry* (2013) 170:59–70. doi: 10.1176/appi.ajp.2012.12070999
11. Pariante CM. Why are depressed patients inflamed? A reflection on 20 years of research on depression, glucocorticoid resistance and inflammation. *Eur Neuropsychopharmacol.* (2017) 27:554–9. doi: 10.1016/j.euroneuro.2017.04.001
12. Simons K. How can Omic Science be improved? *Proteomics* (2018) 18:e1800039. doi: 10.1002/pmic.201800039
13. Shevchenko A, Simons K. Lipidomics: coming to grips with lipid diversity. *Nat Rev Mol Cell Biol.* (2010) 11:593–8. doi: 10.1038/nrm2934
14. Cannistraci CV, Ravasi T, Montevecchi FM, Ideker T, Alessio M. Nonlinear dimension reduction and clustering by minimum curvilinearity unfold neuropathic pain and tissue embryological classes. *Bioinformatics* (2010) 26:531–9. doi: 10.1093/bioinformatics/btq376
15. Lecun Y, Bengio Y, Hinton G. Deep learning. *Nature* (2015) 521:436–44. doi: 10.1038/nature14539
16. Ciucci S, Ge Y, Durán C, Palladini A, Jiménez-jiménez V, Martínez-sánchez LM, et al. Enlightening discriminative network functional modules behind Principal Component Analysis separation in differential-omic science studies. *Sci Rep.*(2017) 7:43946. doi: 10.1038/srep43946
17. Yugi K, Kubota H, Hatano A, Kuroda S. Trans-omics: how to reconstruct biochemical networks across multiple 'Omic' layers. *Trends Biotechnol.* (2016) 34:276–90. doi: 10.1016/j.tibtech.2015. 12.013
18. Drysdale AT, Grosenick L, Downar J, Dunlop K, Mansouri F, Meng Y, et al. Resting-state connectivity biomarkers define neurophysiological subtypes of depression. *Nat Med.* (2016) 23:28–38. doi: 10.1038/nm.4246
19. Hyde CL, Nagle MW, Tian C, Chen X, Paciga SA, Wendland JR, et al. Identification of 15 genetic loci associated with risk of major depression in individuals of European descent. *Nat Genet.* (2016) 48:1031–6. doi: 10.1038/ng.3623
20. Surma MA, Herzog R, Vasilj A, Klose C, Christinat N, Morin-Rivron D, et al. An automated shotgun lipidomics platform for high throughput, comprehensive, and quantitative analysis of blood plasma intact lipids. *Eur J lipid Sci Technol.* (2015) 117:1540–9. doi: 10.1002/ejlt.2015 00145
21. Bowden JA, Heckert A, Ulmer CZ, Jones CM, Koelmel JP, Abdullah L, et al. Harmonizing lipidomics : NIST interlaboratory comparison exercise for lipidomics using SRM 1950–metabolites in frozen human plasma. *J Lipid Res.* (2017) 58:2275–88. doi: 10.1194/jlr.M079012
22. Hannun YA, Obeid LM. Principles of bioactive lipid signalling: lessons from sphingolipids. *Nat Rev Mol Cell Biol.* (2008) 9:139–50. doi: 10.1038/nrm2329
23. Sud M, Fahy E, Cotter D, Brown A, Dennis EA, Glass CK, et al. LMSD: LIPID MAPS structure database. *Nucleic Acids Res.* (2007) 35:D527–32. doi: 10.1093/nar/gkl838
24. Quehenberger O, Dennis EA. The human plasma lipidome. *N Engl J Med.* (2011) 365:1812–23. doi: 10.1056/NEJMra1104901
25. Meer G Van, Voelker DR, Feigenson GW. Membrane lipids: where they are and how they behave. *Nat Rev Mol Cell Biol.* (2008) 9:112–24. doi: 10.1038/nrm2330
26. Schneider M, Levant B, Reichel M, Gulbins E, Kornhuber J, Müller CP. Lipids in psychiatric disorders and preventive medicine. *Neurosci Biobehav Rev.* (2017) 76:336–62. doi: 10.1016/j.neubiorev.2016.06.002

26. Schneider M, Levant B, Reichel M, Gulbins E, Kornhuber J, Müller CP. Lipids in psychiatric disorders and preventive medicine. *Neurosci Biobehav Rev.* (2017) 76:336–62. doi: 10.1016/j.neubiorev.2016.06.002
27. Tsui-Pierchala BA, Encinas M, Milbrandt J, Johnson EM. Lipid rafts in neuronal signaling and function. *Trends Neurosci.* (2002) 25:412–7. doi: 10.1016/S0166-2236(02)02215-4
28. Ledesma MD, Martin MG, Dotti CG. Lipid changes in the aged brain: effect on synaptic function and neuronal survival. *Prog Lipid Res.* (2012) 51:23–35. doi: 10.1016/j.plipres.2011.11.004
29. Tansey MG, Baloh RH, Milbrandt J, Johnson EM. GFRα-mediated localization of RET to lipid rafts is required for effective downstream signaling, differentiation, and neuronal survival. *Neuron* (2000) 25:611–23. doi: 10.1016/S0896-6273(00)81064-8
30. Simons K, Gerl MJ. Revitalizing membrane rafts: new tools and insights. *Nat Rev Mol Cell Biol.* (2010) 11:688–99. doi: 10.1038/nrm2977
31. Hallahan B, Ryan T, Hibbeln JR, Murray IT, Glynn S, Ramsden CE, et al. Efficacy of omega-3 highly unsaturated fatty acids in the treatment of depression. *Br J Psychiatry* (2016) 209:192–201. doi: 10.1192/bjp.bp.114.160242
32. Parekh A, Smeeth D, Milner Y, Thuret S. The Role of lipid biomarkers in major depression. (2017) 5:E5. doi: 10.3390/healthcare5010005.
33. Gulbins E, Palmada M, Reichel M, Lüth A, Böhmer C, Amato D, et al. Acid sphingomyelinase – ceramide system mediates effects of antidepressant drugs. *Nat Med.* (2013) 19:2–9. doi: 10.1038/nm.3214
34. Oliveira TG, Chan RB, Bravo F V, Miranda A, Silva RR, Zhou B, et al. The impact of chronic stress on the rat brain lipidome. *Mol Psychiatry* (2016) 21:80–88. doi: 10.1038/mp.2015.14
35. Aimo L, Liechti R, Hyka-nouspikel N, Kuznetsov D, Niknejad A, Gleizes A, et al. The SwissLipids knowledgebase for lipid biology. *Bioinformatics* (2015) 31:2860–6. doi: 10.1093/bioinformatics/btv285
36. Chan P, Suridjan I, Mohammad D, Herrmann N, Mazereeuw G, Hillyer LM, et al. Novel phospholipid signature of depressive symptoms in patients with coronary artery disease. *J Am Heart Assoc.* (2018) 7:e008278. doi: 10.1161/JAHA.117.008278
37. Demirkan A, Isaacs A, Ugocsai P, Liebisch G, Struchalin M, Rudan I, et al. Plasma phosphatidylcholine and sphingomyelin concentrations are associated with depression and anxiety symptoms in a Dutch family-based lipidomics study Ays. *J Psychiatr Res.* (2013) 47:357–62. doi: 10.1016/j.jpsychires.2012.11.001
38. Hennebelle M, Otoki Y, Yang J, Hammock BD, Levitt AJ, Taha AY, et al. Altered soluble epoxide hydrolase-derived oxylipins in patients with seasonal major depression: an exploratory study. *Psychiatry Res.* (2017) 252:94–101. doi: 10.1016/j.psychres.2017.02.056
39. Kim EY, Lee JW, Lee MY, Kim SH, Mok HJ, Ha K, et al. Serum lipidomic analysis for the discovery of biomarkers for major depressive disorder in drug-free patients. *Psychiatry Res.* (2018) 265:174–82. doi: 10.1016/j.psychres.2018.04.029
40. Knowles EEM, Huynh K, Meikle PJ, Göhring HHH, Olvera RL, Mathias SR, et al. The lipidome in major depressive disorder : shared genetic influence for ether-phosphatidylcholines, a plasma-based phenotype related to inflammation, and disease risk. *Eur Psychiatry* (2017) 43:44–50. doi: 10.1016/j.eurpsy.2017.02.479
41. Kuwano N, Kato TA, Setoyama D, Sato-Kasai M, Shimokawa N, Hayakawa K, et al. Tryptophan-kynurenine and lipid related metabolites as blood biomarkers for first-episode drug-naïve patients with major depressive disorder: an exploratory pilot case-control study. *J Affect Disord.* (2018) 231:74–82. doi: 10.1016/j.jad.2018.01.014
42. Liu X, Zheng P, Zhao X, Zhang Y, Hu C, Li J, et al. Plasma lipidomics reveals potential lipid markers of major depressive disorder. *Anal Bioanal Chem.* (2016) 408:6497–507. doi: 10.1007/s00216-016-9768-5
43. Chen S, Wei C, Gao P, Kong H, Jia Z, Hu C, et al. Effect of *Allium macrostemon* on a rat model of depression studied by using plasma lipid and acylcarnitine profiles from liquid chromatography/mass spectrometry. *J Pharm Biomed Anal.* (2014) 89:122–9. doi: 10.1016/j.jpba.2013.10.045
44. Faria R, Santana MM, Aveleira CA, Maciel E, Melo T, Santinha D, et al. Alterations in phospholipidomic profile in the brain of mouse model of depression induced by chronic unpredictable stress. *Neuroscience* (2014) 273:1–11. doi: 10.1016/j.neuroscience.2014.04.042
45. Lee LHW, Shui G, Farooqui AA, Wenk MR, Tan CH, Ong WY. Lipidomic analyses of the mouse brain after antidepressant treatment: evidence for endogenous release of long-chain fatty acids? *Int J Neuropsychopharmacol.* (2009) 12:953–64. doi: 10.1017/S146114570900995X
46. Lee LHW, Tan CH, Shui G, Wenk MR, Ong WY. Role of prefrontal cortical calcium independent phospholipase A2 in antidepressant-like effect of maprotiline. *Int J Neuropsychopharmacol.* (2012) 15:1087–98. doi: 10.1017/S1461145711001234
47. Moher D, Liberati A, Tetzlaff J, Altman DG. Preferred reporting items for systematic reviews and meta-analyses: the PRISMA statement. *J Clin Epidemiol.* (2009) 62:1006–12. doi: 10.1016/j.jclinepi.2009.06.005
48. Kim W, Lee M, Park M, Jung J, Uhlinger DJ, Kwak J. Dexamethasone enhances phospholipase D activity in M-1 cells. *Exp Mol Med.* (2000) 32:170–7. doi: 10.1038/emm.2000.28
49. Dolinsky VW, Douglas DN, Lehner R, Vance DE. Regulation of the enzymes of hepatic microsomal triacylglycerol lipolysis and re-esterification by the glucocorticoid dexamethasone. *Biochem J.* (2004) 974:967–74. doi: 10.1042/bj20031320
50. Pruzanski W, Wilmore DW, Suffredini A, Martich GD, Hoffman AGD, Browning JL, et al. Hyperphosoholipasemia A2 in human volunteers challenged with intravenous endotoxin. *Inflammation* (1992) 16:561–70. doi: 10.1007/BF00918980
51. Mondelli V, Vernon AC, Turkheimer F, Dazzan P, Pariante CM. Brain microglia in psychiatric disorders. *Lancet Psychiatry* (2017) 4:563–72. doi: 10.1016/S2215-0366(17)30101-3
52. Liu X, Zheng P, Zhao X, Zhang Y, Hu C, Li J, et al. Discovery and validation of plasma biomarkers for major depressive disorder classification based on liquid chromatography–mass spectrometry. *J Proteome Res.* (2015) 14:2322–30. doi: 10.1021/acs.jproteome.5b00144
53. Davis J, Goadrich M. The relationship between precision-recall and roc curves. In: *Proceedings of the 23rd International conference on Machine Learning.* New York, NY (2006) 233–40. doi: 10.1145/1143844.1143874
54. Liu Y, Yieh L, Yang T, Drinkenburg W, Peeters P, Steckler T, et al. Metabolomic biosignature differentiates melancholic depressive patients from healthy controls. *BMC Genomics* (2016) 17:669–86. doi: 10.1186/s12864-016-2953-2
55. Berglund L, Sacks F, Brunzell JD. Risk factors for cardiovascular disease : renewed interest in triglycerides Risk factors for cardiovascular disease : renewed interest in triglycerides. *Clin Lipidol.* (2017) 8:1–4. doi: 10.2217/clp.12.81
56. Cruciani-Guglielmacci C, Magnan C. Brain lipoprotein lipase as a regulator of energy balance. *Biochimie* (2017) 143:51–5. doi: 10.1016/j.biochi.2017.07.012
57. Smedman A, Basu S, Jovinge S, Fredrikson GN, Vessby B. Conjugated linoleic acid increased C-reactive protein in human subjects. *Br J Nutr.* (2005) 94:791–5. doi: 10.1079/BJN20041419
58. Su H, Liu R, Chang M, Huang J, Wang X. Dietary linoleic acid intake and blood inflammatory markers: a systematic review and meta-analysis of randomized controlled trials. *Food Funct.* (2017) 8:3091–103. doi: 10.1039/C7FO00433H
59. Burke JE, Dennis EA. Phospholipase A_2 structure/function, mechanism, and signaling. *J Lipid Res.* (2009) 50:S237–42. doi: 10.1194/jlr.R800033-JLR200
60. Weng R, Shen S, Burton C, Yang L, Nie H, Tian Y, et al. Lipidomic profiling of tryptophan hydroxylase 2 knockout mice reveals novel lipid biomarkers associated with serotonin deficiency. *Anal Bioanal Chem.* (2016) 408:2963–73. doi: 10.1007/s00216-015-9256-3
61. Mocking RJT, Ruhe HG, Assies J, Lok A, Koeter MWJ, Visser I, et al. Relationship between the hypothalamic–pituitary–adrenal-axis and fatty acid metabolism in recurrent depression. *Psychoneuroendocrinology* (2013) 38:1607–17. doi: 10.1016/j.psyneuen.2013.01.013
62. Mocking RJT, Verburg HF, Westerink AM, Assies J, Vaz FM, Koeter MWJ, et al. Fatty acid metabolism and its longitudinal relationship with the hypothalamic–pituitary–adrenal axis in major depression : associations with prospective antidepressant response. *Psychoneuroendocrinology* (2015) 59:1–13. doi: 10.1016/j.psyneuen.2015.04.027
63. Klein J. Functions and pathophysiological roles of phospholipase D in the brain. *J Neurochem.* (2005) 94:1473–87. doi: 10.1111/j.1471-4159.2005.03315.x

64. Mocking RJT, Nap TS, Westerink AM, Assies J, Vaz FM, Koeter MWJ, et al. Biological profiling of prospective antidepressant response in major depressive disorder: associations with (neuro) inflammation, fatty acid metabolism, and amygdala-reactivity. *Psychoneuroendocrinology* (2017) 79:84–92. doi: 10.1016/j.psyneuen.2017.02.019
65. Lozanski G, Berthier F, Kushner I. The sphingomyelin–ceramide pathway participates in cytokine regulation of C-reactive protein and serum amyloid A, but not a-fibrinogen. *Biochem J.* (1997) 328:271–5. doi: 10.1042/bj3280271
66. Huys QJM. Advancing clinical improvements for patients using the theory-driven and data-driven branches of computational psychiatry. *JAMA Psychiatry* (2018) 75:225–6. doi: 10.1001/jamapsychiatry.2017.4246
67. Acevedo A, Duran C, Ciucci S, Gerl M, Cannistraci CV. LIPEA: Lipid Pathway Enrichment Analysis. *bioRxiv* [Preprint] (2018). doi: 10.1101/274969

20

Toward Precision Psychiatry in Bipolar Disorder: Staging 2.0

Estela Salagre[1], *Seetal Dodd*[2,3,4], *Alberto Aedo*[1,5], *Adriane Rosa*[6,7,8], *Silvia Amoretti*[9], *Justo Pinzon*[1], *Maria Reinares*[1], *Michael Berk*[2,3,4,10], *Flavio Pereira Kapczinski*[11], *Eduard Vieta*[1*] and *Iria Grande*[1*]

[1] Barcelona Bipolar Disorders Program, Hospital Clinic, Institute of Neurosciences, University of Barcelona, IDIBAPS, CIBERSAM, Barcelona, Spain, [2] IMPACT Strategic Research Centre, Barwon Health, Deakin University, Geelong, VIC, Australia, [3] Department of Psychiatry, University of Melbourne, Parkville, VIC, Australia, [4] Orygen, The National Centre of Excellence in Youth Mental Health, Melbourne, VIC, Australia, [5] Bipolar Disorders Unit, Department of Psychiatry, School of Medicine, Pontificia Universidad Católica de Chile, Santiago, Chile, [6] Laboratory of Molecular Psychiatry, Hospital de Clínicas de Porto Alegre, Porto Alegre, Brazil, [7] Postgraduate Program: Psychiatry and Behavioral Science, Universidade Federal do Rio Grande do Sul (UFRGS), Porto Alegre, Brazil, [8] Department of Pharmacology and Postgraduate Program: Pharmacology and Therapeutics, Universidade Federal do Rio Grande do Sul (UFRGS), Porto Alegre, Brazil, [9] Barcelona Clínic Schizophrenia Unit, Hospital Clinic de Barcelona, CIBERSAM, Barcelona, Spain, [10] Florey Institute for Neuroscience and Mental Health, Parkville, VIC, Australia, [11] Department of Psychiatry & Behavioral Neurosciences, Mcmaster University, Hamilton, ON, Canada

Correspondence:
Eduard Vieta
evieta@clinic.cat
Iria Grande
igrande@clinic.cat

Personalized treatment is defined as choosing the "right treatment for the right person at the right time." Although psychiatry has not yet reached this level of precision, we are on the way thanks to recent technological developments that may aid to detect plausible molecular and genetic markers. At the moment there are some models that are contributing to precision psychiatry through the concept of staging. While staging was initially presented as a way to categorize patients according to clinical presentation, course, and illness severity, current staging models integrate multiple levels of information that can help to define each patient's characteristics, severity, and prognosis in a more precise and individualized way. Moreover, staging might serve as the foundation to create a clinical decision-making algorithm on the basis of the patient's stage. In this review we will summarize the evolution of the bipolar disorder staging model in relation to the new discoveries on the neurobiology of bipolar disorder. Furthermore, we will discuss how the latest and future progress in psychiatry might transform current staging models into precision staging models.

Keywords: bipolar disorder, staging, biomarkers, personalized psychiatry, prevention

INTRODUCTION

Bipolar disorder is a chronic psychiatric condition characterized by mood swings with both manic and depressive symptoms (1). Despite this general picture, bipolar disorder is a highly heterogeneous condition regarding clinical presentation, response to treatment and functional outcome (2, 3). Subsequent DSM and ICD versions have increasingly reflected this heterogeneity, for instance, by adding diagnosis and course specifiers (4). Still, the focus of current systems of classification remains largely cross-sectional and limited to clinical features (5). Moreover, these criteria apply to people with established disorder, but miss people in the prodromal phases of the illness (4).

Emerging data points to the need of a broader approach to bipolar disorder. There is increasing evidence that bipolar disorder is a neuroprogressive disorder, meaning that longer duration of the disease entails more pronounced changes at the clinical and neuropathological level, which may lead to treatment refractoriness and neuropsychological deficits (6, 7). Moreover, several studies support the notion of a prodromal stage before illness onset (8). In an attempt to introduce a longitudinal perspective of the illness in the diagnostic process which would include the earliest phases of bipolar disorder and guide treatment and prognosis, some authors have suggested incorporating the staging model in psychiatry (9–13).

The staging model is based on the concept that an illness progresses following an identifiable temporal progression, from at-risk or prodromal stages to chronic ones (10). Moreover, considering the neuroprogressive course of psychiatric disorders, the staging model assumes that treatment needs and response may differ according to stage. While early stages of the disease might show a better response to simpler treatment regimens, chronic stages might need more complex treatments and still show less clinical improvement (14). Consequently, defining the stage in which the patient is located may help clinicians to choose the treatment that is better adapted to the patient's needs (14). Additionally, the administration of a timely treatment precisely adapted to the stage in which the patient is located might modify or even prevent the progression to subsequent stages of the disease (10).

The staging model in bipolar disorder has been in constant development since its introduction in psychiatry. As new evidence on bipolar disorder has emerged, staging models were refined according to these new findings. In spite of this, experts supporting the staging model still warn that this model gives a standard vision of the progression of the disorder that might not suit every patient (15, 16).

New advances in the field of biological markers (e.g., molecular and neuroanatomical markers of illness vulnerability and/or progression), genetics (e.g., genetic markers or pharmacogenomics) or computer science (e.g., machine learning approaches) might provide current staging models of a higher level of precision regarding diagnosis, prognosis, and treatment choice (15, 16), allowing a more personalized approach to the patient.

The aim of this review is to summarize the evolution of the staging model in bipolar disorder in relation to the new discoveries on the course and neurobiology of the disease. Furthermore, we will discuss how the latest and ongoing progresses in psychiatry might transform current staging models into precision staging models.

THE EVOLUTION OF STAGING MODELS IN BIPOLAR DISORDER

The Dawn of Staging in Psychiatry: Fava and Kellner Staging Model (1993)

Fava and Kellner, in 1993, first proposed the application of the concept of staging to psychiatric disorders (9), as staging had shown to be useful in other complex diseases potentially severe if untreated, such as diabetes mellitus, cardiovascular diseases and neoplastic diseases. However, their staging model faced a major limitation in psychiatry research, which was the dearth of longitudinal studies assessing the progression of psychiatric disorders and the scarce data available on prodromal symptoms.

As a result, the staging model proposed by Fava and Kellner did not focus on the longitudinal course of bipolar disorder, but described the different stages that can be seen in a manic episode based on symptom severity (**Table 1**). Although their model referred only to the manic phase of the disease, Fava and Kellner provided the basis for future staging models in psychiatry.

The Spread of the Concept of Staging in Psychiatry: McGorry et al. (10)

In 2006, McGorry and colleagues introduced a staging model which highlighted the longitudinal course of psychiatric diseases in the psychotic spectrum, also integrating mood disorders (10). They underlined that the staging model does not imply that every patient needs to go through every stage. The main characteristic of McGorry and colleagues' model is that it is built on evidence on major psychiatric disorders jointly and not exclusively on data on bipolar disorder. Importantly, compiling evidence emerging from research on neurobiological correlates of psychotic disorders, allowed McGorry and colleagues to go one step forward and include some biological and endophenotypic markers in the earlier stages of their model (**Table 1**). They warned, though, that evidence on biological markers arose from studies that evaluated patients with long-established disease, raising the question whether these biological markers were inherent to psychiatric disorders or a consequence of illness duration.

They also incorporated some indicators of illness extent and progression -that is, functioning and cognitive impairment- in their staging model. They defended the importance of addressing social adaptation when assessing patients, as they noted that a person who already presents a great deal of collateral academic or social damage at illness onset may be less likely to respond to treatment and hence is more prone to have a worse prognosis. McGorry and colleagues have continued to progress a transdiagnostic staging model, arguing that the early stages are non-specific, although the later courses of different major psychiatric disorders can have divergent course and outcome patterns (17).

New Insights on Bipolar Disorder Progression: Berk et al. (11)

Although similar to and adapting from McGorry and colleagues' model (10), Berk and colleagues' model focused exclusively on bipolar disorder (11). At that moment, a growing body of evidence on a prodromal state for bipolar disorder started to appear (11). Besides identifying risk factors for bipolar disorder, mainly a positive family history of mood disorder and stressful life events (18–20), emerging studies on high-risk youth described a series of prodromal symptoms (21–23), therefore supporting the notion of a traceable at-risk stage.

TABLE 1 | Stage definition according to each staging model.

	Clinical stage definition				
	Fava and Kellner (9)	**McGorry et al. (10)**	**Berk et al. (11)**	**Kapczinski et al. (12)**	**Duffy (13)**
At-risk stages	**Stage 1:** Prodromal manic symptoms (increased self-confidence, energy and elated mood)	**Stage 0:** Increased risk of psychotic or severe mood disorder without symptoms *BIOMARKERS: Trait marker candidates and endophenotypes,* e.g., *Smooth Pursuit Eye Movements, P 50, Niacin sensitivity, Binocular rivalry, Prepulse Inhibition, Mismatch Negativity, Olfactory deficits, etc.*	**Stage 0:** Increased risk of severe mood disorder (e.g., family history, abuse, substance use) No specific symptoms currently	**Latent Stage:** At risk for developing BD, positive family history, mood or anxiety symptoms without criteria for threshold BD	**Stage 0:** **a) Classical Episodic Bipolar:** asymptomatic individuals + familial risk for classical BD or recurrent affective disorders **b) Spectrum bipolar:** asymptomatic individuals + familial risk for chronic psychotic disorders or atypical bipolar disorder.
		Stage 1a: Mild or non-specific symptoms, mild functional change or decline	**Stage 1a:** Mild or non-specific symptoms of mood disorder		**Stage 1:** **a) Classical Episodic Bipolar:** non-specific syndromes + familial risk for classical BD or recurrent affective disorders. **b) Spectrum bipolar:** non-specific syndromes and neurodevelopmental disorders + familial risk for chronic psychotic disorders or atypical BD.
		Stage 1b: Ultra high risk: moderate but subthreshold symptoms, moderate neurocognitive changes and functional decline (GAF<70) *BIOMARKERS: Niacin sensitivity, folate status, MRI and MRS changes, HPA axis dysregulation*	**Stage 1b:** Prodromal features: ultra-high risk		
Early stages	**Stage 2:** Hypomania	**Stage 2:** First episode of psychotic or severe mood disorder Full threshold disorder with moderate-severe symptoms, neurocognitive deficits and functional decline (GAF 30-50)	**Stage 2:** First-episode threshold mood disorder	**Stage I**: Well-defined periods of euthymia without overt psychiatric symptoms *BIOMARKERS:* ↑ *TNF-α*, ↓ *3-NT*	**Stage 2:** **a) Classical Episodic Bipolar:** minor mood and single episode depressive disorder + familial risk for classical BD or recurrent affective disorders. **b) Spectrum bipolar disorder:** negative syndrome + familial risk for chronic psychotic disorders or atypical BD.
Mid-stages	**Stage 3:** Manic episode without psychotic features	**Stage 3a:** Incomplete remission from first episode	**Stage 3a:** Recurrence of sub-threshold mood symptoms	**Stage II:** Symptoms in interepisodic periods related to comorbidities *BIOMARKERS:* ↓ *TNF-α*, ↓ *BDNF,* ↑ *3-NT*	**Stage 3:** **a) Classical Episodic Bipolar:** recurrent major depressive disorder. **b) Spectrum Bipolar:** attenuated psychotic syndrome

(Continued)

TABLE 1 | Continued

	Clinical stage definition				
	Fava and Kellner (9)	**McGorry et al. (10)**	**Berk et al. (11)**	**Kapczinski et al. (12)**	**Duffy (13)**
		Stage 3b: Recurrence/relapse of psychotic/mood disorder which stabilizes with treatment at a level of GAF, residual symptoms, or neurocognition below the best level achieved following remission from first episode	**Stage 3b:** First threshold relapse		
		Stage 3c: Specialist care services	**Stage 3c:** Multiple relapses		
Late stages	**Stage 4:** Manic episode with psychotic features	**Stage 4:** Severe, persistent or unremitting illness as judged on symptoms, neurocognition and disability criteria.	**Stage 4:** Persistent unremitting illness	**Stage III:** Marked impairment in cognition and functioning *BIOMARKERS: Morphometric changes in brain may be present,* ↑ *TNF-α*, ↓*BDNF*, ↑ *3-NT*	**Stage 4a:** **a) Classical Episodic Bipolar:** classic BD. **b) Spectrum bipolar:** mixed mania, psychotic/cyclic mania **Stage 4b:** **a) Classical Episodic Bipolar:** BD with residual symptoms. **b) Spectrum bipolar:** psychotic disorders.

BD, bipolar disorder; BDNF, brain-derived neurotrophic factor; GAF, Global Assessment of Functioning; HPA, hypothalamic–pituitary–adrenal; MRI, magnetic resonance imaging; MRS, magnetic resonance spectroscopy; TNF-α, tumor necrosis factor alpha; 3-NT, 3-nytrotyrosine.

Moreover, at that moment there was increasing evidence emerging from clinical, neuroimaging and neurocognitive studies that supported a progressive and deteriorating course of bipolar disorder (11). For instance, it had been reported that inter-episode periods were longer after the first episodes, but tended to shorten as the number of episodes increased (24). It had also been found that longer duration of the illness with multiple relapses seemed to be associated with increased medical comorbidities and increased suicidal risk (25). Furthermore, available evidence suggested that response to psychological and pharmacological treatments might not be the same over the illness course (26–29). Response to lithium, for example, seemed to be better if started early after illness onset (30, 31) and before multiple relapses had taken place (32). The number of episodes had also been found to be related to neuroanatomic changes in the brain (33). In 2002, Strakowski et al. (33) described increased lateral ventricular size in bipolar patients with multiple manic episodes, but not in first-episode patients. Likewise, evidence supported that a longer duration of illness and a larger number of episodes was associated with cognitive dysfunction which, in turn, seemed to involve a worse clinical course and functional disability (34). The authors hypothesized that all those alterations observed in the later stages of bipolar disorder were a consequence of progressive changes in the central nervous system due to subsequent mood episodes (6, 7). This phenomenon was called neuroprogression (6). Berk and colleagues suggested several possible pathways involved in neuroprogression including inflammation, oxidative stress, neurotrophins imbalance, mitochondrial dysfunction and epigenetics (6, 7).

Drawing all this evidence together, Berk and colleagues described a staging model with a special focus on the initial phases of the disease and number of episodes (**Table 1**).

The Ascendance of Biological Psychiatry: Kapczinski et al. (12)

Kapczinski and colleagues' model appeared at a moment when biological explanations gained prominence and risk phases were explained based on a gene-environmental (GxE) approach (12). For early stages, the GxE perspective suggested that individual genetic differences determine distinct resilience or vulnerability to environmental stress, placing individuals at different risk levels to develop bipolar disorder (35, 36). For late stages, this approach suggested that every individual has a different neuronal resilience to the deleterious effect of repetitive mood episodes (12). Along this line, Kapczinski et al. (37) adapted McEwens' notion of allostatic load to bipolar disorder (38). This concept implies that the interaction of neuroprogressive changes, somatic comorbidities and substance abuse leads to a dwindling resilience to life stress, especially if coping skills are poor (37). Hence, according to Post's kindling hypothesis (36), while stressful life events are an important trigger for first affective episodes, later on the course of the disease recurrences might take place without a clear environmental factor (37).

At that time, studies focusing on the pathophysiology of bipolar disorder reported a deregulation of oxidative and inflammatory pathways in bipolar disorder, especially during mood episodes (39–43), which came with a decrease in neurotrophic factors, like brain-derived neurotrophic factor (BDNF) (44–46). Importantly, it was also described that levels of neurotrophins, oxidative and inflammatory markers differed depending on illness stage (47, 48). For instance, compared to controls, the serum levels of the pro-inflammatory cytokine IL-6 were increased both in the early and late stages of bipolar disorder, while levels of BDNF and the anti-inflammatory cytokine IL-10 were decreased in late stages (meaning patients with 10–20 years of illness duration) but not in early stages (47). TNF-alpha levels appeared to be elevated throughout the illness course but were even higher in later stages (47). In addition, some parameters of oxidative stress, such as 3-nitrotyrosine, were found to be altered in the early and late stages of bipolar disorder, but not in controls (48). The activity of key enzymes in the glutathione pathway was found to be increased in late-stage patients compared with early-stage patients and controls (48). Hence, these data supported the hypothesis presented by Berk and colleagues indicating that neurotrophic, inflammatory and oxidative pathways may be involved in neuroprogression (6). Furthermore, neuroimaging findings also supported the concept of neuroprogression, as although some cerebral structures were shown to be already altered in early stages (49–51), longitudinal studies indicated that patients with repetitive mood episodes showed a progressive brain gray matter loss (52, 53). All these findings implied the identification of putative biomarkers that could be useful to distinguish between patients in early and late stages of bipolar disorder (54).

Psychosocial functioning was also gaining momentum as an outcome measure in bipolar disorder, since it had been demonstrated that symptomatic recovery is not equivalent to functional recovery (55). Psychosocial functioning involves domains such as work and education, leisure time, social and affective relationships or independent living (56), and it can be negatively affected by clinical variables and neurocognitive impairments (57).

Accordingly, Kapczinski and colleagues presented a model based on functioning that, moreover, incorporated cognition and biomarkers (12) (**Table 1**).

A Broader Vision of Bipolar Disorder: Duffy (13)

Duffy proposed a more integrative clinical staging model which described the natural history of bipolar disorder according to illness subtypes: the classical form of bipolar disorder (alternant manic-depressive episodes) vs. the broader bipolar spectrum (13). Duffy claimed that, while the classical form of bipolar disorder tended to follow the progressive course described in previous staging models (i.e., a recurrent and deteriorating course with an increasingly shorter inter-episodic period), other subtypes of bipolar disorder might present a different evolution (13). Evidence, for instance, supported that lithium non-responders showed a more chronic course and a higher-risk of non-affective disorders in family members (58, 59). Neuroimaging and genetic differences between classical lithium responsive bipolar patients and lithium non-responsive bipolar patients were also reported (60, 61). Moreover, her model was supported by longitudinal data showing differences between offspring of lithium responders and lithium non-responders regarding the prodromal period and longitudinal course of bipolar disorder. Offspring of lithium responders had a personal history of anxiety and sleep disorders before illness onset and, once bipolar disorder was established, tended to show an episodic remitting course with good response to lithium (62–64). In contrast, offspring of lithium non-responders manifested higher rates of early developmental alterations, attention deficits and cluster A personality traits (62–64) and, for those who developed bipolar disorder, illness course tended to be more torpid and response to anticonvulsant or atypical antipsychotic seemed to be better than to lithium (63). Thus, Duffy aimed to present an integrative staging model that describes the expected longitudinal course of classical episodic bipolar disorder and of bipolar spectrum disorder (**Table 1**).

WHEN STAGING IS NOT ENOUGH

Although different staging models have been proposed in bipolar disorder over the last 25 years, they still need to be better operationalized and validated by empirical research (14). The idea behind the different staging models is to allow defining, for every individual, the extent of illness progression in the moment of the evaluation (65). This can help to refine diagnosis, adjust prognosis and choose the best treatment according to illness stage (66). In this regard, authors have suggested some treatment approaches adapted to every stage: most models agree that prodromal stages would benefit from interventions targeted toward reducing stressors and increasing coping skills; early stages would benefit from patient and family psychoeducation and simpler pharmacological regimens; while mid-stages would need more intensive psychotherapies and more complex pharmacotherapies (12, 15). Clozapine or functional remediation therapies would be reserved for more chronic stages (15). Some individuals with highly refractory illness may need more "palliative" approaches focusing on reduction of side-effects and unnecessary polypharmacy, limited symptom control, identifying and targeting psychological and social problems, and setting realistic goals to aim for the best quality of life for people and their families within the envelope of their disability (67).

However, even if the staging model proposes stage-targeted treatments that might provide a better clinical outcome with less side effects, there are still differences among the patients of a particular stage. In consequence, "standard stage-adapted treatments" may not be useful for every patient at a particular stage (15) and increasing the level of precision in every stage would be desirable in order to achieve an even more personalized way of approaching the patient (16) (**Figure 1**).

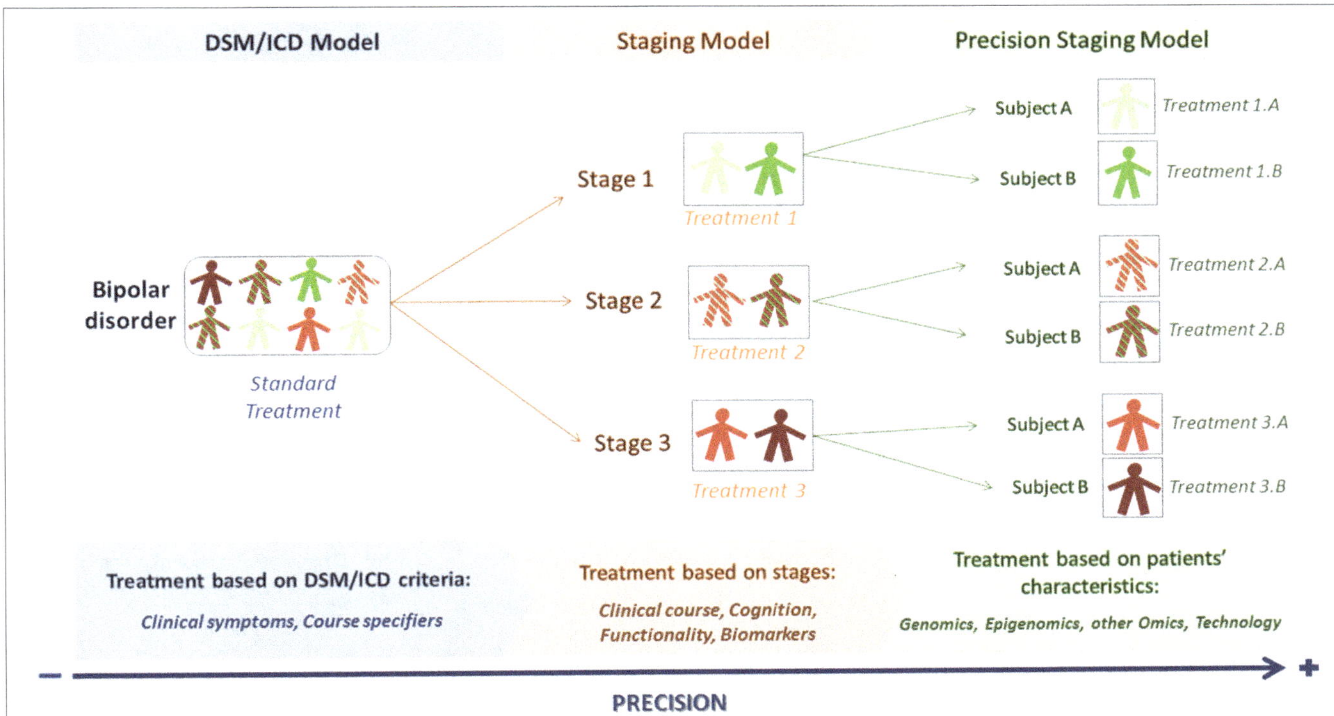

FIGURE 1 | From DSM/ICD to precision staging models. The DSM/ICD model classifies patients into particular conditions according to clinical-based criteria. DSM/ICD diagnosis can be refined by course specifiers. The staging model allows placing the patient in a particular stage according to the extent of illness progression, starting from at-risk stages (stage 1) to more chronic ones (stage 3). However, there can still be differences between patients within a particular stage. A precision staging model would then use the new advances on precision medicine to better characterize the patients and offer them a more personalized treatment.

FROM STAGING TO PRECISION STAGING MODELS

The aim of precision psychiatry is to offer the patient tailored medical decisions and treatments (68). For that purpose, precision psychiatry needs to integrate biographical, clinical and biological information regarding each individual (69). In addition, precision psychiatry is envisaged to benefit from the coming advances in technological, data, and computer science to aid diagnostic processes and treatment provision. A precision staging model would ideally incorporate all these recent progresses into the appropriate stage (**Table 2**).

Many advances in precision medicine are related to genomics. Genomics have led to improvements in staging models in some branches of medicine, especially cancer (70). However, psychiatric disorders are genetically complex conditions and their genetic underpinnings remain to be determined. Still, international consortia that comprise samples from several countries have brought some light on risk loci associated with bipolar disorder (71, 72). These collaborative genome-wide association studies (GWAS) allow overcoming replication difficulties often seen in genetic studies due to small sample sizes. One of these studies analyzed genomic data on a sample of 40,000 bipolar patients and replicated the discoveries of previous GWAS studies regarding several single-nucleotide polymorphisms (SNPs) statistically associated with the disease, including variants within the genes CACNA1C, ANK3, MAD1L1, and SYNE1 (73). Two new risk loci were also identified (73). Moreover, the Psychiatric Genomics Consortium has recently identified specific loci that distinguish between bipolar disorder and schizophrenia (74). Genetic markers promise to be valuable at the earliest stages of bipolar disorder, as the main aim of mental health approaches at at-risk and early stages is to predict disease vulnerability and make accurate diagnosis. So far, though, little of the advances in genomics have translated into clinically useful tools.

Besides genetic markers, screening for risk factors and epigenetic modifications may be another useful tool at at-risk stages of the disease, given that stressful life events, particularly childhood trauma, can alter DNA methylation and may increase the risk of developing mood disorders (75). Concordant with this, childhood verbal, physical, or sexual abuse has been related to a worse illness course (76).

Risk calculators are another promising tool for at-risk stages (77), as the multifactorial and polygenic nature of bipolar disorder makes it improbable that a single factor can accurately predict its onset (78). The Pittsburgh Bipolar Offspring Study group (BIOS) has recently developed a risk calculator to predict the 5-year risk of bipolar disorder onset in offspring of parents with bipolar disorder combining dimensional measures of mania, depression, anxiety, mood lability, psychosocial functioning, and parental age of mood disorder onset (79). Although their findings need to be replicated, the model seemed to be able to predict onset of bipolar disorder with an area under the curve (AUC) in the receiver operating characteristic curve analysis of 0.76 and might be of potential value for youth at ultra-high risk for BD. Machine learning, a field of computer science that studies and constructs

TABLE 2 | Potential precision staging model in bipolar disorder.

Clinical stage	Definition	Potential precision tools and precision interventions	Domains to be assessed and general interventions
At-risk stages	Increased risk of severe mood disorder (e.g., family history, abuse, substance use) Asymptomatic or non-specific symptoms of mood disorder	Individualized evaluation of risk/protective factors Genetic and epigenetic markers	a) Clinical domain b) Cognitive domain c) Functional domain d) Comorbidities domain: - Substance use - Physical comorbidities - Psychological comorbidities
	Prodromal features: ultra-high risk	Genetic and epigenetic markers Risk Calculator Risk biomarkers (molecular, neuroimaging) Machine learning approaches (risk for bipolar disorder) Cognitive enhancers	
Early stages	First-episode threshold mood disorder	Genetic markers of treatment response Epigenetics (illness course) Biomarkers of treatment response and illness progression Machine learning approaches (suicide risk) mHealth (Psychoeducation, monitoring)	Pharmacotherapy and psychological interventions adapted to each individual physical and psychological comorbidities
Mid stages	Clinical relapse	Pharmacogenetic tests Biomarkers of treatment response and illness progression Machine learning approaches (suicide risk) mHealth (psychoeducation, monitoring) Functional remediation tailored to patients' profile, cognitive enhancers	Substance use intervention
Late stages	Persistent unremitting illness	Functional remediation tailored to patients' profile	

algorithms that can learn from large number of data, find patterns and make predictions (80), might also be useful to estimate the individual probability of a particular outcome (80, 81). Mourao-Miranda et al. (82), for instance, found that machine learning approaches using functional magnetic resonance imaging (fMRI) data could differentiate between adolescents genetically at-risk for mood disorders and healthy controls with a 75% accuracy (sensitivity = 75%, specificity = 75%). Moreover, those at-risk adolescents who developed an anxiety or depressive disorder at follow-up showed significantly higher predictive probabilities, therefore suggesting that predictive probabilities could be used as a score to predict which at-risk adolescents would develop a mood disorder in the future (82).

Early and middle stages of bipolar disorder may benefit from progress in the field of pharmacogenomics. This is the study of genetic variations that affects individual response to drugs and vulnerability to adverse effects (83). After the first acute episode, selecting the best treatment for the patient, both in terms of efficacy and tolerability is a necessary but complex task. International consortiums in genetics, such as the International Consortium of Lithium Genetics (ConLiGen) (71), have worked to disentangle genetic variants associated with treatment response, mainly response to lithium. In 2016, the ConLiGen consortium uniformly phenotyped 2,563 bipolar patients and reported a genome-wide significant association with a locus of four linked SNPs on chromosome 21 and lithium response (84). Another recent GWAS performed by the ConLiGen consortium displayed that bipolar patients with a low genetic load for schizophrenia showed a better response to lithium (85). Pharmacogenetic screening for hepatic cytochrome P450 genetic polymorphisms can also be helpful in the near future to predict tolerability and side effects of psychiatric treatments (86). While the precise patient profile that would benefit from these tests remains to be elucidated, pharmacogenetic tests are kept for selected patients with unusual patterns of drug response or unexpected adverse reactions (83, 87).

Less progress has been made in the field of biological markers in the last few years and data on molecular and neuroimaging biomarkers is still contradictory and limited by the heterogeneity between studies and the poor specificity of the putative biomarkers (88). Although evidence is not yet compelling, some biological markers have been suggested to be associated with increased risk of conversion to bipolar disorder, and therefore may be useful when assessing subjects at at-risk stages. fMRI studies report that frontal hyperactivation during working memory paradigms may be associated with genetic risk for bipolar disorder (89, 90). In more established stages, neuroimaging might be useful to monitor treatment response (91). Also, a preliminary study using a voxel-based morphometry-pattern classification approach was able to distinguish between patients with unipolar and bipolar depression based on structural gray matter differences (92). Studies on biological markers have also suggested that peripheral concentrations of BDNF could be used to discriminate unipolar depression from bipolar depression (93, 94), but evidence is not clear (95). This would be of the utmost importance in the earliest stages of the disease, considering that bipolar disorder is often misdiagnosed since the index episode is frequently depressive. In consequence, patients are treated with antidepressants and the introduction of a mood stabilizer is delayed until the first manic episode is detected, which may negatively affect illness course and prognosis (8).

Regarding other molecular markers, hypothalamic-pituitary-adrenal (HPA) axis dysfunction is thought to be one of the pathways involved in neuroprogression in bipolar disorder (96), but it has also been suggested to be a useful trait marker in high-risk individuals (97, 98). Alterations in neurotransmitters transporters have been suggested as markers of bipolar disorder (96), but there is no evidence on changes in neurotransmitters according to illness stage. Regarding later stages of bipolar disorder, recent studies have reported higher levels of TNF-alpha and IL-6 in late stages of bipolar disorder (99, 100). Similarly, Soeiro-de Souza and colleagues described that patients with recurrent episodes showed increased oxidative and inflammatory markers, which were related to the number of manic episodes (101). Further, increased inflammation, increased oxidative stress and reduced telomere length have been suggested as possible mechanistic links between psychiatric diseases like bipolar disorder and other systemic diseases, such as endocrine or cardiovascular diseases (102–105). Hence, the identification of a deregulation on those pathways related to both psychiatric and somatic diseases may have therapeutic implications (106). For instance, bipolar patients exhibiting persistently increased low-grade inflammation (107) might benefit from anti-inflammatory treatment strategies and from periodic screening of systemic conditions like metabolic syndrome (106). Considering these data, screening for physical comorbidities seems especially important in middle and late stages of the disease, albeit protecting against complications like physical comorbidities or substance abuse should be a priority at every stage of the disease.

Cognition is another important domain that needs an individualized evaluation throughout all the stages of bipolar disorder (108). On one hand, cognitive reserve, defined as the ability of a brain to cope with brain pathology in order to minimize symptoms (109), may be useful in early stages to predict neurocognitive performance in patients with bipolar disorder (110), as it has been found that lower estimated cognitive reserve is associated with worse performance in neuropsychological tests and more functional impairment (110, 111). Similarly, a recent study on first-episode psychosis has found that those patients with affective psychosis with a greater cognitive reserve showed a higher socioeconomic status, better functioning and greater verbal memory performance (112). This study also emphasizes the need to explore the impact of specific interventions, like physical activities and hobbies, on cognitive reserve, since it could be useful to guide the development of personalized treatment programs (112). Therefore, cognitive enhancing strategies might be key in the early stages and not necessarily in the late stages of the disease. On the other hand, evidence points to a heterogeneous cognitive profile in bipolar patients both in "cold" and "hot" cognition (113–115). The presence of such heterogeneous cognitive profiles among patients with bipolar disorder might be taken into account to design more tailored cognitive remediation therapies adapted to each individual needs (116–118). Cognitive deficits may also limit long-term psychosocial functioning, which means that patients with greater cognitive impairment are more likely to experience poorer outcomes. Previously, we showed that patients in stage I and healthy controls had similar functioning patterns. In addition, a strong linear association was found between functioning and clinical stages, suggesting a progressive functional decline from stage I through to stage IV of bipolar disorder. These findings provide further support to the clinical staging model in bipolar disorder, indicating that bipolar patients lie on a continuum of disorder progression ranging from periods of favorable functioning to others of incomplete functional recovery (118). The link between variables related to the course of the illness, cognitive deficits and functioning suggests that early intervention is crucial to prevent illness progression and to improve cognitive/functional outcome. Some studies have also found different profiles of psychosocial functioning in patients with bipolar disorder, which should also be taken into consideration in the framework of a personalized approach (3, 119).

All these advances should complement regular clinical practice, which already contains elements of staging and precision psychiatry. The assessment of the patient's particular symptoms, such as his/her distinctive early signs of relapse, predominant polarity (i.e., the "tendency" to present more depressive or manic relapses) (120) or individual suicide risk (121) is regularly done in clinical settings and is essential to monitor the patient evolution and guide treatment selection. Technological advances used in everyday life, encompassed in the concept of mobile Health (mHealth), might be a valuable tool to help clinicians to collect individualized data on illness course and monitor illness progression (122). For instance, changes in activity, geolocation or sleep patterns may help to detect early signs of mood relapse (123, 124). Additionally, smartphone apps can be used to empower patients with bipolar disorder to detect prodromal symptoms of relapse by providing them personalized psychoeducational messages (125, 126). New methods like machine learning approaches might also be useful in the future to help predict suicide risk (127, 128).

DISCUSSION

In this review we describe the evolution of the staging model in bipolar disorder since its introduction into psychiatry. The first staging models in bipolar disorder were initially based on evidence derived from cross-sectional studies, but longitudinal studies and data on neuroimaging, peripheral biomarkers, cognition, psychosocial functioning, and prodromal symptoms have successively enriched the staging models (66). We have also described several elements of precision psychiatry that could be incorporated in future precision staging models.

The main advantage of staging and precision medicine is the recognition that a reductionist clinical approach based on the presence or absence of a series of symptoms is not enough to design an adequate therapeutic strategy. These symptoms need to be considered in the light of the illness progression and, most importantly, of the patient's own clinical evolution. For instance, the presence of a switching or non-switching pattern should be considered when evaluating a patient, as it has prognostic implications and therefore might impact staging. As highlighted in a review by Salvadore et al. (129), patients showing a switching pattern [i.e., patients showing a "sudden transition from a mood episode to another episode of the opposite polarity" (129)] usually spend less time in remission, show higher comorbidity rates and substance abuse and are at a higher risk of suicide attempt (129). While mood symptoms will of course still be the cornerstone of bipolar disorder diagnosis, other elements should be likewise considered as they can be as informative as clinical symptoms (9, 10, 12, 15). As such, everyday difficulties, cognitive complains, substance abuse or comorbidities can be markers of illness severity or stage specifiers and merit an individualized assessment and treatment. Social and personal losses due to the illness and previous personality should also be included in a standard evaluation throughout the stages and be given the attention they deserve (10). Patients' insight and perception of the disease should be carefully assessed, as these are important prognosis and therapeutic factors, especially in early stages (8). Medication load, treatment satisfaction, and compliance should be also carefully assessed, as it might influence disease progression. While this way of approaching the patient is naturally adopted by most clinicians and many guidelines, it remains underrepresented in diagnostic manuals (5). In any case, this approach is more in line with the World Health Organization definition of health: "Health is a state of complete physical, mental and social well-being and not merely the absence of disease or infirmity"[1]. The inclusion of self-report measures of well-being in research and clinical care in bipolar disorder may contribute to take into consideration the patient's perspective when assessing the efficacy and usefulness of pharmacological and psychological interventions (130).

Another important point of clinical staging is the assumption that prodromal phases of the disease can be also identified and targeted. The possibility of making an early diagnosis radically changes the way how bipolar disorder in particular, and psychiatric diseases in general, have hitherto been managed. At-risk stages are rather non-specific, though. In consequence, the prodromal period has also been preferably defined as "at risk mental states" (17), as a prodrome is defined as "any symptom that signals the impending onset of a disease" (131) and evidence does not support this definition. On one hand, data from the field of ultra-high risk in psychosis shows that disease onset is not deterministic and a significant proportion of the at-risk youth show a remission of these early symptoms (132). On the other hand, these early symptoms are not specific to any disease but can progress into several possible psychiatric conditions (64). In the absence of specific genetic markers for bipolar disorder or very precise risk calculators, transdiagnostic preventive interventions aimed to reduce stress, educate on mental-well-being and prevent substance abuse are preferable at these at-risk stages (133). Implementing early interventions that include enhancing

[1] WHO. http://apps.who.int/gb/bd/PDF/bd47/EN/constitution-en.pdf?ua=1. 1946

cognitive reserve by increasing mental stimulation (reading and cognitive exercises), introducing physical exercise and leisure activities or building social skills and social interaction, may provide a set of skills that can help to cope better with the disease (134–136). This kind of preventive interventions or "positive habits" could even be implemented at school or primary care, which could help to reduce stigma on mental health by educating the population on the importance of taking care of mental well-being (133).

In this regard, it has been suggested that a transdiagnostic staging model might be more adequate for the study of at-risk phases, while disorder-specific models are more useful once the fully-develop disorder emerges (15). It is necessary to bear in mind that psychiatric disorders are dynamic and clinical symptoms may evolve over time, requiring a change in diagnosis (137). Nevertheless, the general staging approach supported by stage specifiers should still be useful to assess illness severity regardless of changes in DSM or ICD diagnosis.

Biomarkers also face the problem of lack of specificity. Alterations in the inflammatory or oxidative systems have been found across several psychiatric and medical diagnoses (138). Again, biomarkers could be more stage-specific than illness-specific and be conceived as an additional tool for the assessment of illness risk or treatment outcome. Low sensitivity and replicability seems a bigger handicap. Moreover, most published data on biomarkers are based on the currently commercially available ELISA kits, which is also a limiting factor. State-of-the-art techniques widely used in precision medicine might help to overcome these limitations. A multi-omic approach, meaning using genomic, epigenomics, transcriptomics, proteomics, metabolomics, metagenomics, and lipidomics data, combined with environmental information gathered, for instance, through mobile devices, could help to identify more sensitive biomarkers panels to guide diagnosis and treatment choice (69). However, as these "omic" platforms cannot be used in regular clinical practice, the potential discoveries arising from these platforms need to be translated into an immuno-based assay, which is a more viable option. New strategies with a more integrative approach between clinical factors and biological markers are being proposed in biomarker research of lithium response, which are expected to shed some light on precision drug prescription (139).

Precision in psychiatry implies embracing the multifactoriality of psychiatric diseases and the need to incorporate in the patient's assessment a range of biological and environmental factors that interact with each other in a dynamic way. Moreover, the biological and environmental factors involved in illness onset and progression are particular to every patient, as it is the way they interact (17). The use of personal devices to monitor the trajectories of patients at anytime and anywhere might help to deepen our knowledge on the complex interaction between biological and environmental factors. They can also allow evaluating less studied markers, such as sleep or chronobiological markers, which may turn out to be very informative (140). Moreover, further studies on epigenetics or mitochondrial genomes might identify novel factors involved in this complex disease (141). Similar to what is being developed in the field of psychosis, research on bipolar disorder could benefit from consortia sharing data to develop machine learning algorithms to help the prediction of bipolar disorder onset (17, 142).

A major limitation of current staging models is the absence of an agreement on the definition of stages. Moreover, operationalized cut-off points are lacking, probably due to the lack of longitudinal studies assessing patients according to stages, the absence of clear and reproducible neurobiological markers defining every stage and the intrinsic heterogeneity of psychiatric illnesses (15, 16, 143). Therefore, the current proposed models of staging are mainly theoretical and need to be validated for the moment. Additionally, participants of the available studies assessing differences between early and late stages of bipolar disorder include subjects attending specialized clinics, hence probably representing more severe forms of bipolar disorder (16). Moreover, it should be noted that precision medicine is still in its early beginnings, meaning that findings on genomics, genetic markers, and epigenetics are preliminary and need to be replicated before being integrated in any model of classification.

Until more solid information is available on the biology of the disease, though, the staging models can be based on pragmatic variables, like number of episodes and impact on cognition and functionality. A staging system based on characteristics that can be easily measured allows to standardize it and make it available and applicable in a broader number of clinical settings and countries worldwide (144).

Regardless of what the future brings, personalized medicine means "patient-centered care," therefore the choice among those new diagnostic techniques or treatments should be subject to a consensus between the clinician and the patient, especially considering the new ethical challenges that precision psychiatry brings with it (145). While psychiatrists can offer their expertise, patients opinions and preferences should play a central role in treatment decisions through shared decision-making (145).

AUTHOR CONTRIBUTIONS

ES was responsible for conception and design as well as initial drafting of the manuscript. All other authors (SD, AA, AR, SA, JP, MR, MB, FK, EV, and IG) were responsible for revising the manuscript critically for important intellectual content of the version of the manuscript to be published. All authors read and approved the final manuscript.

ACKNOWLEDGMENTS

AR would like to thank the support of the CNPq PQ Process 305705-2015-9. MB is supported by a NHMRC Senior Principal Research Fellowship (1059660). EV is grateful for the support received from the Instituto de Salud Carlos III, Ministry of Economy and Competitiveness of Spain (PI 12/00912), integrated into the Plan Nacional de I+D+I and cofunded by ISCIII-Subdirección General de Evaluación and Fondo Europeo de Desarrollo Regional (FEDER); Centro para la

Investigación Biomédica en Red de Salud Mental (CIBERSAM), Secretaria d Universitats i Recerca del Departament d'Economia i Coneixement (2014_SGR_398), Seventh European Framework Programme (ENBREC), and the Stanley Medical Research Institute. IG is supported by the Instituto de Salud Carlos III, Ministry of Economy, and Competitiveness of Spain [Juan Rodés Contract (JR15/00012) and a grant (PI16/00187)] integrated into the Plan Nacional de I+D+I and cofunded by ISCIII-Subdirección General de Evaluación and Fondo Europeo de Desarrollo Regional (FEDER).

REFERENCES

1. Grande I, Berk M, Birmaher B, Vieta E. Bipolar disorder. *Lancet* (2016) 387:1561–72. doi: 10.1016/S0140-6736(15)00241-X
2. Solomon DA, Leon AC, Coryell WH, Endicott J, Li C, Fiedorowicz JG, et al. Longitudinal course of bipolar I disorder: duration of mood episodes. *Archi Gene Psychiatry* (2010) 67:339–47. doi: 10.1001/archgenpsychiatry.2010.15
3. Sole B, Bonnin CM, Jimenez E, Torrent C, Torres I, Varo C, et al. Heterogeneity of functional outcomes in patients with bipolar disorder: a cluster-analytic approach. *Acta Psychiatr Scand.* (2018) 137:516–27. doi: 10.1111/acps.12871
4. de Dios C, Goikolea JM, Colom F, Moreno C, Vieta E. Bipolar disorders in the new DSM-5 and ICD-11 classifications. *Revista de Psiquiatria y Salud Mental* (2014) 7: 79–85. doi: 10.1016/j.rpsm.2014.07.005
5. Vieta E. DSM-5.1. *Acta Psychiatr Scand.* (2016) 134:187–8. doi: 10.1111/acps.12624
6. Berk M Neuroprogression: pathways to progressive brain changes in bipolar disorder. *Int J Neuropsychopharmacol.* (2009) 12:441–5. doi: 10.1017/S1461145708009498
7. Berk M, Kapczinski F, Andreazza AC, Dean OM, Giorlando F, Maes M, et al. Pathways underlying neuroprogression in bipolar disorder: focus on inflammation, oxidative stress and neurotrophic factors. *Neuroscience Biobehav Rev.* (2011) 35:804–17. doi: 10.1016/j.neubiorev.2010.10.001
8. Vieta E, Salagre E, Grande I, Carvalho AF, Fernandes BS, Berk M, et al. Early intervention in bipolar disorder. *Am J Psychiatry* (2018) 175:411–426. doi: 10.1176/appi.ajp.2017.17090972
9. Fava GA, Kellner R. Staging: a neglected dimension in psychiatric classification. *Acta Psychiatrica Scand.* (1993) 87:225–30. doi: 10.1111/j.1600-0447.1993.tb03362.x
10. McGorry PD, Hickie IB, Yung AR, Pantelis C, Jackson HJ. Clinical staging of psychiatric disorders: a heuristic framework for choosing earlier, safer and more effective interventions. *Australian N Zeal J Psychiatry* (2006) 40:616–22. doi: 10.1080/j.1440-1614.2006.01860.x
11. Berk M, Conus P, Lucas N, Hallam K, Malhi GS, Dodd S, et al. Setting the stage: from prodrome to treatment resistance in bipolar disorder. *Bipolar Disord.* (2007) 9:671–8. doi: 10.1111/j.1399-5618.2007.00484.x
12. Kapczinski F, Dias VV, Kauer-Sant'Anna M, Frey BN, Grassi-Oliveira R, Colom F, et al. Clinical implications of a staging model for bipolar disorders. *Expert Rev Neurotherapeut.* (2009) 9:957–66. doi: 10.1586/ern.09.31
13. Duffy A. Toward a comprehensive clinical staging model for bipolar disorder: integrating the evidence. *Can J Psychiatry* (2014) 59:659–66. doi: 10.1177/070674371405901208
14. Vieta E, Reinares M, Rosa AR. Staging bipolar disorder. *Neurotoxicity Res.* (2011) 19:279–85. doi: 10.1007/s12640-010-9197-8
15. Berk M, Post R, Ratheesh A, Gliddon E, Singh A, Vieta E, et al. Staging in bipolar disorder: from theoretical framework to clinical utility. *World Psychiatry* (2017) 16:236–44. doi: 10.1002/wps.20441
16. Fernandes BS, Berk M. Staging in bipolar disorder: one step closer to precision psychiatry. *Revista Brasileira de Psiquiatria* (2017) 39:88–9. doi: 10.1590/1516-4446-2017-3902
17. McGorry PD, Hartmann JA, Spooner R, Nelson B. Beyond the "at risk mental state" concept: transitioning to transdiagnostic psychiatry. *World Psychiatry* (2018) 17:133–42. doi: 10.1002/wps.20514
18. Hillegers MH, Burger H, Wals M, Reichart CG, Verhulst FC, Nolen WA, et al. Impact of stressful life events, familial loading and their interaction on the onset of mood disorders: study in a high-risk cohort of adolescent offspring of parents with bipolar disorder. *Br J Psychiatry* (2004) 185:97–101. doi: 10.1192/bjp.185.2.97
19. Kessing LV, Agerbo E, Mortensen PB. Major stressful life events and other risk factors for first admission with mania. *Bipolar Disord.* (2004) 6:122–9. doi: 10.1111/j.1399-5618.2004.00102.x
20. McGuffin P, Rijsdijk F, Andrew M, Sham P, Katz R, Cardno A. The heritability of bipolar affective disorder and the genetic relationship to unipolar depression. *Archi Gener Psychiatry* (2003) 60:497–502. doi: 10.1001/archpsyc.60.5.497
21. Thompson KN, Conus PO, Ward JL, Phillips LJ, Koutsogiannis J, Leicester S, et al. The initial prodrome to bipolar affective disorder: prospective case studies. *J Affect Disord.* (2003) 77:79–85. doi: 10.1016/S0165-0327(02)00100-3
22. Egeland JA, Shaw JA, Endicott J, Pauls DL, Allen CR, Hostetter AM, et al. Prospective study of prodromal features for bipolarity in well Amish children. *J Am Acad Child Adoles Psychiatry* (2003) 42:786–96. doi: 10.1097/01.CHI.0000046878.27264.12
23. Shaw JA, Egeland JA, Endicott J, Allen CR, Hostetter AM. A 10-year prospective study of prodromal patterns for bipolar disorder among Amish youth. *J Am Acad Child Adoles Psychiatry* (2005) 44:1104–11. doi: 10.1097/01.chi.0000177052.26476.e5
24. Kessing LV, Mortensen PB, Bolwig TG. Clinical definitions of sensitisation in affective disorder: a case register study of prevalence and prediction. *J Affect Disord.* (1998) 47:31–9. doi: 10.1016/S0165-0327(97)00081-5
25. Angst F, Stassen HH, Clayton PJ, Angst J. Mortality of patients with mood disorders: follow-up over 34–38 years. *J Affect Disord.* (2002) 68:167–81. doi: 10.1016/S0165-0327(01)00377-9
26. Berk M, Brnabic A, Dodd S, Kelin K, Tohen M, Malhi GS, et al. Does stage of illness impact treatment response in bipolar disorder? empirical treatment data and their implication for the staging model and early intervention. *Bipolar Disord.* (2011) 13:87–98. doi: 10.1111/j.1399-5618.2011.00889.x
27. Scott J, Paykel E, Morriss R, Bentall R, Kinderman P, Johnson T, et al. Cognitive-behavioural therapy for severe and recurrent bipolar disorders: randomised controlled trial. *Br J Psychiatry* (2006) 188:313–20. doi: 10.1192/bjp.188.4.313
28. Colom F, Reinares M, Pacchiarotti I, Popovic D, Mazzarini L, Martinez-Aran A, et al. Has number of previous episodes any effect on response to group psychoeducation in bipolar patients? A 5-year follow-up post hoc analysis. *Acta Neuropsychiatrica* (2010) 22:50–3. doi: 10.1111/j.1601-5215.2010.00450.x
29. Reinares M, Colom F, Rosa AR, Bonnin CM, Franco C, Sole B, et al. The impact of staging bipolar disorder on treatment outcome of family psychoeducation. *J Affect Disord.* (2010) 123:81–6. doi: 10.1016/j.jad.2009.09.009
30. Franchini L, Zanardi R, Smeraldi E, Gasperini M. Early onset of lithium prophylaxis as a predictor of good long-term outcome. *Eur Arch Psychiatry Clin Neurosci.* (1999) 249:227–30. doi: 10.1007/s004060050091
31. Berk M, Daglas R, Dandash O, Yucel M, Henry L, Hallam K, et al. Quetiapine v. lithium in the maintenance phase following a first episode of mania: randomised controlled trial. *Br J Psychiatry* (2017) 210:413–21. doi: 10.1192/bjp.bp.116.186833
32. Swann AC, Bowden CL, Calabrese JR, Dilsaver SC, Morris DD. Differential effect of number of previous episodes of affective disorder on response to lithium or divalproex in acute mania. *Am J Psychiatry* (1999) 156:1264–6.
33. Strakowski SM, DelBello MP, Zimmerman ME, Getz GE, Mills NP, Ret J, et al. Ventricular and periventricular structural volumes in first- versus multiple-episode bipolar disorder. *Am J Psychiatry* (2002) 159:1841–7. doi: 10.1176/appi.ajp.159.11.1841
34. Martinez-Aran A, Vieta E, Colom F, Torrent C, Reinares M, Goikolea JM, et al. Do cognitive complaints in euthymic bipolar patients reflect

objective cognitive impairment? *Psychother Psychosomat.* (2005) 74:295–302. doi: 10.1159/000086320

35. Caspi A, Moffitt TE. Gene-environment interactions in psychiatry: joining forces with neuroscience. *Nat Rev Neurosci.* (2006) 7:583–90. doi: 10.1038/nrn1925
36. Post RM. Kindling and sensitization as models for affective episode recurrence, cyclicity, and tolerance phenomena. *Neurosci Biobehav Rev.* (2007) 31:858–73. doi: 10.1016/j.neubiorev.2007.04.003
37. Kapczinski F, Vieta E, Andreazza AC, Frey BN, Gomes FA, Tramontina J, et al. Allostatic load in bipolar disorder: implications for pathophysiology and treatment. *Neurosci Biobehav Rev.* (2008) 32:675–92. doi: 10.1016/j.neubiorev.2007.10.005
38. McEwen BS. Stress, adaptation, and disease. allostasis and allostatic load. *Ann N York Acad Sci.* (1998) 840:33–44. doi: 10.1111/j.1749-6632.1998.tb09546.x
39. Andreazza AC, Cassini C, Rosa AR, Leite MC, de Almeida LM, Nardin P, et al. Serum S100B and antioxidant enzymes in bipolar patients. *J Psychiatric Res.* (2007) 41:523–9. doi: 10.1016/j.jpsychires.2006.07.013
40. O'Brien SM, Scully P, Scott LV, Dinan TG. Cytokine profiles in bipolar affective disorder: focus on acutely ill patients. *J Affect Disord.* (2006) 90:263–7. doi: 10.1016/j.jad.2005.11.015
41. Gergerlioglu HS, Savas HA, Bulbul F, Selek S, Uz E, Yumru M. Changes in nitric oxide level and superoxide dismutase activity during antimanic treatment. *Progress Neuro-Psychopharmacol Biol Psychiatry* (2007) 31:697–702. doi: 10.1016/j.pnpbp.2006.12.020
42. Ortiz-Dominguez A, Hernandez ME, Berlanga C, Gutierrez-Mora D, Moreno J, Heinze G, et al. Immune variations in bipolar disorder: phasic differences. *Bipolar Disord.* (2007) 9:596–602. doi: 10.1111/j.1399-5618.2007.00493.x
43. Brietzke E, Stertz L, Fernandes BS, Kauer-Sant'anna M, Mascarenhas M, Escosteguy Vargas A, et al. Comparison of cytokine levels in depressed, manic and euthymic patients with bipolar disorder. *J Affect Disord.* (2009) 116:214–7. doi: 10.1016/j.jad.2008.12.001
44. Cunha AB, Frey BN, Andreazza AC, Goi JD, Rosa AR, Goncalves CA, et al. Serum brain-derived neurotrophic factor is decreased in bipolar disorder during depressive and manic episodes. *Neurosci Lett.* (2006) 398:215–9. doi: 10.1016/j.neulet.2005.12.085
45. Machado-Vieira R, Dietrich MO, Leke R, Cereser VH, Zanatto V, Kapczinski F, et al. Decreased plasma brain derived neurotrophic factor levels in unmedicated bipolar patients during manic episode. *Biol Psychiatry* (2007) 61:142–4. doi: 10.1016/j.biopsych.2006.03.070
46. Rosa AR, Frey BN, Andreazza AC, Cereser KM, Cunha AB, Quevedo J, et al. Increased serum glial cell line-derived neurotrophic factor immunocontent during manic and depressive episodes in individuals with bipolar disorder. *Neurosci Lett.* (2006) 407:146–50. doi: 10.1016/j.neulet.2006.08.026
47. Kauer-Sant'Anna M, Kapczinski F, Andreazza AC, Bond DJ, Lam RW, Young LT, et al. Brain-derived neurotrophic factor and inflammatory markers in patients with early- vs. late-stage bipolar disorder. *Int J Neuropsychopharmacol.* (2009) 12:447–58. doi: 10.1017/S1461145708009310
48. Andreazza AC, Kapczinski F, Kauer-Sant'Anna M, Walz JC, Bond DJ, Goncalves CA, et al. 3-Nitrotyrosine and glutathione antioxidant system in patients in the early and late stages of bipolar disorder. *J Psychiatry Neurosci.* (2009) 34:263–71.
49. Farrow TF, Whitford TJ, Williams LM, Gomes L, Harris AW. Diagnosis-related regional gray matter loss over two years in first episode schizophrenia and bipolar disorder. *Biol Psychiatry* (2005) 58:713–23. doi: 10.1016/j.biopsych.2005.04.033
50. Koo MS, Levitt JJ, Salisbury DF, Nakamura M, Shenton ME, McCarley RW. A cross-sectional and longitudinal magnetic resonance imaging study of cingulate gyrus gray matter volume abnormalities in first-episode schizophrenia and first-episode affective psychosis. *Arch Gener Psychiatry* (2008) 65:746–60. doi: 10.1001/archpsyc.65.7.746
51. Rosso IM, Killgore WD, Cintron CM, Gruber SA, Tohen M, Yurgelun-Todd DA. Reduced amygdala volumes in first-episode bipolar disorder and correlation with cerebral white matter. *Biol Psychiatry* (2007) 61:743–9. doi: 10.1016/j.biopsych.2006.07.035
52. Moorhead TW, McKirdy J, Sussmann JE, Hall J, Lawrie SM, Johnstone EC, et al. Progressive gray matter loss in patients with bipolar disorder. *Biol Psychiatry* (2007) 62:894–900. doi: 10.1016/j.biopsych.2007.03.005
53. Frey BN, Zunta-Soares GB, Caetano SC, Nicoletti MA, Hatch JP, Brambilla P, et al. Illness duration and total brain gray matter in bipolar disorder: evidence for neurodegeneration? *Eur Neuropsychopharmacol.* (2008) 18:717–22. doi: 10.1016/j.euroneuro.2008.04.015
54. Kapczinski F, Dias VV, Kauer-Sant'Anna M, Brietzke E, Vazquez GH, Vieta E, et al. The potential use of biomarkers as an adjunctive tool for staging bipolar disorder. *Progress Neuro-psychopharmacol Biol Psychiatry* (2009) 33:1366–71. doi: 10.1016/j.pnpbp.2009.07.027
55. Rosa AR, Reinares M, Michalak EE, Bonnin CM, Sole B, Franco C, et al. Functional impairment and disability across mood states in bipolar disorder. *Value Health* (2010) 13:984–8. doi: 10.1111/j.1524-4733.2010.00768.x
56. Rosa AR, Sanchez-Moreno J, Martinez-Aran A, Salamero M, Torrent C, Reinares M, et al. Validity and reliability of the functioning assessment short test (FAST) in bipolar disorder. *Clin Pract Epidemiol Mental Health* (2007) 3:5. doi: 10.1186/1745-0179-3-5
57. Bonnin CM, Martinez-Aran A, Torrent C, Pacchiarotti I, Rosa AR, Franco C, et al. Clinical and neurocognitive predictors of functional outcome in bipolar euthymic patients: a long-term, follow-up study. *J Affect Disord.* (2010) 121:156–60. doi: 10.1016/j.jad.2009.05.014
58. Grof P, Alda M, Grof E, Zvolsky P, Walsh M. Lithium response and genetics of affective disorders. *J Affect Disord.* (1994) 32:85–95. doi: 10.1016/0165-0327(94)90066-3
59. Passmore MJ, Garnham J, Duffy A, MacDougall M, Munro A, Slaney C, et al. Phenotypic spectra of bipolar disorder in responders to lithium versus lamotrigine. *Bipolar Disord.* (2003) 5:110–4. doi: 10.1034/j.1399-5618.2003.00026.x
60. Kruger S, Alda M, Young LT, Goldapple K, Parikh S, Mayberg HS. Risk and resilience markers in bipolar disorder: brain responses to emotional challenge in bipolar patients and their healthy siblings. *Am J Psychiatry* (2006) 163:257–64. doi: 10.1176/appi.ajp.163.2.257
61. Turecki G, Grof P, Grof E, D'Souza V, Lebuis L, Marineau C, et al. Mapping susceptibility genes for bipolar disorder: a pharmacogenetic approach based on excellent response to lithium. *Mol Psychiatry* (2001) 6:570–8. doi: 10.1038/sj.mp.4000888
62. Duffy A, Alda M, Crawford L, Milin R, Grof P. The early manifestations of bipolar disorder: a longitudinal prospective study of the offspring of bipolar parents. *Bipolar Disord.* (2007) 9:828–38. doi: 10.1111/j.1399-5618.2007.00421.x
63. Duffy A, Alda M, Milin R, Grof P. A consecutive series of treated affected offspring of parents with bipolar disorder: is response associated with the clinical profile? *Can J Psychiatry.* (2007) 52:369–76. doi: 10.1177/070674370705200606
64. Duffy A, Horrocks J, Doucette S, Keown-Stoneman C, McCloskey S, Grof P. The developmental trajectory of bipolar disorder. *Br J Psychiatry* (2014) 204:122–8. doi: 10.1192/bjp.bp.113.126706
65. Berk M, Berk L, Dodd S, Cotton S, Macneil C, Daglas R, et al. Stage managing bipolar disorder. *Bipolar Disord.* (2014) 16:471–7. doi: 10.1111/bdi.12099
66. Kapczinski F, Magalhaes PV, Balanza-Martinez V, Dias VV, Frangou S, Gama CS, et al. Staging systems in bipolar disorder: an International Society for Bipolar Disorders Task Force Report. *Acta Psychiatrica Scand.* (2014) 130:354–63. doi: 10.1111/acps.12305
67. Berk M, Berk L, Udina M, Moylan S, Stafford L, Hallam K, et al. Palliative models of care for later stages of mental disorder: maximizing recovery, maintaining hope, and building morale. *Australian N Zeal J Psychiatry* (2012) 46:92–9. doi: 10.1177/0004867411432072
68. Vieta E. Personalised medicine applied to mental health: Precision psychiatry. *Revista de Psiquiatria y Salud Mental* (2015) 8:117–8. doi: 10.1016/j.rpsm.2015.03.003
69. Fernandes BS, Williams LM, Steiner J, Leboyer M, Carvalho AF, Berk M. The new field of 'precision psychiatry'. *BMC Med.* (2017) 15:80. doi: 10.1186/s12916-017-0849-x
70. Berger MF, Mardis ER. The emerging clinical relevance of genomics in cancer medicine. *Nat Rev Clin Oncol.* (2018) 15:353–65. doi: 10.1038/s41571-018-0002-6

71. Schulze TG, Alda M, Adli M, Akula N, Ardau R, Bui ET, et al. The International Consortium on Lithium Genetics (ConLiGen): an initiative by the NIMH and IGSLI to study the genetic basis of response to lithium treatment. *Neuropsychobiology* (2010) 62:72–8. doi: 10.1159/000314708

72. Patrick F. Sullivan, Arpana Agrawal, Cynthia M. Bulik, Ole A. Andreassen, Anders D. Børglum, Gerome Breen, et al. Psychiatric genomics: an update and an agenda. *Am J Psychiatry* (2017) 175:15–27. doi: 10.1176/appi.ajp.2017.17030283

73. Hou L, Bergen SE, Akula N, Song J, Hultman CM, Landen M, et al. Genome-wide association study of 40,000 individuals identifies two novel loci associated with bipolar disorder. *Hum Mol Genet.* (2016) 25:3383–94. doi: 10.1093/hmg/ddw181

74. Bipolar Disorder and Schizophrenia Working Group of the Psychiatric Genomics Consortium. Genomic Dissection of Bipolar Disorder and Schizophrenia, Including 28 Subphenotypes. *Cell* (2018) 173:1705–15.e16. doi: 10.1016/j.cell.2018.05.046

75. Fries GR, Li Q, McAlpin B, Rein T, Walss-Bass C, Soares JC, et al. The role of DNA methylation in the pathophysiology and treatment of bipolar disorder. *Neurosci Biobehav Rev.* (2016) 68:474–88. doi: 10.1016/j.neubiorev.2016.06.010

76. Post RM, Altshuler LL, Kupka R, McElroy SL, Frye MA, Rowe M, et al. Verbal abuse, like physical and sexual abuse, in childhood is associated with an earlier onset and more difficult course of bipolar disorder. *Bipolar Disord.* (2015) 17:323–30. doi: 10.1111/bdi.12268

77. Dipnall JF, Pasco JA, Berk M, Williams LJ, Dodd S, Jacka FN, et al. Getting RID of the blues: Formulating a Risk Index for Depression (RID) using structural equation modeling. *Australian N Zeal J Psychiatry* (2017) 51:1121–33. doi: 10.1177/0004867417726860

78. Vieta E, Berk M, Schulze TG, Carvalho AF, Suppes T, Calabrese JR, et al. Bipolar disorders. *Nat Rev Dis Primers* (2018) 4:18008. doi: 10.1038/nrdp.2018.8

79. Hafeman DM, Merranko J, Goldstein TR, Axelson D, Goldstein BI, Monk K, et al. Assessment of a person-level risk calculator to predict new-onset bipolar spectrum disorder in youth at familial risk. *JAMA Psychiatry* (2017) 74:841–[illegible]. doi: 10.1001/jamapsychiatry.2017.1763

80. Bzdok D, Altman N, Krzywinski M. Statistics versus machine learning. *Nat Methods* (2018) 15:233. doi: 10.1038/nmeth.4642

81. Luo W, Phung D, Tran T, Gupta S, Rana S, Karmakar C, et al. Guidelines for developing and reporting machine learning predictive models in biomedical research: a multidisciplinary view. *J Med Internet Res.* (2016) 18:e323. doi: 10.2196/jmir.5870

82. Mourao-Miranda J, Oliveira L, Ladouceur CD, Marquand A, Brammer M, Birmaher B, et al. Pattern recognition and functional neuroimaging help to discriminate healthy adolescents at risk for mood disorders from low risk adolescents. *PLoS ONE* (2012) 7:e29482. doi: 10.1371/journal.pone.0029482

83. Foulds JA, Maggo SD, Kennedy MA. Personalised prescribing in psychiatry: has pharmacogenomics delivered on its promise? *Aust N Z J Psychiatry* (2016) 50:509–10. doi: 10.1177/0004867416640099

84. Hou L, Heilbronner U, Degenhardt F, Adli M, Akiyama K, Akula N, et al. Genetic variants associated with response to lithium treatment in bipolar disorder: a genome-wide association study. *Lancet* (2016) 387:1085–93. doi: 10.1016/S0140-6736(16)00143-4

85. Amare AT, Schubert KO, Hou L, Clark SR, Papiol S, Heilbronner U, et al. Association of polygenic score for schizophrenia and hla antigen and inflammation genes with response to lithium in bipolar affective disorder: a genome-wide association study. *JAMA Psychiatry* (2018) 75:65–74. doi: 10.1001/jamapsychiatry.2017.3433

86. Singh AB, Baune BT, Hamilton A, Das P, Outhred T, Morris G, et al. Psychotropic pharmacogenetics - Distraction or destiny? *Aust N Z J Psychiatry* (2017) 51:665–7. doi: 10.1177/0004867417715687

87. Perez V, Salavert A, Espadaler J, Tuson M, Saiz-Ruiz J, Saez-Navarro C, et al. Efficacy of prospective pharmacogenetic testing in the treatment of major depressive disorder: results of a randomized, double-blind clinical trial. *BMC Psychiatry* (2017) 17:250. doi: 10.1186/s12888-017-1412-1

88. Castano-Ramirez OM, Sepulveda-Arias JC, Duica K, Diaz Zuluaga AM, Vargas C, Lopez-Jaramillo C. Inflammatory markers in the staging of bipolar disorder: a systematic review of the literature. *Rev Colomb Psiquiatr.* (2018) 47:119–2[illegible]. doi: 10.1016/j.rcp.2017.01.004

89. Drapier D, Surguladze S, Marshall N, Schulze K, Fern A, Hall MH, et al. Genetic liability for bipolar disorder is characterized by excess frontal activation in response to a working memory task. *Biol Psychiatry* (2008) 64:513–20. doi: 10.1016/j.biopsych.2008.04.038

90. Ladouceur CD, Diwadkar VA, White R, Bass J, Birmaher B, Axelson DA, et al. Fronto-limbic function in unaffected offspring at familial risk for bipolar disorder during an emotional working memory paradigm. *Dev Cogn Neurosci.* (2013) 5:185–96. doi: 10.1016/j.dcn.2013.03.004

91. McDonald C. Brain structural effects of psychopharmacological treatment in bipolar disorder. *Curr Neuropharmacol.* (2015) 13:445–57. doi: 10.2174/1570159X13666150403231654

92. Redlich R, Almeida JJ, Grotegerd D, Opel N, Kugel H, Heindel W, et al. Brain morphometric biomarkers distinguishing unipolar and bipolar depression. A voxel-based morphometry-pattern classification approach. *JAMA Psychiatry* (2014) 71:1222–30. doi: 10.1001/jamapsychiatry.2014.[illegible]100

93. Fernandes BS, Gama CS, Kauer-Sant'Anna M, Lobato MI, Belmonte-de-Abreu P, Kapczinski F. Serum brain-derived neurotrophic factor in bipolar and unipolar depression: a potential adjunctive tool for differential diagnosis. *J Psychiatr Res.* (2009) 43:1200–4. doi: 10.1016/j.jpsychires.2009.04.010

94. Li Z, Zhang C, Fan J, Yuan C, Huang J, Chen J, et al. Brain-derived neurotrophic factor levels and bipolar disorder in patients in their first depressive episode: 3-year prospective longitudinal study. *Br J Psychiatry* (2014) 205:29–35. doi: 10.1192/bjp.bp.113.134064

95. Nuernberg GL, Aguiar B, Bristot G, Fleck MP, Rocha NS. Brain-derived neurotrophic factor increase during treatment in severe mental illness inpatients. *Transl Psychiatry* (2016) 6:e985. doi: 10.1038/tp.2016.227

96. Sigitova E, Fisar Z, Hroudova J, Cikankova T, Raboch J. Biological hypotheses and biomarkers of bipolar disorder. *Psychiatry Clin Neurosci.* (2017) 71:77–103. doi: 10.1111/pcn.12476

97. Duffy A, Lewitzka U, Doucette S, Andreazza A, Grof P. Biological indicators of illness risk in offspring of bipolar parents: targeting the hypothalamic-pituitary-adrenal axis and immune system. *Early Interv Psychiatry* (2012) 6:128–37. doi: 10.1111/j.1751-7893.2011.00323.x

98. Ellenbogen MA, Hodgins S, Linnen AM, Ostiguy CS. Elevated daytime cortisol levels: a biomarker of subsequent major affective disorder? *J Affect Disord.* (2011) 132:265–9. doi: 10.1016/j.jad.2011.01.007

99. Grande I, Magalhaes PV, Chendo I, Stertz L, Panizutti B, Colpo GD, et al. Staging bipolar disorder: clinical, biochemical, and functional correlates. *Acta Psychiatr Scand.* (2014) 129:437–44. doi: 10.1111/acps.12268

100. Tatay-Manteiga A, Balanza-Martinez V, Bristot G, Tabares-Seisdedos R, Kapczinski F, Cauli O. Clinical staging and serum cytokines in bipolar patients during euthymia. *Prog Neuropsychopharmacol Biol Psychiatry* (2017) 77:194–201. doi: 10.1016/j.pnpbp.2017.04.028

101. Soeiro-de-Souza MG, Andreazza AC, Carvalho AF, Machado-Vieira R, Young LT, Moreno RA. Number of manic episodes is associated with elevated DNA oxidation in bipolar I disorder. *Int J Neuropsychopharmacol.* (2013) 16:1505–12. doi: 10.1017/S1461145713000047

102. Hatch JK, Scola G, Olowoyeye O, Collins JE, Andreazza AC, Moody A, et al. Inflammatory markers and brain-derived neurotrophic factor as potential bridges linking bipolar disorder and cardiovascular risk among adolescents. *J Clin Psychiatry* (2017) 78:e286-e93. doi: 10.4088/JCP.[illegible]6m10762

103. Powell TR, Dima D, Frangou S, Breen G. Telomere Length and Bipolar Disorder. *Neuropsychopharmacology* (2018) 43:445–53. doi: 10.1038/npp.2017.125

104. de Melo LGP, Nunes SOV, Anderson G, Vargas HO, Barbosa DS, Galecki P, et al. Shared metabolic and immune-inflammatory, oxidative and nitrosative stress pathways in the metabolic syndrome and mood disorders. *Prog Neuropsychopharmacol Biol Psychiatry* (2017) 78:34–50. doi: 10.1016/j.pnpbp.2017.04.027

105. Barbe-Tuana FM, Parisi MM, Panizzutti BS, Fries GR, Grun LK, Guma FT, et al. Shortened telomere length in bipolar disorder: a comparison of the early and late stages of disease. *Rev Bras Psiquiatr.* (2016) 38:281–6. doi: 10.1590/1516-4446-2016-1910

106. Rosenblat JD, McIntyre RS. Bipolar disorder and immune dysfunction: epidemiological findings, proposed pathophysiology and clinical implications. *Brain Sci.* (2017) 7:E144. doi: 10.3390/brainsci7110144

107. Fernandes BS, Steiner J, Molendijk ML, Dodd S, Nardin P, Goncalves CA, et al. C-reactive protein concentrations across the mood spectrum in bipolar

disorder: a systematic review and meta-analysis. *Lancet Psychiatry* (2016) 3:1147–56. doi: 10.1016/S2215-0366(16)30370-4
108. Miskowiak KW, Burdick KE, Martinez-Aran A, Bonnin CM, Bowie CR, Carvalho AF, et al. Assessing and addressing cognitive impairment in bipolar disorder: the International society for bipolar disorders targeting cognition task force recommendations for clinicians. *Bipolar Disord.* (2018) 20:184–94. doi: 10.1111/bdi.12595
109. Stern Y. What is cognitive reserve? Theory and research application of the reserve concept. *J Int Neuropsychol Soc.* (2002) 8:448–60. doi: 10.1017/S1355617702813248
110. Grande I, Sanchez-Moreno J, Sole B, Jimenez E, Torrent C, Bonnin CM, et al. High cognitive reserve in bipolar disorders as a moderator of neurocognitive impairment. *J Affect Disord.* (2017) 208:621–7. doi: 10.1016/j.jad.2016.10.012
111. Anaya C, Torrent C, Caballero FF, Vieta E, Bonnin Cdel M, Ayuso-Mateos JL. Cognitive reserve in bipolar disorder: relation to cognition, psychosocial functioning and quality of life. *Acta Psychiatr Scand.* (2016) 133:386–98. doi: 10.1111/acps.12535
112. Amoretti S CB, Torrent C, Mezquida G, Lobo A, González-Pinto A, Parellada M, et al. Cognitive reserve as an outcome predictor: first-episode affective versus non-affective psychosis *Acta Psychiatr Scand.* (2018) 138:441–55. doi: 10.1111/acps.12949
113. Roux P, Raust A, Cannavo AS, Aubin V, Aouizerate B, Azorin JM, et al. Cognitive profiles in euthymic patients with bipolar disorders: results from the FACE-BD cohort. *Bipolar Disord.* (2017) 19:146–53. doi: 10.1111/bdi.12485
114. Varo C, Jimenez E, Sole B, Bonnin CM, Torrent C, Valls E, et al. Social cognition in bipolar disorder: focus on emotional intelligence. *J Aff Disord.* (2017) 217:210–7. doi: 10.1016/j.jad.2017.04.012
115. Jimenez E, Sole B, Arias B, Mitjans M, Varo C, Reinares M, et al. Characterizing decision-making and reward processing in bipolar disorder: a cluster analysis. *Eur Neuropsychopharmacol.* (2018) 28:863–74. doi: 10.1016/j.euroneuro.2018.04.001
116. Cotrena C, Damiani Branco L, Ponsoni A, Milman Shansis F, Paz Fonseca R. Neuropsychological clustering in bipolar and major depressive disorder. *J Int Neuropsychol Soc.* (2017) 23:584–93. doi: 10.1017/S1355617717000418
117. Miskowiak KW, Ott CV, Petersen JZ, Kessing LV. Systematic review of randomized controlled trials of candidate treatments for cognitive impairment in depression and methodological challenges in the field. *Eur Neuropsychopharmacol.* (2016) 26:1845–67. doi: 10.1016/j.euroneuro.2016.09.641
118. Rosa AR, Magalhaes PV, Czepielewski L, Sulzbach MV, Goi PD, Vieta E, et al. Clinical staging in bipolar disorder: focus on cognition and functioning. *J Clin Psychiatry* (2014) 75:e450–6. doi: 10.4088/JCP.13m08625
119. Reinares M, Papachristou E, Harvey P, Mar Bonnin C, Sanchez-Moreno J, Torrent C, et al. Towards a clinical staging for bipolar disorder: defining patient subtypes based on functional outcome. *J Affect Disord.* (2013) 144:65–71. doi: 10.1016/j.jad.2012.06.005
120. Popovic D, Reinares M, Goikolea JM, Bonnin CM, Gonzalez-Pinto A, Vieta E. Polarity index of pharmacological agents used for maintenance treatment of bipolar disorder. *Eur. Neuropsychopharmacol.* (2012) 22:339–46. doi: 10.1016/j.euroneuro.2011.09.008
121. Jimenez E, Arias B, Mitjans M, Goikolea JM, Ruiz V, Brat M, et al. Clinical features, impulsivity, temperament and functioning and their role in suicidality in patients with bipolar disorder. *Acta Psychiatrica Scand.* (2016) 133:266–76. doi: 10.1111/acps.12548
122. van Os J, Verhagen S, Marsman A, Peeters F, Bak M, Marcelis M, et al. The experience sampling method as an mHealth tool to support self-monitoring, self-insight, and personalized health care in clinical practice. *Depression Anxiety* (2017) 34:481–93. doi: 10.1002/da.22647
123. Abdullah S, Matthews M, Frank E, Doherty G, Gay G, Choudhury T. Automatic detection of social rhythms in bipolar disorder. *J Am Med Informatics Assoc.* (2016) 23:538–43. doi: 10.1093/jamia/ocv200
124. Faurholt-Jepsen M, Busk J, Frost M, Vinberg M, Christensen EM, Winther O, et al. Voice analysis as an objective state marker in bipolar disorder. *Transl Psychiatry* (2016) 6:e856. doi: 10.1038/tp.2016.123
125. Hidalgo-Mazzei D, Mateu A, Reinares M, Murru A, Del Mar Bonnin C, Varo C, et al. Psychoeducation in bipolar disorder with a SIMPLe smartphone application: Feasibility, acceptability and satisfaction. *J Affect Disord.* (2016) 200:58–66. doi: 10.1016/j.jad.2016.04.042
126. Hidalgo-Mazzei D, Reinares M, Mateu A, Juruena MF, Young AH, Perez-Sola V, et al. Is a SIMPLe smartphone application capable of improving biological rhythms in bipolar disorder? *J Affect Disord.* (2017) 223:10–6. doi: 10.1016/j.jad.2017.07.028
127. Passos IC, Mwangi B, Cao B, Hamilton JE, Wu MJ, Zhang XY, et al. Identifying a clinical signature of suicidality among patients with mood disorders: A pilot study using a machine learning approach. *J Affect Disord.* (2016) 193:109–16. doi: 10.1016/j.jad.2015.12.066
128. Tran T, Luo W, Phung D, Harvey R, Berk M, Kennedy RL, et al. Risk stratification using data from electronic medical records better predicts suicide risks than clinician assessments. *BMC Psychiatry* (2014) 14:76. doi: 10.1186/1471-244X-14-76
129. Salvadore G, Quiroz JA, Machado-Vieira R, Henter ID, Manji HK, Zarate CA, Jr. The neurobiology of the switch process in bipolar disorder: a review. *J Clin Psychiatry.* (2010) 71:1488–501. doi: 10.4088/JCP.09r05259gre
130. Bonnin CM, Yatham LN, Michalak EE, Martinez-Aran A, Dhanoa T, Torres I, et al. Psychometric properties of the well-being index (WHO-5) spanish version in a sample of euthymic patients with bipolar disorder. *J Affect Disord.* (2018) 228:153–9. doi: 10.1016/j.jad.2017.12.006
131. https://www.collinsdictionary.com/dictionary/english/prodrome.
132. Lin A, Wood SJ, Nelson B, Beavan A, McGorry P, Yung AR. Outcomes of nontransitioned cases in a sample at ultra-high risk for psychosis. *Am J Psychiatry* (2015) 172:249–58. doi: 10.1176/appi.ajp.2014.13030418
133. Arango C, Diaz-Caneja CM, McGorry PD, Rapoport J, Sommer IE, Vorstman JA, et al. Preventive strategies for mental health. *Lancet Psychiatry* (2018) 5:591–604. doi: 10.1016/S2215-0366(18)30057-9
134. Vieta E. Staging and psychosocial early intervention in bipolar disorder. *Lancet Psychiatry* (2015) 2:483–5. doi: 10.1016/S2215-0366(15)00205-9
135. Amoretti S, Bernardo M, Bonnin CM, Bioque M, Cabrera B, Mezquida G, et al. The impact of cognitive reserve in the outcome of first-episode psychoses: 2-year follow-up study. *Eur Neuropsychopharmacol.* (2016) 26:1638–48. doi: 10.1016/j.euroneuro.2016.07.003
136. Sole B, Jimenez E, Torrent C, Reinares M, Bonnin CDM, Torres I, et al. Cognitive impairment in bipolar disorder: treatment and prevention strategies. *Int J Neuropsychopharmacol.* (2017) 20:670–80. doi: 10.1093/ijnp/pyx032
137. Salvatore P, Baldessarini RJ, Tohen M, Khalsa HM, Sanchez-Toledo JP, Zarate CA, Jr, et al. McLean-Harvard International First-Episode Project: two-year stability of ICD-10 diagnoses in 500 first-episode psychotic disorder patients. *J Clin Psychiatry* (2011) 72:183–93. doi: 10.4088/JCP.09m05311yel
138. Goldsmith DR, Rapaport MH, Miller BJ. A meta-analysis of blood cytokine network alterations in psychiatric patients: comparisons between schizophrenia, bipolar disorder and depression. *Mol Psychiatry* (2016) 21:1696–709. doi: 10.1038/mp.2016.3
139. Scott J, Etain B, Bellivier F. Can an Integrated Science Approach to Precision medicine research improve lithium treatment in bipolar disorders? *Front Psychiatry* (2018) 9:360. doi: 10.3389/fpsyt.2018.00360
140. Ritter PS, Schwabedal J, Brandt M, Schrempf W, Brezan F, Krupka A, et al. Sleep spindles in bipolar disorder - a comparison to healthy control subjects. *Acta Psychiatrica Scand.* (2018) 138:163–72. doi: 10.1111/acps.12924
141. Ryu E, Nassan M, Jenkins GD, Armasu SM, Andreazza A, McElroy SL, et al. A genome-wide search for bipolar disorder risk loci modified by mitochondrial genome variation. *Mol Neuropsychiatry* (2018) 3:125–34. doi: 10.1159/000464444
142. Chung Y, Addington J, Bearden CE, Cadenhead K, Cornblatt B, Mathalon DH, et al. Use of machine learning to determine deviance in neuroanatomical maturity associated with future psychosis in youths at clinically high risk. *JAMA Psychiatry* (2018) 75:960–8. doi: 10.1001/jamapsychiatry.2018.154
143. Duffy A, Malhi GS, Grof P. Do the trajectories of bipolar disorder and schizophrenia follow a universal staging model? *Can J Psychiatry* (2017) 62:115–22. doi: 10.1177/0706743716649189
144. Cadiz F, Gormaz JG, Burotto M. Breast cancer staging: is TNM ready to evolve? *J Global Oncol.* (2018) 4:1–3. doi: 10.1200/JGO.17.00004
145. Salari P, Larijani B. Ethical issues surrounding personalized medicine: a literature review. *Acta Medica Iranica* (2017) 55:209–17.

Permissions

All chapters in this book were first published by Frontiers; hereby published with permission under the Creative Commons Attribution License or equivalent. Every chapter published in this book has been scrutinized by our experts. Their significance has been extensively debated. The topics covered herein carry significant findings which will fuel the growth of the discipline. They may even be implemented as practical applications or may be referred to as a beginning point for another development.

The contributors of this book come from diverse backgrounds, making this book a truly international effort. This book will bring forth new frontiers with its revolutionizing research information and detailed analysis of the nascent developments around the world.

We would like to thank all the contributing authors for lending their expertise to make the book truly unique. They have played a crucial role in the development of this book. Without their invaluable contributions this book wouldn't have been possible. They have made vital efforts to compile up to date information on the varied aspects of this subject to make this book a valuable addition to the collection of many professionals and students.

This book was conceptualized with the vision of imparting up-to-date information and advanced data in this field To ensure the same, a matchless editorial board was set up. Every individual on the board went through rigorous rounds of assessment to prove their worth. After which they invested a large part of their time researching and compiling the most relevant data for our readers.

The editorial board has been involved in producing this book since its inception. They have spent rigorous hours researching and exploring the diverse topics which have resulted in the successful publishing of this book. They have passed on their knowledge of decades through this book. To expedite this challenging task, the publisher supported the team at every step. A small team of assistant editors was also appointed to further simplify the editing procedure and attain best results for the readers.

Apart from the editorial board, the designing team has also invested a significant amount of their time in understanding the subject and creating the most relevant covers. They scrutinized every image to scout for the most suitable representation of the subject and create an appropriate cover for the book.

The publishing team has been an ardent support to the editorial, designing and production team. Their endless efforts to recruit the best for this project, has resulted in the accomplishment of this book. They are a veteran in the field of academics and their pool of knowledge is as vast as their experience in printing. Their expertise and guidance has proved useful at every step. Their uncompromising quality standards have made this book an exceptional effort. Their encouragement from time to time has been an inspiration for everyone.

The publisher and the editorial board hope that this book will prove to be a valuable piece of knowledge for researchers, students, practitioners and scholars across the globe.

List of Contributors

Jaana Suvisaari and Maija Lindgren
Mental Health Unit, National Institute for Health and Welfare, Helsinki, Finland

Outi Mantere
Mental Health Unit, National Institute for Health and Welfare, Helsinki, Finland
Department of Psychiatry, McGill University, Montreal, QC, Canada
Bipolar Disorders Clinic, Douglas Mental Health University Institute, Montreal, QC, Canada
Department of Psychiatry, Faculty of Medicine, University of Helsinki, Helsinki, Finland

Jaakko Keinänen and Tuula Kieseppä
Mental Health Unit, National Institute for Health and Welfare, Helsinki, Finland
Department of Psychiatry, Faculty of Medicine, University of Helsinki, Helsinki, Finland

Teemu Mäntylä and Eva Rikandi
Mental Health Unit, National Institute for Health and Welfare, Helsinki, Finland
Department of Neuroscience and Biomedical Engineering, and Advanced Magnetic Imaging Center Aalto NeuroImaging, Aalto University School of Science, Espoo, Finland
Department of Psychology and Logopedics, University of Helsinki, Helsinki, Finland

Tuukka T. Raij
Mental Health Unit, National Institute for Health and Welfare, Helsinki, Finland
Department of Neuroscience and Biomedical Engineering, and Advanced Magnetic Imaging Center Aalto NeuroImaging, Aalto University School of Science, Espoo, Finland

Rune A. Kroken and Erik Johnsen
Psychiatric Division, Haukeland University Hospital, Bergen, Norway
Norwegian Centre for Mental Disorders Research, Haukeland University Hospital, Bergen, Norway
Department of Clinical Medicine, University of Bergen, Bergen, Norway

Iris E. Sommer
Department of Neuroscience and Department of Psychiatry, University Medical Center Groningen, University of Groningen, Groningen, Netherlands
Department of Biological and Medical Psychology, University of Bergen, Bergen, Norway

Vidar M. Steen
Department of Clinical Science, Norwegian Centre for Mental Disorders Research, KG Jebsen Centre for Psychosis Research, University of Bergen, Bergen, Norway
Dr. E. Martens Research Group of Biological Psychiatry, Department of Medical Genetics, Haukeland University Hospital, Bergen, Norway

Ingrid Dieset
Norwegian Centre for Mental Disorders Research, KG Jebsen Centre for Psychosis Research. Oslo University Hospital and University of Oslo, Oslo, Norway
Division of Mental Health and Addiction, Acute Psychiatric Department, Oslo University Hospital, Oslo, Norway
Faculty of Medicine, Institute of Clinical Medicine, University of Oslo, Oslo, Norway

Adriano Aquino and Paul C. Guest
Laboratory of Neuroproteomics, Department of Biochemistry and Tissue Biology, Institute of Biology, University of Campinas, Campinas, Brazil

Guilherme L. Alexandrino and Fabio Augusto
Gas Chromatography Laboratory, Chemistry Institute, University of Campinas, Campinas, Brazil

Alexandre F. Gomes and Michael Murgu
Mass Spectrometry Applications & Development Laboratory, Waters Corporation, São Paulo, Brazil

Johann Steiner
Department of Psychiatry and Psychotherapy, University of Magdeburg, Magdeburg, Germany
Center for Behavioral Brain Sciences, Magdeburg, Germany

Daniel Martins-de-Souza
Laboratory of Neuroproteomics, Department of Biochemistry and Tissue Biology, Institute of Biology, University of Campinas, Campinas, Brazil
UNICAMP's Neurobiology Center, Campinas, Brazil Instituto Nacional de Biomarcadores em Neuropsiquiatria (INBION), Conselho Nacional de Desenvolvimento Científico e Tecnológico, São Paulo, Brazil

Ben J. A. Palanca
Department of Anesthesiology, Washington University School of Medicine in St. Louis, St Louis, MO, United States
Division of Biology and Biomedical Sciences, Washington University School of Medicine in St. Louis, St Louis, MO, United States

Hannah R. Maybrier, Angela M. Mickle, Emma R. Trammel, J. Wylie Spencer and Troy S. Wildes
Department of Anesthesiology, Washington University School of Medicine in St. Louis, St Louis, MO, United States

Nuri B. Farber, Donald D. Bohnenkamp and Eric Lenze
Department of Psychiatry, Washington University School of Medicine in St. Louis, St Louis, MO, United States

R. Edward Hogan
Department of Neurology, Washington University School of Medicine in St. Louis, St Louis, MO, United States

ShiNung Ching
Division of Biology and Biomedical Sciences, Washington University School of Medicine in St.Louis, St Louis, MO, United States
Department of Electrical Systems and Engineering, Washington University, St Louis, MO, United States

Mathias Basner
Department of Psychiatry, University of Pennsylvania Perelman School of Medicine, Philadelphia, PA, United States

Max B. Kelz
Department of Anesthesiology, University of Pennsylvania Perelman School of Medicine, Philadelphia, PA, United States

Michael S. Avidan
Department of Anesthesiology, Washington University School of Medicine in St. Louis, St Louis, MO, United States
Department of Surgery, Washington University School of Medicine in St. Louis, St Louis, MO, United States

Frauke Schultze-Lutter
Department of Psychiatry and Psychotherapy, Medical Faculty, Heinrich-Heine University, Düsseldorf, Germany

Stefanie J. Schmidt
Department of Clinical Psychology and Psychotherapy, University of Bern, Bern, Switzerland

Anastasia Theodoridou
Department of Psychiatry, Psychotherapy and Psychosomatics, Psychiatric Hospital, University of Zürich, Zürich, Switzerland

Ida Seeberg and Kamilla W. Miskowiak
Neurocognition and Emotion in Affective Disorders Group, Copenhagen Affective Disorder Research Centre, Psychiatric Centre Copenhagen, Rigshospitalet, Copenhagen University Hospital, Copenhagen, Denmark
Department of Psychology, University of Copenhagen, Copenhagen, Denmark

Hanne L. Kjaerstad
Neurocognition and Emotion in Affective Disorders Group, Copenhagen Affective Disorder Research Centre, Psychiatric Centre Copenhagen, Rigshospitalet, Copenhagen University Hospital, Copenhagen, Denmark

Karl Bechter
Department Psychiatry and Psychotherapy II, Bezirkskrankenhaus Günzburg, Ulm University, Ulm, Germany

Julia Maruani and Pierre Alexis Geoffroy
Inserm, U1144, Paris, France
Université Paris Descartes, UMR-S 1144, Paris, France
Université Paris Diderot, Sorbonne Paris Cité, UMR-S 1144, Paris, France
AP-HP, GH Saint-Louis–Lariboisière–F. Widal, Pôle de Psychiatrie et de Médecine Addictologique, Paris, France

Alice Pisoni, Rebecca Strawbridge and Stephani Hatch
Department of Psychological Medicine, Institute of Psychiatry, Psychology and Neuroscience, King's College London, London, United Kingdom

John Hodsoll
Department of Biostatistics, Institute of Psychiatry, Psychology and Neuroscience, King's College London, London, United Kingdom

Timothy R. Powell and Gerome Breen
Social, Genetic and Developmental Psychiatry Centre, Institute of Psychiatry, Psychology and Neuroscience, King's College London, London, United Kingdom

Matthew Hotopf, Allan H. Young, and Anthony J. Cleare
Department of Psychological Medicine, Institute of Psychiatry, Psychology and Neuroscience, King's College London, London, United Kingdom
South London and Maudsley NHS Foundation Trust, London, United Kingdom

Tushar Kanti Das
Department of Psychiatry, University of Western Ontario, London, ON, Canada
Robarts Research Institute, London, ON, Canada
Lawson Health Research Institute, London, ON, Canada

Avyarthana Dey
Department of Psychiatry, University of Western Ontario, London, ON, Canada
Robarts Research Institute, London, ON, Canada

Priyadharshini Sabesan and Alborz Javadzadeh
Department of Psychiatry, University of Western Ontario, London, ON, Canada

Jean Théberge
Lawson Health Research Institute, London, ON, Canada
Department of Medical Biophysics, University of Western Ontario, London, ON, Canada

Joaquim Radua
FIDMAG Germanes Hospitalàries, CIBERSAM, Sant Boi de Llobregat & Institut d'Investigacions Biomediques August Pi i Sunyer (IDIBAPS), Barcelona, Spain

Lena Palaniyappan
Department of Psychiatry, University of Western Ontario, London, ON, Canada
Robarts Research Institute, London, ON, Canada
Lawson Health Research Institute, London, ON, Canada
Department of Medical Biophysics, University of Western Ontario, London, ON, Canada

Dominique Endres, Bernd Feige, Simon J. Maier, Kathrin Nickel, Sabine Hellwig, Jördis Rausch and Ludger Tebartz van Elst
Section for Experimental Neuropsychiatry, Department of Psychiatry and Psychotherapy, Medical Center – University of Freiburg, Faculty of Medicine, of Freiburg, Freiburg, Germany
Department of Psychiatry and Psychotherapy, Medical Center – University of Freiburg, Faculty of Medicine, University of Freiburg, Freiburg, Germany

Dirk-M. Altenmüller
Department of Neurosurgery, Medical Center – University of Freiburg, Faculty of Medicine, University of Freiburg, Freiburg, Germany

Christiane Ziegler, Katharina Domschke and John P. Doerr
Department of Psychiatry and Psychotherapy, Medical Center – University of Freiburg, Faculty of Medicine, University of Freiburg, Freiburg, Germany

Karl Egger
Department of Neuroradiology, Medical Center – University of Freiburg, Faculty of Medicine, University of Freiburg, Freiburg, Germany

Jan Scott
Institute of Neuroscience, Newcastle University, Newcastle upon Tyne, United Kingdom
Faculté de Médecine, Université Paris Diderot, Paris, France

Bruno Etain
Faculté de Médecine, Université Paris Diderot, Paris, France
AP-HP, Groupe Hospitalier Saint-Louis-Lariboisière-Fernand Widal, Paris, France
INSERM, Unité UMR-S 1144, Variabilité de Réponse Aux Psychotropes, Université Paris Descartes-Paris Diderot, Paris, France
AP-HP, Groupe Henri Mondor-Albert Chenevier, Pôle de Psychiatrie, Créteil, France
INSERM, Unité 955, IMRB, Equipe de Psychiatrie Translationnelle, Créteil, France

Frank Bellivier
Faculté de Médecine, Université Paris Diderot, Paris, France
AP-HP, Groupe Hospitalier Saint-Louis-Lariboisière-Fernand Widal, Paris, France
INSERM, Unité UMR-S 1144, Variabilité de Réponse aux Psychotropes, Université Paris Descartes-Paris Diderot, Paris, France
AP-HP, Groupe Henri Mondor-Albert Chenevier, Pôle de Psychiatrie, Créteil, France
INSERM, Unité 955, IMRB, Equipe de Psychiatrie Translationnelle, Créteil, France

Mu-N Liu
Institute of Brain Science, National Yang-Ming University, Taipei, Taiwan
Department of Psychiatry, Taipei Veterans General Hospital, Taipei, Taiwan
Department of Neurology, Memory and Aging Centre, University of California, San Francisco, San Francisco, CA, United States

Chi-Ieong Lau
Department of Neurology, Shin Kong Wu Ho-Su Memorial Hospital, Taipei, Taiwan
Applied Cognitive Neuroscience Group, Institute of Cognitive Neuroscience, University College London, London, United Kingdom
College of Medicine, Fu-Jen Catholic University, Taipei, Taiwan

Ching-Po Lin
Institute of Brain Science, National Yang-Ming University, Taipei, Taiwan
Institute of Neuroscience, National Yang-Ming University, Taipei, Taiwan,
Aging and Health Research Center, National Yang Ming University, Taipei, Taiwan

Rachael Horne
Department of Psychiatry & Behavioural Neurosciences, McMaster University, Hamilton, ON, Canada

Jane A. Foster
Department of Psychiatry & Behavioural Neurosciences, McMaster University, Hamilton, ON, Canada
Department of Psychiatry, St. Michael's Hospital, Toronto, ON, Canada

Dorothee Maria Gescher
Department of Psychiatry and Psychotherapy, Ottovon-Guericke University of Magdeburg, Magdeburg, Germany

Kai G. Kahl and Helge Frieling
Department of Psychiatry, Social Psychiatry and Psychotherapy, Hanover Medical School, Hanover, Germany

Thomas Hillemacher
Department of Psychiatry, Paracelsus Medical University, Nuremberg, Germany

Jens Kuhn
Department of Psychiatry and Psychotherapy, University of Cologne, Cologne, Germany

Thomas Frodl
Department of Psychiatry and Psychotherapy, Ottovon-Guericke University of Magdeburg, Magdeburg, Germany
German Centre for Neurodegenerative Diseases, Magdeburg, Germany

Azmeraw T. Amare and Bernhard T. Baune
Discipline of Psychiatry, School of Medicine, University of Adelaide, Adelaide, SA, Australia

Klaus Oliver Schubert
Discipline of Psychiatry, School of Medicine, University of Adelaide, Adelaide, SA, Australia
Northern Adelaide Local Health Network, Mental Health Services, Adelaide, SA, Australia

Fasil Tekola-Ayele
Epidemiology Branch, Division of Intramural Population Health Research, National Institute of Child Health and Human Development, National Institutes of Health, Bethesda, MD, United States

Yi-Hsiang Hsu
HSL Institute for Aging Research, Harvard Medical School, Boston, MA, United States
Program for Quantitative Genomics, Harvard School of Public Health, Boston, MA, United States
Broad Institute of MIT and Harvard, Cambridge, MA, United States

Katrin Sangkuhl, Ryan M. Whaley and Teri E. Klein
Biomedical Data Science, Stanford University, Stanford, CA, United States

Poulami Barman, Anthony Batzler and Gregory Jenkins
Department of Health Sciences Research, Mayo Clinic, Rochester, NY, United States

Russ B. Altman
Department of Bioengineering, Stanford University, Stanford, CA, United States

Volker Arolt
Department of Psychiatry and Psychotherapy, University of Muenster, Muenster, Germany

Jürgen Brockmöller
Department of Clinical Pharmacology, University Göttingen, Göttingen, Germany

Chia-Hui Chen
Department of Psychiatry, Taipei Medical University-Shuangho Hospital, New Taipei City, Taiwan

Katharina Domschke
Department of Psychiatry and Psychotherapy, Faculty of Medicine, University of Freiburg, Freiburg, Germany

Daniel K. Hall-Flavin, Michelle K. Skime and William V. Bobo
Department of Psychiatry and Psychology, Mayo Clinic, Rochester, NY, United States

Joanna M. Biernacka
Department of Health Sciences Research, Mayo Clinic, Rochester, NY, United States
Department of Psychiatry and Psychology, Mayo Clinic, Rochester, NY, United States

Chen-Jee Hong, Ying-Jay Liou and Shih-Jen Tsai
Department of Psychiatry, Taipei Veterans General Hospital, Taipei, Taiwan,
Division of Psychiatry, School of Medicine, National Yang-Ming University, Taipei, Taiwan

Ari Illi
Department of Psychiatry, Faculty of Medicine and Life Sciences, University of Tampere, Tampere, Finland

Yuan Ji, Liewei Wang and Richard M. Weinshilboum
Department of Molecular Pharmacology and Experimental Therapeutics, Mayo Clinic Rochester, Rochester, MN, United States

Olli Kampman
Department of Psychiatry, Faculty of Medicine and Life Sciences, University of Tampere, Tampere, Finland
Department of Psychiatry, Seinäjoki Hospital District, Seinäjoki, Finland

Toshihiko Kinoshita and Masaki Kato
Department of Neuropsychiatry, Kansai Medical University, Osaka, Japan

Esa Leinonen
Department of Psychiatry, Faculty of Medicine and Life Sciences, University of Tampere, Tampere, Finland
Department of Psychiatry, Tampere University Hospital, Tampere, Finland

Taisei Mushiroda and Michiaki Kubo
RIKEN Center for Integrative Medical Sciences, Kanagawa, Japan

Shinpei Nonen
Department of Pharmacy, Hyogo University of Health Sciences, Hyogo, Japan

Yu-Li Liu
Center for Neuropsychiatric Research, National Health Research Institutes, Miaoli, Taiwan

Verayuth Praphanphoj
Center for Medical Genetics Research, Rajanukul Institute, Department of Mental Health, Ministry of Public Health Bangkok, Bangkok, Thailand

Julia C. Stingl
Research Division Federal Institute for Drugs and Medical Devices, Bonn, Germany

Cathy Davies
Early Psychosis: Interventions and Clinical-Detection Lab, Department of Psychosis Studies, Institute of Psychiatry, Psychology and Neuroscience, King's College London, London, United Kingdom

Joaquim Radua
Early Psychosis: Interventions and Clinical-Detection Lab, Department of Psychosis Studies, Institute of Psychiatry, Psychology and Neuroscience, King's College London, London, United Kingdom
FIDMAG Germanes Hospitalàries, CIBERSAM, Barcelona, Spain
Department of Clinical Neuroscience, Centre for Psychiatry Research, Karolinska Institutet, Stockholm, Sweden

Andrea Cipriani
Department of Psychiatry, University of Oxford, Oxford, United Kingdom
Oxford Health NHS Foundation Trust, Oxford, United Kingdom

Daniel Stahl
Department of Biostatistics, Institute of Psychiatry, Psychology and Neuroscience, King's College London, London, United Kingdom

Umberto Provenzani
Department of Brain and Behavioral Sciences, University of Pavia, Pavia, Italy

Philip McGuire
Department of Psychosis Studies, Institute of Psychiatry, Psychology and Neuroscience, King's College London, London, United Kingdom
National Institute for Health Research Maudsley Biomedical Research Centre, London, United Kingdom
OASIS Service, South London and Maudsley NHS Foundation Trust, London, United Kingdom

Paolo Fusar-Poli
Early Psychosis: Interventions and Clinical-Detection Lab, Department of Psychosis Studies, Institute of Psychiatry, Psychology and Neuroscience, King's College London, London, United Kingdom
Department of Brain and Behavioral Sciences, University of Pavia, Pavia, Italy
National Institute for Health Research Maudsley Biomedical Research Centre, London, United Kingdom
OASIS Service, South London and Maudsley NHS Foundation Trust, London, United Kingdom

Yash B. Joshi
Department of Psychiatry, University of California, San Diego, La Jolla, CA, United States

Gregory A. Light
Department of Psychiatry, University of California, San Diego, La Jolla, CA, United States
VISN-22 Mental Illness, Research, Education and Clinical Center (MIRECC), VA San Diego Health Care System, San Diego, CA, United States

Andreas Walther, Susanne Wehrli and Clemens Kirschbaum
Biological Psychology, TU Dresden, Dresden, Germany

Carlo Vittorio Cannistraci
Biomedical Cybernetics Group, Biotechnology Center (BIOTEC), Center for Molecular and Cellular Bioengineering (CMCB), Center for Systems Biology Dresden (CSBD), Department of Physics, TU Dresden, Dresden, Germany
Brain Bio-Inspired Computing (BBC) Lab, IRCCS Centro Neurolesi "Bonino Pulejo", Messina, Italy

Timothy R. Powell and Gerome Breen
Social, Genetic and Developmental Psychiatry Centre, Institute of Psychiatry, Psychology and Neuroscience, King's College London, London, United Kingdom

Kai Simons and Mathias J. Gerl
Lipotype GmbH, Dresden, Germany

Estela Salagre, Justo Pinzon, Maria Reinares, Eduard Vieta and Iria Grande
Barcelona Bipolar Disorders Program, Hospital Clinic, Institute of Neurosciences, University of Barcelon a,IDIBAPS, CIBERSAM, Barcelona, Spain

Seetal Dodd
IMPACT Strategic Research Centre, Barwon Health, Deakin University, Geelong, VIC, Australia
Department of Psychiatry, University of Melbourne, Parkville, VIC, Australia
Orygen, The National Centre of Excellence in Youth Mental Health, Melbourne, VIC, Australia

Alberto Aedo
Bipolar Disorders Unit, Department of Psychiatry, School of Medicine, Pontificia Universidad Católica de Chile, Santiago, Chile

Adriane Rosa
Laboratory of Molecular Psychiatry, Hospital de Clínicas de Porto Alegre, Porto Alegre, Brazil
Postgraduate Program: Psychiatry and Behavioral Science, Universidade Federal do Rio Grande do Sul (UFRGS), Porto Alegre, Brazil
Department of Pharmacology and Postgraduate Program : Pharmacology and Therapeutics, Universidade Federal do Rio Grande do Sul (UFRGS), Porto Alegre, Brazil

Silvia Amoretti
Barcelona Clínic Schizophrenia Unit, Hospital Clinic de Barcelona, CIBERSAM, Barcelona, Spain

Michael Berk
IMPACT Strategic Research Centre, Barwon Health, Deakin University, Geelong, VIC, Australia
Department of Psychiatry, University of Melbourne, Parkville, VIC, Australia
Orygen, The National Centre of Excellence in Youth Mental Health, Melbourne, VIC, Australia
Florey Institute for Neuroscience and Mental Health, Parkville, VIC, Australia

Flavio Pereira Kapczinski
Department of Psychiatry & Behavioral Neurosciences, Barcelona Bipolar Disorders Program, Hospital Clinic, Mcmaster University, Hamilton, ON, Canada
Institute of Neurosciences, University of Barcelona, IDIBAPS, CIBERSAM, Barcelona, Spain

Index